Medical Microbiology

For Churchill Livingstone

Publisher: Timothy Horne
Project Editor: Jane Starling
Editorial Co-ordination: Editorial Resources Unit
  Copy Editor: Rich Cutler
  Indexer: J. R. Sampson
Production Controller: Lesley W. Small
Design: Design Resources Unit
Sales Promotion Executive: Hilary Brown

Medical Microbiology

A Guide to Microbial Infections: Pathogenesis, Immunity, Laboratory Diagnosis and Control

Edited by

David Greenwood BSc PhD DSc FRCPath

Professor of Antimicrobial Science, Department of
Microbiology, University of Nottingham Medical School,
Nottingham, UK; Honorary Microbiologist, Public Health
Laboratory Service

Richard C. B. Slack MA MB BChir MRCPath DRCOG

Senior Lecturer, Department of Microbiology, University of
Nottingham Medical School, Nottingham, UK; Consultant in
Communicable Disease Control, Nottingham Health
Authority; Honorary Consultant, Public Health Laboratory
Service

John F. Peutherer BSc MB ChB MD FRCPath FRCPE

Senior Lecturer, Department of Medical Microbiology,
University of Edinburgh Medical School; Honorary
Consultant, Lothian Health Board, Edinburgh, UK

FOURTEENTH EDITION

CHURCHILL LIVINGSTONE
EDINBURGH LONDON MADRID MELBOURNE NEW YORK AND TOKYO 1992

CHURCHILL LIVINGSTONE
Medical Division of Longman Group UK Limited

Distributed in the United States of America by Churchill
Livingstone Inc., 650 Avenue of the Americas, New York,
N.Y. 10011, and by associated companies, branches and
representatives throughout the world.

First edition 1925
Second edition 1928
Third edition 1931
Fourth edition 1934
Fifth edition 1938
Sixth edition 1942
Seventh edition 1945
Eighth edition 1948
Ninth edition 1953

Tenth edition 1960
Eleventh edition 1965
Twelfth edition (Vol. 1) 1973
ELBS edition of Twelfth edition
         (Vol. 1) 1974
Twelfth edition (Vol. 2) 1975
Thirteenth edition (Vol. 1) 1978
Thirteenth edition (Vol. 1)
Fourteenth edition 1992

ISBN 0-443-04256-X

British Library Cataloguing in Publication Data
A catalogue record for this book is available from the British
Library.

Library of Congress Cataloging in Publication Data
Medical microbiology: a guide to microbial infections:
    pathogenesis, immunity, laboratory diagnosis and control
    /edited by David Greenwood, Richard C.B. Slack, John
    Forrest Peutherer. – 14th ed.
        p.   cm.
    Rev. ed. of: Mackie & McCartney medical microbiology.
13th ed. 1978.
    Includes index.
    Contents: v. 1 Microbial infections.
    ISBN 0-443-04256-X
    1. Medical microbiology. I. Greenwood, David, 1935–
II. Slack, Richard C. B. III. Peutherer, J. F.
    [DNLM: 1. Diagnosis, Laboratory. 2. Microbiology.
QW 4 M487]
QR46. M35 1992
616'.01--dc20
DNLM/DLC
for Library of Congress   91-23263 CIP

Printed in Hong Kong

Preface

The original 'Mackie and McCartney', published in 1925 under the title *An Introduction to Practical Bacteriology as Applied to Medicine and Public Health*, was a slim octavo volume of less than 300 pages. Although it was written primarily for students of the University of Edinburgh, its fame quickly spread and it became the standard bacteriological textbook for two generations of medical students and trainee bacteriologists throughout the English-speaking world. Expansion of the subject and the inclusion of the burgeoning topics of immunology and virology inevitably increased the size of the book so that, by the time the 11th edition appeared in 1965 under the editorship of Professor Robert Cruickshank, it had become an unwieldy volume of over 1000 pages.

When the 12th edition was being prepared in the early 1970s, the decision was taken to publish it in two parts: volume 1, devoted to medical microbiology in its relation to disease; and volume 2, concerned primarily with laboratory aspects of the practice of medical microbiology. The two volumes have become progressively independent (and unsynchronized in publication) and it became impossible for a single editorial team to cope realistically with the demands of managing both volumes.

Consequently, the present edition, which is in the tradition of volume 1 of the two-volume descendant of 'Mackie and McCartney', has a new editorial team and many new contributors. The basic structure has, however, been retained, although each chapter has been thoroughly revised; indeed, the vast majority has been completely rewritten. Several new chapters have been included to take account of new developments in microbiology and some parts of the book have been re-arranged to provide a more logical presentation of the subject. Helminths are included for the first time.

Despite the considerable progress that has been made in our ability to recognize and control the microbial agents of disease, infection continues to exact an enormous toll of suffering in both the developing and the industrially developed worlds. It is, therefore, as important now as it ever was that medical students should acquire a firm grasp of the basic properties of pathogenic microbes; of their relation to disease; of the response of the body to their presence; and of the measures that are available for their control. In preparing this new edition for the press, we have been very conscious of the need to fulfil these requirements and, thanks to the untiring efforts of our panel of expert contributors, we believe that we have been able to achieve our aim while retaining the tradition of erudition and readability that has been the enduring hallmark of previous editions of 'Mackie and McCartney'. It is our sincere hope that this new text will, like its predecessors, provide a firm grounding in the understanding of infection and its control for a new generation of medical students and microbiologists.

Nottingham and Edinburgh, 1992

D.G.
R.C.B.S.
J.F.P.

Contributors

John P. Arbuthnott ScD FIBiol
Principal and Vice Chancellor, University of
Strathclyde, Glasgow

Sheila M. Burns MBChB MRCPath
Consultant, Regional Virus Laboratory, City
Hospital, Edinburgh

E. Owen Caul FIMLS PhD MRCPath
Clinical Scientist; Honorary Consultant
Virologist, Regional Virus and Public Health
Laboratory, Bristol

Alan Cockayne BSc PhD
SmithKline Beecham Lecturer in Infectious
Disease, Department of Microbiology,
Nottingham

Joyce D. Coghlan BSc PhD
Formerly Director, Leptospira Reference
Laboratory, Public Health Laboratory Service,
London; Formerly Lecturer in Bacteriology,
University of Edinburgh Medical School,
Edinburgh

Dulcie V. Coleman MBBS(Lon) MD(Lon) MRCPath
Professor of Cell Pathology, St Mary's Hospital,
London

J. Gerald Collee MD FRCPath FRCP
Professor and Head, Department of Medical
Microbiology, University of Edinburgh Medical
School; Chief Bacteriologist, Royal Infirmary of
Edinburgh; Consultant Adviser in Microbiology,
Scottish Home and Health Department,
Edinburgh

W. David Cubitt BTech MSc PhD MIBiol FIMLS
Top Grade Virologist, Department of Microbiology, Hospitals for Sick Children, London

J. Mervyn Darville BSc PhD MRCPath
Lecturer in Medical Virology, University of
Bristol; Consultant Virologist, Public Health
Laboratory, Bristol

Ulrich Desselberger MD MRCPath MRCPG
Consultant Virologist and Director, Regional
Virus Laboratories, Birmingham

E. G. V. Evans BSc PhD MIBiol
Senior Lecturer in Medical Mycology, University
of Leeds and General Infirmary, Leeds

R. J. Fallon BSc MD FRCPath FRCPG
Consultant in Laboratory Medicine, Ruchill
Hospital; Honorary Senior Clinical Lecturer in
Bacteriology and Infectious Diseases, University
of Glasgow, Glasgow

R. G. Finch MB ChB FRCP MRCPath
Professor of Infectious Diseases, The City
Hospital, Nottingham

Kenneth L Gage PhD
IRTA Postdoctoral Fellow, Laboratory of
Vectors and Pathogens, Rocky Mountain
Laboratories, Hamilton, Montana, USA

James Cameron Gould BSc(Hons) MD FRCPE
FRCPath FFCM FIBiol FRSE
Consultant Microbiologist; Formerly Director
and Consultant in Charge, Central
Microbiological Laboratories, Edinburgh

John R. W. Govan BSc PhD
Reader, Department of Medical Microbiology,
University of Edinburgh Medical School,
Edinburgh

John M. Grange MSc MD
Reader in Clinical Microbiology, National Heart
and Lung Institute, London

David Greenwood BSc PhD DSc FRCPath
Professor of Antimicrobial Science, Department
of Microbiology, University of Nottingham,
Nottingham; Honorary Microbiologist, Public
Health Laboratory Service

Roger J. Gross MA MSc CBiol DSc
Top Grade Microbiologist, Division of Enteric
Pathogens, Central Public Health Laboratory
Service, London

J. M. Hardie BDS PhD DipBact MRCPath
Reader in Oral Microbiology, The London
Hospital Medical College, London

A. J. Howard MB BS MSc FRCPath
Consultant Medical Microbiologist, Gwynedd
Hospital, Gwynedd

J. M. Inglis BSc PhD MRCPath
Director, Regional Virus Laboratory, City
Hospital, Edinburgh

Richard H. Kimberlin BSc PhD
Independent Consultant on Scrapie and Related
Diseases, Edinburgh

M. J. Lewis MD DipBact
Director, Nottingham Area Public Health
Laboratory; Senior Lecturer, University of
Nottingham, Nottingham

Alasdair P. MacGowan BMedBiol (Hons) MB ChB
Senior Registrar in Medical Microbiology,
Departments of Microbiology, Southmead
Hospital and Bristol Royal Infirmary; Honorary
Clinical Tutor in Medical Microbiology,
University of Bristol, Bristol

Alastair D. Macrae MD FRCPath DipBact
Formerly Consultant Virologist, Public Health
Laboratory Service, Nottingham; Senior
Lecturer, Department of Microbiology,
University of Nottingham, Nottingham

Donald M. McLean MD FRCPC FRCPath
Professor, Division of Medical Microbiology,
University of British Columbia, Vancouver,
Canada

C. R. Madeley MD FRCPath
Professor and Head of Department of Virology,
Royal Victoria Infirmary, Newcastle upon Tyne

Peter Morgan-Capner BSc MBBS MRCPath
Consultant Virologist, Department of Virology,
Preston Infirmary, Preston

Mary Norval BSc PhD DSc
Senior Lecturer, Department of Medical
Microbiology, University of Edinburgh Medical
School, Edinburgh

Marie M. Ogilvie MD BSc
Senior Lecturer in Virology, Department of
Medical Microbiology, Edinburgh University
Medical School, Edinburgh; Honorary
Consultant, Lothian Health Board

J. R. Pattison MA BSc DM FRCPath
Professor, Department of Medical Microbiology,
University College and Middlesex School of
Medicine, London

J. S. M. Peiris MB BS MRCPath DPhil(Oxon)
Consultant Virologist, Department of Virology,
Royal Victoria Infirmary, Newcastle upon Tyne

T. Hugh Pennington MB BS PhD MRCPath
Professor and Head of Department of Medical
Microbiology, University of Aberdeen Medical
School, Aberdeen

John F. Peutherer BSc MB ChB MD FRCPath
FRCPE
Senior Lecturer, Department of Medical
Microbiology, University of Edinburgh Medical
School, Edinburgh; Honorary Consultant,
Lothian Health Board, Edinburgh

Noel W. Preston MD DipBact FRCPath LRCP LRCS
LRFPS
Formerly: Director of Pertussis Reference
Laboratory; Reader in Bacteriology, University of
Manchester; Honorary Consultant
Microbiologist, Public Health Laboratory

Service; WHO Expert Adviser on Bacterial
Diseases

Daniel Reid OBE MD FRCP(Glas) FFCM DPH
Director, Communicable Diseases (Scotland)
Unit, Ruchill Hospital; Honorary Clinical
Lecturer, Department of Infectious Diseases,
University of Glasgow, Glasgow

Philip W. Ross TD MD FRCPath FRCP(Ed) FIBiol
Reader, Department of Medical Microbiology,
University of Edinburgh Medical School;
Honorary Consultant Bacteriologist, Royal
Infirmary, Edinburgh

Haroun N. Shah BSc PhD
Senior Lecturer in Oral Microbiology,
Department of Oral Microbiology, The London
Hospital Medical College, University of London,
London

Rosemary A. Simpson PhD MRCPath
Top Grade Microbiologist, Division of Hospital
Infection, Central Public Health Laboratory,
Colindale, London

M. B. Skirrow MB ChB PhD FRCPath DTM & H
Consultant, Public Health Laboratory Service,
Gloucestershire Royal Hospital, Gloucester

Richard C. B. Slack MA MB BChir MRCPath
DRCOG
Senior Lecturer, Department of Microbiology,
Queen's Medical Centre, Nottingham; Honorary
Consultant Microbiologist, Public Health
Laboratory Service, Nottingham, UK

Isabel W. Smith BSc PhD
Senior Lecturer, Department of Medical
Microbiology, University of Edinburgh Medical
School, Edinburgh

John Stewart BSc PhD
Lecturer, Department of Medical Microbiology,
University of Edinburgh Medical School,
Edinburgh

David Taylor-Robinson MD FRCPath
Professor and Head, Division of Sexually
Transmitted Diseases, Medical Research Council
Clinical Research Centre, Harrow, Middlesex

K. J. Towner BSc PhD
Principal Microbiologist, Department of
Microbiology, and Public Health Laboratory
University Hospital, Nottingham

David H. Walker MD
Professor and Chairman, Department of
Pathology, University of Texas Medical Branch,
Galveston, USA

Penelope Ward MB BS MRCOG
Clinical Research Registrar, St Mary's Hospital,
London

D. M. Weir MD FRCPE
Professor of Microbial Immunology, Department
of Medical Microbiology, University of
Edinburgh Medical School, Edinburgh

J. F. Wilkinson MA PhD
Professor of Microbiology, Department of
Microbiology, University of Edinburgh,
Edinburgh

Acknowledgements

We are most grateful to Linda Bowering, Geraldine Holmes and Marilyn Cole for secretarial help, and to the staff of Churchill Livingstone for their unfailing help and advice at all stages of the preparation of this book.

D.G.
R.C.B.S.
J.F.P.

Contents

PART 1
Microbial biology

1

Microbiology and medicine

D. Greenwood

Applications of microbiology have given medicine its greatest successes in the diagnosis, prevention and cure of disease. Along with the improved nutrition and living conditions achieved in developed communities in the last century, they have brought about a revolutionary betterment in human health and security — a doubling in the average length of life and the safe upbringing of most children born, where before only a minority survived.

The conquest of epidemic and fatal infections has seemed to be so conclusive that the main challenge in medicine is now often seen to lie in other fields, such as those of the mental illnesses and degenerative diseases, but a major shift of attention away from the problems of infection could be dangerous. The relative freedom of society from fatal infections depends on the continued, informed deployment of complex counter-measures: on correct diagnosis and treatment of infections, full implementation of immunization programmes, alert epidemiological surveillance and rigorous environmental sanitation.

Moreover, on a global scale, infection is far from defeated. In the developing nations of the world, an estimated 10 million people (predominantly young children) die each year from the effects of infectious diarrhoeas, measles, malaria, tetanus, diphtheria and whooping cough alone. The tragedy is that we have the means to hand to prevent nearly all these deaths.

Even in the developed world infective illnesses are still extremely common and make up much of the work of family and hospital doctors. At least a quarter of all illness for which patients consult their doctors are infective, and a substantial proportion of patients acquire infection while in hospital. Intensive farming methods and a shift in eating habits to pre-prepared 'fast foods' have led to a sharp increase in food-related infection. In hospitals, new approaches to therapy that deplete the competence of the patient's immune system to cope with infection, as well as the increasing use of shunts, intravenous cannulae and prosthetic devices, all provide the ever-resourceful microbes with new opportunities to invade the host. Surprisingly, 'new' agents of infectious disease continue to be recognized (Table 1.1). The most notorious of these is undoubtedly the human immunodeficiency virus (HIV), the causative

Table 1.1 Some newly recognized infectious agents, 1970–90.

Agent	Disease
Borrelia burgdorferi	Lyme disease
Campylobacter jejuni	Enteritis
Clostridium difficile	Pseudomembranous colitis
Cryptosporidium parvum	Diarrhoea
Gardnerella vaginalis	Bacterial vaginosis
Helicobacter pylori	Gastritis
Hepatitis C virus	Hepatitis
Human herpesvirus 6	Exanthum subitum
Human immunodeficiency virus	Acquired immune deficiency syndrome (AIDS)
Legionella pneumophila	Legionnaires'disease
Mobiluncus spp.	Bacterial vaginosis
Parvovirus	Fifth Disease
Rotavirus	Infantile diarrhoea
'Small round' viruses	Gastro-enteritis

agent of acquired immune deficiency syndrome (AIDS). The rise and spread of this condition provides a sobering reminder of the potential impact of microbial disease. It is as essential now as it ever was that medical personnel should be well trained in matters relating to infection.

Microbiology is the study of living organisms of microscopic size. The term was introduced by the French chemist Louis Pasteur, whose demonstration that fermentation was caused by the growth of bacteria and yeasts (1857–60) provided a main impetus for the development of the science. The term *microbe* was first used by Sédillot in 1878, but is now commonly replaced by that of *micro-organism*.

The microbes of medical interest include *protozoa*, the smallest animals, *fungi*, including moulds and yeasts, *bacteria*, which have much smaller, simpler cells, and *viruses*, the smallest and simplest of all. Most viruses are less than 0.2 micrometres (μm) in diameter and so are not resolvable with the light microscope. Because they lack a cellular structure and can replicate only within a living host cell, viruses are sometimes regarded as components of their host rather than as micro-organisms, but since they are organized bodies, capable of reproducing themselves in different hosts, and of surviving outside their hosts, it is justifiable as well as convenient to classify them as micro-organisms. Although *helminths* (parasitic worms) are macroscopic, they cause infection and their study falls within the province of microbiologists. Students should, therefore, be familiar with their properties.

DEVELOPMENT OF MICROBIOLOGY

Micro-organisms were first seen about 1675 by the Dutchman Antony van Leeuwenhoek. His microscopes consisted of a single biconvex lens that magnified about × 200 and resolved bodies with diameters down to about 1 μm. He found many micro-organisms in materials such as water, mud, saliva and the intestinal contents of healthy subjects, and he recognized them as living creatures ('animalcules') because they swam about actively. That he saw bacteria as well as the larger microbes is known from his measurements of

their size ('one-sixth the diameter of a red blood corpuscle') and his drawings of the forms we now recognize as cocci (spheres), bacilli (rods) and spirochaetes (spiral filaments).

Leeuwenhoek observed that very large numbers of bacteria appeared in watery infusions of animal or vegetable matter which were left to stand for a week or two at room temperature. He believed that these huge populations were the progeny of a few parental organisms, or seeds, that were originally present in the materials of the infusion or had entered it from the air. Other scientists suggested that the organisms arose by *spontaneous generation*, i.e. by the spontaneous conversion of dead organic matter into living microbes, and this suggestion began a controversy that lasted for 200 years. The prototype of the experiment that ultimately was to settle the matter was first described by the French microscopist Louis Joblot in 1718. Joblot boiled a flask of an infusion of hay for 15 min to kill any microbes originally present in it, covered it with a parchment cap to prevent the later entry of other microbes from the air and showed that, on subsequent standing, it remained free from microbial growth. Other workers, notably John Needham (1749), made similar, though not identical, experiments in which, by contrast, the heated, covered infusions gave a growth of organisms and so appeared to demonstrate the occurrence of spontaneous generation. It was not at first realized how exacting were the conditions needed for *sterilization*, i.e. the killing of all micro-organisms, and the maintenance of sterility. The necessary techniques were perfected only after much further work, particularly that by Lazzaro Spallanzani (1765, 1776) and Louis Pasteur (1860–64). Pasteur's flasks of infusions, sterilized by autoclaving at 115–120°C, always remained sterile despite the entry of unheated air through a dust-stopping 'swan neck' or cotton-wool stopper, and so finally proved the absence of spontaneous generation.

Although this conclusion was long delayed, the work on spontaneous generation had the valuable outcome of establishing many of the basic techniques of bacteriology. Convenient nutrient media for preparing growths, or *cultures*, of bacteria in the laboratory were derived from Leeuwenhoek's meat and vegetable infusions, and reliable methods were developed for the sterilization and maintenance of sterility of culture media and equipment. The mechanism of bacterial reproduction by asexual fission was discovered by De Saussure (1760) and the need for high temperatures for sterilization was explained by Ferdinand Cohn's (1876) discovery that certain bacteria form heat-resistant spores. Other techniques essential for the rapid progress of bacteriology were developed by the German bacteriologist Robert Koch, who in 1877 described methods for the easy microscopic examination of bacteria in dried, fixed films stained with aniline dyes, and in 1881 devised the simple method for isolating *pure cultures* of bacteria by plating out mixed material on a solid culture medium on which the progeny of single bacteria grow in separate colonies.

MICRO-ORGANISMS AND DISEASE

Only a small proportion of the micro-organisms that abound in nature are disease-producing, or *pathogenic*, for man. Most are *free-living* in soil, water and similar habitats, and are unable to invade the living body. Some free-living micro-organisms obtain their energy from daylight or by the oxidation of inorganic matter, but the majority feed on dead organic matter and are termed *saprophytes*. In contrast, a *parasite* lives in or on, and obtains its nourishment from, a living host. In medical usage, the term 'parasite' is nowadays usually reserved for parasitic protozoa, helminths and arthropods. The last usually affect the outside of the body and are termed *ectoparasites*. *Commensal* micro-organisms constitute the normal flora of the healthy body. They live on the skin and on the mucous membranes of the upper respiratory tract, intestines and vagina, and obtain nourishment from the secretions and food residues. Since normally they do not invade the blood or tissues, they are generally harmless, but under certain circumstances, as when the body's defences are impaired, they may invade the tissues and cause disease, thus acting as *opportunistic pathogens*. True pathogens are the micro-organisms that are adapted to overcoming the normal defences of the body and invading the tissues;

their growth in the tissues, or their production of poisonous substances (*toxins*), damages the tissues and causes the manifestations of disease. The process of microbial invasion of the body is called *infection*, and a microbial disease is often called an *infective disease*. Those infective diseases that are readily communicable from person to person are called *infectious* or *contagious*.

The *germ theory* of disease was slow in gaining acceptance, though it was early recognized that epidemic diseases such as smallpox, measles, typhus and syphilis were probably spread from person to person. The Italian scholar Girolamo Fracastoro, in his book *De Contagione* (1546), distinguished three modes of transmission: (i) by direct contact, i.e. touching a patient's body; (ii) by contact with fomites, i.e. clothing and household goods contaminated by a patient; and (iii) at a distance through the air. He explained contagion as being due to the transmission of invisible *seeds*, or *germs*, different kinds of which were the specific causes of the different diseases. It is unclear whether he regarded the germs as living, but their ability to multiply in successive hosts would certainly be necessary for their continued spread.

Fracastoro's views were largely forgotten by the time Leeuwenhoek discovered micro-organisms, but speculations then began that these organisms might be the cause of certain diseases. The first clear demonstration of a pathogenic role was made by the Italian civil servant Agostino Bassi (1835), who showed that the calcino disease of silkworms was invariably associated with an invasion of their tissues by a fungus and that the disease could be transmitted by the inoculation of material from the tissues of an infected worm into those of a healthy one.

Despite Bassi's work, the germ theory of disease did not become firmly established until 1876, when Robert Koch, a country doctor in East Prussia, reported his observations on anthrax. 10 years earlier, C. J. Davaine had shown that the blood of sheep dying from anthrax contained numerous non-motile filaments and that its inoculation into healthy sheep caused them to develop anthrax. These findings, however, did not exclude the possibility that the filaments were inanimate products of the disease rather than its cause. Koch began his work by transmitting anthrax from infected sheep and cattle to the mouse, an unnatural but convenient laboratory host. He observed filaments in the blood and tissues of the infected mouse, and proved that they were living bacteria by watching them grow and form spores in drops of sterile ox serum or aqueous humour seeded with fragments of infected tissue. He showed that the bacteria alone were the cause of the disease by growing them in a series of eight pure cultures in aqueous humour, each seeded with a small proportion of the preceding one, and then reproducing the disease by inoculation of the final culture into a mouse. He thus provided the evidence, now described as *Koch's postulates*, which Jacob Henle had earlier stated would be needed to prove that the particular micro-organism was the cause of a particular disease: namely, that the microbe be found in the body in all cases of the disease, that it be isolated from a case and grown in a series of pure cultures in vitro and that it reproduce the disease on the inoculation of a late pure culture into a susceptible animal.

Through the good offices of Professors Cohn and Cohnheim, to whom he demonstrated his experiments at Breslau, Koch obtained a research appointment in Berlin and there built up a successful school of bacteriology. In addition to many discoveries by his pupils, he himself demonstrated the pathogenic roles of the tubercle bacillus (1882) and cholera vibrio (1883), and established the general principle that different specific micro-organisms cause different kinds of disease. This principle is not absolute, and in 1883 some exceptions were demonstrated by the Scottish surgeon Alexander Ogston, who showed that each of two bacteria, *Staphylococcus aureus* and *Streptococcus pyogenes*, were the cause of various suppurative infections, such as abscesses and wound sepsis.

Once the pathogenic role of bacteria had been established, the larger pathogenic protozoa and fungi were soon recognized, e.g. the protozoon of malaria by the French army surgeon Charles Laveran in 1880. The *viruses* were more difficult to demonstrate, for most kinds were too small to be seen with the light microscope and none could be grown on an inanimate culture medium. At first they could be demonstrated only by observation of the disease they produced when infected tissue was inoculated into a susceptible animal. Thus, in studies of rabies, the fatal disease caused by the bite of a rabid animal, such as a dog or wolf, Pasteur and his colleagues in 1881 failed to isolate any micro-organism capable of causing the disease. They were able to reproduce the disease in dogs and rabbits by the intracerebral injection of brain tissue or saliva from a fatal case and they suggested that the causal agent was an organism too small to be seen. Their experiments, however, did not exclude the possibility that the agent might be a bacterium, or a larger microbe which was present but undetected in the inoculum. The means of excluding such a possibility was devised by Ivanowski (1892) in experiments with the viral mosaic disease of tobacco; he transmitted the disease to healthy plants by the inoculation of juice from a diseased plant after it had been filtered through a porcelain filter fine enough to prevent the passage of bacteria. *Filter-passing viruses* were soon similarly demonstrated in foot-and-mouth disease of cattle by Loeffler and Frosch (1898), in yellow fever by Reed, Carroll, Agramonte and Lazear (1900), who had to test their inoculations in human volunteers, and in other diseases. Virology did not progress rapidly, however, until after the Second World War, when the availability of the electron microscope enabled viruses to be visualized and the use of living human and animal tissue cells for the in-vitro culture of viruses was developed by John Enders (1949) and others from the earlier work of pioneers such as Alexis Carrel.

IMMUNITY AND IMMUNIZATION

It was an ancient observation, reported for instance by Fracastoro, that persons who had suffered from a distinctive disease, such as smallpox or measles, resisted it on subsequent exposures and rarely contracted it a second time. Such an acquired immunity is *specific*, i.e. effective only against the same type of infection as that previously suffered (or, exceptionally, a closely related one, as when cowpox immunizes against smallpox).

Artificial immunization against smallpox was practised in various communities by the unsafe method of inoculating smallpox exudate through the skin (variolation), until, in 1796, the safer method of inoculating cowpox exudate (vaccination) was discovered by the Gloucestershire doctor Edward Jenner.

Present day vaccinia virus has been shown to be different from cowpox virus and its origin is obscure. Nevertheless, it is highly effective and has been instrumental in the world eradication of natural smallpox, the last case of which occurred in Somalia in 1977. The natural existence of a safe immunizing agent such as vaccinia virus is exceptional, and we owe to Pasteur the development of immunizing strains of pathogenic microbes which are artificially attenuated (reduced in virulence) by prolonged or repeated culture under unnatural conditions in the laboratory. Pasteur derived such *attenuated live vaccines* for fowl cholera, anthrax, swine erysipelas and rabies, and called them 'vaccines' in honour of Jenner's work with cowpox, or vaccinia (from Latin 'vacca', a cow). In 1881 he made a convincing controlled trial of his anthrax vaccine, in which a vaccinated group of cows and sheep survived a later challenge by the inoculation of virulent anthrax bacilli, while a control group of unvaccinated animals perished from the same challenge. Today, attenuated live vaccines are used with outstanding success against such diseases as tuberculosis, poliomyelitis, measles and yellow fever.

The efficacy of vaccines consisting of killed bacteria was discovered by Salmon and Smith in 1886 in experiments on salmonellosis in pigeons, and today *killed vaccines* are used against, for example typhoid fever, whooping cough and influenza. About 1900, Loewenstein in Vienna and Glenny in London discovered that bacterial toxins rendered non-poisonous by treatment with formaldehyde were effective in immunizing against diphtheria and tetanus, diseases in which the serious effects are due to the toxin. The *toxoids* are now used routinely for the immunization of children.

The first step in elucidating the mechanisms of acquired immunity was the discovery of *antibodies* by Behring and Kitasato in 1890. They found that the injection of sublethal doses of diphtheria or tetanus toxin into guinea-pigs rendered the animals immune to the later injection of large doses of the same toxin. The immunity was associated with the appearance in the animal's blood of a substance, *antitoxin*, that specifically neutralized the toxin both in vitro and in vivo. These diphtheria and tetanus antitoxins were the first known antibodies, but protective antibodies which reacted directly with bacteria and viruses were soon demonstrated by other workers. Antibodies have a highly specific affinity for the microbial substances, or *antigens*, that have induced their formation, and this property is exploited in the common use of blood serum containing antibodies (*antiserum*) in laboratory tests for the precise identification of micro-organisms. Discovery of the means of perpetuating the growth of single antibody-producing cells has enabled these techniques to be further refined by the use of *monoclonal antibodies* that exhibit absolute specificity for the target antigens.

SEROTHERAPY AND CHEMOTHERAPY

The work of Behring and Kitasato led to the successful use of antisera raised in animals for the treatment of patients with diphtheria, tetanus, pneumonia and other diseases. Because, however, the antisera contained animal proteins foreign to the human body, and were given by injection, serotherapy often caused unpleasant allergic responses, called serum sickness. For this reason, and also because serotherapy was unsuccessful against many kinds of infection, further progress depended on the development of drugs that exhibited *selective toxicity*—the ability to inhibit or kill the microbe without harming the patient.

Although agents active against bacteria now form the most abundant group of antimicrobial agents, with over 200 different compounds in use throughout the world for the treatment of systemic human disease, the earliest therapeutic successes were achieved with antiprotozoal and anthelminthic agents. Indeed, effective treatment for malaria (cinchona bark), amoebic dysentery (ipecacuanha root), tapeworm (male fern) and roundworm (wormseed) have been known for centuries. In contrast, effective therapy for systemic bacterial disease was unknown before the use of hexamine (methenamine) at the turn of the 20th century and Paul Ehrlich's development of the arsenical Salvarsan (arsphenamine) for spirochaetal disease in 1909. Even these discoveries were of limited value. The true beginning of the therapeutic revolution in infection dates from Gerhard Domagk's description of Prontosil (the forerunner of sulphonamides) in 1935, the development of Alexander Fleming's penicillin by Howard Florey and his colleagues in 1940, and Selman Waksman's exploitation of the potential for antibiotic production among soil micro-organisms in the 1940s. Within 25 years of these discoveries, most of the major groups of antimicrobial agents had been recognized and more recent developments have chiefly involved chemical alteration of existing molecules.

Progress in the development of antiviral, antifungal and antiparasitic compounds has been much slower and therapeutic options in non-bacterial infection consequently remain severely limited.

LABORATORY DIAGNOSIS OF INFECTIONS

The signs and symptoms of some infective diseases may be specific for a particular micro-organism, e.g. the circumscribed boil of the staphylococcus and the characteristic rash of chickenpox, but those of many infections are unspecific, and any of several different pathogenic organisms may be the cause of an illness such as sore throat, bronchitis, pneumonia, meningitis, diarrhoea, wound sepsis and fever. In these cases, laboratory help is required to elucidate the cause. The reliability of that help depends on the correct techniques being used in collecting the appropriate specimens from the patient, and doctors must be properly instructed in these procedures. The precise indentification of the patient's pathogenic organisms is generally necessary for the effective use of a selective chemotherapeutic drug. In other words, the doctor has to identify and treat specific infections rather than clinical syndromes. Since, moreover, different strains of many bacterial species differ in their

susceptibility to particular drugs, it is usually desirable for the bacterium isolated from the patient to be tested for its drug sensitivity in the laboratory.

EPIDEMIOLOGY AND THE PREVENTION OF INFECTION

A knowledge of the sources, mechanisms of transmission and predisposing conditions of an infection makes it possible to devise preventive measures such as neutralization of the sources, interference with the mechanisms of transmission and removal of the predisposing conditions. Microbiology is thus closely concerned with *epidemiology*, which is the study of the factors that influence the prevalence and distribution of diseases in the community. The reporting of laboratory diagnoses of specific communicable infections to the health officer concerned with preventive measures plays an important part in guiding his day-to-day activities, and the collection of records of laboratory findings helps to guide national policies for immunization and environmental hygiene.

Sources of infection are the habitats in which the pathogenic microbes ordinarily grow and from which they are disseminated to susceptible hosts. Inanimate objects which carry the pathogens through the environment in a surviving, but non-growing, condition are known as *vehicles* of infection. Many species of pathogens are derived exclusively or mainly from *ill patients* as their source, but many others grow in, and are disseminated from, healthy persons, known as *carriers*, in whom they cause only a limited, subclinical infection. The existence of carriers was first demonstrated about 1900 in studies of typhoid fever initiated by Koch, and their importance as sources of infection is due to their mobility and lack of recognition in the community. Some infections, called *zoonoses*, have their sources in animals, which are the natural hosts of the pathogen, e.g. rabies, bubonic plague, brucellosis and leptospirosis. They are transmissible from animal to man, but not ordinarily from man to man, so that prevention depends on the control of human contact with the infected animals. As well as these kinds of *exogenous* infections from external sources, there are also many infections, termed *endogenous*, which are due to the opportunistic invasion of tissues by a commensal, or 'carried', organism that hitherto grew harmlessly elsewhere in the body, e.g. infections of the lung with pneumococci previously resident in the throat. The prevention of endogenous infections depends on the avoidance of predisposing conditions that impair the tissue defences.

Epidemiological observations may suggest by what mechanisms an infection is transmitted and so lead to the formulation of preventive measures even when the causal micro-organism is still unknown. In 1846, for instance, in a maternity clinic in Vienna, Ignaz Semmelweis deduced that puerperal fever was caused by a putrefactive agent which doctors picked up on their hands when attending patients or performing necropsies and then transferred into the birth canal when assisting women at childbirth. He reduced the number of deaths from 8.3 to 2.3% of mothers by requiring staff regularly to wash their hands in hypochlorite solution until they were free from the smell of putrefaction.

In comparable work, the anaesthetist John Snow (1849, 1854) showed that the geographical distribution of cholera in London was related to the sources of the supplies of drinking water, and concluded that the 'peculiar poison of the disease' was spread in patients' faeces, which contaminated water later drunk by other persons (faecal–oral transmission). Measures subsequently taken to ensure the purity of drinking water by protection, filtration and chlorination have led to the decline of cholera, typhoid fever and other water-borne infections.

The development of the techniques of antiseptic and aseptic surgery for the prevention of wound sepsis had its origin in the conception by Joseph Lister (1867) that if, as shown by Pasteur, bacteria were the cause of the fermentation and putrefaction of dead organic matter, they might well also be the cause of suppuration in living tissues. By covering operation wounds with dressings soaked in carbolic acid to kill any bacteria present in them and to exclude others from entry, and by disinfecting his hands and instruments, he greatly reduced the incidence of sepsis in his patients.

The discovery that blood-sucking arthropods spread certain diseases led to prevention by measures for the control of these *vectors*. In 1893 Theobald Smith and F. L. Kilborne first showed that Texas fever of cattle was spread by ticks that bite an infected cow and transmit its blood to another animal. Subsequently, it was shown that malaria was transmitted by anopheles mosquitoes (Ronald Ross, 1898), yellow fever by aedes mosquitoes (Reed and co-workers, 1900), bubonic plague by the rat flea (Liston and co-workers, 1905) and typhus fever by lice (Charles Nicolle, 1909). Campaigns of vector control by the use of insecticides and other means have since been conducted for the prevention of these diseases.

A major group of infections that have proved largely insusceptible to control by environmental sanitation are those of the respiratory tract, e.g. common colds, sore throats, influenza, whooping cough, pneumonia, tuberculosis, measles, and chickenpox. Organisms that enter and leave the body via the respiratory tract may be transmitted by a variety of means, including contact and airborne secretion droplets. It is probably this versatility in their means of spread, as well as the frequency with which urban dwellers share and breathe indoor air polluted by others, that explains the continuing high prevalence of respiratory infections.

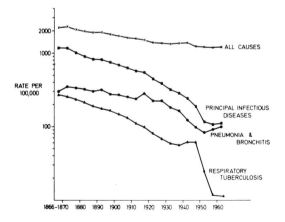

Fig. 1.1   Crude death rates in Scotland per 100 000 members of the population for all causes, principal infectious diseases, pneumonia and bronchitis, and respiratory tuberculosis. Five year averages between 1866 and 1965.

Although infective illness has remained common during the last 100 years, developed countries have seen a phenomenal decrease in the death rate from infections. In Scotland, deaths from the principal infectious diseases contributed, at a rate of 1167 per 100 000 of the population per annum, more than a half of all deaths, in the quinquennium 1861–65, whereas in 1961–65 they were reduced to the rate of 111 per 100 000 and contributed only one-tenth of all deaths (see Fig. 1.1). A similar decline in deaths from infectious disease occurred in England and Wales and predated the availability of effective chemotherapy. Since the steep decline in deaths began more than a century before preventive and curative medicine became significantly effective, the earlier reduction in deaths must have been due to improvements in nutrition and living conditions which increased the resistance of individuals to the point that they generally recovered from their many infections. Subsequently, and particularly with the introduction of immunization programmes and antimicrobial therapy in the last 50 years, medicine has made a more substantial contribution to the saving of life.

RECOMMENDED READING

Brock T D 1961 *Milestones in Microbiology*. Prentice-Hall, Engelwood Cliffs, N J. Reprinted 1975 by the American Society for Microbiology, Washington

Bulloch W 1960 *The History of Bacteriology*. Oxford University Press, Oxford

Burnet F M 1972 *Natural History of Infectious Disease*, 4th edn. Cambridge University Press, Cambridge

Collard P 1976 *The Development of Microbiology*. Cambridge University Press, Cambridge

Dubos R J 1950 *Louis Pasteur, Free Lance of Science*. Little Brown, Boston. Reprinted 1986 by Da Capo Press, New York

Foster W D 1970 *A History of Medical Bacteriology and Immunology*. Cox and Wyman, London

Grant J P 1991 *The State of the World's Children, 1991*. Oxford University Press (for UNICEF), Oxford,

Macfarlane G 1984 *Alexander Fleming; the Man and the Myth*. Chatto and Windus, London

Waterson A P, Wilkinson L 1978 *An Introduction to the History of Virology*. Cambridge University Press, Cambridge

Zinsser H 1935 *Rats, Lice and History*. Routledge, London

2

Morphology and nature of micro-organisms

D. Greenwood

Living material is organized in units known as *cells*. Each cell consists of a body of protoplasm, the *protoplast*, enclosed by a thin semipermeable membrane, the *cytoplasmic membrane* or *plasma membrane*, and also in some cases, by an outer, relatively rigid *cell wall*. The protoplast is differentiated into a major part, the *cytoplasm*, and an inner body, the *nucleus*, which contains the hereditary determinants of character, the *genes*, borne on thread-like *chromosomes*.

Micro-organisms are generally regarded as living forms that are microscopical in size and relatively simple, usually unicellular, in structure. The diameter of the smallest body that can be resolved and seen clearly with the naked eye is about 100 µm. All but a few of the bacteria are smaller than this and a microscope is therefore necessary for their observation. Viruses are even smaller and in most cases an electron microscope is needed to visualize them.

However, when bacteria or fungi are allowed to grow on a nutritive, solid supporting medium, their numerous progeny form *colonies* that are readily visible to the naked eye. Many viruses can be grown within cultures of living cells (*tissue cultures*) in the laboratory and many cause characteristic *cytopathic effects* visible in the light microscope.

It is useful to draw a clear distinction between relatively primitive (*prokaryotic*) cells and more advanced (*eukaryotic*) cells. The bacteria and related organisms (rickettsiae, chlamydiae and mycoplasmas) are prokaryotic cells whereas the cells of fungi, protozoa, plants and animals are eukaryotic.

Viruses fall into neither category; they are not cells in the accepted sense and rely on the biochemical processes of the host cell for their replication and propagation.

The main distinguishing features of the prokaryotic cell are:

1. Its nucleus appears as a simple, homogeneous body not possessing a nuclear membrane separating it from the cytoplasm, nor a nucleolus, nor a spindle, nor a number of separate non-identical chromosomes.

2. It lacks the internal membranes isolating the respiratory and photosynthetic enzyme systems in specific organelles, comparable with the membrane-bound mitochondria and chloroplasts of eukaryotic cells. Thus, the respiratory enzymes in bacteria are located mainly in the peripheral cytoplasmic membrane and their effective functioning is dependent upon the integrity of the cell protoplast as a whole.

3. Its rigid cell wall contains as its main strengthening element a specific peptidoglycan substance not found in eukaryotic organisms.

The bodies of higher plants and animals including helminths (see Chapter 62) are multicellular, with interdependence and specialization of function amongst the cells, the different kinds of cells being segregated in separate tissues. Many micro-organisms, on the other hand, are unicellular, existing as single cells, unattached to their fellows. Other micro-organisms grow as aggregates of cells joined together by their cell walls in clusters, chains, rods, filaments (hyphae) or mycelia (i.e.

meshworks of branching filaments). Generally, these morphologically multicellular microbes are physiologically unicellular, each cell being self-sufficient and, if isolated artificially, able to nourish itself, grow and reproduce the species. Some specialization of cell function, approaching that of true multicellular organisms, is encountered in colonies of moulds and filamentous 'higher' bacteria in which certain cells form an aerial mycelium and are specialized for the formation and dissemination of spores; these cells are dependent for their nutrition on the activities of other cells comprising a vegetative mycelium.

Most fungi form an aerial mycelium, but some (*yeasts* and *yeast-like fungi*) grow by budding, or by germ-tube formation. Others (*dimorphic fungi*) can exist in the yeast or mycelial form depending on the environmental conditions (see Chapter 60).

Protozoa are all unicellular, but encompass a wide diversity of morphological forms. Some (e.g. *Entamoeba* spp. and *Giardia lamblia*) have the capacity to enter a resting phase (*cyst*) by secretion of an external wall. This enables them to survive outside the host. Other protozoa (e.g. malaria parasites) exist as very diverse morphological and metabolic types at different stages in a complex life cycle (see Chapter 61). Bacterial cells are smaller (usually between 0.4 and 1.5 μm in short diameter, than those of fungi and protozoa, and in most cases they have relatively rigid cell walls

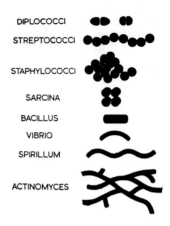

Fig. 2.1 The shapes and characteristic groupings of various bacterial cells.

that maintain their characteristic shape; this may be spherical (coccus), rod-shaped (bacillus), comma-shaped (vibrio), spiral (spirillum and spirochaete) or filamentous (Fig. 2.1). They show little structural differentiation when examined by ordinary microscopical methods.

ANATOMY OF THE BACTERIAL CELL

The principal structures of the bacterial cell are shown in Fig. 2.2. The *protoplast*, i.e. the whole body of living material (*protoplasm*), is bounded peripherally by a very thin, elastic and semiperme-

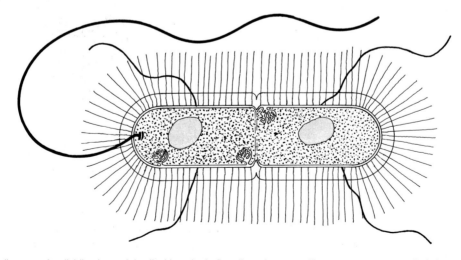

Fig. 2.2 A diagram of a dividing bacterial cell with a single flagellum, four sex pili, numerous common fimbriae, a cell wall, a cytoplasmic membrane, two nuclear bodies, three mesosomes and numerous ribosomes.

able cytoplasmic membrane. Outside, and closely covering this, lies the rigid, supporting *cell wall*, which is porous and relatively permeable. Cell division occurs by the development, from the periphery inwards, of a transverse cytoplasmic membrane and a transverse cell wall, or *cross wall*.

The *cytoplasm*, or main part of the protoplasm, consists of a watery sap packed with large numbers of small granules called *ribosomes* and a few convoluted membranous bodies called *mesosomes* (see below). The nuclear material, nucleus or *chromatin*, is not normally seen with the light microscope. Fig. 2.3 is an electron micrograph of a thin section of a dividing bacterial cell.

In addition to these essential structures, other intracellular and extracellular structures may be present in some species of bacteria; their occurrence sometimes depends upon particular conditions of growth. *Inclusion granules* of storage products such as volutin (polyphosphate), lipid (poly-*β*-hydroxybutyrate), glycogen or starch may occur in the cytoplasm. Outside the cell wall, there may be a protective gelatinous covering layer called a *capsule* or, when it is too thin to be resolved with the light microscope (< 0.2 µm), a *microcapsule*. Soluble large-molecular material may be dispersed by the bacterium into the environment as *loose slime*. Some bacteria bear, protruding outwards from the cell wall, one or more kinds of filamentous appendages: *flagella*, which are organs of locomotion; *fimbriae*, which appear to be organs of adhesion; and *pili*, which are involved in the transfer of genetic material. Because they are exposed to contact and interaction with the cells and humoral substances of the body of the host, the surface structures of bacteria are the structures most likely to have special roles in the processes of infection.

Bacterial nucleus (DNA)

The genetic information of a bacterial cell is contained in a single, long molecule of double-stranded deoxyribonucleic acid (DNA) which can be extracted in the form of a closed circular thread about 1 mm long. The cell solves the problem of packaging this enormous macromolecule

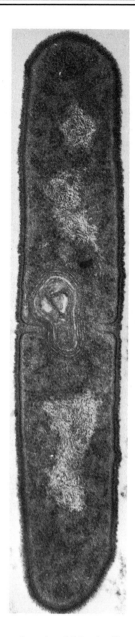

Fig. 2.3 A thin section of a dividing bacillus showing cell wall, cytoplasmic membrane, ribosomes, a developing crosswall, and a mesosome. (By courtesy of Dr P J Highton and editors of *Journal of Ultrastructure Research*.) x 50 000.

by condensing and looping it into a *supercoiled* state. As well as the chromosome, the bacterium may contain one or more additional fragments of DNA, known as *episomes* or *plasmids*. As the bacterial chromosome is not bound to proteins, it does not stain like a eukaryotic chromosome and in unstained bacteria examined normally with the light microscope, or in bacteria stained by the usual methods, there is no obvious differentiation into nucleus and cytoplasm. Only a single nuclear body is present in some cells, whilst in others, as a result of nuclear division preceding cell division, two or more may be present. These can be revealed by special staining procedures. Unlike the intracellular storage granules described below, they are constantly present in all cells and under all conditions of culture. The nuclear bodies replicate by growth and simple fission, and not by mitosis; they show no outer nuclear membrane separating them from the cytoplasm, and they have no nucleolus.

Cytoplasm of bacteria

The cytoplasm of the bacterial cell is a viscous watery solution, or soft gel, containing a variety of organic and inorganic solutes, and numerous small granules called *ribosomes*. The cytoplasm of bacteria differs from that of the higher eukaryotic organisms in not containing an endoplasmic reticulum or membrane bearing microsomes, in not containing mitochondria and in not showing signs of internal mobility such as cytoplasmic streaming, the formation, migration and disappearance of vacuoles, and amoeboid movement.

Ribosomes

Bacterial ribosomes are slightly smaller (10-20 nm) than those of eukaryotic cells and they have a sedimentation constant of 70S, being composed of a 30S and a 50S subunit (cf. 40S and 60S in the 80S eukaryotic counterparts). They may be seen with the electron microscope and number tens of thousands per cell. They are strung together on strands of messenger RNA (mRNA) to form *polysomes* and it is at this site that the code of the mRNA is translated into peptide sequences. Thus the ribosomal components link up and travel along the mRNA strand and here determine the sequence of amino acids brought to the site on transfer RNA (tRNA) molecules and built into specific polypeptides.

Inclusion granules

In many species of bacteria, round granules are observed in the cytoplasm. These are not permanent or essential structures, and may be absent under certain conditions of growth. They appear to be aggregates of substances concerned with cell metabolism, e.g. an excess metabolite stored as a nutrient reserve. Generally, they are present in largest amount when the bacteria have access to an abundance of energy-yielding nutrients, and diminish or disappear under conditions of energy source starvation. They consist of volutin (polyphosphate), lipid, glycogen, starch or sulphur.

Volutin and lipid granules, 0.1–1.0 μm in diameter, are seen in many parasitic and saprophytic bacteria, and their demonstration may assist in the identification of certain organisms; thus, the diphtheria bacillus may be distinguished from related bacilli found in the throat by its content of volutin granules.

Volutin granules (syn. metachromatic granules). These granules have an intense affinity for basic dyes. With toluidine blue or methylene blue, they stain a red-violet colour contrasting with the blue staining of the bacterial protoplasm. By special methods such as those of Neisser and Albert the granules can be demonstrated with even greater colour contrast. Their metachromatic staining is thought to be due to their content of polymerized inorganic polyphosphate, an energy-rich compound that may act as a reserve of energy and phosphate for cell metabolism or may be a by-product. Volutin granules are slightly acid-fast, resisting decoloration by 1% sulphuric acid; they are more refractile than the protoplasm and are sometimes distinguishable in unstained wet films. By electron microscopy they appear as very opaque, clearly demarcated bodies.

Lipid granules. These granules have an affinity for fat-soluble dyes such as Sudan black; they are then coloured black in contrast to the remaining protoplasm, which can be counterstained pink with water-soluble basic fuchsin. The granules are spherical, of varying size and highly refractile, being easily seen in unstained preparations. They appear as unstained spaces in bacteria treated with simple stains or by Gram's method. In the bacteria so far subjected to chemical analysis, the granules appear to consist mainly of polymerized β-hydroxybutyric acid. The manner in which the lipid content of bacteria, e.g. in the *Bacillus* genus, varies with the conditions of culture suggests that this substance may act as a carbon and energy storage product.

Polysaccharide granules. These granules are of either glycogen (red-brown) or starch (blue) and can be seen in the cytoplasm of certain bacteria when they are stained with iodine. Many other species, e.g. *Escherichia coli*, do not form granules visible with the light microscope but they can be seen with the electron microscope.

Mesosomes

These are convoluted or multilaminated membranous bodies visible in the electron microscope. They develop by complex invagination of the cytoplasmic membrane into the cytoplasm, sometimes in relation to the nuclear body and often from the sites of cross-wall formation in Gram-positive bacteria. Similar structures have been noted in Gram-negative bacteria where they are not so common. Mesosomes are thought to be involved in mechanisms responsible for the compartmenting of DNA at cell division and at sporulation. They may also have a function analogous to the mitochondria of the eukaryotic cell — providing a membranous support for respiratory enzymes.

Cytoplasmic membrane

The bacterial protoplast is limited externally by a thin, elastic cytoplasmic membrane, which is 5–10 nm thick, consists mainly of lipoprotein and is visible in some ultrathin sections examined with the electron microscope. *Membranes* generally

appear in suitably stained electron microscope preparations as two dark lines about 2.5 nm wide separated by a lighter area of similar width. The classical model of a 'unit membrane' is shown in Fig 2.4: lipid molecules are arrayed in a double layer with their hydrophilic polar regions externally aligned and in contact with a layer of protein at each surface. The functions of membranes differ widely in nature and it is clear that this simplified model cannot account for all of the variations of function that are already known. More complex membrane architecture is gradually being revealed by special electron microscope techniques such as freeze etching which uses heavy-metal shadowing to reveal details of the faces of fractured frozen membranes imprinted on a carbon replica. In bacteria, the cytoplasmic membrane lacks cholesterol, which is a normal constituent of animal cell membranes. The cytoplasmic membrane constitutes an osmotic barrier that is impermeable to many small molecular solutes and is responsible for maintaining the differences in solute content between the cytoplasm and the external environment. It permits the passive diffusion inwards and outwards of water and certain other small molecular substances, especially lipid-soluble ones, and it actively effects the selective transport of specific nutrient solutes into the cell and that of waste products out of it. In addition to the enzymes, or *permeases*, responsible for the active uptake of nutrients, the cytoplasmic membrane contains many other kinds of enzymes, notably respiratory enzymes and pigments (cytochrome system), certain enzymes of the tricarboxylic acid cycle and, probably, polymerizing enzymes that manufacture the substances of the cell wall and extracellular structures. It has little mechanical strength and is supported on the outside by the cell wall (Fig. 2.5).

Fig. 2.4 A diagram of a unit membrane. A lipid bilayer with polar (hydrophilic) regions externally orientated towards a layer of protein at each surface has a characteristic appearance when stained and seen in cross-section in the electron microscope.

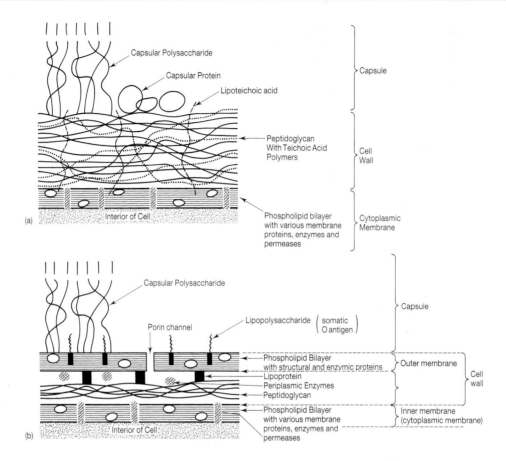

Fig. 2.5 a The envelope of the Gram-positive cell wall.
     b The envelope of the Gram-negative cell wall.

Cell wall

The cell wall encases the protoplast and lies immediately external to the cytoplasmic membrane. It is 10–25 nm thick, strong and relatively rigid, though with some elasticity, and openly porous, being freely permeable to solute molecules smaller than 10 000 Da in mass and 1 nm in diameter. It supports the weak cytoplasmic membrane against the high internal osmotic pressure of the protoplasm (usually between 5 and 25 atm) and maintains the characteristic shape of the bacterium in its coccal, bacillary, filamentous or spiral form.

The integrity of the cell wall is essential to the viability of the bacterium. If the wall is weakened or ruptured, the protoplasm may swell from osmotic inflow of water and burst the weak cyto-

plasmic membrane. This process of lethal disintegration and dissolution is termed *lysis*.

The cell wall plays an important part in *cell division*. A transverse partition of cell wall material grows inwards, like a closing iris diaphragm, from the lateral wall at the equator of the cell and forms a complete *cross-wall* separating two daughter cells. The cell wall is not seen in conventionally stained smears examined with the light microscope. It can be demonstrated by special staining methods but most readily and clearly by electron microscopy; it is seen both in ultrathin sections and, as an empty fold surrounding the shrunken protoplast, in whole-cell preparations shadow-cast with heavy metal.

The chemical composition of the cell wall differs considerably between different bacterial species, but in all species the main strengthening component is *peptidoglycan* (syn. *mucopeptide* or *murein*). Peptidoglycan is composed of *N*-acetylglucosamine and *N*-acetylmuramic acid molecules linked alternately in a chain (Fig. 2.6). The *N*-acetylmuramic acid units each carry a short peptide, usually consisting of L-alanine, D-glutamic acid, either *meso*-diaminopimelic acid (in Gram-negative bacteria) or L-lysine (in Gram-positive bacteria) and D-alanyl-D-alanine. The wall is given its strength by cross-links that form between adjacent strands. These may be formed directly between the *meso*-diaminopimelic acid or L-lysine of one strand and the penultimate D-alanine of the next, or (the usual form in Gram-positive organisms) through an interpeptide bridge composed of up to five amino acids; in either case, the terminal D-alanine is lost in the cross-linking reaction (Fig. 2.7). Several antibiotics interfere with the construction of the cell wall peptidoglycan (see Chapter 6).

The walls of Gram-positive bacteria contain more peptidoglycan and are thicker and stronger (more extensively cross-linked) than those of Gram-negative bacteria. This difference is associated with a higher internal osmotic pressure in Gram-positive cells.

The presence of peptidoglycan has been demonstrated in rickettsiae and chlamydiae, and this is

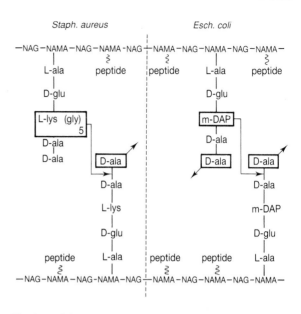

Fig. 2.7 Schematic representation of the peptidoglycan of a representative Gram-positive organism (*Staphylococcus aureus*) and a representative Gram-negative organism (*Escherichia coli*). Note that in the Gram-positive organism cross-linking occurs through a peptide bridge (pentaglycine in *Staph. aureus*) whereas direct cross-linking occurs in *Esch. coli*. In both cases the terminal D-alanine is lost. Not all peptides are engaged in cross-linking in *Esch. coli* and carboxypeptidases remove redundant D-alanine residues.

taken to indicate that these organisms are phylogenetically related to the bacteria rather than to the viruses, in which muramic acid has not been found.

The bacterial cell wall also contains other components whose nature and amount vary with the species. Many Gram-positive bacteria contain relatively large amounts of *teichoic acid* (a polymer of ribitol or glycerol phosphate complexed with sugar residues) interspersed with the peptidoglycan; some of this material (*lipoteichoic acid*) is linked to lipids buried in the cell membrane. Gram-negative bacteria possess a complex membrane-like structure external to the peptidoglycan layer. In *Esch. coli* this comprises lipid, polysaccharide, lipoprotein and lipopolysaccharide and makes up over 80% of the wall weight. This outer membrane confers several important properties on Gram-negative bacteria: it protects the peptidoglycan from the effects of lysozyme; it impedes the ingress of many antibiotics that are thus rendered impotent;

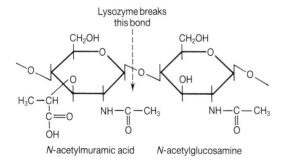

Fig. 2.6 The basic building block of bacterial cell wall peptidoglycan. *N*-acetylmuramic acid is derived from *N*-acetylglucosamine by the addition of a lactic acid moiety. Each *N*-acetylmuramic acid molecule is substituted with a pentapeptide; an *N*-acetylglucosamine molecule is joined to the muramylpentapeptide within the cell membrane and the unit is transferred to growth points in the existing peptidoglycan, where adjacent strands are cross-linked. See also Figs 2.7 and 6.1.

components of the lipopolysaccharide, in particular the core structure, lipid A, forms *endotoxin*, which when released in the bloodstream, may give rise to *endotoxin shock*.

Lysozyme is a natural body defence substance which lyses bacteria of many species. It cleaves the link between *N*-acetylglucosamine and *N*-acetylmuramic acid (Fig. 2.6). Bacteriophages possess a lysozyme-like enzyme that allows their initial penetration into the bacterium and, after they have reproduced, causes lysis of the bacterium.

It should be noted, moreover, that bacteria themselves possess enzymes, called *autolysins*, able to hydrolyse their own cell wall substances. Under normal conditions their action is confined to re-modelling of the cell wall in the course of growth.

Weakening, removal or defective formation of the cell wall is involved in the production of the various abnormal forms called *spheroplasts*, *protoplasts*, *pleomorphic involution forms*, and *L-forms* (see below).

Capsules, microcapsules and loose slime

Many bacteria are surrounded by a discrete covering layer of a relatively firm gelatinous material that lies outside and immediately in contact with the cell wall. When this layer, in the wet state, is wide enough (0.2 μm or more) to be resolved with the light microscope, it is called a *capsule*. When it is narrower, and detectable only by indirect, serological means, or by electron microscopy, it may be termed a *microcapsule*. The capsular gel consists largely of water and has only a small content (e.g. 2%) of solids. In most species, the solid material is a complex polysaccharide, though in some species its main constituent is polypeptide or protein.

Loose slime, or *free slime*, is an amorphous, viscid colloidal material that is secreted extracellularly by some non-capsule bacteria and also, outside their capsules, by many capsulate bacteria. In capsulate bacteria the slime is generally similar in chemical composition and antigenic character to the capsular substance. When slime-forming bacteria are grown on a solid culture medium, the slime remains around the bacteria as a matrix in which they are embedded and its presence confers on the growths a watery and sticky 'mucoid' character. The slime is freely soluble in water and, when the bacteria are grown or suspended in a liquid medium, it passes away from them and disperses through the medium.

Demonstration. Capsules and slime are usually invisible in films stained by ordinary methods except as clear haloes surrounding the stained bacteria. Since capsules consist largely of water, they shrink very greatly on drying. For this reason, dry-film methods of demonstrating capsules are unreliable; the capsules may shrink so much that they become invisible or, on the other hand, shrinkage artefacts may give the appearance of capsules on non-capsulate bacteria. The most reliable method of demonstration is by 'negative' staining in wet films with India ink; the carbon particles of the ink make a dark background in the film, but cannot penetrate the capsule, which thus appears as a clear halo around the bacterium (Fig. 2.8). When bacteria that have been grown on solid medium are being examined for capsules, it is important that they should first be washed or suspended for a sufficient time in water to ensure the removal of any loose slime which can be observed when films are made directly from the solid medium.

Microcapsules may not be seen at all and for this reason their presence has generally to be

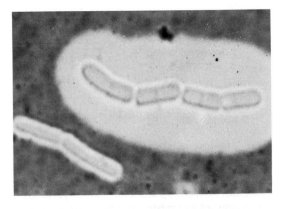

Fig. 2.8 *Bacillus megaterium.* Chain of bacilli with large capsule and pair with very small capsule in wet film with India ink. × 3500.

deduced from serological evidence that the cell wall antigen (e.g. the O, or somatic, antigen in Enterobacteriaceae) is masked by a covering layer (e.g. of K, or 'capsular', antigen).

In attempts to demonstrate capsules it should be remembered that their development is often dependent on the existence of favourable environmental conditions. Thus, their size may vary with the amount of carbohydrate in the culture medium available for nutrition of the bacteria. In the later stages of growth in artificial culture (e.g. 12–24 h) they may become reduced in size due to carbon and energy starvation or they may disappear due to the accumulation in the medium of capsule-degrading enzymes (e.g. hyaluronidase in the case of *Streptococcus pyogenes*).

Function It is not known with certainty what are the functions of capsules and microcapsules, but it is probable that their principal action is in protecting the cell wall against attack by various kinds of antibacterial agents, e.g. bacteriophages, colicines, complement, lysozyme and other lytic enzymes, that otherwise would more readily damage or destroy it. In the case of certain capsulate pathogenic organisms (e.g. pneumococcus, pyogenic streptococci, anthrax bacillus and plague bacillus) good evidence has been obtained to show that the capsule protects the bacteria against ingestion by the phagocytes of the host. The capsule is thus an important agent determining virulence, and non-capsulate mutants of these bacteria are found to be non-virulent. In some organisms the capsule contains more than one functional component. Thus, *Str. pyogenes*, which under favourable conditions of growth may form an anti-phagocytic capsule composed of hyaluronic acid, also possesses a second surface substance, M protein, which inhibits either the ingestion or the intracellular digestion of the cocci by the phagocytes; the M protein occurs in association with the hyaluronic acid capsule or, when the latter is absent, by itself in the form of a microcapsule. In *Bacillus anthracis* the capsule is a polymer of D-glutamic acid and protects the bacteria not only against phagocytosis but also, to some extent, against the action of a bactericidal basic polypeptide present in animal tissues.

The capsular substance is usually antigenic and the capsular antigens play a very important part in determining the antigenic specificity of bacteria. When capsulate pneumococci are treated with type-specific antiserum, the sharpness of outline of the capsule is greatly enhanced. This is referred to as the '*capsule-swelling reaction*'.

Flagella and motility

Motile bacteria possess filamentous appendages known as *flagella*, which act as organs of locomotion. The flagellum is a long, thin filament, twisted spirally in an open, regular wave form. It is about 0.02 µm thick and is usually several times the length of the bacterial cell. It originates in the bacterial protoplasm and is extruded through the cell wall. According to the species, there may be one or several (e.g. 1–20) flagella per cell, and in elongated bacteria the arrangement of the flagella may be *peritrichous*, or *lateral*, when they originate from the sides of the cell, or *polar*, when they originate from one or both ends. Where several occur on a cell, they may function coiled together as a single 'tail'. Flagella consist largely or entirely of a protein, *flagellin*, belonging to the same chemical group as myosin, the contractile protein of muscle. They can be demonstrated easily and clearly with the electron microscope, usually appearing as simple fibrils without internal differentiation (Fig. 2.9). In some preparations the flagellum appears as a hollow tube formed of helically twisted fibrils, and the flagella of some bacteria, e.g. vibrios, have an outer sheath; but bacterial flagella do not have the complex structure of the flagella and cilia of plants and animals, which in all cases consist of two central and nine peripheral fibrils contained in a tube-like sheath. They are invisible in ordinary preparations by the light microscope, but may be shown by the use of special staining methods, and in special circumstances by dark-ground illumination. Because of the difficulties of these methods, the presence of flagella is commonly inferred from the observation of motility.

Motility may be observed either microscopically or by noting the occurrence of spreading growth in semi-solid agar medium. On microscopical observation of wet films, motile bacteria are seen

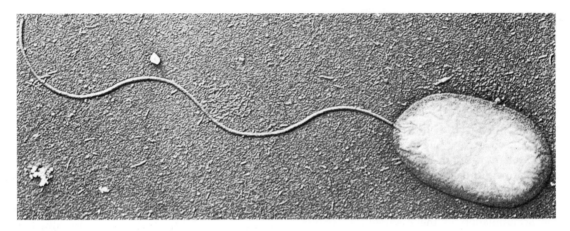

Fig. 2.9 *Pseudomonas aeruginosa*. Bacillus with a single polar flagellum, dried and shadow-cast. Electron microscope × 38 000. (From Wilkinson J F, Duguid J P 1960 The influence of cultural conditions on bacterial cytology. *International Review of Cytology* 9:1–76.)

swimming in different directions across the field, with a darting, wriggling or tumbling movement. True motility must be distinguished from a drifting of the bacteria in a single direction due to a current in the liquid, and also from Brownian movement, which is a rapid oscillation of each bacterium within a very limited area due to bombardment by water molecules.

Among the spirochaetes, motility appears to be a function of the cell body, since flagella do not occur. The most characteristic movement is a fast spiral rotation on the long axis with slow progression in the axial line; movements of flexion and lashing movements may be observed. Some spirochaetes possess an axial filament and others a band of fibrils wound around their surface from pole to pole. It has been suggested that these structures may contribute to motility, either through being themselves contractile or by acting as stiffeners for recoil against the contractile protoplast.

Function. It is not known with certainty what advantage a bacterium derives from its ability to move actively. Motility may be beneficial in increasing the rate of uptake of nutrient solutes by continuously changing the environmental fluid in contact with the bacterial cell surface. Random movement and dispersion through the environment may be beneficial ensuring that at least some cells of a strain reach every locality suitable for colonization. There is, moreover, good evidence that the movement of many bacteria is *directed* by responses of the organism towards localities favourable to growth and away from unfavourable regions. Thus, bacteria tend to migrate towards regions where there is a higher concentration of nutrient solutes (a process known as *chemotaxis*) and away from regions containing higher concentrations of disinfectant substances (*negative chemotaxis*). Motile aerobic bacteria show positive *aerotaxis* and migrate towards regions where there is a higher concentration of dissolved oxygen; anaerobes migrate away from such regions.

It might be supposed that the power of active locomotion would assist pathogenic bacteria in penetrating through viscid mucous secretions and epithelial barriers, and in spreading throughout the body fluids and tissues, but it must be noted that many non-motile pathogens (e.g. brucellae and streptococci) are no less invasive than motile ones.

Fimbriae

Certain Gram-negative bacilli, including intestinal commensal and pathogenic species, possess filamentous appendages of a different kind from the flagella. These are called *fimbriae* and they occur in non-motile, as well as in motile strains. They are far more numerous than flagella (e.g. 100–500 being borne peritrichously by each cell) and are much shorter and only about half as thick (e.g. varying from 0.1 to 1.5 μm in length and having a uniform width between 4 and 8 nm). They do not have the smoothly curved spiral form of flagella and are mostly more or less straight. They cannot be seen with the light microscope but are clearly seen with the electron microscope in preparations that have been metal-shadowed or negatively stained with phosphotungstic acid (see Fig. 2.10).

Most genetically fimbriate strains of bacteria readily undergo a reversible variation between a fimbriate phase and a non-fimbriate phase that is affected by the conditions of growth. The majority of bacilli in the culture become fimbriate, as a result of prolonged culture or serial (48-hourly)

subculture, in static liquid medium incubated aerobically. The non-fimbriate phase predominates when subcultures are made serially on a solid culture medium.

Function. There is evidence that fimbriae may function as organs of adhesion. The possession of fimbriae confers on bacilli the power of adhering firmly to solid surfaces of various kinds, including those of the cells of animals, plants and fungi. Comparable non-fimbriate bacilli do not adhere when they collide with such surfaces. The adhesive property may be of value to the bacteria in holding them in nutritionally favourable micro-environments. Moreover, bacteria growing in stagnant liquid medium under air are assisted by the possession of fimbriae to grow attached together in the form of a *pellicle* that floats on the surface of the medium where the growth is greatly

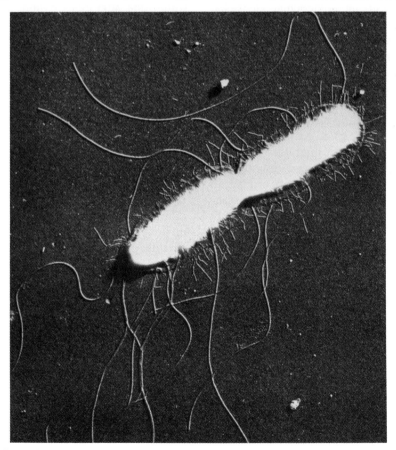

Fig. 2.10 *Salmonella typhi.* Dividing bacillus from log-phase culture bears about 15 long wavy flagella and over 100 short fimbriae. Note dense (white) shrunken protoplast surrounded by an empty fold of cell wall. Whole bacillus dried and shadow-cast. Electron microscope × 16 000. (From Duguid J P, Wilkinson J F 1961 Environmentally induced changes in bacterial morphology. *Symposia of the Society of General Microbiology* **11**: 69–99.)

enhanced by the free supply of atmospheric oxygen.

Haemagglutination. The majority of fimbriate bacteria bear fimbriae of a type that enables them to adhere to, among other kinds of tissue cells, the red blood cells of many animal species (e.g. to guinea-pig, fowl, horse and pig red cells very strongly, to human cells moderately strongly, to sheep cells weakly and to ox cells scarcely at all). If a drop of a concentrated suspension of fimbriate bacilli is mixed for a few minutes with a drop of a suspension of guinea-pig red cells, the adhering bacilli bind the red cells together in clumps visible to the naked eye. A simple haemagglutination test can thus be used to determine whether a culture contains fimbriate bacilli.

There exist different types of fimbriae having different adhesive properties. The commonest kind, type 1, which occurs in escherichia, klebsiella, serratia, salmonella and shigella organisms is about 8 nm in width, and it may be recognized by the observation that its adhesive and haemagglutinating actions are completely and specifically inhibited by the addition of a small amount (0.1–0.5%) of D-mannose to the test mixture (i.e. its activities are mannose-sensitive). A few salmonella organisms (e.g. *S. gallinarum* and *S. pullorum* possess a kind of fimbriae (type 2), apparently devoid of all haemagglutinating and adhesive properties. In addition to, or instead of, type 1 fimbriae, some klebsiella and serratia organisms possess type 3 fimbriae, about 5 nm in width; these do not agglutinate red cells unless the cells are first heated or tanned, and their adhesive properties are unaffected by mannose. Proteus organisms possess a kind of fimbriae (type 4) which have mannose-resistant haemagglutinating activity against untreated red cells of certain species. It should be noted also that some bacteria, e.g. many strains of *Esch. coli*, possess mannose-resistant haemagglutinating factors that are not associated with fimbriae.

Pili (sex pili)

These structures are similar to fimbriae, but are functionally different. They are longer than fimbriae and confer the ability to attach specifically to other bacteria that lack these appendages. Pili appear to be involved in the transfer of DNA during conjugation (Chapter 7); they also act as receptor sites for certain bacteriophages described as being 'donor-specific'.

BACTERIAL REPRODUCTION

Among the 'lower' or true bacteria, multiplication takes place by *simple binary fission*. The cell grows in size, usually elongating to twice its original length, and the protoplasm becomes divided into two approximately equal parts by the ingrowth of a transverse septum from the plasma membrane and cell wall. In some species, the cell wall septum, or cross-wall, splits in two and the daughter cells separate almost immediately. In others, the cell walls of the daughter cells remain continuous for some time after cell division and the organisms grow adhering in pairs, clusters, chains or filaments. If cross-wall splitting is thus delayed in an organism in which the cross-walls of successive cell divisions are all formed in parallel planes, the cells will be grouped in pairs, chains, rods or filaments. If it is delayed in an organism that forms successive cross-walls in different planes, e.g. ones at right angles to each other, the cells will be grouped in pairs, forming either cubic or irregular clusters. Under favourable conditions, growth and division are repeated with great rapidity, e.g. every half-hour or less, so that one individual cell may reproduce thousands of millions of new organisms in less than a day (see Chapter 3).

In the 'higher', or mycelial, bacteria, growth takes place by extension of the vegetative filaments, and multiplication by transverse division of these into shorter forms, or by the liberation of numerous conidia (see below) which later germinate and give rise to fresh mycelia.

Bacterial spores

Some species, notably those of the genera *Bacillus* and *Clostridium*, develop a highly resistant resting phase or *endospore*, whereby the organism can survive in a dormant state through a long period of starvation or other adverse environmental condition. The process does not involve multiplication: in *sporulation*, each vegetative cell forms only one spore, and in subsequent *germination* each spore gives rise to a single vegetative cell. Certain specific antigens develop in the spore that are not found in the vegetative cells.

Sporulation. Sporulation occurs as a response to starvation or, at least, the exhaustion of a limiting substance. It does not take place as long as conditions continue to favour maximal vegetative growth. In certain species, sporulation may be induced by depletion of nutrients necessary for vegetative growth, e.g. the carbon and energy source, the nitrogen source, sulphate, phosphate or iron salt; at the same time, the process requires a continued supply of other minerals (potassium, magnesium, manganese and calcium salts), and favourable conditions of moisture, temperature, pH, oxygen tension, etc. The spore is formed inside the parent vegetative cell (hence the name 'endospore'). It develops from a portion of protoplasm near one end of the cell (the 'forespore'), incorporates part of the nuclear material (equivalent to one genome) of the cell and acquires a thick covering layer, the 'cortex', and a thin, but tough, outer 'spore coat' consisting of several layers. Spores of some species have an additional, apparently rather loose covering known as the exosporium. The appearance of the mature spores varies according to the species, being spherical, ovoid or elongated, occupying a terminal, subterminal or central position, and being narrower than the cell, or broader and bulging it (Fig. 2.11). Finally, the remainder of the parent cell disintegrates and the spore is freed. Figure 2.12 shows a cross-section of a typical spore.

Viability. Spores are much more resistant than the vegetative forms to injurious chemical and physical influences, including exposure to disinfectants, drying and heating. Thus, application of moist heat at 100–120°C for a period of 10–20 min may be needed to kill spores, whereas heating at 60°C suffices to kill vegetative cells. Spores may remain viable for many years, either in the dry state or in moist conditions unfavourable to growth.

The marked resistance of spores has been attributed to several factors in which they differ from vegetative cells: the impermeability of their

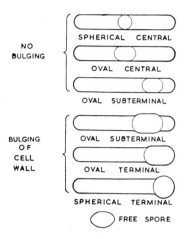

Fig. 2.11 The shape and situation of the spore in the bacterial cell.

cortex and outer coat, their high content of calcium and dipicolinic acid, their low content of water and their very low metabolic and enzymic-activity.

Germination. Germination of the spore occurs when the external conditions become favourable to growth by access to moisture and nutrients. It is irreversible and involves rapid degradative changes. The spore successively loses its heat resistance and its dipicolinic acid; it loses calcium, it becomes permeable to dyes and its refractility changes. Spores that have survived exposure to severe adverse influences such as heat are much

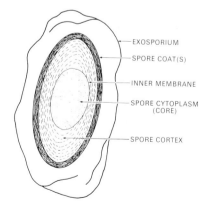

Fig. 2.12 Cross-section of a bacterial spore. The core is surrounded by the inner spore membrane. The cortex, a laminated structure, is protected by a more resistant layer or multiple layers forming the spore coat. In some cases, a loose outer covering (exosporium) can be defined.

more exacting than normal spores in their requirements for germination. For this reason, specially enriched culture media are used when testing the sterility of materials, such as surgical catgut, that have been exposed to disinfecting procedures. In the process of germination, the spore swells, its cortex disintegrates, its coat is broken open and a single vegetative cell emerges.

The initiation of germination is incompletely understood. It is clear that the degree of dormancy of spores may be altered by various treatments, including transient exposure to heat at 80°C for example, so that germination can then proceed more rapidly in the individual cells or more completely in a spore population. This alteration of the degree of dormancy is distinct from germination and is reversible if germination does not proceed. It is called *activation*.

Outgrowth. This term is used to denote the stage from germination up to the formation of the first vegetative cell and prior to the first cell division. The conditions required for successful outgrowth may differ markedly from those that allow germination.

Demonstration. In unstained preparations the spore is recognized within the parent cell by its greater refractility. It is larger than lipid inclusion granules and is often ovoid, in contrast to the spherical shape of the lipid granules. Mature ungerminated spores are 'phase-bright' in the phase-contrast microscope; immature or germinated spores are 'phase-dark'. When mature, the spore resists coloration by simple stains, appearing as a clear space within the stained cell protoplasm. Spores are slightly acid-fast and may be stained differentially by a modification of the Ziehl-Neelsen method.

Conidia (exospores)

Some of the mycelial bacteria (*Actinomycetales*) and many filamentous fungi form *conidia*, resting spores of a kind different from endospores. The conidia are borne *externally* by abstriction from the ends of the parents cells (conidiophores) and are disseminated by the air or other means to fresh habitats. They are not specially resistant to heat and disinfectants.

Pleomorphism and involution

During growth, bacteria of a single strain may show considerable variation in size and shape, forming a proportion of cells that differ grossly from the normal, e.g. swollen, spherical and pear-shaped forms, elongated filaments and filaments with localized swellings. This pleomorphism occurs most readily in certain species (e.g. *Streptobacillus moniliformis*, *Yersinia pestis*) in ageing cultures on artificial medium and especially in the presence of antagonistic substances such as penicillin, glycine, lithium chloride, sodium chloride in high concentrations, and organic acids at low pH. The abnormal cells are generally regarded as degenerate or *involution* forms; some are non-viable, whilst others may grow and revert to the normal form when transferred to a suitable environment. In many cases the abnormal shape seems to be the result of defective cell wall synthesis; the growing protoplasm expands the weakened wall to produce a grotesquely swollen cell comparable to a spheroplast (see below) that later usually bursts and lyses.

Spheroplasts and free protoplasts

If bacteria have their cell walls removed or weakened while they are held in a sufficiently concentrated solution such as 0.2–1.0 M sucrose with 0.01 M Mg^{2+} to prevent them imbibing water by osmosis, they may escape being lysed and, instead, may become converted into viable spherical bodies. If all the cell wall material has been removed from them, the spheres are *free protoplasts*. If they remain enclosed by an intact, but weakened residual cell wall, they are called *spheroplasts*. Protoplasts, for example, are readily liberated from the Gram-positive *Bacillus megaterium*, by dissolution of the cell walls with egg-white lysozyme. Spheroplasts are readily produced from Gram-negative bacilli such as *Esch. coli* by growing the organism in the presence of penicillins or other β-lactam antibiotics that specifically inhibit synthesis of the peptidoglycan component of the cell wall. A similar result may be obtained by culturing certain bacteria on media lacking a nutrient, e.g. diaminopimelic acid, lysine or a hexosamine derivative, that they require specifically for cell wall synthesis.

Protoplasts and spheroplasts are osmotically sensitive; they vary in size with the osmotic pressure of the suspending medium and, if the medium is much diluted, they swell up, burst and perish by lysis. If maintained in an osmotically protective nutrient medium, they remain viable and continue to metabolize, synthesize and grow. Protoplasts do not multiply (but see L-forms below). Spheroplasts, when kept in suitable conditions, may multiply by fission or budding and reproduce through many serial subcultures. The spheroplasts of Gram-negative bacilli, because they retain a residual wall structure, are not as osmotically sensitive as free protoplasts and are capable of growing on an ordinary agar culture medium. Protoplasts have not been found capable of reforming their cell walls and reverting to normal bacterial morphology, but spheroplasts commonly revert en masse when transferred to culture medium lacking the cell wall inhibitor.

L-forms of bacteria (or L-phase organisms)

These are abnormal growth forms that may arise spontaneously (e.g. in *Streptobacillus moniliformis* and *Bacteroides* spp.) or by the inhibition of cell wall synthesis in bacteria of normal morphology. They may be stable in the sense that special conditions of culture, such as the presence of penicillin, are not required to prevent their reversion to the parental bacterial forms. They differ from the parent bacteria in lacking a rigid cell wall and, in consequence, regular size and shape, but they are nevertheless viable and capable of growing and multiplying on a suitable nutrient medium. They range in size from minute bodies about 0.1 μm in diameter to large ones of 10–20 μm. The smallest viable forms are about 0.3 μm in diameter and may pass through bacteria-stopping filters. Some L-forms may be entirely devoid of a cell wall, and others, like spheroplasts, possess an intact cell wall that is weakened by absence of peptidoglycan.

Colonies of L-phase organisms on agar media are small and have a characteristic 'fried egg' appearance, rather like mycoplasmas. Because of their fragility, microscopical examination of L-forms is best done in situ on the agar medium, a coverslip being applied to a block of agar bearing the growth. If desired, the organisms can be stained after fixation by a fixative that is allowed to diffuse through the agar.

Reversion to the bacterial form. True L-forms, even if their origin was induced by exposure to penicillin or other cell wall inhibitor, continue to reproduce as L-forms through repeated subcultures in the absence of cell wall inhibitor, and give rise to revertants of normal bacterial morphology only occasionally.

Role. Although they have many resemblances to mycoplasmas, L-forms should probably be regarded as laboratory artefacts that do not occur or survive to any important extent in natural habitats. It is possible that L-forms could account for bacterial persistence during therapy with certain antibiotics. L-forms are non-pathogenic to laboratory animals.

MORPHOLOGICAL STUDY OF BACTERIA

Microscopical examination is usually the first step taken in the identification of an unknown bacterium. The bacterium may be allocated to one or other of the major groups when its *morphology* and *staining reactions* have been observed. The morphological features of importance are the size, shape and grouping of the cells, and their possession of any distinctive structures such as endospores, flagella (sometimes inferred from the simple observation of motility), capsules and intracellular granules. Staining reactions are observed after treatment by special procedures such as the Gram and Ziehl–Neelsen stains. A preparation stained by one of these methods usually suffices for observation of the general morphology of the bacterium, but some morphological features can be demonstrated only by the application of further special stains.

The optical, or light microscope is generally sufficient for making the observations of shape, staining reaction and special morphology that are required for the identification of a bacterium. The electron microscope, which has contributed much new information about the fine structure of the bacterial cell, is rarely required for bacteriological diagnostic work, but is essential for the visualization of viruses.

Unstained preparations of living organisms

The morphology of bacteria can be studied in the first place by examining them microscopically, suspended in a thin film of fluid between a glass slide and coverslip in an 'unstained wet film'. In this way their general shape can be seen and their motility determined. Certain very slender bacteria, however, such as the spirochaetes, are so feebly refractile that they cannot be seen by the ordinary microscopic methods, and *dark-ground illumination* or *phase-contrast microscopy* is necessary for their demonstration. Phase-contrast microscopy may also be used to demonstrate motility, spores and intracellular granules.

Stained preparations

Bacteria are more readily studied when immobilized by fixation and darkly stained in contrast with the bright background. Methods for simple staining impart the same colour to all bacteria and other biological material, whereas methods for differential staining impart a distinctive colour only to certain types of bacteria.

Simple staining is effected by the application of a watery solution of a basic dye, e.g. methylene blue, methyl violet or basic fuchsin, sometimes along with a mordant to allow better penetration. The coloured, positively charged cation of the basic dye combines with negatively charged groups in the bacterial protoplasm, especially with the phosphate groups in the abundant nucleic acids. The stain is retained through a subsequent washing with water for the removal of excess dye from the slide. Acidic dyes, having coloured anions, do not stain bacteria strongly except at very acid pH values, and thus can be used for 'negative staining' (see below). Cells or structures that stain with basic dyes at normal pH values are described as *basophilic* and those that stain with acidic dyes as *acidophilic*.

Before staining, the film or smear of bacteria must be fixed on the slide, usually by heat; the slide is first thoroughly dried in air and then heated gently in a flame. Vegetative bacteria are thereby killed, rendered permeable to the stain, stuck to the surface of the slide and preserved from undergoing autolytic changes. Chemical fixatives are used for sections of infected tissue and films of infected blood, since they cause less damage to the tissue cells; fixatives include formalin, mercuric chloride, methyl alcohol and osmic acid.

It should be noted that the bacterial cell wall is not stained by ordinary methods and the coloured body seen corresponds to the cell protoplasm only. This is usually much shrunken as a result of drying. Chains of stained bacteria thus show the coloured bodies separated by gaps that are the sites of unstained, connecting cell walls.

Certain bacteria do not colour evenly with simple stains. Thus, the diphtheria bacillus shows a 'beaded' appearance, with alternating dark and light bars. The plague bacillus shows 'bipolar staining', the ends being more deeply coloured than the centre. The uneven staining may be due to the manner in which the protoplasm shrinks when the cell is dried and fixed.

'*Negative*' or *background staining* is of value as a rapid method for the simple morphological study of bacteria and yeasts. The bacteria are mixed with a substance such as India ink, or nigrosin, which after spreading as a film, yields a dark background in which the organisms stand out as bright, unstained objects.

Silver impregnation methods are used to stain spirochaetes, especially in tissues. The slender cells are thickened by a dark deposit of silver on their surface.

Differential staining reactions. *Gram's stain* has the widest application, distinguishing all bacteria as 'Gram-positive' or 'Gram-negative', according to whether or not they resist decoloration with acetone, alcohol or aniline oil after staining with a triphenyl methane dye, e.g. methyl violet, and subsequent treatment with iodine. The Gram-positive bacteria resist decoloration and remain stained a dark purple colour. The Gram-negative bacteria are decolorized, and are then counterstained light pink by the subsequent application of basic fuchsin, safranin, neutral red or dilute carbol fuchsin. In routine diagnostic work a Gram-stained smear is often the only preparation examined microscopically, since it shows clearly the general morphology of the bacteria as well as revealing their Gram-reaction. It should be noted that characteristically Gram-positive species may sometimes appear Gram-negative under certain conditions of growth; thus, some show an increasing proportion of Gram-negative cells in ageing cultures on nutrient agar. On the other hand, characteristically Gram-negative species do not produce cells that stain Gram-positively in correctly treated smears. Gram reactivity appears to reflect a fundamental aspect of cell structure and is correlated with many other biological properties. Thus, the different species of a single genus generally show the same reaction. Gram-positive bacteria are more susceptible than Gram-negative bacteria to the antibacterial actions of penicillin, acids, iodine, basic dyes, detergents and lysozyme, and less susceptible to alkalies, azide, tellurite, proteolytic enzymes, lysis by antibody and complement, and plasmolysis in solutes of high osmotic pressure.

The mechanism of the Gram stain is not fully understood. The more acidic character of the protoplasm of Gram-positive species, which is enhanced by treatment with iodine, may partly explain their stronger retention of basic dye. Probably, however, the more important difference is in the permeability of the cell wall during the staining process. After staining with methyl violet and treatment with iodine, a dye–iodine complex or 'lake' is formed within the cell; this is insoluble in water but moderately soluble and dissociable in the acetone or alcohol used as the decolorizer. Under the action of the decolorizer, the dye and iodine diffuse freely out of the Gram-negative cell, but not from the Gram-positive cell, presumably because the latter's cell wall is less permeable. Gram positive bacteria become Gram-negative when their cell wall is ruptured or removed.

The *acid-fast staining reaction*, as revealed by the Ziehl–Neelsen method is of value in distinguishing a few bacterial species, e.g. the tubercle bacillus,

from all others. These 'acid-fast' bacteria are relatively impermeable and resistant to simple stains, but when stained with a strong reagent such as hot basic fuchsin in aqueous 5% phenol, subsequently resist decolorization by 20% sulphuric acid. Any decolored non-acid-fast organisms are counterstained in a contrasting colour with methylene blue or malachite green.

The acid-fast bacteria have an exceptionally rich and varied content of lipids, fatty acids and higher alcohols. Acid fastness depends on the structural integrity of the cell, its content of lipids and, possibly, on a special anatomical disposition of the lipids.

COMPOSITION OF VIRUSES
Structure

The basic infectious particle of a virus is known as the *virion*. In the simplest viruses this consists of nucleic acid and a surrounding coat of protein called the *capsid*. Some viruses are enclosed within an *envelope* usually derived from host cell membranes, but modified by the inclusion of viral glycoproteins. The capsid is composed of distinct morphological units or *capsomeres* which are assembled from viral proteins. Depending on the arrangement of these proteins, the capsomeres may be spherical, cylindrical or ring-like in appearance. The *nucleocapsid* is the combination of nucleic acid and capsid. The arrangement of the capsomeres around the nucleic acid determines the *symmetry* of the virion. When the capsomeres are applied directly to the helical nucleic acid this forms a coil-like structure with the appearance of a hollow tube. Viruses with this arrangement are said to have *helical symmetry*. Most helical viruses enclose the nucleocapsid within an envelope and thus do not have a rigid appearance. The other major type is shown by the viruses with *icosahedral symmetry* (Fig. 2.13) in which the capsomeres are arranged as if they lay on the faces of an icosahedron which has 20 equilateral triangular faces and 12 corners or apices (Fig. 2.14). Capsomeres on the faces and edges of this figure are called hexons as they always link with six adjacent capsomeres; those positioned at the

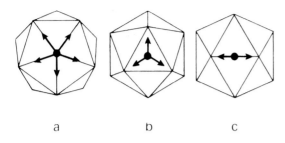

Fig. 2.13 An icosahedron viewed along its **a** five-fold, **b** three-fold and **c** two-fold axes of symmetry.

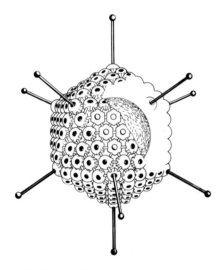

Fig. 2.14 A diagram of an icosahedron of an adenovirus. The core of DNA is represented by a circular mass. Some of the pentamers at the 12 vertices have been indicated with protruding fibres and terminal knobs. The remaining 240 hexamer capsids are, for the most part, shown as compressed into hollow spheres linked to each other by divalent bonds. The hexagonal shape of a few of the capsomeres is seen in the centre of the diagram.

apices are the pentons as they always join to five capsomeres. Viruses with icosahedral symmetry have a rigid structure and in the electron microscope have a characteristic hexagonal outline with triangular faces. However, if the diameter of the virion is less than about 50 nm the particle will appear spherical. Many viruses with icosahedral symmetry are enclosed by an outer envelope. The poxviruses are large and complex and do not show either type of symmetry; they are referred to as complex. The size of virions varies considerably, from 25 to 300 nm, in different families (Fig. 2.15).

Viral nucleic acid

The commonest types of nucleic acid in viruses of man are single-stranded RNA and double-stranded DNA. However, both double-stranded RNA and single-stranded DNA occur in the reoviruses and parvoviruses, respectively. The genomes of RNA viruses may be present as a single strand as in paramyxoviruses, or as two copies as in the retroviruses, or exist as a specific number of fragments as in the orthomyxoviruses and reoviruses. Circular molecules of DNA are present in the virions of papovaviruses and hepadnaviruses. The amount of nucleic acid in virions is constant for a particular virus but shows considerable variation; thus the molecular weight can vary from about 1.5 million in the parvo-and hepadnaviruses to 80–240 million for the poxviruses.

Virion enzymes

Several viruses carry essential enzymes in the virion. As discussed in Chapter 9, an RNA-dependent RNA polymerase or transcriptase is an essential component of the virion in several virus families, including the negative-strand RNA viruses. Among DNA viruses only the poxviruses carry a DNA-dependent RNA polymerase. The hepadnaviruses have a virion polymerase complex that has some similarity to the reverse transcriptase complex found in the retroviruses.

Viral proteins

Analysis of the proteins produced in a cell during viral infection shows that some are essential components of the virion; these are the structural proteins and include capsid proteins and enzymes as well as basic core proteins which may be necessary to package the nucleic acid within the capsid. Other proteins such as enzymes are needed for the production of viral components but are not part of the virion; these are the non-structural proteins. The essential steps of virus attachment and penetration of the host cell are known to depend on regions of the outer capsid such as the apical fibres and knobs of adenoviruses or on parts of the envelope glycoproteins of viruses such as influenza A and B and the human immuno-deficiency virus.

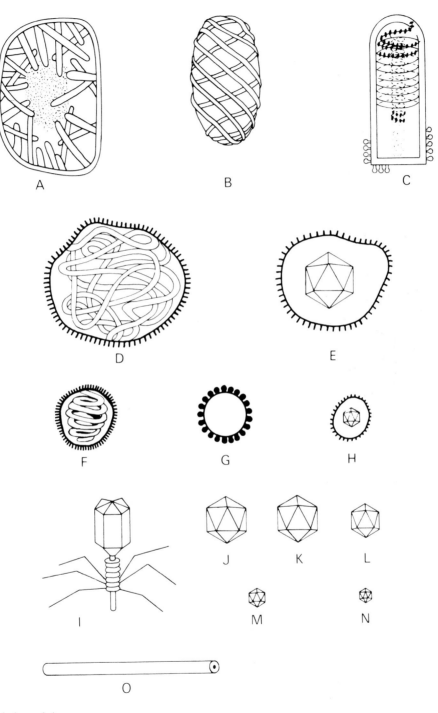

Fig. 2.15   Morphology of viruses.

A	Orthopoxvirus	E	Herpesvirus	I	T-even coliphage	M	Picornavirus
B	Parapox virus	F	Orthomyxovirus	J	Adenovirus	N	Parvovirus
C	Rhabdovirus	G	Coronavirus	K	Reovirus	O	Tobacco mosaic virus
D	Paramyxovirus	H	Togavirus	L	Papovavirus		

RECOMMENDED READING

Actor P, Daneo-Moore L, Higgins M L Salton M R J, Shockman G D 1988 *Antibiotic Inhibition of Bacterial Cell Surface Assembly and Function.* American Society for Microbiology, Washington

Fields B N, Knipe D M (eds) 1990 *Virology*, 2nd edn. Raven Press, Newford

Frey D, Oldfield R J, Bridger R C 1979 *A Colour Atlas of Pathogenic Fungi.* Wolfe Medical, London

Gillies R R 1984 *Gillies and Dodds Bacteriology Illustrated*, 5th edn. Churchill Livingstone, Edinburgh.

Lugtenberg B, van Alphen L 1983 Molecular architecture and functioning of the outer membrane of *Escherichia coli* and other bacteria. *Biochimica et Biophysica Acta* 737: 51–115

Madeley C R, Field A M 1988 *Virus Morphology*, 2nd edn. Churchill Livingstone, Edinburgh

Mandelstam J, McQuillen K, Dawes I W 1982 *Biochemistry of Bacterial Growth*, 3rd edn. Blackwell Scientific, Oxford.

Mendelson N H 1982 Bacterial growth and division: genes structures, forces, and clocks. *Microbiological Reviews* 46: 341–375

Nikaido H, Vaara M 1985 Molecular basis of bacterial outer membrane permeability. *Microbiological Reviews* 49:1–32

Olds R J 1975 *A Colour Atlas of Microbiology.* Wolfe Medical Publications, London

Rogers H J, Perkins H R, Ward J B 1980 *Microbial Cell Walls and Membranes.* Chapman and Hall, London

Shockman G D, Barrett J F 1983 Structure, function and assembly of cell walls from Gram-positive bacteria. *Annual Review of Microbiology* 37: 501–527

3

Growth and nutrition of micro-organisms

J. F. Wilkinson

This chapter will be largely concerned with the growth and nutrition of prokaryotes (bacteria), but most of the principles concerned apply equally well to many eukaryotic micro-organisms. The growth of viruses is discussed elsewhere (Chapter 9).

MICROBIAL GROWTH

When an inoculum of cells from a pure culture of bacteria is introduced into a suitable nutrient medium and incubated under appropriate conditions, almost all of the cells have the potential to grow at a very rapid rate. This growth, by which is meant an orderly increase in all the components of an organism, is normally associated with multiplication. The method of division of most bacteria is by binary fission — a new cell grows until it doubles its size, at which point it divides into two halves. Some eukaryotic micro-organisms multiply by budding or by hyphal growth. Very large populations of cells are normally involved and the individual cells do not all divide simultaneously. Equal proportions of the total population divide successively in unit periods of time so that growth and multiplication can be considered as synonymous in relation to time. This is not so for each single bacterium in which cell growth and cell division are clearly separately controlled variables. It is possible to produce a synchronously dividing population by artificial means but such situations are not normally encountered in nature and methods that measure an increase in numbers or in mass are used as indices of 'growth'. It is important to realize the rapidity of growth under favourable circumstances when a cell may double every 20 min. If this rate were maintained for 24 h, the progeny of a single cell would be about 1×10^{21} cells and would have a mass of approximately 4000 tons! The conditions used for culture never permit such a rate of multiplication for more than a short time, generally because of an insufficiency of nutrients or of special growth factors. In microbial disease, the various host defence mechanisms may further limit the potential for growth.

Batch culture

When a small number of organisms are taken from a culture and inoculated into a fresh growth medium, the number of cells inoculated may multiply a million-fold or more during growth. If the number of cells present at different times after inoculation is measured, and the number is plotted in relation to the period of growth, the resultant plot is referred to as a *batch growth curve*. Two types of growth curve can be drawn according to the measurement of cell numbers that is used:

1. A *total count* is based on the number of cells present, irrespective of whether they are living or not. An organism is considered living or viable if it is capable of continued multiplication; if it is not so capable it is called dead or non-viable.

2. A *viable count* measures only those cells capable of growing and hence of producing a colony on a suitable growth medium. With organisms like streptococci or staphylococci that grow as linked chains or clumps, each group of several bacteria will produce only one colony. Viable counts are thus expressed as *colony-forming units*, not absolute numbers of bacteria.

Figure 3.1 shows the four main phases of growth.

Lag phase

In this period there is no appreciable multiplication of cells although they may increase considerably in size and show marked metabolic activity. The duration of this phase varies according to the condition and number of cells in the inoculum and it can be looked upon as representing the time taken for the organism to adapt itself to growth in the fresh medium. The cells in an inoculum may be so depleted of enzymes, metabolic intermediates, and other factors, that some time is required for these materials to build up to their optimal levels. Alternatively, if the composition of the new medium differs significantly in composition from that in which the inoculum was growing previously, entirely new enzymes may require to be synthesized by the process of induction or by the selection of mutants.

Logarithmic (log) or exponential phase

In this period, the cells grow at a constant rate and, as a result of division by binary fission, there is a linear relationship between time and the logarithm of the number of cells. It is important to realize the potential of exponential growth. If the number of bacterial cells in a culture increases 10-fold they will increase 100-fold in twice that time, 1000-fold in three times the given period and so on, although the rate of division is usually much slower in vivo. Once an infection overwhelms the body defences and gets out of control, it becomes increasingly difficult to eradicate it as time goes on. The actual rate of growth is directly related to the generation time (the time between divisions) of the bacterium under the particular environ-

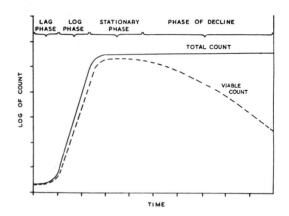

Fig. 3.1 Continuous line, total number of bacteria alive and dead. Interrupted line, total number of living bacteria.

mental factors that prevail. Some of the environmental factors that affect the rate of growth are considered later in this chapter.

Stationary phase

In due course, exponential growth is no longer possible and the rate of multiplication decreases until it ceases altogether and the cells pass into the stationary phase. It is theoretically possible to reach a stable number of cells by the establishment of an equilibrium between the rates of growth and death but the common situation is one in which neither growth nor death occurs but the cells remain in a state of suspended animation. Although the normal metabolism associated with biosynthesis and growth no longer occurs, there is usually some metabolic activity going on; this is known as endogenous metabolism and it probably acts to provide the cell with energy and intermediates required to maintain life. The cessation of growth in the stationary phase is most commonly caused by the exhaustion of an essential nutrient in the medium, or the accumulation of toxic waste products; for example, organic acids are common end-products of fermentation and their accumulation can lead to a lowering of pH to a value inimical to growth.

Since a variety of factors can bring about the onset of the stationary phase, cells in this phase can exhibit a corresponding variation in morphology and physiology, both between themselves and in comparison with exponential-phase cells. Thus stationary-phase cells may have a high level of intracellular storage polymers such as polysaccharide (usually glycogen in bacteria) and lipid (usually poly-β-hydroxybutyrate in bacteria); these substances are often virtually absent in exponential-phase cells. Similarly a Gram-positive organism may become Gram-negative in the stationary phase. In routine studies of morphological characteristics it is best to observe young cells that are in a growing phase.

At the onset of the stationary phase, many species of bacteria produce *secondary metabolites,* i.e. natural products formed mainly or only by cells that have stopped dividing. These secondary metabolites are diverse in nature and each kind has a restricted taxonomic distribution. They include many antibiotics and exotoxins. In spore-forming species the initiation of sporulation typically occurs at the end of the exponential phase or early in the stationary phase.

Death or decline phase

After a variable period of time in the stationary phase, the cells in a culture become incapable of growth when transferred to a fresh medium. This is reflected in Fig. 3.1 as an increasing divergence between the total count (living and dead cells) and the viable count (living cells only). The causes of this loss of viability are various, the main determinant being the nature of the factor that caused the cessation of growth at the onset of the stationary phase. If it is due to the accumulation of toxic products, there may be a very brief stationary phase followed by a rapid death rate. In some cases, there may be a rapid fall in the total count as well as the viable count because micro-organisms are very prone to digest themselves so that they eventually lyse and liberate their cytoplasmic contents into the environment; this process is known as *autolysis.* Not all bacteria are subject to such rapid degeneration and death; some organisms under appropriate environmental conditions may stay in the stationary phase for days. Clearly the rapidity of the onset of the death phase is an important factor that may influence the spread of infection.

Continuous culture

Batch culture is the usual method of growing bacteria in the laboratory. However, it is possible to use an 'open' system in which there is a continuous supply of fresh nutrients into the culture vessel and a continuous removal of grown bacteria by means of a constant-level device. This method of culture — called *continuous culture* — may correspond more truly with the situation occurring in some diseases of man and animals. The basis for most continuous culture systems in the laboratory is the *chemostat* (Fig. 3.2). In this system, the rate of growth is controlled by the rate of addition of fresh nutrient that is pumped from the medium vessel. This, in turn, controls the rate of removal of cells via the overflow device into the collector vessel. When equilibrium is reached, the rate of production of new

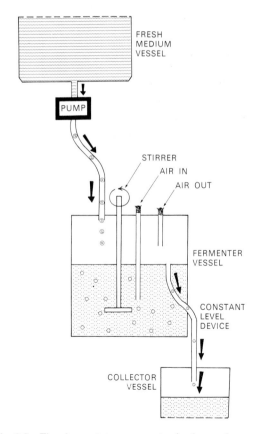

Fig. 3.2 The chemostat: an apparatus for the continuous culture of bacteria.

cells by multiplication is equal to the rate of removal of grown cells into the collector vessel. This state can be continued indefinitely so as to provide a source of reproducible cells from an environment which can itself be varied by altering the nature or rate of addition of fresh medium. Although continuous culture is too cumbersome for routine use, it is employed in research and for large-scale industrial systems.

Growth requirements

In order to identify and study a bacterial species, it is necessary to grow the organism under laboratory conditions and it is therefore essential to know its growth requirements. Two conditions must be fulfilled: (1) suitable nutrients must be supplied; and (2) the physical conditions must be as near optimum as possible for the organism under consideration.

MICROBIAL PHYSIOLOGY

Micro-organisms differ widely in the nutritional factors and the physical conditions needed for their growth; these differences reflect the physiological characteristics of the organisms concerned. It is important, therefore, to understand some of the principles underlying microbial physiology.

Chemical composition

The basic chemical composition of all micro-organisms is essentially similar. Water is the major component, making up about 80% of the cell's weight. Typical figures for the other components are given in Table 3.1.

It must be emphasized that these figures are average and typical ones, the actual value varying with both the micro-organism and the cultural conditions employed. For example, the mycobacteria are characterized by a high lipid content irrespective of the growth conditions, whereas most micro-organisms grown in the presence of an excess of a carbon and energy source will have a high polysaccharide content due to the accumulation of storage polymers.

Table 3.1 The composition of a typical prokaryotic and eukaryotic micro-organism given as percentages of the dry weight.

Component	Prokaryote	Eukaryote
Nucleic acid	10	5
Protein	40	45
Polysaccharide	15	15
Peptidoglycan	10	0
Lipid	15	20
Low mol.wt compounds	10	15

It is evident that polymers of high molecular weight make up a large proportion of the dry weight of micro-organisms, as indeed they do with all living organisms. This fact is even more striking in prokaryotes where an appreciable amount of lipid may be in the form of poly-β-hydroxybutyrate. Apart from normal lipid, the other low molecular-weight components are co-enzymes, prosthetic groups, intermediary metabolites and inorganic salts.

The study of comparative biochemistry has shown that living organisms are similar in their component chemical units as well as in the mechanisms by which these components are formed — the process of metabolism. Thus the nucleotide and amino acid components of nucleic acids and proteins are the same in bacteria as in mammals or higher plants. The types of enzymic reaction carried out and the co-enzymes involved in them are virtually identical and in all organisms the adenosine diphosphate $\rightleftharpoons$ adenosine triphosphate (ADP $\rightleftharpoons$ ATP) system is used for most energy conversions. The study of molecular biology has shown an even more striking picture of unity in the synthesis of protein and nucleic acid where the methods of transcription, translation and coding are almost identical. It is true that there are exceptions to this basic unity, a fortunate fact for the development of chemotherapy. As can be seen in Table 3.1, the peptidoglycan component of the bacterial cell wall is unique to prokaryotes as are its characteristic monomer components — N-acetylmuramic acid, diaminopimelic acid and some D-amino acids. Certain monosaccharides may also be specific and micro-organisms are characterized by the wide variety of these that can occur in cell wall or capsular polysaccharides. The variety and the different methods of linkage involved partly explains why such a wide range of different antigenic types of organism can be seen in nature. There are also substances unique to eukaryotic cells such as sterols that are almost always absent from prokaryotes.

Microbial metabolism

Granted that all micro-organisms have a remarkable resemblance in basic chemical composition, how far do they show a similar metabolism? A cell's metabolism can be conveniently divided into the following sections:

1. The conversion of the carbon of nutrients into basic 'building blocks' to be used in biosynthesis.
2. The conversion of ADP to ATP by the energy-yielding metabolism.

These two processes can be considered together as comprising catabolism. Some non-parasitic micro-organisms are able, like plants, to use carbon dioxide as the main source of carbon and are called *autotrophs* (or *lithotrophs*). Energy is obtained in these organisms by the oxidation of inorganic compounds (*chemosynthetic autotrophs* or *chemolithotrophs*) or from sunlight (*photosynthetic autotrophs* or *photolithotrophs*). However, the majority of micro-organisms, including all those that are directly important in medicine, obtain their energy by the breakdown of suitable organic nutrients; they are called *heterotrophs* or *chemo-organotrophs*. In them, stages 1 and 2 are combined, the carbon and energy source being partly used to produce ATP and partly used to provide building blocks.

3. The building blocks are converted to monomers, eventually in an activated form.
4. These activated monomers are polymerized.

These two biosynthetic processes comprising anabolism require energy mainly provided as ATP.

5. The polymers are transported to the appropriate area of the cell for their proper functioning. For example, some proteins must be incorporated into the cytoplasmic membrane, others into the nucleus, others into ribosomes and so on. We are only beginning to understand this process, but there is no reason to believe that the basic mechanism in micro-organisms differs from that in higher organisms.

Catabolism

Micro-organisms differ widely in the range of organic compounds that can be used as a source of carbon and energy. Some bacteria are remarkably versatile, such as species of the genus *Pseudomonas*, and can utilize any one of many organic compounds (sugars, acids alcohols, etc.) as the sole source of carbon and energy, whereas many bacteria are much more specific in their requirement. In general, all micro-organisms seem to have certain fundamental metabolic pathways concerned in the interconversions necessary for the production of the basic 'building blocks' for growth. Examples are the enzymes concerned in the glycolytic pathway, pentose phosphate cycle and tricarboxylic acid cycle; such enzymes are synthesized irrespective of the environmental conditions and form a group called *constitutive enzymes*. On the other hand, leading into these general metabolic sequences there are specific pathways concerned with the breakdown of a particular substrate. The enzymes concerned in these pathways are usually *inducible*; i.e. they are produced only in the presence of an inducer, generally the substrate itself. The obvious advantage of such a system to an organism is one of economy; as there are hundreds of such specific enzymes that may be required it would be very wasteful to produce them all irrespective of what chemical compounds are present in the environment. Another regulatory process is that of *catabolite repression* in which a common carbon and energy source such as glucose actually represses the synthesis of a wide variety of enzymes that are not concerned with glucose breakdown.

Such regulatory processes are useful in the evolutionary struggle because they give the organism the necessary versatility to adapt to changing environments.

Aerobic and anaerobic growth

Micro-organisms differ considerably in the way in which the carbon and energy source is broken down to provide energy. This difference mainly concerns the involvement of oxygen as a terminal electron acceptor in the system. The majority of bacteria are described as *facultative anaerobes* because they are able to grow either aerobically, i.e. in the presence of air and free oxygen, or anaerobically, in its absence. Certain other species grow only in the presence of air or free oxygen and are described as s*trict* or *obligate aerobes,* whereas others that grow only in the absence of free oxygen and may be killed in its presence are known as *strict anaerobes.* For the anaerobes the ultimate determining factor for growth is the state of oxidation of the environment, this being best described in terms of the oxidation– reduction, or *redox* potential. In the presence of oxygen, a strict anaerobe is liable to produce peroxides and superoxides that it cannot destroy; strict anaerobes lack catalase, peroxidase and superoxide dismutase, enzymes present in aerobes and facultative anaerobes that break down these potentially toxic compounds.

Finally, there is a group of organisms that grow best in the presence of a trace only of free oxygen and often prefer an increased concentration of carbon dioxide; these are called *micro-aerophilic.*

Aerobic respiration*.* Aerobes obtain most of their energy by a series of coupled oxido-reductions in which the ultimate electron acceptor is atmospheric oxygen; in this *aerobic respiration,* the carbon and energy source may be completely oxidized to carbon dioxide and water. Energy is obtained by the production of energy-rich phosphate bonds and their transfer to ADP to form ATP during the passage of electrons through the electron transport system, a process known as *oxidative phosphorylation.* The electron transport systems of micro-organisms are often very similar to those occurring in higher organisms and involve pyridine nucleotide co-enzymes, flavoproteins, cytochromes and cytochrome oxidases.

Anaerobic respiration*.* Anaerobes can only oxidize compounds at the expense of some electron acceptor other than oxygen. In some instances, an inorganic compound capable of reduction, such as nitrate or sulphate, acts as the electron acceptor; this process is known as *anaerobic respiration* and energy is again produced mainly during the passage of electrons from the substrate to the inorganic electron acceptor. Anaerobic growth probably occurs more commonly by a process in which the carbon and energy source provides both an electron donor and an electron acceptor in a series of coupled oxido-reductions. This process is known as *fermentation* and it leads to the formation of a variety of waste products such as ethanol in cultures of yeasts, and organic acids and alcohols in cultures of bacteria; thus, lactic acid is produced by lactobacilli and streptococci, and a mixture of lactic, acetic, formic and succinic acids by the enterobacteria. Carbon dioxide and, in some cases, hydrogen are commonly produced and therefore fermentation is usually accompanied by the production of both acid and gas. The nature of the fermentation product is also of significance in the classification of bacteria. During the process of fermentation, energy-rich phosphate bonds are produced by the introduction of inorganic phosphate into intermediates on the fermentation pathway, a process known as *substrate-level phosphorylation.* The energy-rich phosphate groups so produced are transferred to ADP to form ATP under the influence of the appropriate phosphorylation enzyme. It should be noted that the amount of energy produced from a given source under anaerobic conditions is considerably less than that produced under aerobic conditions so that growth of a facultative anaerobe is usually much more abundant under aerobic conditions.

Anabolism

The end-products of biosynthesis are very similar for all micro-organisms. However, there are wide differences in the ability of cells to carry out the individual biosyntheses of essential monomers and co-enzymes. Some are capable of synthesizing all their amino acids, nucleotides, monosaccharides, co-enzymes, and so on from the building blocks produced by catabolism. Others almost completely lack such biosynthetic powers and depend entirely on their nutrient environment for the provision of such substances in ready-made form. Within these two extremes there is a wide spectrum of different biosynthetic abilities. With respect to the actual enzymes involved in particular pathways, there is very little difference in the intermediates and reactions involved in the whole range of living organisms. Just as the enzymes concerned in the specific utilization of carbon sources are subject to control by induction, enzymes catalysing biosynthesis are subject to *feedback inhibition* and to *repression*. In feedback inhibition, the end-product inhibits the action of the *first enzyme* of the *specific* pathway and thus exerts a fine control over the action of enzymes already present. In repression the end-product inhibits the production of *all* the enzymes concerned in its specific biosynthesis. These two control processes between them prevent the synthesis of the enzymes and their products when the end-product is already present as a nutrient in the environment and they therefore contribute significantly to the economy of the cell.

Although micro-organisms vary widely in their ability to synthesize essential low molecular-weight compounds, all cellular forms of life must have a certain range of enzymes to catalyse required polymerizations because it is not possible to incorporate an extracellularly provided polymer directly into the cell structure. In general, substances of high molecular weight cannot penetrate the cytoplasmic membrane.

MICROBIAL NUTRITION

The growth of micro-organisms is dependent on an adequate supply of suitable nutrients. Some species are able to grow under a wide range of conditions, but others, especially the more strictly parasitic such as the gonococcus, are very exacting and restrictive in their requirements. Whilst it is hardly possible to reproduce exactly the natural environmental conditions of pathogenic bacteria in the laboratory, suitable artificial culture media have been devised for the majority.

Major nutrient requirements

In view of the similarity of the chemical components of all micro-organisms, the different nutrient requirements that are recognized must reflect different biosynthetic abilities. It is possible to view these different nutrient requirements in terms of the provision of bulk elements or in terms of the requirements for specific organic compounds.

The main elements required for growth are carbon, hydrogen, oxygen and nitrogen, with sulphur and phosphorus required in somewhat smaller amounts, and other elements such as sodium, potassium, magnesium, iron and manganese in considerably smaller amounts. Since hydrogen and oxygen can be supplied in the water that is essential for any growth, it is evident that carbon and nitrogen are the main bulk elements required.

Carbon and energy source

A heterotroph must be supplied with an organic compound or compounds that can be broken down to provide suitable building blocks and to convert ADP to ATP. The organic compounds that can be used generally reflect the normal environment of an organism; parasitic micro-organisms will normally use organic compounds such as carbohydrates and amino acids present in the tissue fluids of their hosts.

Nitrogen source

The main inorganic form of nitrogen used in biosynthesis is ammonia, usually in the form of an ammonium salt. It can be provided directly in the environment or it can be produced indirectly by the de-amination of organic nitrogenous nutrients such as amino acids or by the reduction of nitrates. A few bacteria can use gaseous nitrogen as a nitrogen source and reduce it to ammonia by the process of nitrogen fixation. These nitrogen-fixing micro-organisms are of no direct importance in medicine but their occurrence is of critical importance to the natural ecosystem.

Other inorganic salts

Micro-organisms require a supply of inorganic salt for growth, particularly the anions phosphate and sulphate, and the cations sodium, potassium, magnesium, iron, manganese and calcium. Some ions such as cobalt are needed in such trace amounts that it is difficult in practice to demonstrate a requirement.

Organic compounds

Certain organic compounds such as amino acids, nucleotides, monosaccharides, lipids and co-enzymes must be either synthesized by the micro-organism or provided as nutrients in the environ-ment. Micro-organisms vary widely in their bio-synthetic capacity and this variation is reflected in their nutrient requirements. Consider the amino acids as an example. Twenty amino acids must be provided for protein synthesis and several more for peptidoglycan synthesis in prokaryotes. Some micro-organisms can synthesize all of their amino acids for themselves from the carbon and energy source together with ammonium and sulphate ions. Other micro-organisms are unable to carry out the biosynthesis of any of their amino acids and these therefore become essential nutrients that must be supplied in the growth medium. A complete range of biosynthetic abilities and, therefore, of nutrient requirements is found be-tween these two extremes. It is interesting to note that man comes about midway on such a scale, being able to synthesize about half the total number of amino acids. A similar range of biosynthetic ability and nutrient requirement in the bacteria can be found for nucleotides and their com-ponent purines and pyrimidines and for co-enzymes. If a co-enzyme or an essential part of a co-enzyme is required as a nutrient, it is usually required in small catalytic amounts and is some-times known as a *growth factor* or *microbial vitamin*. Many of these substances are, of course, identical to the vitamins required for mammalian nutrition, e.g. thiamine, riboflavine, nicotinic acid, pyridoxine, *p*-aminobenzoic acid, folic acid, biotin, coba-mide, etc. Monosaccharides and lipids, however, are usually synthesized from the bulk carbon and energy source.

Permeability of the cell to various nutrients

Any compound that is going to be used as a nutrient has to pass through the cytoplasmic membrane in order to reach the cytoplasm where most further metabolism occurs. Transport or translocation of soluble nutrients is achieved through the action of carrier mechanisms referred to as *permeases* or *porters*. In bacteria and fungi all nutrients must be soluble since endocytosis cannot occur. Moreover, high molecular-weight polymers must be hydrolysed by extracellular enzymes before they can be used.

Nutritional evolution

Some bacteria have comprehensive synthetic abilities and are therefore *non-exacting* nutrition-ally; they are able to synthesize all their structural units from the carbon and energy source and inorganic salts. Other bacteria, in the course of evolution towards a strictly parasitic mode of life, have increasingly obtained their amino acids, nucleotides and growth factors from the tissues of their host, and have lost the power of synthe-sizing these compounds. Nutritionally exacting species (e.g. *Streptococcus pyogenes*) can grow in a synthetic medium only if it contains a wide range of different amino acids, nucleotides and growth factors. Certain obligate intracellular parasites (rickettsiae and chlamydiae) have special cyto-plasmic membranes that allow the passage of nucleoside triphosphates from the host cell; these 'energy parasites' have come to depend on the uptake of preformed ATP. This process of nu-tritional evolution can be paralleled in the labora-tory by the selection of mutants. An enzyme catalysing a step in the synthesis of an amino acid, nucleotide or growth factor may be lost as a result of gene mutation and the variant strain thus becomes nutritionally exacting in respect of the substance which the parent strain can synthesize for itself.

MEDIA FOR MICROBIAL GROWTH

General laboratory media

The purposes of a general laboratory medium are two-fold. Firstly, it should support the growth of as wide a range of micro-organisms as possible; in other words, it should contain a sufficiency of the generally required microbial nutrients. Second-ly, it should be cheap and easy to produce. In practice, the most important substances required for microbial growth are amino acids, nucleotides, growth factors, a bulk source of carbon, energy and nitrogen and certain inorganic ions. In order to provide these components, most general laboratory media contain the following:

1. A hydrolysate of a cheap protein, preferably prepared by the use of a proteolytic enzyme to prevent amino acid destruction, which can occur during acid hydrolysis. Such hydrolysates are called peptones and should contain all the essential amino acids.

2. A source of growth factors and inorganic salts. This is usually provided by an extract of meat or of yeast. Sometimes a further enrichment is provided by the addition of special sources of growth factors such as blood, serum or egg.

3. Usually sodium chloride is added for the growth of parasitic micro-organisms to bring the osmotic pressure up to a figure comparable with that of host tissues.

It should be noted that such media have no single carbon and energy source, but instead a series of organic compounds such as amino acids are catabolized to produce building blocks and energy; the remainder of these compounds may be incorporated directly into the cell.

Synthetic media

A synthetic medium is one in which all of the nutrients are specified and added separately to give a chemically defined product. Media of this type are used for various experimental purposes. A simple synthetic medium contains a suitable carbon and energy source (e.g. glucose or lactate), an inorganic nitrogen source (e.g. an ammonium salt) and various inorganic salts in a buffered aqueous solution. Such media provide the basic essentials for the growth of many non-parasitic heterotrophs but they will not support the growth of most parasitic micro-organisms, which require complex synthetic media. Synthetic media are designed to meet the particular requirements of the micro-organism concerned; they are expensive and tedious to make and are therefore only used for special purposes.

Special media

Various media have been developed for special purposes in microbiology. *Selective* media contain substances that inhibit or poison all but a few types of micro-organism, thus facilitating the isolation of a particular species from a mixed inoculum. If a liquid medium favours the multiplication of a particular species, either by containing additional materials that selectively favour it or inhibiting substances that suppress competitors, it is called an *enrichment* medium, and is commonly a first stage in the isolation of pure cultures by conventional plating-out methods. Clearly these cultures will not indicate the proportion of the species originally present in an inoculum. Certain media are referred to as *indicator* media; they contain some substance that is changed visibly as a result of the metabolic activity of particular organisms. Combinations of enriched media with selective agents and indicator systems are frequently used in the diagnostic laboratory.

PHYSICAL CONDITIONS REQUIRED FOR GROWTH

A bacterial cell may double its size and divide within 30 min and it must be capable of synthesizing its own weight of cell material within that period. Accordingly, it must have a very rapid rate of metabolism together with a correspondingly rapid uptake of nutrients and disposal of waste products. It can do this only because of its small size, which gives it a very large surface for absorption and excretion in relation to its volume. But the very rapid growth that occurs in the log phase is possible only under certain restricted environmental conditions.

Influence of oxygen and carbon dioxide

It is necessary to provide the correct atmosphere for the growth of strict aerobes and anaerobes. A sufficiently low redox potential for the growth of strict anaerobes can be obtained in liquid or semi-solid media by the use of a reducing agent such as thioglycollate. Alternatively, the culture can be incubated in an oxygen-free atmosphere in an anaerobic jar or cabinet.

All bacteria require a small amount of carbon dioxide for growth. This is normally provided by the atmosphere, or by the cell's own metabolism. Some bacteria (e.g. *Brucella abortus* on first isolation from blood) require a much higher concentration of carbon dioxide (5–10%) and this must be provided during laboratory cultivation.

Influence of temperature

Growth. For each species there is a definite temperature range within which growth takes place. The limits are the maximum and minimum temperatures, and an intermediate *optimum* temperature can usually be recognized at which growth is most rapid. In the laboratory, bacteria are grown at this optimum temperature in a thermostatically controlled incubator. The optimum temperature of a bacterium is approximately that of its natural habitat, e.g. about 37°C in the case of organisms that are parasitic on man and warm-blooded animals. These, and many saprophytes of soil and water that grow best at between 25 and 40°C, are termed *mesophilic*). Some mesophiles have a wide growth temperature range (e.g. 5–43°C for *Pseudomonas aeruginosa*), whereas others are more restricted (e.g. 30–39°C for *Neisseria gonorrhoeae*). Few grow appreciably at temperatures below 5°C (as in a domestic refrigerator) or at temperatures above 45°C.

A group of soil and water bacteria, the *psychrophiles*, grow best at temperatures below 20°C, usually quite well at 0°C and in some cases down to -7°C on unfrozen media. Their importance lies in their ability to cause spoilage of refrigerated and frozen food.

Another group of non-parasitic bacteria, the *thermophiles*, grow best at high temperatures between 55 and 80°C, and have minimum growth temperatures ranging from 20 to 40°C (facultative thermophiles), or even above 40°C (strict thermophiles).

Viability. Heat is an important agent in the artificial destruction of micro-organisms, the effect depending under moist conditions on the coagulation and denaturation of cell proteins, and under dry conditions, on oxidation and charring. Among the bacteria that are parasites of mammals, non-sporing forms in moist conditions generally cannot withstand temperatures above 45°C for any length of time. The time of exposure to heat that is necessary for killing is shorter the higher the temperature, and various other factors influence the exact amount of heating required. Thus, bacteria are more susceptible to 'moist heat', e.g. in hot water or saturated steam, than to 'dry heat', e.g. in a hot-air oven. They are rendered more susceptible to the lethal effect of heat by the presence of acid, alkali or any chemical disinfectant, and less susceptible by the presence of organic substances such as proteins, sugars and fats, and also by their own occurrence in large numbers. The *thermal death point* of a particular organism is the lowest temperature that kills it under standard conditions, and within a given time, e.g. 10 min. Under moist conditions, it lies between 50 and 65°C for most non-sporing mesophilic bacteria, and between 100 and 120°C for the spores of most sporing species. The extreme limit of resistance to moist heat is shown by the spores of a non-pathogenic, strictly thermophilic bacillus, *Bacillus stearothermophilus*, which is killed only after exposure to 121°C for 10–35 min. With dry heat, the 10 min thermal death points of sporing bacteria are mostly between 140 and 180°C.

At low temperatures some species die rapidly, but most survive well, and may be preserved for long periods at between 3 and 5°C in a refrigerator, or in the frozen state in a deep freeze or in liquid nitrogen. The process of freezing kills a proportion of the bacterial cells present, and this is least if freezing is effected rapidly, or if a stabilizer such as glycerol is added.

Influence of moisture and of desiccation

Four-fifths by weight of the bacterial cell consists of water and, as in the case of other organisms, moisture is absolutely necessary for growth. Microbes vary widely in their ability to survive when dried under natural conditions, as in infected exudate smeared on clothing or furniture, and converted to dust. Thus, the gonococcus, *Treponema pallidum* and the common cold virus appear to die quickly, whereas the tubercle bacillus, *Staphylococcus aureus* and the smallpox virus may survive for weeks or months. Bacterial endospores survive drying especially well; for instance the spores of *Bacillus anthracis*, when dried on threads, have survived for over 60 years.

Even delicate, non-sporing organisms may survive drying for a period of years if they are desiccated rapidly and completely, preferably while frozen, and thereafter maintained in a high vacuum in a sealed glass ampoule stored at room temperature in the dark. This is the basis of the *lyophilization* or *freeze-drying* process of preserving bacterial cultures in the laboratory.

Influence of hydrogen ion concentration

A suitable environmental pH is an essential factor in microbial metabolism and growth. The majority of commensal and pathogenic bacteria grow best at a neutral or very slightly alkaline reaction (pH 7.2–7.6). Some bacteria, however, flourish in the presence of a considerable degree of acidity and are termed *acidophilic*, e.g. *Lactobacillus* species. Others are very sensitive to acid, but tolerant of alkali, e.g. *Vibrio cholerae*. Strong acid or alkali, e.g. 5% hydrochloric acid or sodium hydroxide, are rapidly lethal to most bacteria, the mycobacteria being exceptional in resisting them.

Influence of light and other radiations

Darkness provides a favourable condition for growth and viability. Ultraviolet rays are rapidly bactericidal, e.g. direct sunlight or radiation from a mercury vapour lamp. Even diffuse daylight, as it enters a room through window glass, signi-

ficantly shortens the survival of micro-organisms and may be of hygienic importance. Bacteria are also killed by ionizing radiations.

Influence of osmotic pressure

Bacteria resemble other cells in being subject to osmotic phenomena. However, they are relatively tolerant of changes in the osmotic pressure of their environment and can grow in media with widely varying contents of salt, sugar and other solutes. This is partly a reflection of the mechanical strength of their cell walls. For most species the maximum concentration of sodium chloride permitting growth lies between 5 and 12%, though *halophilic* species occur that can grow at higher concentrations up to saturation. The latter are saprophytes whose importance lies in their ability to cause spoilage of food preserved with salt or sugar; they are not pathogenic. Sudden exposure of bacteria to solutions of high salt concentration (e.g. 2–25% sodium chloride) may cause *plasmolysis*, i.e. temporary shrinkage of the protoplast and its retraction from the cell wall due to the osmotic withdrawal of water; this occurs much more readily in Gram-negative than in Gram-positive bacteria. Sudden transfer from a concentrated to a weak solution, or to distilled water, may cause *plasmoptysis* — i.e. swelling and bursting of the cell as a result of excessive uptake of water.

Influence of mechanical and sonic stresses

Although their cell walls have considerable strength and some elasticity, it is possible to rupture and kill bacteria by exposure to mechanical stresses. A bacterial suspension may be largely disintegrated by subjection to very vigorous shaking with fine glass beads, or to supersonic or ultrasonic vibration. These measures are used in separating the large molecular components of the cell.

RECOMMENDED READING

Dawes I W, Sutherland I W 1991 *Microbial Physiology*, 2nd edn. Blackwell, Oxford
Ingraham J L, Maaløe O, Neidhardt F C 1983 *Growth of the*

Bacterial Cell. Sinauer, Sunderland, Mass.
Mandelstam J, McQuillen K, Dawes I W 1982 *Biochemistry of Bacterial Growth*, 3rd edn. Blackwell, Oxford

4

Classification and identification of micro-organisms

D. Greenwood

Micro-organisms may be classified in the following large biological groups:

1. Algae
2. Protozoa
3. Slime moulds
4. Fungi
5. Bacteria
6. Archaebacteria
7. Viruses.

The algae (excluding the blue–green algae), the protozoa, slime moulds and fungi include the larger and more highly developed micro-organisms; their cells have the same general type of structure and organization, described as *eukaryotic*, that is found in higher plants and animals. The bacteria, including organisms of the mycoplasma, rickettsia and chlamydia groups, together with the related blue–green algae, comprise the smaller micro-organisms with a simpler form of cellular organization described as *prokaryotic*. The archaebacteria are a distinct phylogenetic group of prokaryotes, which bear only a remote ancestral relationship to other organisms.

The viruses are the smallest of the infective agents; they have a relatively simple structure that is not comparable with that of a cell, and their mode of reproduction is fundamentally different from that of cellular organisms. Even simpler are *viroids*, protein-free fragments of single-stranded circular RNA that cause disease in plants. Other types of infectious particle have been postulated: *prions* are described as infectious proteins devoid

of nucleic acid, while *virinos* are said to consist of a small amount of nucleic acid complexed with protein derived from the host cell. There is considerable debate about the true status of prions and virinos and of the relationship, if any, between them.

Helminths (parasitic worms) are too big to be regarded as micro-organisms, but they cause infection and are appropriately considered among other infective agents. They are dealt with in Chapter 62.

Since the algae, slime moulds and archaebacteria are not thought to contain species of medical or veterinary importance they will not be considered further. Blue-green algae do not cause infection, but certain species produce potent peptide toxins that may affect persons or animals ingesting polluted water.

CLASSIFICATION AND TAXONOMY

Classification is the orderly grouping of things — in the present context, micro-organisms. *Taxonomy* raises classification to the level of a science and has its own agreed rules. *Nomenclature* concerns the naming of things and also requires agreement so that the same name is used unambiguously by everyone. Changes in nomenclature have the potential to cause much confusion and should not be introduced without clear justification. In routine clinical practice, microbiologists are generally more concerned with *identification* — the correct naming of isolates according to agreed systems of taxonomy and nomenclature — than with the science of taxonomy itself.

Protozoa, fungi and helminths are classified and named according to the standard rules of biological taxonomy and nomenclature that have been developed following the pioneering work of the 18th century Swedish botanist Linnaeus (Carl von Linné). Large subdivisions (class, order, family, etc.) are finally classified into individual *species* designated by a Latin binomial, the first term of which is the *genus*, e.g. *Plasmodium* (genus) *falciparum* (species). Occasionally it is useful to recognize a biological variant with particular properties: thus *Trypanosoma* (genus) *brucei* (species) *gambiense* (variant) differs from the variant *T. brucei brucei* in being pathogenic for humans.

Bacteria are also classified along these lines, but the infinite variety of microbial life and the natural capacity of bacteria for variation and adaptation make the problems of rigid classification difficult. Moreover, species of bacteria cannot be defined by the criterion of continued fertile interbreeding used for higher plants and animals, since they do not reproduce sexually. At present no standard classification of bacteria is universally accepted and applied, although *Bergey's Manual of Systematic Bacteriology* (published by Williams and Wilkins) is widely used as an authoritative source.

Bacterial nomenclature is governed by an international code prepared by the *International Committee on Systematic Bacteriology* and published as *Approved Lists of Bacterial Names* in the *International Journal of Systematic Bacteriology*; most new species are also first described in this journal. However, the journal is not ordinarily among the first to be regularly scanned by practising medical microbiologists, and usage often lags behind official precept.

Attempts have been made to classify viruses according to classic Linnaean principles, but these organisms do not lend themselves easily to such an approach and virologists have generally resisted adoption of binomial designations in medical virology.

METHODS OF CLASSIFICATION

In most systems of bacterial classification, the major groups are distinguished by characters, such as cell shape, Gram reaction and spore formation, that are considered to be of special importance; genera and species are distinguished by properties considered of less importance, such as fermentation reactions, nutritional requirements and pathogenicity. This system suffers from the weakness that decisions about the relative 'importance' of different characters, thus about their priority in defining the major and minor groupings, are often purely arbitrary.

Adansonian or numerical classification

The uncertainties of arbitrary choices are avoided in the Adansonian system of taxonomy. This system determines the degrees of relationship between strains by a statistical coefficient that takes account of the widest range of characters, all of which are considered of equal weight. It is clear, of course, that some characters, e.g. cell shape or Gram reaction, represent a much wider and permanent genetic commitment than other characters which, being dependent on only one or a few genes, are relatively mutable. For this reason, the Adansonian method is most useful for the classification of strains within a larger-grouping that shares major characters.

By scoring a large number of phenotypic characters it is possible to estimate a *similarity coefficient* when shared positive characters are considered, or a *matching coefficient* when both negative and positive shared characters (matches) are taken into account. The observations can be analysed by computer to indicate degrees of similarity for a group of different organisms by the preparation of a *similarity matrix* (Fig. 4.1) or a dendrogram (Fig. 4.2).

DNA composition

The hydrogen bonding between guanine and cytosine (G-C) base pairs in DNA is stronger than that between adenine and thymine (A-T). Thus the melting or denaturation temperature of DNA (at which the two strands separate) is primarily determined by the G + C content. At

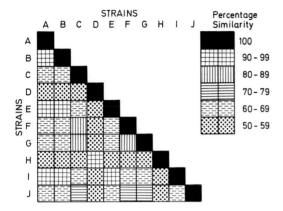

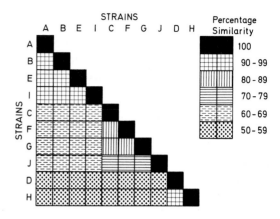

Fig. 4.1   A similarity matrix for 10 strains A–J. In the left-hand panel the strains are arranged in alphabetical order. To emphasize similarities, the matrix is redrawn according to a process called cluster analysis and this is shown in the right hand panel. This shows that strains A, B, E and I are highly similar phenons; strains D and H form a separate group that are closely related to each other, but not to the other strains. (slightly modified from Sneath P H A 1962 The construction of taxonomic groups. In: Ainsworth G C, Sneath P H A (eds). Cambridge University Press, Cambridge).

the melting temperature, the separation of the strands brings about a marked change in the light absorption characteristics at a wavelength of 260 nm and this is readily detected by spectrophotometry.

By measuring the G+C content of a bacterial preparation in this way it can be shown that there is a very wide range in the G + C component of DNA varying from about 25 to 80 moles% in different genera. However, for any one species, the G + C content is relatively fixed, or falls within a very narrow range, and this provides a basis for classification.

DNA homology

Another approach to classification is to arrange individual organisms into groups on the basis of the *homology* of their DNA base sequences. Tests of DNA homology exploit the fact that double strands re-form from separated strands during controlled cooling of a heated preparation of DNA. This 'annealing' process can be readily demonstrated with suitably heated homologous DNA extracted from a single species, but it can also occur when a mixture of DNA from two related species is used; in the latter case, hybrid pairs of DNA strands are produced. These hybrid pairings occur with high frequency between complemen-

tary regions of DNA and the degree of hybridization can be assessed if labelled DNA preparations are used. Binding studies with mRNA can also give information to complement these observations, which provide genetic evidence of relatedness among bacteria.

Organisms with different G + C ratios are very unlikely to show DNA homology. However, organisms with the same, or close, G + C ratios do not necessarily show homology.

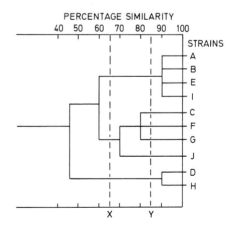

Fig. 4.2   A hierarchic taxonomic tree (*dendrogram*) prepared from the similarity matrix data shown in Fig. 4.1. The broken lines X and Y indicate levels of similarity at which separation into genera and species might be possible. (Slightly modified from Sneath (1962) – see Fig. 4.1 for reference.)

Ribosomal RNA sequencing

The structure of ribosomal RNA (rRNA) appears to have been highly conserved during the course of evolution and close similarities in nucleotide sequences reflect phylogenetic relationships. Advances in technology have made nucleotide sequencing relatively simple, so that investigation of similarities in oligonucleotides derived from rRNA are increasingly used in taxonomic studies.

CLASSIFICATION IN CLINICAL PRACTICE

The identification of micro-organisms in laboratories of medical microbiology requires a pragmatic approach to taxonomy. Table 4.1 outlines a simple, but practical, classification scheme in which organisms are grouped according to a few shared characteristics. Within these groups, organisms may be further identified, sometimes to species level, by a few supplementary tests. Protozoa, helminths and fungi can often be definitively identified on morphological criteria alone (see appropriate chapters).

Protozoa

These are non-photosynthetic unicellular organisms with protoplasm clearly differentiated into nucleus and cytoplasm. They are relatively large with transverse diameters mainly in the range 2–100 µm. Their surface membranes vary in complexity and rigidity from a thin, flexible membrane in amoebae, which allows major changes in cell shape and the protrusion of pseudopodia for the purposes of locomotion and ingestion, to a relatively stiff pellicle in ciliate protozoa, which preserves a characteristic cell shape. Most free-living and some parasitic species capture, ingest and digest internally solid particles of food material; many protozoa, for instance, feed on bacteria. Protozoa, therefore, are generally regarded as the lowest forms of animal life, though certain flagellate protozoa are closely related in their morphology and mode of development to photosynthetic flagellate algae in the plant kingdom. Protozoa reproduce asexually by binary fission or by multiple fission (*schizogony*), and some also by a sexual mechanism (*sporogony*).

The most important groups of medical protozoa are the *sporozoa* (malaria parasites etc.), amoebae and flagellates (see Chapter 61).

Fungi

These are non-photosynthetic organisms possessing relatively rigid cell walls. They may be saprophytic or parasitic and take in soluble nutrients by diffusion through their cell surfaces.

Moulds grow as branching filaments (*hyphae*), usually between 2 and 10 µm in width, which interlace to form a meshwork (*mycelium*). The hyphae are coenocytic (i.e. have a continuous multinucleate protoplasm), being either non-septate or else septate with a central pore in each cross wall. Moulds reproduce by the formation of various kinds of sexual and asexual spores that develop from the vegetative (feeding) mycelium, or from an aerial mycelium that effects their airborne dissemination.

Yeasts are ovoid or spherical cells that reproduce asexually by budding and also, in many cases, sexually, with the formation of sexual spores. They do not form a mycelium, although the intermediate *yeast-like fungi* from a pseudomycelium consisting of chains of elongated cells. The *dimorphic fungi* produce a vegetative mycelium in artificial culture, but are yeast-like in infected lesions. The higher fungi of the class *Basidiomycetes* (mushrooms), which produce large fruiting structures for aerial dissemination of spores, play no part in infection of man or animals, although some species are poisonous.

Bacteria

The main groups of bacteria are distinguished by microscopical observation of their morphology and staining reactions. The Gram staining procedure, which reflects fundamental differences in cell wall structure, separates most bacteria into two great divisions: *Gram-positive bacteria* and *Gram-negative bacteria* (see Chapter 2).

Details of structure provide a basis for a separate division into:

1. *Filamentous bacteria (Actinomycetes)*, most of which are capable of true branching and which may produce a type of mycelium

Table 4.1   A simple classification of some micro-organisms of medical importance

---

EUKARYOTIC GENERA

PROTOZOA

Sporozoa: *Plasmodium, Isospora, Toxoplasma, Cryptosporidium*

Flagellates: *Giardia, Trichomonas, Trypanosoma, Leishmania*

Amoebae: *Entamoeba, Naegleria, Acanthamoeba*

Others: *Babesia, Balantidium, Pneumocystis*[a]

FUNGI

Mould-like: *Epidermophyton, Trichophyton, Microsporum, Aspergillus*

Yeast-like: *Candida*

Dimorphic: *Histoplasma, Blastomyces, Coccidioides*

True yeast: *Cryptococcus*

PROKARYOTIC GENERA

FILAMENTOUS BACTERIA

Actinomyces, Nocardia, Streptomyces, Mycobacterium

'TRUE BACTERIA'

Gram-positive bacilli: Aerobes — *Corynebacterium, Listeria, Bacillus*

Anaerobes — *Clostridium, Lactobacillus, Eubacterium*

Gram-positive cocci: *Staphylococcus, Streptococcus, Enterococcus*

Gram-negative cocci: Aerobes — *Neisseria*

Anaerobes — *Veillonella*

Gram-negative bacilli: Aerobes

Enterobacteria — *Escherichia, Klebsiella, Proteus, Salmonella, Shigella*

Pseudomonads — *Pseudomonas, Alcaligenes*

Parvobacteria — *Haemophilus, Bordetella, Brucella, Pasteurella, Yersinia*

Anaerobes — *Bacteroides, Fusobacterium*

Gram-negative vibrios: *Vibrio, Spirillum, Campylobacter, Helicobacter*

SPIROCHAETES

Borrelia, Treponema, Leptospira

MYCOPLASMAS

Mycoplasma, Ureaplasma

RICKETTSIAE AND CHLAMYDIAE

Rickettsia, Coxiella, Rochalimaea, Chlamydia

---

[a] May be a fungus.

2. *'True' bacteria*, which multiply by simple binary fission
3. *Spirochaetes*, which divide by transverse binary fission
4. *Mycoplasmas* which lack a rigid cell wall
5. *Rickettsiae* and *chlamydiae*, which are strict intracellular parasites.

Filamentous bacteria

These are sometimes referred to as 'higher bacteria'. A few are of medical interest as pathogens and some produce antibiotics.

1. *Actinomyces.* Gram-positive, non-acid-fast, tend to fragment into short coccal and bacillary forms and not to form conidia; anaerobic (e.g. *Actinomyces israelii*).
2. *Nocardia.* Similar to *Actinomyces*, but aerobic and mostly acid-fast (e.g. *Nocardia asteroides*).
3. *Streptomyces.* Vegetative mycelium does not fragment into short forms; conidia form in chains from aerial hyphae (e.g. *Streptomyces griseus*).
4. *Mycobacterium.* Acid-fast; Gram-positive, but does not readily stain by the Gram method; usually bacillary, rarely branching; aerobic (e.g. *Mycobacterium tuberculosis*).

True bacteria

Most medically important bacteria fall into this group. They are classified on the basis of their shape:

1. Cocci — spherical, or nearly spherical cells
2. Bacilli — relatively straight, rod-shaped (cylindrical) cells
3. Vibrios and spirilla — curved or twisted rod-shaped cells.

Cocci. The main groups of cocci are distinguished by their predominant mode of cell grouping and their reaction to the Gram stain. The different cocci are relatively uniform in size (usually about 1 μm in diameter). Some species are capsulate and a very few are motile.

1. *Streptococcus.* Gram-positive; cells mainly adherent in chains, due to successive cell divisions occurring in the same axis (e.g. *Streptococcus pyogenes*); sometimes predominantly diplococcal (e.g. *Streptococcus pneumoniae*).
2. *Staphylococcus* and *Micrococcus.* Gram-positive; cells mainly adherent in irregular clusters, due to successive divisions occurring irregularly in different planes (e.g. *Staphylococcus aureus*).
3. *Sarcina.* Gram-positive cells mainly adherent in cubical arrays of eight, or multiples thereof, due to division occurring successively in three planes at right angles (e.g. *Sarcina lutea*).
4. *Neisseria.* Gram-negative; cells mainly adherent in pairs and slightly elongated at right angles to axis of pairs (e.g. *Neisseria meningitidis*).
5. *Veillonella.* Gram-negative; generally very small cocci arranged mainly in clusters and pairs; anaerobic (e.g. *Veillonella parvula*).

Bacilli. The primary subdivision of the rod-shaped bacteria is made according to their staining reaction by the Gram method and the presence or absence of endospores.

1. *Gram-positive spore-forming bacilli.* Apart from some rare saprophytic varieties, the only bacteria to form endospores are those of the genera *Bacillus* (aerobic) and *Clostridium* (anaerobic). They are Gram-positive, but liable to become Gram-negative in ageing cultures. The size, shape and position of the spore may assist recognition of the species; e.g. the bulging, spherical, terminal spore ('drum stick' form) of *Clostridium tetani*.
2. *Gram-positive non-sporing bacilli.* These include several genera. *Corynebacterium* is distinguished by a tendency to slight curving, a club-shaped or ovoid swelling of the bacilli, and their arrangement in parallel or angular clusters due to the snapping mode of cell division. *Erysipelothrix* and *Lactobacillus* are distinguished by a tendency to grow in chains and filaments, and *Listeria* by flagella that confer motility.
3. *Gram-negative bacilli.* This large grouping includes numerous genera such as the pseudomonads and the family Enterobacteriaceae ('coliform bacilli') as well as small, often pleomorphic bacilli represented by *Haemophilus*, *Brucella*, etc. ('parvobacteria'), and anaerobes such as *Bacteroides*.
4. *Vibrios and spirilla.* Vibrios and the related campylobacters are recognized as short, non-

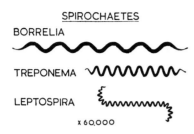

Fig. 4.3 Morphology of spirochaetes.

flexuous, comma-shaped rods (e.g. *Vibrio cholerae*) and spirilla as non-flexuous spiral filaments (e.g. *Spirillum minus*). They are Gram-negative and mostly motile, having polar flagella and showing very active 'darting' motility.

Spirochaetes

These organisms differ from the 'true' bacteria in being slender flexuous spiral filaments which, unlike the spirilla, are motile without possession of flagella. The staining reaction, when demonstrable, is Gram-negative. The different varieties are recognized by their size, shape, wave form and refractility, observed in the natural state in unstained wet films by dark-ground microscopy (Fig. 4.3).

1. *Borrelia*. Larger and more refractile than the other pathogenic spirochaetes and more readily stained by ordinary methods; coils large and open, with a wavelength of 2–3 µm; by electron microscopy a leash of 8–12 fibrils, each about 0.02 µm thick, is seen twisted round the whole length of the protoplast (e.g. *Borrelia recurrentis*).

2. *Treponema*. Thinner filaments in coils of shorter wavelength (e.g. 1.0–1.5 µm), typically presenting a regular 'corkscrew' form; feebly refractile and difficult to stain except by silver impregnation methods; by electron microscopy, a leash of four fibrils is seen wound round the protoplast within the cell wall (e.g. *Treponema pallidum*).

3. *Leptospira*. The coils are so fine and close (wavelength about 0.5 µm) that they are barely discernible by dark-ground microscopy, though clearly seen winding round two axial filaments by electron microscopy. One or both extremities of the organism are hooked, or recurved, so that it may take the shape of a walking-stick, an S or a C (e.g. *Leptospira interrogans*).

Mycoplasmas

These are prokaryotes that differ from 'true' bacteria in their smaller size and their lack of a rigid cell wall, which leads to extreme pleomorphism and sensitivity to external osmotic pressure. The viable elements range from 0.15 to over 1 µm in diameter, the smallest being capable of passing through filters that retain conventional bacteria. Mycoplasmas can be cultivated on cell-free nutrient media and are the smallest and simplest organisms capable of autonomous growth.

Rickettsiae and chlamydiae

The rickettsiae are rod-shaped, spherical or pleomorphic Gram-negative organisms. They are generally smaller than 'true' bacteria, but are still resolvable in the light microscope. Most are strict parasites that can grow only in the living tissues of a suitable animal host, usually intracellularly (e.g. *Rickettsia prowazekii*). Chlamydiae are similar to rickettsiae, but have a more complex intracellular cycle (e.g. *Chlamydia trachomatis*).

Viruses

Viruses usually consist of little more than a strand of DNA or RNA (never both) enclosed in a simple protein shell known as a *capsid*. Sometimes the complete nucleocapsid may be enclosed in a lipoprotein envelope largely derived from the host cell. Viruses are capable of growing only within the living cells of an appropriate animal, plant or bacterial host; none can grow in an inanimate nutrient medium. The viruses that infect and parasitize bacteria are named *bacteriophages* or *phages*.

A simple classification of the viruses that are involved in human disease is shown in Table 4.2.

IDENTIFICATION OF MICRO-ORGANISMS

Precise identification of bacteria is time consuming and contentious and is best carried out in specialized reference centres. For most clinical purposes

Table 4.2 Principal types of virus causing human disease

Type of virus	Examples
RNA viruses	
Orthomyxoviruses	Influenza A, B, C viruses
Paramyxoviruses	Parainfluenza viruses
	Mumps virus
	Measles virus
	Respiratory syncytial virus
Rhabdoviruses	Rabies virus
Arenaviruses	Lassa virus
Filoviruses	Marburg and Ebola viruses
Togaviruses	Many arboviruses
	Rubella virus
Flaviviruses	Yellow fever virus
Bunyaviruses	Hantaan virus
Coronaviruses	Coronavirus
Caliciviruses	Calicivirus
Picornaviruses	Enteroviruses
	Poliovirus, 3 types
	Echovirus, 31 types
	Coxsackie A virus, 24 types
	Coxsackie B virus, 6 types
	Enterovirus types 68–71
	Hepatitis A virus (type 72)
	Rhinovirus, many serotypes
Retroviruses	Human immunodeficiency viruses
	HTLV-1, -2
Reoviruses	Rotaviruses
DNA viruses	
Poxviruses	Variola, Vaccinia
	Molluscum contagiosum virus
	Orf
Herpesviruses	Herpes simplex virus
	Varicella–zoster virus
	Cytomegalovirus
	Epstein–Barr virus
	Human herpes virus 6
Adenoviruses	Many serotypes
Papovaviruses	Papilloma viruses (warts)
Hepadnaviruses	Hepatitis B virus
Parvoviruses	B 19 virus

what is required is clear guidance on the likely cause of an infection, not a rigorously accurate, but belated description of what the patient has already recovered (or possibly died) from. Consequently, medical microbiologists usually rely on a few simple procedures, notably microscopy and culture, backed up, when necessary, by a few supplementary tests.

Microscopy is the most rapid test of all, but culture inevitably takes at least 24 h, and sometimes longer. More rapid tests are constantly being sought, and some progress has been achieved with antigen detection methods and specific *gene probes* (see below).

Most specimens for bacteriological examination, whether from humans, animals or the environment, contain mixtures of bacteria and it is essential to obtain *pure cultures* of individual isolates before embarking on identification. Non-cultural methods, such as antigen detection or gene probes, do not have this disadvantage; however they do have the potential limitation of being highly specific so that the investigator must know beforehand what is to be looked for.

Microscopy

Morphology and staining reactions of individual organisms generally serve as preliminary criteria to place an unknown species in its appropriate biological group. A Gram stain smear suffices to show the Gram reaction, size, shape and grouping of the bacteria, and the arrangement of any endospores.

An unstained wet film may be examined with the dark-ground microscope to observe the morphology of delicate spirochaetes; an unstained wet film, or 'hanging-drop' preparation is examined with the ordinary microscope for observation of motility.

To identify mycobacteria, or other acid-fast organisms, a preparation is stained by the Ziehl–Neelsen method or one of its modifications.

The microscopic characters of certain organisms in pathological specimens may be sufficient for presumptive identification, e.g. tubercle bacilli in sputum, or *Treponema pallidum* in exudate from a chancre. However, many bacteria share similar morphological features and further tests must be applied to differentiate them.

Cultural characteristics

The appearance of colonial growth on the surface of a solid medium, such as nutrient agar, is often

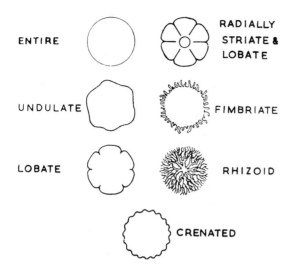

Fig. 4.4 Edges of bacterial colonies.

very characteristic. Attention is paid to the diameter of the colonies, their outline (Fig. 4.4), their elevation (Fig. 4.5), their translucency (clear, translucent or opaque) and colour. Changes brought about in the medium (e.g. haemolysis in a blood agar medium) may also be significant.

The range of conditions that support growth is characteristic of particular organisms. The ability or inability of the organism to grow on media containing selective inhibitory factors. (e.g. bile salt, specific antimicrobial agents, low or high pH) may also be of diagnostic significance.

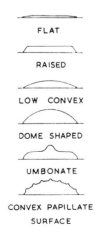

FLAT

RAISED

LOW CONVEX

DOME SHAPED

UMBONATE

CONVEX PAPILLATE
SURFACE

Fig. 4.5 Elevations of bacterial colonies

Biochemical reactions

Species that cannot be distinguished by morphology and cultural characters may exhibit metabolic differences that can be exploited. Is is usual to test the ability of the organism to produce acidic and gaseous end-products, when presented with individual carbohydrates (glucose, lactose, sucrose, mannitol, etc.) as the sole carbon source. Other tests determine whether the bacterium produces particular end-products (e.g. indole, hydrogen sulphide) when grown in suitable culture media, and whether it possesses certain enzyme activities, such as oxidase, catala e, urease, gelatinase or lecithinase.

Traditionally, such tests have been performed selectively and individually according to the recommendations of standard guides, such as the invaluable *Cowan and Steele's Manual for the Identification of Medical Bacteria* (published by Cambridge University Press). For practical reasons many workers are now turning to the commercially prepared galleries of identification tests which, though expensive, combine simplicity and accuracy. Test kits are now available for a number of different groups of organisms, including enterobacteria, staphylococci, streptococci and anaerobes.

Sometimes more elaborate procedures may be used for the analysis of metabolic products. For example, gas-liquid chromatography is widely used to recognize characteristic volatile fatty acids and alcohols produced by anaerobic bacteria.

Gene probes

These are cloned fragments of DNA that recognize complementary sequences within micro-organisms; binding is detected by tagging the DNA with a radio-active label, or with a reagent that can be developed to give a colour reaction. By selecting DNA fragments specific for features characteristic of individual organisms, gene probes can be tailored to the rapid identification of individual species in clinical material. One disadvantage of this approach is that the organism itself is not made available for subsequent tests of susceptibility to antimicrobial agents, toxin production or epidemiological investigation. However, probes able to detect genes for antibiotic resistance, toxin production or epidemiological markers are also being developed.

Antigenic characters

Antibody reactions

Species and types of micro-organism can often be identified by specific 'antibody reactions'. These reactions depend on the fact that the serum of an animal immunized against a micro-organism contains specific antibodies for the homologous species or type that reacts in a characteristic manner (e.g. agglutination or precipitation) with the particular micro-organism. Such simple in-vitro tests have been used for many years in microbiology, notably in the formal identification of presumptive isolates of pathogens (e.g. salmonellae) from clinical material. More refined methods of antigen detection, some of which can be directly applied to clinical specimens without prior culture, are gaining in popularity.

The specificity and range of antibody tests have been greatly improved by the availability of highly specific *monoclonal antibodies*. These are produced by the *hybridoma* technique in which individual antibody-producing spleen cells are fused with 'immortal' tumour cells in vitro. The progeny of these hybrid cells produce only the type of antibody appropriate to the spleen cell precursor.

Counterimmuno-electrophoresis

This technique has been widely used for the detection of pneumococcal and certain other antigens. The specimen to be tested for the particular antigen and the homologous antibody are placed in separate wells in an agar gel and subjected to an electric current. Antigens that carry a negative charge migrate towards the anode, and the positively charged antibody towards the cathode. A line of precipitation is formed at the point at which the two meet.

Enzyme-linked immunosorbent assay (ELISA)

In this test a specific antibody is attached to the surface of a plastic well and material containing the test antigen is added. After washing, more of the specific antibody is added, this time labelled with an enzyme which can initiate a colour reaction when provided with the appropriate substrate.

The ELISA method may also be used in the reverse manner for the quantitative detection of antibodies, by adsorbing purified antigen to the well before adding test serum; in this case the enzyme-linked system used to detect the antigen-antibody reaction is a labelled anti-human globulin.

Latex agglutination

By adsorbing specific antibody to inert latex particles, a visible agglutination reaction can be induced in the presence of homologous antigen. Once again, this principle can be applied in reverse to detect serum antibodies.

Haemagglutination and haemadsorption

Certain viruses, notable the influenza viruses, have the property of attaching to specific receptors on the surface of appropriate red blood cells. In this manner the virus particles act as bridges linking the red cells in visible clumps.

In tissue culture, such haemagglutinins may appear on the surface of cells infected with a virus. If red cells are added to the tissue culture, they adhere to the surface of infected cells, a phenomenon known as *haemadsorption*.

Red blood cells can also be coated with specific antibody so that they agglutinate in the presence of the homologous virus particle in a manner similar to that described for latex agglutination above.

Fluorescence microscopy and immunofluorescence

When certain dyes are exposed to ultraviolet light, they absorb energy and emit visible light (i.e. they fluoresce). Tissues or organisms stained with such a dye and examined with ultraviolet light in a specially adapted microscope are seen as fluorescent objects; for example, auramine can be used in this way to stain *Mycobacterium tuberculosis*.

Antibody molecules can be labelled by conjugation with a fluorochrome dye such as fluorescein isothiocyanate (which fluoresces green) or rhodamine (orange-red). When fluorescent antibody is allowed to react with homologous antigen exposed at a cell surface, this *direct immunofluorescence* procedure affords a highly sensitive method for the identification of the particular antigen. For this procedure it is necessary to have a specific antibody conjugate for each antigen; however, unconjugated antibody can be used and the reaction then detected by addition of an antiglobulin conjugate which will react with any antibody from the species in which the antibody was raised.

Typing of bacteria

A population of bacteria presumed to descend from a single bacterium as found in a natural habitat, in primary cultures from the habitat, and in subcultures from the primary cultures, is called a *strain*. Each primary culture from a natural source is called an *isolate*. The distinction between strains and isolates may be important; for example, cultures of typhoid bacilli isolated from 10 different patients should be regarded simply as 10 different *isolates* unless epidemiological or other evidence indicates that the patients have been infected from a common source with the same *strain*.

The ability to discriminate between similar strains may be of great epidemiological value in tracing sources or modes of spread of infection in a community, and various typing methods have been devised.

Strains may be distinguishable only in minor characters and it is usually simpler to establish differences between isolates from a common source than unequivocally to prove their identity. Demonstration of an identical response by a single reproducible typing method is not proof that two strains are the same. However, the confidence with which similarity can be inferred is greatly increased if more than one typing method is used.

Biotyping and serotyping

Special biochemical or serological tests may be used to distinguish particular *biotypes* or *serotypes* that show variations in metabolic behaviour or antigenic structure.

Phage typing

Bacteria often show differential susceptibility to lysis by certain bacteriophages. The *phage type* of the culture is identified according to the pattern of susceptibility to a set of lytic phages. Phage typing is widely used to discriminate among strains of salmonella and of staphylococci.

Bacteriocine typing

Bacteriocines are naturally occurring antibacterial substances elaborated by members of the family Enterobacteriaceae and some other bacteria. They are active mainly against strains of the same genus as the producer strain. For example, indicator strains for the pyocine typing of *Pseudomonas aeruginosa* are also members of the genus *Pseudomonas*.

Patterns of susceptibility to bacteriocines produced by the indicator strains allow the division of serologically homogeneous species into *bacteriocine types*.

Animal pathogenicity and toxigenicity

Animal pathogenicity tests were formerly much used in the diagnosis of tuberculosis and certain other diseases. They have now been almost entirely replaced by cultural methods.

Similarly, animal tests for the demonstration of bacterial toxins have largely been superseded by in-vitro tests.

Antibiotic sensitivity tests

The organism is tested for its ability to grow in the presence of different concentrations of antimicrobial agents. Dilutions of the agent can be made in nutrient broth or incorporated into agar during the preparation of agar plates. In the latter case, many different isolates can be tested at the same time by spot inoculation of the plate. The *minimum inhibitory concentration* (MIC) is the lowest concentration of the antimicrobial agent that prevents the development of visible growth during overnight incubation.

In the *disc diffusion test*, the culture to be examined is seeded confluently, or semi-confluently, over the surface of an agar plate and paper discs individually impregnated with different antibiotics are spaced evenly over the inoculated plate. Antibiotic diffuses outwards from each disc into the surrounding agar and produces a diminishing gradient of concentration. On incubation the bacteria grow on areas of the plate except those around the drugs to which they are sensitive. The width of each *zone of inhibition* is a rough measure of the degree of sensitivity to the drug.

Information about the sensitivity pattern of strains (*antibiograms*) isolated from patients is required as a guide to therapy and may also be used as an epidemiological marker in tracing hospital cross-infections.

RECOMMENDED READING

Cowan S T 1974 *Cowan and Steele's Manual for the Identification of Medical Bacteria*, 2nd edn. Cambridge University Press, Cambridge.

Holt J G (editor-in-chief) (1984–89) *Bergey's Manual of Systematic Bacteriology*. Williams and Wilkins, Baltimore, vols 1–4

Moore W E C, Moore L V H 1989 *Index of the Bacterial and Yeast Nomenclatural Changes*. American Society for Microbiology, Washington, DC

Skerman V B D, McGowan V, Sneath P H A 1989 *Approved Lists of Bacterial Names*, amended edn. American Society for Microbiology, Washington, DC

Woese C R 1987 Bacterial evolution. *MIcrobiological Reviews* 51: 221–271

5

Sterilization and disinfection

R. A. Simpson

Procedures that kill micro-organisms have important applications in practical microbiology and in the practice of medicine and surgery. Laboratory work with pure cultures requires the use of apparatus and culture media that have been rendered sterile, while the need to avoid infecting the patient requires the use of equipment, instruments, dressings and parenteral drugs that are free from all living micro-organisms, or at least from those which may give rise to infection.

General definitions

Two distinct terms, *sterilization* and *disinfection* are used to describe processes for the killing or removal of micro-organisms and it is important to recognize the difference in meaning.

Sterilization is a process used to achieve sterility, an absolute term meaning the absence of all micro-organisms.

Disinfection is used to describe a process which reduces the number of contaminating micro-organisms, particularly those liable to cause infection, to a level which is deemed no longer harmful to health.

Cleaning is a soil-removing process which removes a high proportion of micro-organisms present. The reduction in contamination by cleaning processes is difficult to quantify other than visually. However, cleaning processes have wide application in the hospital environment and as the necessary prerequisite to sterilization and disinfection.

Antisepsis is the term used to describe disinfection applied to living tissue such as a wound. The term *sanitization* is also used to describe disinfection, particularly in the USA, and is generally used in conjunction with catering and food equipment.

Decontamination is a general term for the treatment used to make equipment safe to handle, including microbiological, chemical, radio-active and other contamination.

STERILIZATION

Definition

Sterilization means the freeing of an article from all living organisms, including viruses, bacteria and their spores, and fungi and their spores. In practice, all processes of sterilization have a finite probability of failure. An article may be regarded as sterile if it can be demonstrated that there is a probability of less than 1 in a million of there being viable micro-organisms on it.

Uses

Sterilization is required in medical practice for instruments and materials used in procedures that involve penetration into normally sterile parts of the body, e.g. in surgical operations, intravenous infusions, hypodermic injections and diagnostic aspirations. It is also required for media, reagents and equipment used in laboratory practice.

Methods

Five main methods are used for sterilization.

Heat. The only method of sterilization that is both reliable and widely applicable is by heating under carefully controlled conditions at temperatures above 100°C to ensure that bacterial spores are killed.

Ionizing irradiation. Both beta (electrons) and gamma (photons) irradiation are employed industrially for the sterilization of single-use disposable items such as needles and syringes, latex catheters and surgical gloves.

Filtration. Filters are used to remove bacteria and all larger micro-organisms from liquids that are liable to be spoiled by heating, e.g. blood serum and antibiotic solutions in which contamination with filter-passing viruses is improbable or unimportant.

Sterilant gases. Ethylene oxide is used mainly by industry for the sterilization of thermolabile material, such as plastics which cannot withstand heating. Formaldehyde in combination with sub-atmospheric steam is more commonly used in hospitals for reprocessing thermolabile equipment. For either process, care should be taken to avoid toxic and other hazards both for the user and the patient.

Sterilant liquids. Use of liquids such as glutaraldehyde is generally the least effective and the most unreliable method. Such methods should be regarded as 'high-grade disinfection' only, to be applied only when no other sterilization method is available.

DISINFECTION

Definition

Disinfection, the freeing of an article from some or all of its burden of contaminating micro-organisms, is a relative term embracing a wide range of efficacy against particular viruses, vegetative bacteria and fungi, but not usually including bacterial spores.

Uses

Disinfection, rather than sterilization, is applied in circumstances in which sterility is unnecessary or sterilizing procedures are impracticable. Thus, in the absence of demonstrable clinical need, it is uneconomic to sterilize bed-pans, eating utensils, bed linen and other items of everyday living which may spread infection within hospitals. Moreover, the pathogens likely to be present on these articles rarely include those that form spores.

Similarly, it is a valuable precaution to treat the skin around the site of an invasive procedure, such as an injection or surgical operation, with an antiseptic that will kill many of the vegetative micro-organisms and reduce the chance of some of them being carried into the wound.

Methods

Disinfection is achieved by means of processes similar to, although less severe than, those used for sterilization.

Heat. A variety of methods are available using steam or water, some of which incorporate a cleaning stage within an automatic controlled process.

Ultraviolet radiation. This has limited application for the disinfection of surfaces and some piped-water supplies, but lacks penetrative power for more widespread application.

Gases. Formaldehyde is used as a fumigant in laboratory environments, e.g. before changing a filter in a safety cabinet or in the event of a gross spillage.

Filtration. Air supplied to operating theatres and other critical environments is filtered to remove potentially hazardous micro-organisms.

Chemical. Various chemicals with antimicrobial properties are used as disinfectants. They are all liable to be inactivated by excessive dilution and contact with organic materials such as dirt or blood, or a variety of other materials, Nevertheless they may provide a convenient method for environmental disinfection and other specific applications.

CHOICE OF METHOD

The choice of method of sterilization or disinfection depends on the nature of the item to be treated, the likely microbial contamination, and the risk of transmitting infection to patients or staff in contact with the item. The choice may be

Table 5.1 Risks to patients from equipment and the environment

Risk group	Examples	Choice of process
I. High risk (critical)		
Direct contact with a break in skin or mucous membrane or entering a sterile body area.	Surgical instruments; needles, syringes; parenteral fluids; arthroscopes	Must be sterile: heat sterilization, irradiation
II. Intermediate risk (semi-critical)		
Direct contact with mucous membrane but tissue is intact	Endotracheal tubes; aspirators; gastroscopes	Need not be sterile: disinfection acceptable; thorough cleaning with liquid chemicals
III. Low risk (non-critical)		
No direct contact with the patient other than via unbroken skin	Bed-pans, urinals; furniture; sinks, drains; walls, floors	Thorough cleaning (with disinfection as necessary) by washer or disinfector with detergents

based on an assessment of risk according to different categories of patient (e.g. immunocompromised) and equipment and their application (Table 5.1). The selection of sterilization, disinfection or simple cleaning processes for individual items of equipment and the environment should be agreed as part of the infection control policy of a hospital (see Chapter 67). The preferred option wherever possible, for both sterilization and disinfection, is heat rather than chemicals. This relates not only to the antimicrobial efficacy but to safety considerations, which are more difficult to control in some chemical processes. Wherever chemicals are to be used for disinfection and sterilization, the safety of persons involved directly or indirectly in the procedure must be considered. It should be remembered that all sterilizing and disinfecting agents will have some action on human cells. No method should be assumed to be safe unless appropriate precautions are taken.

MEASUREMENT OF MICROBIAL DEATH

Every method used must be validated to demonstrate the required degree of microbial kill. With heat sterilization and irradiation, a biological test may not be required if the physical conditions are sufficiently well-defined and controlled. For practical purposes a micro-organism may be regarded as 'dead' when it has lost the ability to reproduce. When micro-organisms are subjected to a lethal process, the number of viable cells decreases exponentially in relationship to the extent of exposure. If the logarithm of the number of survivors is plotted against the lethal dose received (e.g. time of heating at a particular temperature) the resulting curve is described as the *survivor curve*. This is independent of the size of the original population and is approximately linear.

It should be noted that the linear survivor curve is an idealized concept and, in practice, minor variations from this condition, such as an initial shoulder or final tail, are found to occur (see Fig. 5.1).

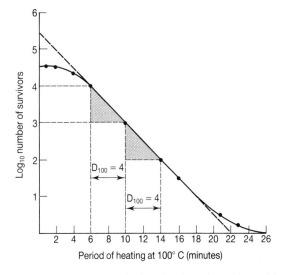

Fig. 5.1 The rate of inactivation of an inoculum of bacterial spores showing the decimal reduction time (D value) at 100°C and the non-linear 'shoulder and tail' effects.

D value. The D value or decimal reduction value is the lethal dose required to inactivate 90% of the initial population. From Fig. 5.1, it can be seen that the time (dose) required to reduce the population from 1 000 000 to 100 000 is the same as the time (dose) required to reduce the population from 100 000 to 10 000, i.e. the D value remains constant over the full range of the survivor curve. Extending the treatment beyond the point where there is one surviving cell does not give rise to fractions of a surviving cell but rather to a statement of the probability of finding one survivor. Thus by extrapolation from the experimental data it is possible to determine the lethal dose required to give a probability of less than 10^{-6} which is required to meet the pharmacopoeial definition of 'sterile'.

FACTORS INFLUENCING THE RESISTANCE OF MICRO-ORGANISMS

Many common factors affect the ability of micro-organisms to withstand the lethal effects of sterilization or disinfection processes. Factors specific to individual processes are considered in the description of those processes.

Species or strain of micro-organism

In general, vegetative bacteria and viruses are more susceptible, and bacterial spores the most resistant, to sterilizing and disinfecting agents. However, within different species and strains of species there may be wide variation in intrinsic resistance. For example, within the Enterobacteriaceae D values at 60°C range from a few minutes (*Escherichia coli*) to 1 h (*Salmonella senftenberg*). The typical D value for *Staphylococcus aureus* at 70°C is less than 1 min compared with 3 min for *Staph. epidermidis*. However, an unusual strain of *Staph. aureus* has been isolated with a D value of 14 min at 70°C. Such variations may be attributed to a variety of morphological or physiological changes such as alterations in cell proteins or specific targets in the cell envelope affecting permeability.

Inactivation data obtained for one micro-organism should not be extrapolated to another; thus it should not be assumed that bactericidal disinfectants are also potent against viruses. The inactivation data for scrapie and Creutzfeldt-Jakob disease suggest a highly resistant agent requiring six times the normal heat sterilization cycle (134°C for 18 min).

Physiological state

The conditions under which the micro-organisms were grown before exposure to the lethal process have a marked effect on their resistance. Organisms grown under nutrient-limiting conditions are typically more resistant than those grown under nutrient-rich conditions. Vegetative cells usually show increasing resistance through the late logarithmic phase of growth which declines erratically during the stationary phase.

Ability to form spores

Bacterial endospores, formed principally by *Bacillus* and *Clostridium* spp. are the forms most resistant to most processes. Similarly, fungal spores are more resistant than the vegetative mycelium, although they are not usually as resistant as bacterial spores. Bacterial spores were used to define the sterilization processes in current use and preparations of bacterial spores (biological indicators) are still used to monitor the efficacy of processes such as ethylene oxide sterilization, in which physical monitoring may be inadequate. In general, disinfection processes have little or no activity against bacterial spores.

Suspending menstruum

The micro-environment of the organism during exposure to the lethal process has a profound effect on its resistance. Thus, micro-organisms occluded in salt have greatly enhanced resistance to ethylene oxide; the presence of blood or other organic material will reduce the effectiveness of hypochlorite solution.

Number of micro-organisms

The higher the initial 'bioburden', the more extensive must be the process to achieve the same assurance of sterility.

STERILIZATION BY HEAT

Moist heat is much more effective than dry heat because it kills micro-organisms by coagulating and denaturing their enzymes and structural proteins, a process in which water participates. It is therefore necessary for all parts of the load to be sterilized to be in direct contact with water molecules or steam. Sterilization requires exposure to moist heat at 121°C for 15 min.

Dry heat is believed to kill micro-organisms by causing a destructive oxidation of essential cell constituents. Killing of the most resistant spores by dry heat requires a temperature of 160°C for 2 h. This high temperature causes slight charring of paper, cotton and other organic materials.

Factors influencing sterilization by heat

The factors to be considered include:

1. The temperature
2. The time of exposure
3. The number of vegetative micro-organisms and spores present
4. The species
5. The strain and spore-forming ability of the micro-organisms
6. The nature of the contaminated material.

Temperature and time. These are inversely related, shorter times sufficing at higher temperatures. The recommended combinations of temperature and time are listed in Table 5.2. These minimum times are for holding at the given temperature and do not include time for heating up or cooling the load for safe handling. Thus the total cycle time for processing a sterilized article will be much longer.

Microbial load. The number of micro-organisms and spores affects the rapidity of sterilization. The number of survivors diminishes exponentially with the duration of heating (see Fig. 5.1) and the time of complete sterilization increases in relation to the numbers initially present. In practice it is usual to minimize the number of contaminating bacteria by prior cleaning. Where this is not possible, e.g. contaminated laboratory

Table 5.2 Minimum recommended hold times for heat sterilization

Process	Temperature (°C)	Hold time (min)
Dry heat	160	120
	170	60
	180	30
Moist heat	121	15
	126	10
	134	3

cultures, an extended period of heating to achieve the required temperature will be needed.

Sterilization by moist heat

Moist heat sterilization requires attainment of temperatures above that of boiling water. Such conditions are attained under controlled conditions by raising the pressure of steam in a pressure vessel (*autoclave*). Thus, at sea-level, boiling water at atmospheric pressure (1 bar) will produce steam at 98–100°C, whereas raising the pressure to 2.4 bar increases the temperature to 125°C and at 3.0 bar to 134°C. Conversely, at subatmospheric pressures, including those at higher altitude, water will boil at lower temperatures.

The quality of steam for sterilization

Steam is a non-toxic, non-corrosive and highly effective sterilizing agent. The quality of steam for sterilization is critical; it must be *saturated*, which means that it holds all the water it can in the form of a transparent vapour, and it must be *dry*, which means that it does not contain water droplets.

Saturated steam is a more efficient sterilizing agent than dry heat, partly because of the greater lethal action of moist heat but also because it is quicker in heating up the article to be sterilized. When dry saturated steam meets a cooler surface it condenses into a small volume of water and liberates the latent heat of vaporization. The energy available from this latent heat is considerable, e.g. 6 litres of steam at a temperature of 134°C (and a corresponding pressure of 3 bar absolute) will condense into 10 ml of water and liberate 2162 J of heat energy. By comparison, less than 100 J of heat energy is released to an article by the sensible heat from air at 134°C.

If steam is at a higher temperature than the corresponding pressure would allow, it is referred to as *superheated steam* and behaves in a similar manner to hot air. Conversely, steam which contains suspended droplets of water at the same temperature is referred to as *wet steam* and is also less efficient. The presence of air in steam affects the sterilizing efficiency by changing the pressure-temperature relationship.

Types of steam sterilizer

Sterilizers for porous loads. These are intended to deal with dressings, textiles, wrapped instruments and wrapped utensils. Such loads are liable to trap air within the fabric, packaging or within narrow lumen instruments. This type of sterilizer must have a vacuum-assisted air removal stage to ensure that adequate air is removed from the load before admission of steam for sterilization. The vacuum pulsing of air also ensures that the load is dry on completion of the cycle.

Sterilizers for fluids in sealed containers. Sterilizers for pharmaceutical fluids and laboratory media in sealed containers and ampoules must have a safety feature to ensure that the door cannot be opened until the contents of the glass containers have fallen below 80°C. Otherwise the thermal stress of cold air on opening the door may cause the bottles to explode under pressure, causing serious injury.

Sterilizers for unwrapped instruments and utensils. These simple machines should not be used for wrapped articles and are recommended for use in dental clinics and in general practice.

Laboratory sterilizers. These machines are needed for a variety of different types of load, such as culture media in containers, laboratory glassware and equipment.

Monitoring of steam sterilizers

Physical measurements of temperature, pressure and time with thermometers and pressure gauges are recorded for every load and periodic detailed tests are undertaken with temperature-sensitive probes (thermocouples) inserted into standard test packs. Biological indicators comprising dried spore suspensions of a reference heat-resistant bacterium, *Bacillus stearothermophilus*, are no longer considered appropriate for routine testing, although spore indicators are essential for low-temperature gaseous processes in which the physical measurements are not reliable.

Sterilizers incorporating a vacuum-assisted air removal cycle are fitted with an air detector. In addition, the *Bowie-Dick* test is performed. This test monitors penetration of steam into a wrapped pack and will detect a blockage of even and rapid steam penetration by a 'bubble' of residual air in the pack. In the original test, an adhesive indicator tape, in the shape of a cross, was stuck onto a sheet of paper which was placed at the centre of a stack of towels (the test pack). The indicator shows a colour change from colourless to black, which should be even along the entire cross of the tape.

Sterilization by dry heat

Incineration

This is an efficient method for the sterilization and disposal of contaminated materials at a high temperature. It has a particular application for pathological waste materials, surgical dressings, sharp needles and other clinical waste.

Red heat

Inoculating wires, loops and points of forceps are sterilized by holding them in the flame of a Bunsen burner until they are red hot.

Flaming

Direct exposure for a few seconds may be used for scalpels and the necks of flasks, but it is of uncertain efficacy. Inoculating loops and needles are sometimes treated by immersing them in methylated spirit and burning off the alcohol, but this method does not produce a sufficiently high temperature for sterilization and care must be taken to avoid the flammable risk of alcohol.

Hot air sterilizer

Hot air sterilizers are used to process materials which can withstand high temperatures for the

restrict the term *antiseptic* to preparations applied to open wounds or abraded tissue and would prefer the term *skin disinfection* for the removal of organisms from hands and intact skin surfaces.

Factors influencing the performance of chemical disinfectants

Many factors influence the activity of disinfectants. These include:

1. The concentration of the disinfectant
2. The number, type and location of micro-organisms
3. The temperature and pH of treatment
4. The presence of extraneous material such as organic or other interfering substances.

In general, the rate of inactivation of a susceptible microbial population in the presence of an antimicrobial chemical is dependent on the relative concentration of the two reactants, the micro-organism and the chemical. The optimum concentration required to produce a standardized microbial effect in practice is described as the *in-use* concentration. Care must always be taken in preparing an accurate in-use dilution of concentrated product. Accidental or arbitrary overdilution may result in failure of disinfection.

The velocity of the reaction depends upon the number and type of organisms present. In general, Gram-positive bacteria are more sensitive to disinfectants than Gram-negative bacteria; mycobacteria and fungal spores are relatively resistant and bacterial spores are highly resistant. Enveloped or lipophilic viruses are relatively sensitive, whereas hydrophilic viruses such as poliovirus and other enteroviruses are less susceptible. Although difficult to test in vitro, there is evidence that hepatitis B virus is more resistant than other viruses (including human immunodeficiency virus) and most vegetative bacteria to the action of chemical disinfectants and heat.

Glutaraldehyde is highly active against bacteria, viruses and spores. Other disinfectants such as hexachlorophane have a relatively narrow range of activity, predominantly against Gram-positive cocci. Some disinfectants are more active or stable at a particular pH value, e.g. glutaraldehyde is more stable at acidic pH values but is used for preference at a higher pH value (8.0) to improve the antimicrobial effect.

Inactivation of disinfectants may be caused by many common circumstances such as hard tap-water, cork, plastics, blood, urine, soaps and detergents, or another disinfectant. Information should be sought from the manufacturer or from reference authorities to confirm that the disinfectant will remain active in the circumstances of use.

Alcohols

Isopropanol, ethanol and industrial methylated spirits have optimal bactericidal activity in aqueous solution at concentrations of 70–90% and have little bactericidal effect outside this range. They have limited activity against mycobacteria and are not sporicidal. Action against viruses is generally good. Because of their volatile nature, alcohols have been widely recommended as rapidly drying disinfectants for skin and surfaces. However, in many instances, particularly where organic matter such as blood or other protein-based contamination is present, the contact time may be insufficient to achieve adequate penetration and kill. Alcohols should therefore be used on physically clean surfaces such as washed thermometers or trolley tops but are unsuitable for dirty surfaces. Care must be taken when used on the skin in conjunction with diathermy and other instances of flammable risk. Alcohols or alcohol-based formulations with chlorhexidine or povidone iodine are good choices for hand disinfection, applied as handrubs on the dry skin, often with added emollient to counteract the drying effect.

Aldehydes

Most aldehyde disinfectants are based on glutaraldehyde or fomaldehyde formulations, alone or in combination. *Glutaraldehyde* has a broad-spectrum action against vegetative bacteria, fungi and viruses, but acts more slowly against spores. It is often used for equipment such as endoscopes that cannot be sterilized or disinfected by heat. It is an irritant to eyes, skin and respiratory mucosa and must be used with adequate protection of staff and ventilation of the working environment. It must be thoroughly rinsed from treated equipment with sterile water to avoid carry-over of toxic residues and recontamination. The alkaline buffered solution is claimed to remain active for a specific number of days, according to the manufacturer's instructions, but will vary depending on the 'in-use' situation, including the amount of organic material.

Biguanides

Chlorhexidine. Disinfection of the skin and mucous membranes is commonly carried out using chlorhexidine. It is less active against Gram-negative bacteria such as *Pseudomonas* and *Proteus* spp. and in aqueous solution has limited virucidal, tuberculocidal and negligible sporicidal activity. It is often combined with a compatible detergent for handwashing or with alcohol as a handrub. Chlorhexidine has a low irritancy and toxicity, which enable effective action as an antiseptic even on exposed healing surfaces. It is inactivated by organic matter, soap, anionic detergents, hard water and some natural materials such as the cork liners of bottle closures.

Halogens

Hypochlorites. These are broad-spectrum, inexpensive chlorine-releasing disinfectants. They are the disinfectants of choice against viruses, including hepatitis B virus. Their main disadvantages are the serious inactivation by organic matter and corrosion of metals. For circumstances of heavy soilage such as blood spillage, the higher concentration of 10 000 p.p.m. available chlorine is recommended.

The corrosion risk of hypochlorites means that contact with metallic instruments and equipment should be avoided. The bleaching action of hypochlorites may have a detrimental effect on fabrics, e.g. in treating a spillage on a carpet.

Chlorine-releasing disinfectants are relatively stable in concentrated form as liquid bleach or as tablets (sodium dichloroisocyanurates) but should be stored in well-sealed containers in a cool, dark place. On dilution to the required concentration for use, activity is rapidly lost.

Hypochlorites have widespread application as laboratory disinfectants on bench surfaces and in discard pots. Care should be taken to remove all chlorine-releasing agents from laboratory areas before the use of formaldehyde fumigation to avoid the production of carcinogenic reaction products.

Iodine. Like chlorine, iodine is inactivated by organic matter and has the additional disadvantages of staining and hypersensitivity. The *iodophors*, which contain iodine complexed with an anionic detergent, or *povidone iodine*, a water-soluble complex of iodine and polyvinyl pyrrolidone, are less irritant and cause less staining. Aqueous and alcohol-based povidone iodine preparations are widely used in skin disinfection, including preoperative preparation of the skin.

Phenolics

These have been widely used as general-purpose environmental disinfectants in hospital and laboratory practice. They exhibit broad-spectrum activity and are relatively cheap. Clear soluble phenolics have been used to disinfect environmental surfaces and spillages if organic soil and transmissible pathogens may be present. As hospital disinfection policies are rationalized, the phenolics are gradually being replaced by a detergent for cleaning and a hypochlorite for disinfection of contaminated sources. Most phenolics are stable and not readily inactivated by organic matter, with the exception of the chloroxylenols ('Dettol'), which are also inactivated by hard water and are not recommended for hospital use. Phenolics are incompatible with cationic detergents. Contact should be avoided with rubber and plastics, such as mattress covers, into which the phenolics are absorbed and which may increase the permeability of the material to body fluids. The slow release of phenol fumes in closed environments and the need to avoid skin contact are other reasons for care in situations where the phenolics are still used.

The bis-phenol *hexachlorophane* has been used as a skin disinfectant in powder or emulsion formulations, notably for prophylaxis against staphylococcal infection in nurseries. This disinfectant has particular activity against Gram-positive cocci. Concern has been expressed about the possible toxic effect of absorption across the neonatal skin barrier on repeated exposure, promoted in part by the observations of ill-effects when a hexachlorophane formulation was manufactured in error at excessively high concentration. An alternative, which has been used in the control of methicillin-resistant *Staph. aureus* (MRSA) outbreaks is *triclosan*.

Oxidizing agents and hydrogen peroxide

Various agents, including chlorine dioxide, peracetic acid and hydrogen peroxide, have good antimicrobial properties but are corrosive to skin and metals. Hydrogen peroxide is a highly reactive chemical which has limited application for the treatment of wounds.

Surface-active agents

Anionic, cationic, non-ionic and amphoteric *detergents* are generally used as cleaning agents. The cationic (*quaternary ammonium compounds*) and amphoteric agents have limited antimicrobial activity against vegetative bacteria and some viruses but not mycobacteria and bacterial spores. Quaternary ammonium compounds act by disrupting the membrane of the micro-organisms, leading to cell lysis. Care must be taken to avoid overgrowth by Gram-negative contaminants and inactivation by mixing cationic and anionic agents. Disinfection may be enhanced by the appropriate combination of a surface-active agent with disinfectant to improve contact spread and cleansing properties.

Disinfectant testing

A wide range of testing methods have been developed for different products and different applications in the medical, food and veterinary areas. Standardization of test methods within Europe is currently in progress, which will include:

1. Simple screening tests of the rate of kill
2. Laboratory tests simulating in-use conditions (skin disinfection tests, inanimate surface tests)
3. In-use tests on equipment and solutions.

The purpose of the 'in-use' test is to monitor not only the performance of a particular disinfectant but also how it is being used. Samples of the disinfectant dilutions in use around the hospital are taken to determine the survival and multiplication of contaminating pathogens in a stale or over-diluted formulation.

STERILIZATION AND DISINFECTION POLICY

Each hospital, through the infection control team, should agree a policy to ensure that staff responsible for sterilization and disinfection are familiar with the agents to be used and the procedures involved. The policy should consider:

1. The sources (equipment, skin, environment) for which a choice of process is required.
2. The processes and products available for sterilization and disinfection. An effective policy may include a limited number of process options; restrictions on the range of chemical disinfectants will eliminate unnecessary costs, confusion and chemical hazards.
3. The category of process required for each item: sterilization for surgical instruments and needles; heat disinfection for laundry, crockery, bed-pans; cleaning for floors, walls and furniture.
4. The specific products and method to be used for each item of equipment, the site of use and the staff responsible for the procedure.

Effective implementation of the policy requires liaison and training of staff and updating the policy. Safety considerations for staff and patients require a careful assessment of specific procedures to minimize risks, e.g. to avoid skin contact and fumes from disinfectants by the use of protective clothing and local ventilation.

RECOMMENDED READING

Ayliffe G A J, Coates D, Hoffman P N 1984 *Chemical Disinfection in Hospitals*, Public Health Laboratory Service, London
Gardner JF, Peel MM 1986 *Introduction to Sterilization and Disinfection*. Churchill Livingstone, Edinburgh
Maurer IM 1985 *Hospital Hygiene*, 3rd edn. Edward Arnold, London
Medical Research Council 1959 Sterilization by steam under increased pressure. A report to the Medical Research Council by the Working Party on Pressure-Steam Sterilizers. *Lancet* i: 427–435
Russell AD, Hugo WB, Ayliffe GAJ (eds) 1982 *Principles and Practice of Disinfection, Preservation and Sterilisation*. Blackwell Scientific, Oxford,
Spalding EH 1968 Chemical disinfection of medical and surgical materials. In: Lawrence CA, Block SS (eds) *Disinfection, Sterilization and Preservation*. Lea and Febiger, Philadelphia

6

Antimicrobial agents

D. Greenwood

The study of antimicrobial agents embraces not only antibacterial compounds, but also antiviral, antifungal, antiprotozoal and even anthelminthic agents. The term *chemotherapy* is usually used more generally to include the use of antitumour drugs. The strategy of antimicrobial chemotherapy is covered in Chapter 65.

The term *antibiotic* strictly refers to naturally occurring products of one organism that are inhibitory to others. According to this definition, chemical compounds such as sulphonamides, quinolones, nitrofurans and imidazoles should be referred to as *chemotherapeutic agents*. However, since some antibiotics can be manufactured synthetically while others are the products of chemical manipulation of naturally occurring antibiotics (*semi-synthetic antibiotics*) the distinction has become blurred and of doubtful value. Antimicrobial substances that are too toxic to be used other than in topical therapy or for environmental decontamination are referred to as *antiseptics* or *disinfectants* (Chapter 5).

ANTIBACTERIAL AGENTS

The principal types of antibacterial agent are listed in Table 6.1. Because there are so many of them it is convenient to group them according to their site of action.

Inhibitors of bacterial cell wall synthesis

Since most bacteria possess a rigid cell wall that is lacking in mammalian cells, this structure is a prime target for agents that exhibit *selective toxicity*, the ability to inhibit or destroy the microbe without harming the host. However, the bacterial cell wall can also prevent access of agents that would otherwise be effective. Thus, the complex outer envelope of Gram-negative bacteria is impermeable to large hydrophilic molecules, which may be prevented from reaching an otherwise susceptible target.

Inhibitors of bacterial cell wall synthesis act on the formation of the peptidoglycan layer (Fig. 6.1). Bacteria that lack peptidoglycan, such as mycoplasmas, are, of course, resistant to these agents.

β-Lactam agents

Penicillins, cephalosporins and other compounds that feature a β-lactam ring in their structure fall into this group (Fig. 6.2). All these compounds bind to proteins situated at the cell wall–cell membrane interface. These penicillin-binding proteins are involved in cell wall construction, including the cross-linking of the peptidoglycan strands that gives the wall its strength.

Penicillins. Benzylpenicillin (penicillin G) exhibits unrivalled activity against staphylococci, streptococci, neisseriae, spirochaetes and certain other organisms. However, resistance, normally due to the production of β-lactamase (penicillinase), has undermined its activity against staphylococci and, to a lesser extent, gonococci. In some parts of the world, strains of pneumococci that exhibit

Table 6.1 Principal types of antibacterial agent (other than agents used exclusively in mycobacterial infection)

Agent	Site of action	Usual activity[a] against					
		Staphylococci	Streptococci	Enterobacteria	*Pseudomonas aeruginosa*	*Mycobacterium tuberculosis*	Anaerobes
Penicillins	Cell wall	(+)	+	V	V	−	+[b]
Cephalosporins	Cell wall	+	+	+	V	−	+[b]
Other β-lactams	Cell wall	V	V	+	V	−	V
Glycopeptides	Cell Wall	+	+	−	−	−	+[c]
Tetracyclines	Ribosome	(+)	(+)	(+)	−	−	(+)
Chloramphenicol	Ribosome	+	+	+	−	−	−
Aminoglycosides	Ribosome	+	−	+	V	V	−
Macrolides	Ribosome	+	+	−	−	−	+
Lincosamides	Ribosome	+	+	−	−	−	+
Fusidic acid	Ribosome	+	+	−	−	+	+
Rifamycins	RNA synthesis	+	+	+	−	+	+
Sulphonamides	Folate metabolism	(+)	(+)	(+)	−	−	−
Diaminopyrimidines	Folate metabolism	+	+	(+)	−	−	−
Quinolones	DNA synthesis	V	V	+	V	V	−
Nitrofurans	DNA synthesis	−	−	+	−	−	+
Nitro-imidazoles	DNA synthesis	−	−	−	−	−	+

[a] Usual spectrum of intrinsic activity; parentheses indicate that resistance is common.
[b] Poor activity against anaerobes of the *Bacteroides fragilis* group.
[c] Poor activity against most Gram-negative anaerobes.
V = variable activity among different agents of the group.

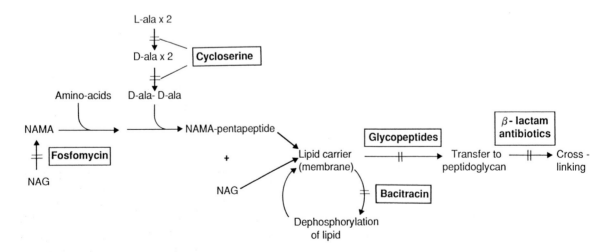

NAG = *N*-acetylglucosamine

NAMA = *N*- acetylmuramic acid

Fig. 6.1 Sites of action of inhibitors of bacterial cell wall synthesis.

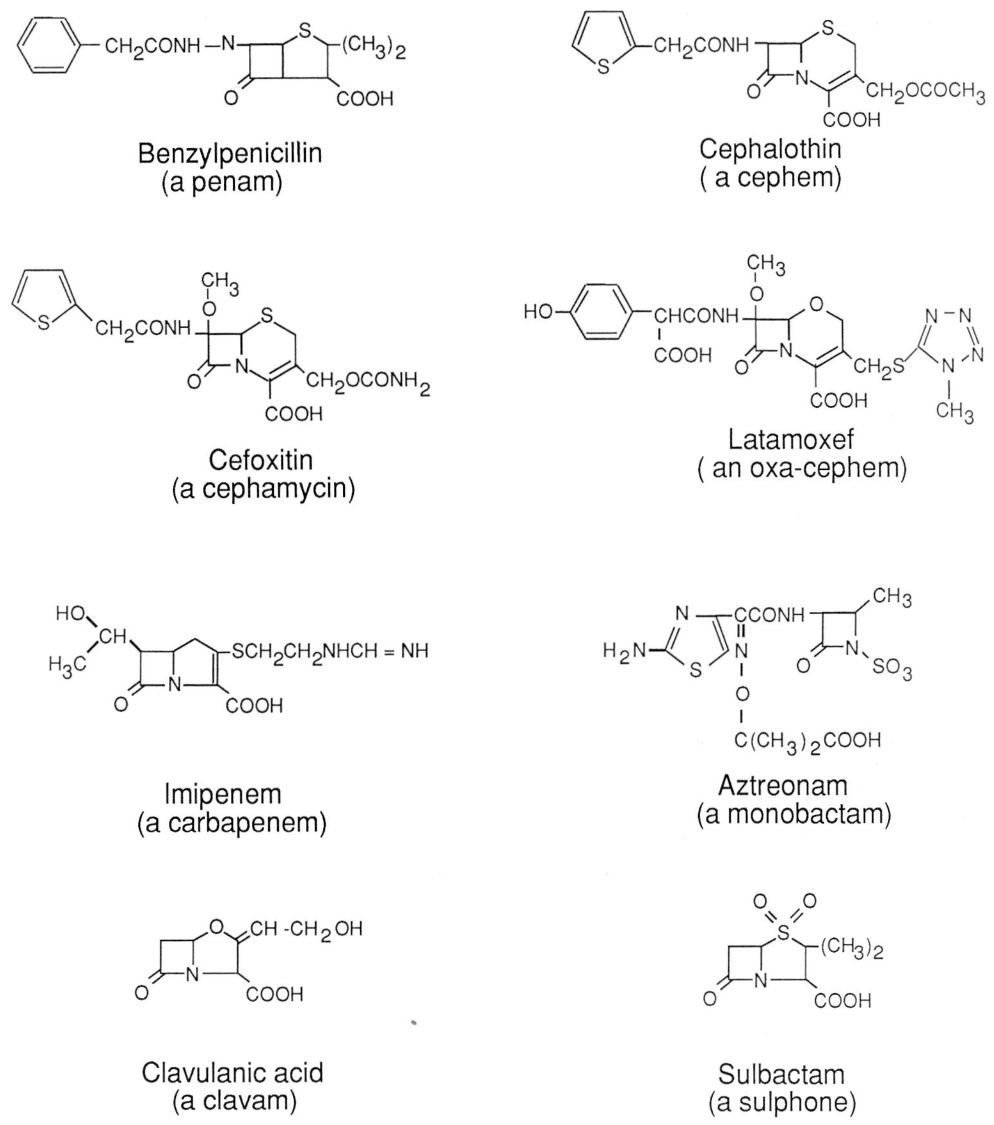

Fig. 6.2 Examples of different types of molecular structure among β-lactam antibiotics.

reduced susceptibility to penicillin by a non-enzymic mechanism may be encountered.

Benzylpenicillin revolutionized the treatment of infection caused by some of the most virulent bacterial pathogens, but it also suffered from a number of shortcomings:

1. Breakdown by gastric acidity when given orally
2. Very rapid excretion by the kidney
3. Susceptibility to penicillinase
4. A restricted spectrum of activity.

Further development of the penicillin family has been directed towards improving these properties. Crucial to this was the discovery that removal of the phenylacetic acid side chain left intact the core structure, 6-aminopenicillanic acid, the starting point for the numerous semi-synthetic penicillins that have been produced (Table 6.2).

Cephalosporins. Cephalosporins are close cousins of the penicillins, but the β-lactam ring is fused to a six-membered dihydrothiazine ring rather

Table 6.2 Development of penicillins

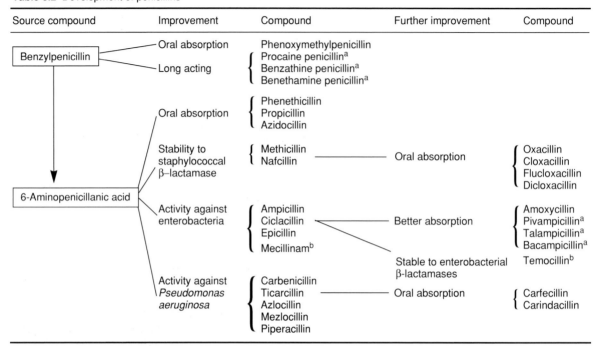

Source compound	Improvement	Compound	Further improvement	Compound
Benzylpenicillin	Oral absorption	Phenoxymethylpenicillin		
	Long acting	Procaine penicillin[a] Benzathine penicillin[a] Benethamine penicillin[a]		
6-Aminopenicillanic acid	Oral absorption	Phenethicillin Propicillin Azidocillin		
	Stability to staphylococcal β–lactamase	Methicillin Nafcillin	Oral absorption	Oxacillin Cloxacillin Flucloxacillin Dicloxacillin
	Activity against enterobacteria	Ampicillin Ciclacillin Epicillin Mecillinam[b]	Better absorption	Amoxycillin Pivampicillin[a] Talampicillin[a] Bacampicillin[a]
			Stable to enterobacterial β-lactamases	Temocillin[b]
	Activity against *Pseudomonas aeruginosa*	Carbenicillin Ticarcillin Azlocillin Mezlocillin Piperacillin	Oral absorption	Carfecillin Carindacillin

[a] Pro-drugs that release, or are converted to, active penicillins.
[b] Inactive against Gram-positive bacteria.
'Improvement' means a qualitative improvement and is not intended to indicate that compounds listed together are necessarily equivalent.

than the five-membered thiazolidine ring of penicillins. The additional carbon offers the possibility of additional substitutions that may alter the pharmacological behaviour of the molecule, and sometimes its antibacterial activity. Some cephalosporins (e.g. cephalothin, cefotaxime) carry an acetoxymethyl group on the extra carbon. This can be deacetylated by hepatic enzymes in the body to produce a less active derivative, but it is doubtful whether this has any therapeutic significance. Other cephalosporins (e.g. cephamandole, cefoperazone, cefotetan and the oxa-cephem latamoxef) possess a methyltetrazole substituent. Use of compounds with this feature has been associated with hypoprothrombinaemia and bleeding in some patients.

Cephalosporins have some apparent advantages over penicillins in that they are generally stable to staphylococcal penicillinase; they normally exhibit a broader spectrum; and they are less prone to cause hypersensitivity reactions. On the other hand, the more active compounds can only be administered parenterally and the group lacks activity against enterococci. The most important cephalosporin derivatives are shown in Table 6.3.

Other β-lactam agents. Various agents with diverse properties share the structural feature of a β-lactam ring with penicillins and cephalosporins (Table 6.4). *Latamoxef* (moxalactam) is an oxa-cephem with properties similar to those of broad-spectrum, β-lactamase-stable cephalosporins. *Imipenem* is a carbapenem with an unusually broad spectrum of activity embracing most Gram-positive and Gram-negative aerobic and anaerobic bacteria. In contrast, *aztreonam*, which is a monocyclic β-lactam antibiotic (monobactam), possesses a spectrum that is restricted to aerobic Gram-negative bacteria. The clavam *clavulanic acid* and the sulphone *sulbactam* exhibit poor antibacterial activity, but have proved useful as β-lactamase inhibitors when used in combination with β-lactamase-susceptible compounds (e.g. co-amoxiclav).

Table 6.3 Development of cephalosporins

Source compound	Route of administration	Compound	Improvement	Compound	Further improvement	Compound
Cephalosporin C → 7-Aminocephalosporanic acid	Oral	Cephalexin Cephradine Cefaclor Cephaloglycin Cefroxadine	Enzyme stability / Longer plasma half-life	Cefuroxime axetil / Cefadroxil Cefatrizine	More active	Cefixime
	Parenteral	Cephalothin Cephaloridine Cephazolin Cephacetrile Cefapirin Ceftezole Cefazedone	Improved stability to enterobacterial β-lactamases	Cefuroxime Cefoxitin Cefotetan Cephamandole Cefotiam	More active / More active and longer half-life	Cefotaxime Ceftizoxime Cefmenoxime / Ceftriaxone
			Longer plasma half-life	Cefonicid Ceforanide		
			Activity against *Pseudomonas aeruginosa*	Cefsulodin Cefoperazone	More active	Ceftazidime

'Improvement' means a qualitative improvement and is not intended to indicate that compounds listed together are necessarily equivalent.

Table 6.4 Clinically useful β-lactam compounds other than penicillins and cephalosporins

Compound	Structure[a]	Chief properties
Aztreonam	Monobactam	Narrow spectrum
Imipenem	Carbapenem	Very broad spectrum
Latamoxef	Oxa-cephem	Broad spectrum
Clavulanic acid	Clavam	β-Lactamase inhibitor
Sulbactam	Sulphone	β-Lactamase inhibitor

[a]See Fig. 6.2.

Other inhibitors of bacterial cell wall synthesis

Vancomycin and teicoplanin. These are glycopeptide antibiotics with a spectrum restricted to Gram-positive bacteria. Resistance among susceptible species is presently uncommon although resistant enterococci have been described; these agents have been successfully used in infections caused by multiresistant staphylococci.

Fosfomycin. This is a broad-spectrum agent that has been widely used in some countries, notably for the treatment of urinary tract infection. Resistance arises readily in vitro.

Bacitracin. This antibiotic is active against Gram-positive bacteria, but is too toxic for systemic use. It is found in many topical preparations and is also used in the laboratory in the presumptive identification of haemolytic streptococci of Lancefield group A.

Cycloserine. This enjoyed brief popularity as a second-line agent for the treatment of tuberculosis, but has largely fallen into disuse with the availability of more active, less toxic compounds.

Inhibitors of bacterial protein synthesis

The ribosomes of bacteria are sufficiently different from those of mammalian cells to allow selective inhibition of bacterial protein synthesis. Most of these agents are true antibiotics (or derivatives thereof) produced by *Streptomyces* or other soil organisms.

Tetracyclines

These are extremely broad-spectrum agents with important activity against chlamydiae, rickettsiae and mycoplasmas as well as most conventional Gram-positive and Gram-negative bacteria. The various members of the tetracycline group are closely related and differ more in their pharmacological behaviour than in antibacterial activity. Doxycycline and minocycline are the tetracyclines in most common use. Resistance has limited the value of tetracyclines against many Gram-positive and Gram-negative bacteria.

Chloramphenicol

This compound and the related thiamphenicol also possess a very broad antibacterial spectrum. Use of chloramphenicol has been limited to a few clinical indications, including typhoid fever and meningitis, because of the occurrence of a rare but fatal side-effect, aplastic anaemia. Thiamphenicol is said to lack this disadvantage, but is more likely to cause a reversible type of bone marrow toxicity.

Aminoglycosides

Streptomycin, the first antibiotic to be discovered by random screening of soil organisms, is predominantly active against enterobacteria and *Mycobacterium tuberculosis*. Like all members of the aminoglycoside family it has no useful activity against streptococci or anaerobes. The group also has in common a tendency to damage the eighth cranial nerve (ototoxicity) and the kidney (nephrotoxicity). The chief properties of aminoglycosides in clinical use are shown in Table 6.5. The aminoglycosides are bactericidal compounds that have been widely used, often in combination with β-lactam antibiotics, with which they interact synergically, in the 'blind' treatment of sepsis in immunocompromised patients. Resistance may arise from ribosomal changes (streptomycin), alterations in drug uptake, or modification by bac-

terial enzymes (phosphorylation, acetylation or adenylation).

Macrolides

The first macrolide, erythromycin, established itself as a useful antistaphylococcal and antistreptococcal agent, chiefly for use in patients who are allergic to penicillins. More recently it has found extended use in Legionnaires' disease and in those cases of campylobacter enteritis that require antimicrobial therapy. Erythromycin and other macrolides have no useful activity against enteric Gram-negative bacilli. Erythromycin is usually administered orally as the stearate salt or as esterified *pro-drugs* (pharmacological preparations that improve absorption and deliver the active drug into the circulation). Salts suitable for intravenous administration are also available.

Other macrolides include spiramycin, which is generally less active than erythromycin against Gram-positive cocci, but has some useful activity against the protozoan parasite *Toxoplasma gondii*, and oleandomycin, which exhibits properties similar to that of erythromycin. Some newer macrolides, such as azithromycin, roxithromycin and clarithromycin, may offer improved pharmacological properties.

Lincosamides

The original lincosamide antibiotic, lincomycin, has been virtually superseded by the 7-deoxy-7-chloro derivative, clindamycin, which is better

Table 6.5. Summary of the important differential properties of aminoglycoside antibiotics

| Aminoglycoside | Activity against | | Susceptibility to inactivation by bacterial enzymes | Relative degrees of | |
	Pseudomonas aeruginosa	Mycobacterium tuberculosis		Ototoxicity	Nephrotoxicity
Amikacin	+	+	±	++	+
Gentamicin	+	−	++	++	++
Kanamycin	−	+	++	++	++
Neomycin	−	±	++	+++	++
Netilmicin	+	−	+	+	+
Sissomicin	+	−	++	++	++
Streptomycin	−	+	++	+++	±
Tobramycin	+	−	++	++	++

absorbed after oral administration and is more active against the organisms within its spectrum. These include staphylococci, streptococci and most anaerobic bacteria, against which clindamycin exhibits outstanding activity. Enthusiasm for the use of clindamycin has been tempered by an association with the occasional development of severe diarrhoea which sometimes progresses to a life-threatening pseudomembranous colitis (see *Clostridium difficile*, Chapter 23).

Fusidic acid

The structure of fusidic acid is related to that of steroids, but the antibiotic is devoid of steroid-like activity. It has an unusual spectrum of activity that includes corynebacteria, nocardia and *M. tuberculosis*, but the antibiotic is usually regarded simply as an antistaphylococcal agent. It penetrates well into bone and has been widely used (generally in combination with a β-lactam antibiotic to prevent the selection of resistant variants) in the treatment of staphylococcal osteomyelitis.

Inhibitors of nucleic acid synthesis

Nucleic acids are ubiquitous in living cells and it is perhaps surprising that a number of important antibacterial agents act directly or indirectly on DNA or RNA synthesis.

Sulphonamides and diaminopyrimidines

These agents act indirectly on DNA synthesis because of their effect on folic acid metabolism. Folic acid is used in many one-carbon transfers in living cells, including the conversion of deoxyuridine to thymidine. During this process the active form of the vitamin, tetrahydrofolate, is oxidized to dihydrofolate and this must be reduced before it can function in further reactions.

Sulphonamides are analogues of *p*-aminobenzoic acid and prevent the condensation of this compound with dihydropteridine during the formation of folic acid. Diaminopyrimidines, which include trimethoprim and the antimalarial compounds pyrimethamine and cycloguanil (the metabolic product of proguanil), interfere with the re-

duction of dihydrofolate to tetrahydrofolate. Sulphonamides and diaminopyrimidines thus act at sequential stages of the same metabolic pathway. This results in a synergic interaction which is exploited therapeutically in the trimethoprim-sulphamethoxazole (co-trimoxazole) and pyrimethamine-sulfadoxine combinations.

Sulphonamides are broad-spectrum antibacterial agents, but resistance is common and the group also suffers from problems of toxicity. They are now little used outside urinary tract infection. The numerous members of the group exhibit similar, but not identical, antibacterial activity, but differ widely in their pharmacokinetic behaviour. Sulphadiazine and sulphadimidine (also known as sulfamethazine) are most commonly used.

Trimethoprim is also broad-spectrum and, in most clinical situations, is probably as effective alone as when combined with a sulphonamide.

Quinolones

These drugs act on the α-subunit of DNA gyrase. Two groups are presently available (Table 6.6). Nalidixic acid and its early congeners are narrow-spectrum agents active only against Gram-negative bacteria. Their use is virtually restricted to urinary tract infection, although they have also been used in enteric infections and, in the case of acrosoxacin, in gonorrhoea. Newer fluoro-quinolones, including ciprofloxacin, norfloxacin, enoxacin and ofloxacin, display much enhanced activity which brings *Pseudomonas aeruginosa* and many Gram-positive bacteria within the spectrum.

Table 6.6 Types of quinolone antibacterial agent

Older, narrow-spectrum quinolones	Newer, broad-spectrum quinolones
Acrosoxacin	Ciprofloxacin
Cinoxacin	Enoxacin
Flumequine	Norfloxacin
Nalidixic acid	Ofloxacin
Oxolinic acid	Pefloxacin
Pipemidic acid	Temafloxacin
Piromidic acid	

Quinolones are quite well absorbed when given orally and are widely distributed throughout the body. Extensive metabolization may occur, particularly with nalidixic acid and the older derivatives. Ciprofloxacin and the newer fluoroquinolones have been successfully used in a wide variety of infections, but the development of resistance to the rather modest concentrations achievable in tissues may eventually limit their value outside urinary tract infection.

Nitro-imidazoles

Azole derivatives feature prominently among antifungal, antiprotozoal and anthelminthic agents. Those that exhibit antibacterial activity are 5-nitro-imidazoles that, at the low redox (E_h) values produced intracellularly in anaerobic organisms, are reduced to a short-lived intermediate which causes strand breakage in DNA. Because of the requirement for low E_h values, 5-nitro-imidazoles are active only against anaerobic (and certain micro-aerophilic) bacteria and anaerobic protozoa. The representative of the group most commonly used clinically is metronidazole, but similar derivatives include tinidazole, ornidazole and nimorazole.

Nitrofurans

The most familiar nitrofuran derivative is nitrofurantoin, an agent used exclusively in urinary tract infection. A related compound, furazolidone, has been used with variable success in enteric infections. Nifurtimox, one of the few agents to exhibit activity against the protozoan parasite *Trypanosoma cruzi* (see below) is also a nitrofuran derivative.

The mode of action of nitrofurans has not been elucidated, but it is probable that a reduced metabolite acts on DNA in a manner analogous to that of the nitro-imidazoles.

Novobiocin

This compound acts on the β-subunit of DNA gyrase (cf. quinolones). It was once widely used as a reserve antistaphylococcal agent, but is no longer favoured because of problems of resistance and toxicity.

Rifamycins

This group of antibiotics is characterized by excellent activity against mycobacteria, although other bacteria are also susceptible; staphylococci in particular are exquisitely sensitive. These compounds act by inhibiting transcription of RNA from DNA. Rifampicin, the best known member of the group, has been widely used in tuberculosis and leprosy. Wider use has been discouraged on the grounds that it might inadvertently foster the emergence of resistance in mycobacteria.

Rifapentine has similar properties, but exhibits a longer plasma half-life. Rifabutin (ansamycin) has been used in infections caused by atypical mycobacteria of the avium-intracellulare group, but results have been disappointing.

Miscellaneous antibacterial agents

Hexamine (methenamine)

Hexamine decomposes to formaldehyde and ammonia under mildly acidic conditions. It is sometimes used in the form of the hippuric acid or mandelic acid salt in the prophylaxis of recurrent urinary tract infection.

Polymyxins

Two members of this family are in use: polymyxin B and colistin (polymyxin E). They act like cationic detergents to disrupt the cell membrane. Polymyxins exhibit potent antipseudomonal activity, but toxicity has limited their usefulness except in topical preparations. If systemic use is contemplated, a sulphomethylated derivative, colistin sulphomethate, is preferred.

Pristinamycin

This is a naturally occurring antibiotic complex consisting of two synergic components, a macrolide and a depsipeptide. Pristinamycin, which is only available in certain countries, is predominantly an antistaphylococcal agent.

Antimycobacterial agents

As well as streptomycin and rifampicin (see above)

Table 6.7 Summary of the spectrum of activity of antifungal agents

Agent	Candida albicans	Cryptococcus neoformans	Dermatophytes	Aspergillus fumigatus	Dimorphic fungi
Amphotericin B	+	+	−	+	+
Flucytosine	+	+	−	−	−
Griseofulvin	−	−	+	−	−
Imidazoles	+	+	+	−	+
Itraconazole	+	+	+	+	+
Nystatin[a]	+	−	+	−	−
Terbinafine	−	−	+	+[b]	+[b]

[a] For topical use only; [b] clinical efficacy not yet established

a number of other agents are used exclusively for the treatment of mycobacterial infection. These include isoniazid, ethambutol and pyrazinamide, which are commonly found in antituberculosis regimens, and diaminodiphenylsulphone (dapsone) and clofazimine, which are used in leprosy. *p*-Aminosalicylic acid (PAS), which was formerly used in tuberculosis, has now been largely abandoned. Fluoroquinolones, such as ciprofloxacin, exhibit quite good activity against mycobacteria and may have a role in treatment if their value is confirmed in clinical trials.

ANTIFUNGAL AGENTS

Although superficial fungal infections can be effectively treated with a number of topical agents, including benzoic acid (Whitfield's ointment), tolnaftate and polyenes such as nystatin, these are too toxic for systemic use. One polyene, amphotericin B, is widely used, despite its toxicity, for the treatment of intractable systemic disease caused by yeasts and other fungi. Dermatophyte infections can often be cured by oral therapy with griseofulvin or terbinafine, antifungal agents that are deposited in newly formed keratin.

Antifungal agents with the broadest spectrum of activity, embracing yeasts, filamentous fungi and dimorphic fungi, are all azole derivatives; either 2-nitroimidazoles, such as clotrimazole, miconazole and ketoconazole, or triazoles, such as itraconazole and fluconazole. Itraconazole is unique in exhibiting useful activity against *Aspergillus fumigatus*; fluconazole is particularly

well-distributed after oral administration and has been used successfully in cryptococcal meningitis. The spectrum of activity of the common antifungal compounds is shown in Table 6.7.

ANTIVIRAL AGENTS

Relatively few agents are available for the treatment of viral infection (Table 6.8); most are nucleoside analogues. Of these, only acyclovir

Table 6.8 Antiviral agents in clinical use

Compound	Mode of action	Indication
Acyclovir	Nucleoside analogue	Herpes simplex
Amantadine (and rimantadine)	Viral uncoating and assembly	Influenza A
Foscarnet	Inhibition of polymerase	Cytomegalovirus retinitis
Ganciclovir	Nucleoside analogue	Cytomegalovirus
Idoxuridine	Nucleoside analogue	Herpes simplex (topical)
Inosine pranobex[a]	Immunomodulator	(Herpes simplex)
Tribavirin[b]	Nucleoside analogue	Respiratory syncytial virus
Trifluridine	Nucleoside analogue	Herpes simplex (topical)
Vidarabine	Nucleoside analogue	Herpes viruses
Zidovudine	Nucleoside analogue	Human immuno-deficiency virus

[a] Also known as isoprinosine
[b] Also known as ribavirin

exhibits true selective toxicity. All nucleoside analogues must be phosphorylated within the cell before they can interrupt viral nucleic acid synthesis, but, uniquely, acyclovir is preferentially phosphorylated by a thymidine kinase enzyme produced by the herpes simplex virus. Consequently, acyclovir is activated only in cells infected with the virus.

The acquired immune deficiency syndrome (AIDS) pandemic has generated an enormous interest in potential antiviral agents. One, zidovudine (azidothymidine), has now been in use for several years and a number of other compounds, notably dideoxynucleosides, are showing promise. Further details of antiviral compounds can be found in Chapter 9.

Table 6.9 Agents useful against the major protozoan parasites of man

Species	Agent
Cryptosporidium parvum	None
Entamoeba histolytica	Metronidazole
	Emetine
	Diodoquin
	Chloroquine
	Diloxanide furoate
Giardia lamblia	Metronidazole
	Mepacrine
Leishmania spp.	Sodium stibogluconate
Plasmodium spp.	Chloroquine
	Quinine
	Pyrimethamine
	Proguanil
	Mefloquine
	Halofantrine
Pneumocystis carinii [a]	Co-trimoxazole
	Pentamidine
Toxoplasma gondii	Pyrimethamine + sulphadiazine
Trichomonas vaginalis	Metronidazole
Trypanosoma rhodesiense and *T. gambiense*	Melarsoprol
	Suramin
	Pentamidine
	Eflornithine[b]
Trypanosoma cruzi	Nifurtimox
	Benznidazole

[a]Taxonomy uncertain; may be a fungus.
[b]Not active against *T. rhodesiense*.

ANTIPARASITIC AGENTS

Progress in the development of new agents for the treatment of protozoal and helminthic infections has been slow and the choice remains extremely limited.

Part of the problem is that protozoa and helminths encompass a wide range of biological types, reflecting diverse solutions to the problems of their specialized parasitic existence. Consequently, there are few 'broad-spectrum' antiprotozoal or anthelminthic agents, although some compounds, notably the benzimidazoles, thiabendazole, mebendazole and albendazole, exhibit a surprising range of activity against intestinal helminths.

Antimicrobial agents commonly used against pathogenic protozoa and helminths are shown in Tables 6.9 and 6.10

Table 6.10 Spectrum of activity of some anthelminthic agents

Agent	Active against
Benzimidazoles[a]	Intestinal nematodes
Diethylcarbamazine	Filariae
Ivermectin	*Onchocerca volvulus*
	Other filariae
Niclosamide	Tapeworms
Niridazole	*Schistosoma haematobium*
	Dracunculus medinensis
Metriphonate	*Schistosoma haematobium*
Oxamniquine	*Schistosoma mansoni*
Piperazine	*Ascaris lumbricoides*
	Enterobius vermicularis
Praziquantel	*Schistosoma* spp.
	Other trematodes
	Tapeworms
Pyrantel pamoate	Intestinal nematodes
Tetrachloroethylene	*Necator americanus*
Trivalent antimonials	*Schistosoma* spp.

[a]Includes mebendazole, thiabendazole and albendazole.

RECOMMENDED READING

Franklin T J, Snow GA 1989 *Biochemistry of Antimicrobial Action* 4th edn. Chapman and Hall, London

Greenwood D (ed) 1989 *Antimicrobial Chemotherapy*, 2nd edn. Oxford University Press, Oxford

Greenwood D, O'Grady F 1985 *The Scientific Basis of Antimicrobial Chemotherapy*. Cambridge University Press, Cambridge

Kucers A, Bennett N McK 1987 *The Use of Antibiotics*, 4th edn. Heinemann, London

Lambert H P, O'Grady F W 1992 *Antibiotic and Chemotherapy*, 6th edn. Churchill Livingstone, Edinburgh

Pratt W B, Fekety R 1986 *The Antimicrobial Drugs*. Oxford University Press, Oxford

Russell A D, Chopra I 1990 *Understanding Antibacterial Action and Resistance*. Ellis Horwood, Chichester

7

Bacterial genetics

K. J. Towner

GENETIC ORGANIZATION AND REGULATION OF THE BACTERIAL CELL

All properties of a bacterial cell, including those of medical importance such as virulence, pathogenicity and antibiotic resistance, are ultimately determined by the genetic information contained within the cell *genome*. This information is normally encoded by the specific sequence of nucleotide bases comprising the cell's deoxyribonucleic acid (DNA). There are four common nucleotide bases in DNA: adenine, guanine, cytosine and thymine; it is the linear order in which these bases are arranged which determines the properties of the cell. In all bacteria so far studied, most of the genetic information required by the cell is arranged in the form of a single circular double-stranded chromosome. In *Escherichia coli* the chromosome is about 1300 μm long and occurs in an irregular coiled bundle lying free in the cytoplasm. The DNA is not associated with protein or histone molecules as it is in eukaryotic cell chromosomes.

In addition to the single main chromosome, bacterial cells may also carry one or more small circular extrachromosomal elements. These were originally called episomes, but are now termed *plasmids*. Plasmids replicate independently of the main chromosome in the cell. Although dispensible, they often carry supplementary genetic information coding for beneficial properties (e.g. resistance to antibiotics) which enable the host cell to survive under a particular set of environmental conditions.

A third source of genetic information in a bacterial cell can be provided by the presence of certain types of bacterial viruses, *bacteriophages*. Bacteriophages essentially consist of just a protein coat enclosing the virus genome and, since they are unable to multiply in the absence of their bacterial host, they are generally lethal to their host cell. In some instances, they can enter a potentially long-term state of controlled replication, *lysogeny*, within the bacterial cell without causing lysis. In such a state the bacteriophage genome effectively becomes a temporary part of the total genetic information available to the cell and may consequently bestow additional properties on the cell.

Not all genetic material consists of double-stranded DNA. Some bacteriophages contain single-stranded molecules of either DNA or RNA which can be either circular or linear in configuration. Within the prokaryotic kingdom, and including bacteriophages, genome size varies over more than three orders of magnitude from about 3 to 5000 kilobases (kb) (Table 7.1).

Processes leading to protein synthesis

The character of a bacterial cell is essentially determined by the specific polypeptides which comprise its enzymes and other proteins. The DNA acts as a template for the *transcription* of

Table 7.1 Examples of prokaryotic genetic elements

Genetic element	Type	Configuration	Size (kb)
Bacterial chromosome			
Escherichia coli	DNA	ds circular	3.8×10^3
Bacillus subtilis	DNA	ds circular	2.0×10^3
Plasmids			
R300B	DNA	ds circular	9.0
RK2	DNA	ds circular	60.0
Bacteriophages			
MS2	RNA	ss linear	3.6
Φ174	DNA	ss circular	5.4
T7	DNA	ds linear	40.4

Abbreviations: ss, single-stranded; ds, double-stranded; kb, kilobase.

RNA by RNA polymerase for subsequent protein production within the cell. In the transcription process the specific sequence of nucleotides in the DNA determines the corresponding sequence of nucleotides in the messenger RNA (mRNA). This, in turn, is then *translated* into the appropriate sequence of amino acids by ribosomes. Finally, the sequence of amino acids in the resulting polypeptide chain determines the configuration into which the polypeptide chain folds itself, which in many cases determines the enzymic properties of the completed protein. A segment of DNA that specifies the production of a particular polypeptide chain is called a *gene*, while the processes of transcription and translation leading to protein synthesis are collectively termed the *central dogma* of molecular biology. These processes are illustrated schematically in Fig. 7.1.

Gene regulation

Most bacteria contain enough DNA to code for the production of between 1000 and 3000 different polypeptide chains, i.e. 1000 to 3000 different genes. However, during normal bacterial life, some polypeptides will only be required at particular stages, while others will be needed only when the cell is provided with a new or unusual growth substrate. Protein production is an energy-intensive process and therefore the expression of many genes is actively controlled within the cell to prevent wasteful energy consumption.

In prokaryotic bacteria the process of gene expression is regulated mainly at the transcriptional level, thereby conserving the energy supply and the transcription–translation apparatus. This is achieved by means of regulatory elements that either inhibit or enhance the rate of RNA chain initiation and termination for a particular gene. There are numerous regulatory mechanisms involved in co-ordinating the many biochemical reactions that proceed inside a cell, but the classic example of the sort of molecular mechanism involved in gene regulation is the control of β-galactosidase production in *Esch. coli*.

Most strains of *Esch. coli* can utilize lactose as a source of energy. The enzyme used to split the disaccharide, β-galactosidase, is produced only in the presence of lactose and its production is switched off when not required. Lactose is described as an *inducer* and β-galactosidase is termed an *inducible* enzyme. The gene for β-galactosidase, termed *lacZ*, is clustered on the chromosome with three other genes that enable *Esch. coli* to utilize lactose (Fig. 7.2): *lacI*, which codes for the *repressor*, a regulatory protein; *lacY*, which codes for a permease required for active transport of lactose into cells; and *lacA*, which codes for a transacetylase enzyme that reduces the toxicity of some galactosides by transferring acetyl groups. These genes are all involved in a common regulatory system, and this functional unit is known as the lactose (*lac*) operon. In bacteria it is quite common to find that groups of related genes are clustered on the chromosome and regulated by a common mechanism.

For transcription to occur as the first stage in protein synthesis, RNA polymerase has to attach to the DNA at a specific *promoter* region and transcribe the DNA in a fixed direction. The *lac* operon can be switched off by the attachment of a repressor molecule to a specific region of the DNA, known as the *operator*, which lies between the promoter and the *lacZ* gene (Fig. 7.2); the repressor then blocks the movement of the RNA polymerase molecule so that *lacZ* and the following genes are not transcribed.

The repressor is an allosteric molecule with two active sites. One recognizes the operator region of the *lac* operon so that the repressor can bind to it to prevent transcription. The other recognizes the inducer — i.e. a lactose molecule or a closely

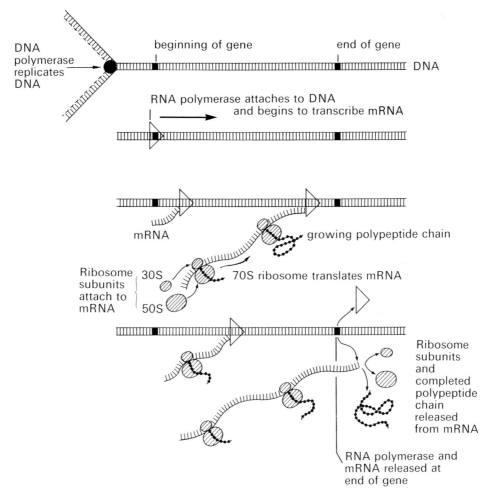

Fig. 7.1   The central dogma of molecular biology.

related derivative. When the inducer is present it binds to the repressor and simultaneously alters the binding specificity at the other site, so that the repressor no longer binds to the operator and transcription can resume. When the inducer has been metabolized by the enzymes produced, the repressor is then free to attach again to the operator site and production of β-galactosidase is once more repressed. This type of transcriptional regulation is particularly effective as bacterial mRNA is short-lived and enzyme production ceases rapidly when transcription is stopped.

There are many different variations on this basic regulatory system. For example, a repressor may be normally inactive, but activated by the end-product of a biosynthetic pathway; thus only when the end-product is present in adequate concentration will the repressor combine with the operator and switch off transcription of the operon.

Other more complicated systems are known to exist. Regulation of the *ara* (arabinose) operon involves a series of proteins that bind to the DNA and assist RNA polymerase to initiate transcription, while the *trp* (tryptophan) operon is partly regulated by involvement of the translation apparatus in determining whether transcription of the operon will continue once begun. Other regulatory systems display both minor and major differences. Finally, it should be stressed that

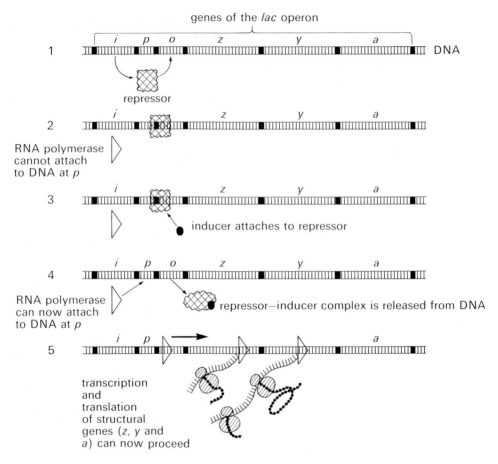

Fig. 7.2 The *lac* operon of *Esch. coli.*
1 The *lac* repressor is produced from the *i* gene
2 Binding of the repressor to the operator site (*o*) prevents transcription of the genes *z* (β-galactosidase), *y* (galactoside permease) and *a* (transacetylase)
3 The inducer (lactose, or a closely related derivative) can bind specifically to the repressor
4 The repressor molecule is thereby altered at its operator-binding site and the repressor–inducer complex is released from the DNA
5 RNA polymerase can now attach to the promoter site (*p*) and transcribe the structural genes of the *lac* operon.

prokaryotic gene regulation frequently involves interwoven regulatory circuits that respond to a variety of different stimuli.

MUTATION

As bacteria reproduce by asexual binary fission, the genome is normally identical in all the progeny. The DNA replication process is therefore very accurate, but occasional rare inaccuracies produce a slightly altered nucleotide sequence in one of the progeny cells. Such a *mutation* is heritable and will be stably passed on to subsequent generations. One of the fundamental requirements for evolution is that, although gene replication must normally be completely accurate to ensure stability, there must also be occasional variation to produce new or altered characters that could prove to be of selective value to the organism. Mutations may not produce any observable effect on the structure or function of the corresponding protein, but in a small proportion of cases an enzyme with altered specificity for substrates, inhibitors or regulatory molecules may be produced. This is the kind of mutation that is most likely to be of evolutionary value to an organism; indeed, many examples of acquired antibiotic resistance have been shown to be of this type. Other mutations may alter a gene so that a non-functional protein is formed; if this protein is essential to the cell then the mutation will be lethal.

Since mutation may occur in any of the cell's several thousand genes, and different mutations in the same gene may produce different effects in the cell, the number of possible mutations is very large. Particular mutations occur at fairly constant rates, normally between once per 10^4 and once per 10^{10} cell divisions. As a large bacterial colony contains at least 10^9 cells, even a 'pure' bacterial culture will contain many thousands of different mutations affecting many of the genes in the cell. Some of these mutations will be viable and could be selected by particular environmental conditions during subculture. For the same reason, in an infected patient, a variety of mutants will appear spontaneously in the population that grows from the few bacteria originally entering the body. Such mutations may enhance the ability of an organism to grow in the body, e.g. by conferring antibiotic resistance, enhanced virulence, or altered surface antigens. In such a situation, cells with the mutation will rapidly outgrow cells without the mutation, so that *selection* of the mutant cells occurs and they soon become the predominant type.

Phenotypic variation

The properties of a bacterial cell at a particular time are referred to as the cell's *phenotype*. These properties are determined not only by its genome (*genotype*), but also by its environment. *Phenotypic variation* occurs when the *expression* of genes is changed in response to the environment, e.g. by the induction or repression of synthesis of particular enzymes. The distinction is important: genotypic mutation is heritable and maintained through changes in environmental conditions, whereas phenotypic variation is reversible, being dependent on environmental conditions and altering when

these change. Phenotypic variation is therefore *not* a form of mutation.

Types of mutation

Mutations can conveniently be divided into *multisite mutations*, involving extensive chromosomal rearrangements such as inversions, duplications and deletions, and *point mutations*, which are defined as only affecting one, or very few, nucleotides. The structure of DNA is such that point mutations can be divided into one of three basic types: the substitution of one nucleotide for another, the deletion of one or more nucleotides, and the insertion of one or more nucleotides (Fig. 7.3).

Mutations occur spontaneously during replication of DNA, but most are immediately corrected by the cell's editing apparatus. The frequency of stable spontaneous mutation is often too low for convenient experimentation and *mutagens* are therefore used to increase the frequency of mutants in cultures. Common mutagens include irradiation (X-rays or ultraviolet light) and chemicals (5-bromouracil, 2-aminopurine, nitrous acid, hydroxylamine) that interfere with DNA replication either by acting as base analogues or by altering DNA bases in situ.

Mutations are normally stably inherited by the progeny, but secondary mutations can occasionally restore the original nucleotide sequence. It is important to distinguish this relatively rare event of *back-mutation* from the separate process of *phase variation*, which is readily reversible and occurs with relatively high frequency in either direction, e.g. once per 10^3 cell divisions. The variation of certain Gram-negative bacteria between a fimbriate and a non-fimbriate phase, and the variation of flagellar antigens in *Salmonella* species are examples of phase variation. These seem to involve special genetic regions that are specifically inverted to yield alternative gene products and different phenotypes. In some cases it is known that promoters initiate RNA transcription in different directions to give a flip-flop type of action. The number of such switching systems is probably quite limited, but they have value to the organism in providing a mechanism

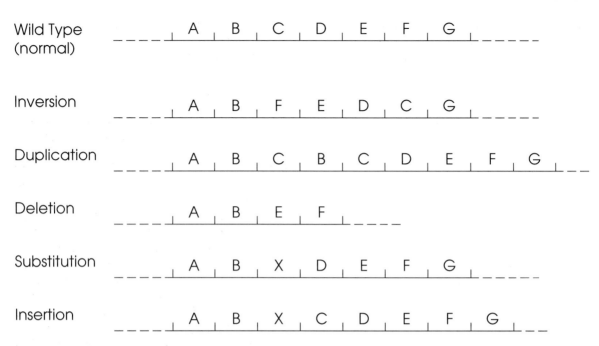

Fig. 7.3 Examples of types of mutations. The top sequence represents a portion of the wild-type chromosome from which the different mutational rearrangements shown below are derived.

to switch to a reversible alternative, as opposed to an irreversible change.

Isolation of mutants

The study of bacterial genetics is dependent upon the isolation and characterization of mutants in particular genes. Mutations may occur in any gene, but many individual mutations are lethal. Other mutations affect gene products that are essential only under particular cultural conditions. Considerable ingenuity may be required to devise laboratory conditions that promote growth of mutants defective in a particular function and that allow selection of small numbers of these mutants from the large numbers of normal (wild-type) cells in the culture. A few general principles are described below.

Drug-resistant mutants

Mutations can be found that produce increased resistance to almost any antimicrobial agent and these can be readily isolated in the laboratory since resistant mutants grow in the presence of drug concentrations that inhibit the growth of drug-sensitive cells. Study of such mutants is an essential step in understanding the modes of action of antibiotic agents and mechanisms of resistance to them.

Auxotrophic mutants

Many organisms can grow in simple defined culture media because they have the ability to synthesize all of their own essential metabolites; such cells are termed *prototrophic*. Mutants that have lost the ability to make a particular essential metabolite, such as an amino acid, are called auxotrophic mutants (*auxotrophs*). To select an auxotrophic mutant from a prototrophic population, colonies resulting from a large number of cells on a complex medium must be tested for the ability to grow on media with and without the specific metabolite of interest. A common short cut is to use the technique of *replica plating* to test simultaneously all the colonies from one plate. This is done with a circular pad of sterile velvet that is first pushed against the master plate of colonies. The velvet picks up an imprint of the original colonies which can then be used to inoculate several replica plates containing combinations of different metabolites. The ability of the original colonies to grow on the different sets of media can then be directly compared. Studies of auxotrophs with mutations affecting different enzymes in a biosynthetic pathway are very valuable in the elucidation of such pathways.

Metabolic mutants

Other commonly studied mutations affect enzymes involved in the fermentation of sugars and the breakdown of a variety of other substances in the bacterial environment. Mutations in some of these genes can be detected by growing the cells on special media which produce a distinctive colour in or around colonies producing the enzyme. For example, the production of β-galactosidase can be demonstrated on media containing lactose as the only sugar and an indicator such as neutral red. Colonies producing β-galactosidase turn red following the production of acid, whereas colonies of mutants unable to ferment lactose remain colourless.

The detailed function and regulation of processes in the bacterial cell can be analysed only by searching systematically for mutations that affect each separate step in a process. Many different types of regulation occur in the coordination of all the biochemical reactions that proceed inside a cell and the isolation of specific mutants is fundamental to their understanding.

GENE TRANSFER

A change in the genome of a bacterial cell may be due either to mutation in the cell's own DNA or result from the acquisition of additional DNA from an external source. DNA may be transferred between bacteria by three mechanisms: *transformation, conjugation* and *transduction*. Each of these mechanisms probably occurs at a low frequency in nature and has therefore probably been of value in bacterial evolution. It should, however, be noted that the acquisition by bacteria of new properties following gene transfer is significant, as with mutation, only if the new

genetic end-product is subject to favourable selection by the conditions under which the bacteria are growing.

Transformation

Most species of bacteria are unable to take-up exogenous DNA from the environment; indeed, most bacteria produce nucleases that recognize and break down foreign DNA. However, bacteria in some genera, notably pneumococci, *Haemophilus influenzae* and certain *Bacillus* species, have been shown to be capable of taking up DNA either extracted artificially or released by lysis from cells of another strain. Cells are 'competent' for transformation only under certain conditions of growth, usually in late log phase or, in *Bacillus* species, during sporulation. The classic experiments on transformation studied the genes of specific capsular polysaccharides specifying virulence in pneumococci. Griffith demonstrated in 1928 that live, avirulent, non-capsulate ('rough') cells derived from one capsular type (type 2) were transformed by mixing with killed virulent capsulate ('smooth') cells of a second type (type 1) in the peritoneal cavity of the mouse. The animals subsequently died of pneumococcal infection following the acquisition by the live type 2 cells of the gene for type 1 capsule production from the killed cells.

Bacterial geneticists have also developed treatments by means of which organisms can be made artificially competent. In the case of *Esch. coli* the treatment involves incubation at a low temperature (4°C) in the presence of calcium ions, followed by a short exposure to a temperature of 42°C. Several other factors, including other metal ions, also stimulate the process. The absolute requirement for calcium ions in producing competent cells of *Esch. coli* indicates that structural alterations in the cell wall, sufficient to allow the passage of DNA molecules, are probably taking place.

Once a piece of DNA has entered the cell by transformation, it has to become incorporated into the existing chromosome of the cell by a process of *recombination* in order to survive. This is a complex molecular process for which the transformed DNA must have been derived from a closely related strain, since pieces of DNA can normally recombine with the chromosome only when there is a high degree of nucleic acid similarity (*homology*).

Any gene may be transferred by transformation, as any fragment of a donor chromosome may be taken up by the recipient cells. However, a piece of DNA introduced into a cell by transformation will normally be relatively short, and will only contain a very small number of genes. For this reason transformation is only of limited use for studying the organization of genes in relation to one another (*genetic mapping* — see later).

Conjugation

Conjugation is a process in which one cell, the *donor* or male cell, makes contact with another, the *recipient* or female cell, and DNA is transferred directly from the donor into the recipient. Certain types of plasmids, known as *transfer factors* or *sex factors*, carry the genetic information necessary for conjugation to occur. Only cells that contain such a plasmid can act as donors; those lacking a sex factor act as recipients.

Transfer of DNA between cells by conjugation requires direct contact between the donor and the recipient cell. Plasmids capable of mediating conjugation carry genes coding for the production of a 1–2 μm-long protein appendage, termed a *pilus*, on the surface of the donor cell. The tip of the pilus attaches to the surface of a recipient cell and holds the two cells together. DNA can then pass into the recipient cell, but it is not absolutely certain whether transfer actually occurs through the pilus, or whether the pilus simply acts as a mechanism by which the donor and female cells can be drawn together. Different types of pilus are specified by different types of plasmid and can therefore be used as an aid to plasmid classification.

In the vast majority of cases, the only DNA which is transferred during the conjugation process is the sex factor (plasmid) which mediates the process. It is thought that one strand of the circular DNA of the sex factor is nicked open at a specific site and the free end is passed into the recipient cell. The DNA is replicated during transfer so that each cell receives a copy (Fig. 7.4). As donor ability is dependent upon having a copy of the sex factor, the recipient strain becomes converted into a donor, able to conjugate with further recipients and convert them in turn! In this way a sex factor may rapidly spread through a whole population of recipient cells; this process is sometimes described as infectious spread of a plasmid.

Mobilization of chromosomal genes

Many plasmids have the ability to act as sex factors and transfer themselves. Some plasmids also have the ability to mobilize the chromosomal genes of bacteria. The prototype plasmid of this type is the 'F factor' (fertility factor) of *Esch. coli*. The F factor is a sex factor that contains the basic genetic information for extrachromosomal existence and for self-transfer. Cells that contain the F plasmid free in the cytoplasm (*F⁺ cells*) have no unusual characteristics apart from the ability to produce F pili and to transfer F to *F⁻ cells* by conjugation. In a very small proportion of F⁺ cells, the F plasmid becomes inserted into the bacterial chromosome. Once inserted, the entire chromosome behaves like an enormous F plasmid, and hence chromosomal genes can be transferred in the normal sex factor manner to a recipient cell at a relatively high frequency. Cultures of cells in which F has inserted into the chromosome are consequently termed *high-frequency recombination (Hfr)* strains. One important difference is that the chromosome tends to break randomly during the longer time period required for complete transfer. Only the very rare recipient cell that receives the whole chromosome, complete with the entire integrated F plasmid, will also become F⁺.

There is an additional mechanism by which chromosomal genes may be mobilized by conjugation to a recipient cell. In any culture of Hfr cells there are a few in which the F plasmid has excised itself from the chromosome and reverted to the free state. F is not always excised accurately and occasionally an F plasmid is excised together

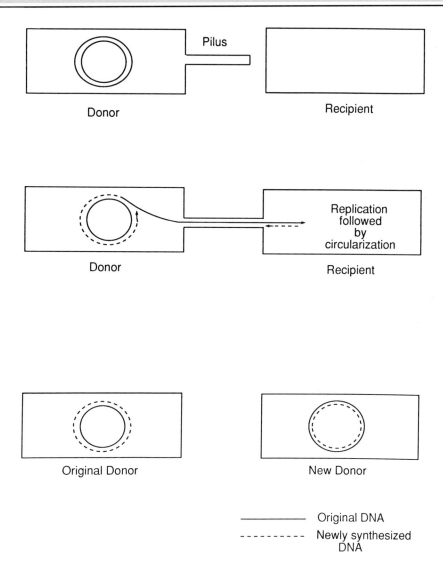

Fig. 7.4 Schematic representation of the process of plasmid transfer. Transfer of a single DNA strand is followed by replication and circularization in the recipient cell. Simultaneous replication of the remaining strand in the donor cell also occurs. Note that for simplicity the bacterial chromosome is not shown in this representation.

with some of the neighbouring chromosomal genes. An F plasmid that has picked up a small portion of the chromosome in this way is known as an *F-prime* (F'). A well-known example is the F-*lac* plasmid, which is an F' carrying the genes of the *Esch. coli* lactose operon. When an F' transfers itself into a recipient cell, its associated genes function normally on the plasmid in the new host. Thus non-lactose-fermenting organisms become lactose fermenters when they receive

F-*lac*. When F-*lac* is transferred into *Esch. coli*, the cells become diploid for the *lac* genes. The particular value of this partial diploidy is that it allows the study of interactions between different *lac* operon mutations within the same cell. This led to the discovery of the mechanisms of control for inducible enzymes described earlier. It is important to emphasize that the F plasmid system is confined to *Esch. coli* and other closely related enteric bacteria. Many other plasmids are capable of mediating conjugation, and sometimes chromosome mobilization, not only in *Esch. coli*, but also in other bacteria. For example, plasmid RP4 and its relatives have been used to mediate conjugation in a wide range of Gram-negative bacteria, while more recently there have been reports of conjugation systems in Gram-positive bacteria, such as *Enterococcus faecalis*, and several *Streptomyces* species. Although most conjugation systems in bacteria that have been elucidated have been shown to be plasmid-determined, many plasmids have transfer systems unrelated to that of the F plasmid. The extent to which unrelated systems share common conjugation mechanisms is unknown.

Transduction

The third known mechanism of gene transfer in bacteria involves the transfer of DNA between cells by bacteriophages. Most bacteriophages carry their genetic information (the phage genome) as a length of double-stranded DNA coiled up inside a protein coat. Other phages are known in which the phage genome consists of single-stranded DNA or RNA but, as far as is known, transducing phages all contain double-stranded DNA. Two major types of transduction are known to occur in bacteria: *generalized* transduction and *specialized* transduction.

Generalized transduction

When bacteriophages multiply inside an infected bacterial cell, each phage head is normally filled with a copy of the replicated phage genome. However, with certain types of phage a new phage particle is formed, at a frequency of about 1 in 10^6, which accidentally contains a length of bacterial chromosome DNA instead of phage DNA. When such a phage particle subsequently infects a second bacterial cell, the DNA that enters the cell is a short segment of chromosome from the original host. Bacterial genes have been *transduced* by the phage into the second cell. Since phages of this type pick up any portion of the bacterial chromosome entirely at random, they can transduce any chromosomal gene at approximately the same frequency, and are termed *generalized transducing phages*. Genes can be transduced only between fairly closely related strains as particular phages usually only attack a limited range of bacteria. As well as chromosomal genes, generalized transducing bacteriophages may also pick up and transfer plasmid DNA. As an example, the penicillinase gene in staphylococci is usually located on a plasmid and it may be transferred into other staphylococcal strains by transduction.

Specialized transduction

Bacteriophages that lyse the host cell are known as *virulent* phages and are said to produce a lytic cycle of infection. In contrast, *temperate* phages are able to infect a cell without necessarily causing immediate cell lysis and death. The surviving bacterial cell (carrying a copy of the bacteriophage genome) is termed a *lysogen*. The cells are said to be *lysogenic* and the latent phage is called a *prophage*.

The molecular mechanism by which lysogens are formed has been intensively studied with λ-phage of *Esch. coli*. The λ-phage DNA is linear inside the phage protein coat, but after it enters the bacterial cell the two ends are joined to form a circle. Usually the DNA is then replicated as the phage follows the normal lytic cycle resulting in the death of a cell. However, in a small proportion of infected cells the multiplication of the phage DNA is repressed by a mechanism similar to that involved in the regulation of the *lac* operon of *Esch. coli*. The phage DNA codes for the production of a specific repressor molecule that can attach to the phage DNA and switch off transcription of other genes that are essential for normal multiplication. Under these conditions the phage DNA can insert into the host cell DNA and is then stably replicated as part of the host cell chromosome. This is a symbiotic relationship in which the integrated phage DNA imparts *immunity* to the lysogenized cell against superinfection by genetically related phages, as well as certain unrelated phages.

The lysogenic state is stable but not permanent. The prophage may become excised from the chromosome by a process that is the reverse of integration: phage proteins are produced, the phage DNA is replicated and the cell is lysed in the normal way. This process of phage *induction* occurs spontaneously at low frequency (10^{-2} to 10^{-5} per cell per generation), but the frequency can be increased artificially, e.g. using ultraviolet light.

Following induction, excision of prophage is usually exact. However, occasionally the prophage picks up DNA adjacent to the phage integration site (Fig. 7.5). Since the phage protein coat can contain only a fixed amount of DNA, a transducing phage that contains a few bacterial genes at one end of its DNA often lacks a few phage genes at the other end. When the defective phage genome is transduced into a second cell, the phage can still integrate into its normal site on the chromosome, but is unable to replicate normally and lyse the cell. The result is that the added piece of bacterial DNA is transduced to the chromosome of the new host cell by the defective phage DNA. Since a temperate phage normally has a specific insertion site on the chromosome, it can pick up and transduce only a short length of DNA containing a few genes on either side of this site. The process is therefore termed *specialized* or *restricted transduction*.

Lysogenic conversion

The presence of prophage DNA constitutes a genetic alteration to the host cell. Usually only the phage repressor gene is expressed, but in certain cases it can be demonstrated that other genes are also expressed by the host cell. For example, *Corynebacterium diphtheriae* only produces diphtheria toxin when it is lysogenized by β phage; the toxin is specified by one of the phage genes. This process is termed *lysogenic conversion*. It is probable that the production of many toxins by staphylococci, streptococci and clostridia is also dependent upon lysogenic conversion by specific bacteriophages. In such cases, lysogenic conversion not only gives the cell superinfection immunity, but also actively influences the virulence of the bacterium for man.

GENETIC MAPPING

The location of genes with reference to each other and to their respective control regions by mapping techniques is an essential part of genetic analysis and requires the transfer of genetic material between different mutants by the mechanisms described in the previous sections. By far the most extensive genetic map available is that

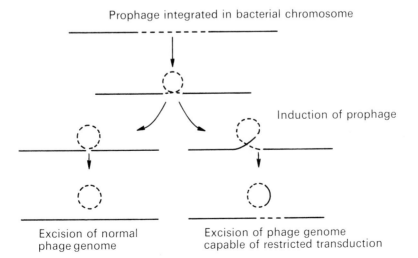

Prophage integrated in bacterial chromosome

Induction of prophage

Excision of normal phage genome

Excision of phage genome capable of restricted transduction

Fig. 7.5   Restricted transduction.

of *Esch. coli* K12. It is now a relatively simple matter to map an 'unknown' gene on the chromosome of *Esch. coli* K12, but is much more difficult for less intensively studied genera.

The first step involves a procedure termed *interrupted mating*. The bacterial chromosome of an Hfr strain is transferred at a uniform rate to the recipient cell; the origin of transfer depends upon the position on the chromosome at which the F plasmid integrated, but all cells of a particular Hfr strain have F integrated at the same site. Approximately 100 min (at 37°C) are required to transfer the entire chromosome. When Hfr donor cells conjugate with F⁻ recipient cells, the recipients acquire the donor chromosome genes in the order in which they occur on the chromosome. Mating cells can be broken apart mechanically by vigorous shaking, so that the piece of DNA that is being transferred is broken. If conjugation is interrupted at different times the order of the genes in the donor cell determines the time that each gene first becomes detectable in the recipient.

Different Hfr strains can have the F factor inserted at different sites. During conjugation, the genes are in the same order on the circular chromosome, but transfer starts at different points and may proceed in either direction. As shown in Fig. 7.6, one Hfr strain may transfer genes in the order *ABCDE* . . . while another transfers *PQRST* . . . and a third transfers *JIHGF* . . . . In this way an unknown mutation can be rapidly mapped within known segments of the bacterial chromosome.

Mapping by interrupted mating is not particularly accurate, and serves chiefly as a means to locate the approximate position of an unknown gene on the bacterial chromosome. Once this has been done, *fine-structure mapping* can be carried out by generalized transduction.

In *Esch. coli*, the generalized transducing bacteriophage P1 packages random fragments of chromosomal DNA following infection. Only about 91.5 kb of DNA can be contained within the phage, which means that only closely linked genes can be transferred together in a single transducing particle. Moreover, there is an inverse correlation between the frequency at which two

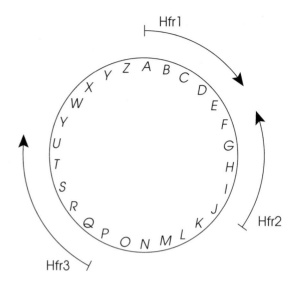

Fig. 7.6 Chromosome mapping by the use of Hfr strains. Circular chromosome of *Escherichia coli* with hypothetical genes *A–Z*. Different Hfr strains (1, 2, 3, ...) have the F factor integrated at different sites and transfer the chromosome into the recipient from different starting points. Different Hfr strains may transfer the genes in different directions.

markers are transduced together and genetic distance. A mathematical formula allows co-transduction frequency to be converted to separation distances expressed in minutes of genetic map. Mapping by P1 transduction allows rapid ordering of genes that are located closely together and can, in certain instances, allow the ordering of different mutations *within* a single gene.

Recent advances in molecular biology mean that particular genes can be isolated, cloned and their complete nucleotide sequences determined. It is therefore now possible to elucidate the relationship between gene structure and function in the cell at the most fundamental molecular level.

PLASMIDS

Properties encoded by plasmids

Plasmids are circular extrachromosomal genetic elements that may encode a variety of supplementary genetic information, including the information for self-transfer to other cells by conjugation. Not all plasmids can transfer themselves: the *non-conjugative* class of plasmids encodes neither donor pili nor transfer. They can, however, be *mobilized* by other conjugative plasmids present in the same donor cell. Apart from this optional transfer ability, all bacterial plasmids contain the basic genetic information necessary for self-replication and segregation into daughter cells at cell division. Plasmids seem to be ubiquitous in bacteria; many encode genetic information for such properties as resistance to antibiotics, bacteriocin production, resistance to toxic metal ions, enterotoxin production, enhanced pathogenicity, reduced sensitivity to mutagens, or the ability to degrade complex organic molecules.

Plasmid classification

Because of the vast range of plasmids, it is necessary to have a means of classification so that their distribution and epidemiology can be studied.

Plasmids can initially be grouped according to the properties which they encode, but other methods are needed in order to study their spread and distribution. These methods can be conveniently subdivided into physical and genetic methods.

Physical methods

Since all plasmids are relatively small structures that are normally separate from the bacterial cell chromosome, it is possible to isolate them from the chromosome by physical techniques. Centrifugation and electrophoresis techniques allow the sizes of different plasmids to be directly compared. Plasmids of similar size which confer identical phenotypes on the host cells may, however, be totally unrelated from a molecular viewpoint. Such relationships can be examined by generating *restriction endonuclease fingerprints* from purified plasmid DNA. A restriction endonuclease is an enzyme which breaks the DNA molecule at, or near to, a specific nucleotide sequence to produce discrete DNA fragments which can be separated by gel electrophoresis. The pattern ('fingerprint') of fragments produced is dependent on the

distribution of the specific DNA sequences recognized by the enzyme. Closely related plasmids will produce the same, or very similar, fingerprints, while unrelated plasmids will produce different fingerprints (Fig. 7.7). Restriction endonucleases of different specificities may be needed to generate distinctive fingerprints.

Genetic methods

An initial genetic test will distinguish groups of plasmids which are self-transmissible from those that are not. Linked with the question of transferability is the question of host range: some groups can be transferred only between members of the enterobacteria, others can be transferred from the enteric bacteria to the *Pseudomonas* family, while others can be transferred between almost any Gram-negative bacteria. Similar host range relationships exist amongst plasmids of Gram-positive bacteria.

Once a plasmid's host range has been determined, plasmids may be classified by *incompati-*

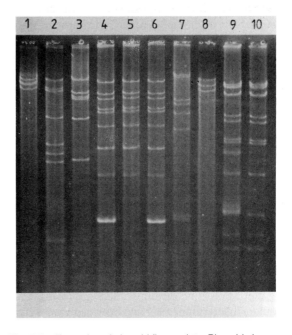

Fig. 7.7 Examples of plasmid fingerprints. Plasmids in tracks **4**, **5** and **6** are closely related to each other. Similarly, plasmids in tracks **9** and **10** are closely related. Plasmids in the other tracks appear to be unrelated.

bility testing. This method relies on the fact that closely related plasmids are unable to coexist stably in the same bacterial cell. Plasmids which are sufficiently closely related to interfere with each other's replication in this manner are said to be *incompatible* and to belong to the same *incompatibility group*. In contrast, unrelated plasmids *can* coexist stably and are therefore said to belong to different incompatibility groups.

If the introduction of an unknown plasmid into a host that contains a plasmid of *known* incompatibility group results in the elimination of the resident plasmid, this is evidence that they are incompatible; the unknown plasmid belongs to the same group as the known plasmid.

For reproducible results, plasmids must be classified by incompatibility in one chosen host since incompatibility relationships may differ in different hosts. The most widely used classification system for plasmids from Gram-negative bacteria depends on experiments with *Esch. coli* K12, into which plasmids from naturally occurring strains of many Gram-negative genera can be transferred by conjugation. However, most plasmids from Gram-positive genera such as *Streptococcus* and *Staphylococcus*, and some of those in Gram-negative genera such as *Pseudomonas*, *Proteus* and *Serratia*, are not transferable to *Esch. coli* K12 and cannot be included in this scheme. Even so, about 20 incompatibility groups have been identified in *Esch. coli* K12.

Examination of incompatibility relationships of plasmids in other host genera has also been used as a method of classification of plasmids that do not transfer readily to *Esch. coli*. About nine different incompatibility groups have been identified in *Pseudomonas aeruginosa*, but other systems are less advanced.

A final method for plasmid classification involves the use of specific virulent bacteriophages. All members of the same plasmid incompatibility group produce the same type of pilus for conjugation. For some incompatibility groups, specific virulent bacteriophages have been isolated which will only adhere to the type of pilus produced by that particular group of plasmids. Lysis by such a phage shows that a particular type of pilus is being produced, which in turn allows the identi-

fication of the group to which the plasmid contained in the cell belongs.

Plasmid epidemiology and distribution

Some plasmid groups have been identified in many different countries of the world, while others have so far been found only in a single bacterial species isolated from a solitary ecological niche. There seem to be two major ways in which plasmids spread: (i) by direct transfer from one bacterium to another in a particular micro-environment; (ii) by being carried in a particular host from one environment, e.g. a hospital, to another. The epidemiological tracing of these pathways requires identification not just of the plasmids involved, but also of their host bacterial strains.

THE GENETIC BASIS OF ANTIBIOTIC RESISTANCE

All of the properties of a micro-organism are ultimately determined by genes that can be either located on the chromosome or on plasmids. With regard to antibiotic resistance it is important to distinguish between *intrinsic* and *acquired* resistance. Intrinsic resistance is dependent upon the natural insusceptibility of an organism. In contrast, acquired resistance involves changes in the DNA content of a cell, such that the cell acquires a phenotype (i.e. antibiotic resistance) which is not inherent in that particular species.

Intrinsic resistance

Organisms that are naturally insensitive to a particular drug will always exist. The most obvious determinant of bacterial response to an antibiotic is the presence or absence of the target for the drug's action. Thus polyene antibiotics such as amphotericin B kill fungi by binding tightly to the sterols in the fungal cell membrane and altering the permeability of the fungal cell. Since bacterial membranes do not contain sterols they are intrinsically resistant to this class of antibiotics. Similarly, the presence of a permeability barrier provided by the cell envelopes of Gram-negative bacteria is important in determining sensitivity patterns to many antibiotics. Intrinsic resistance is usually predictable in a clinical situation and should not pose problems provided that an informed and judicious choice is made of appropriate antimicrobial therapy.

Acquired resistance

A problem of chemotherapy has been the appearance of resistance to particular drugs in a normally sensitive microbial population. An organism may lose its sensitivity to an antibiotic during a course of treatment. In some cases the loss of sensitivity may be slight, but often organisms become resistant to clinically achievable concentrations of a drug. Once resistance has appeared, the continuing presence of an antibiotic exerts a *selective pressure* in favour of the resistant organisms. Three main factors affect the frequency of acquired resistance: the amount of antibiotic which is being used; the frequency with which bacteria can undergo spontaneous mutations to resistance; and the prevalence of plasmids able to transfer resistance from one bacterium to another.

Chromosomal mutations

Random spontaneous mutations continuously occur at a low frequency in all bacterial populations and some mutations may confer resistance to a particular antibiotic. The rate at which these mutations occur is not influenced by the antibiotic, but in the presence of the drug the resistant mutant can survive, grow and eventually become the predominant, or only, member of the population. The degree of resistance conferred by chromosomal mutation depends upon the biological consequences of the mutation. With *single large-step mutations* the drug target is altered by mutation so that it is totally unable to bind a drug, although it can still carry out its normal biological function sufficiently well to permit the continued survival of the cell. This type of mutation occurs with streptomycin, but is otherwise not very common clinically. More commonly, the target is altered so that it can no longer bind a drug as efficiently, although it still has some resi-

dual affinity. In such a case a higher concentration of antibiotic would be required to produce the same antimicrobial effect: the *minimum inhibitory concentration* (MIC) of the antibiotic for the organism would be increased. Once a slightly resistant organism has been produced, additional mutational events — each conferring an additional small degree of resistance — can eventually lead to the production of organisms that are highly resistant to antibiotic. This is called the *multistep* pattern of resistance. Spontaneous chromosomal mutation is of clinical importance in tuberculosis in which mutants resistant to any single drug, e.g. streptomycin, rifampicin or isoniazid, are likely to be present in the patient before the start of treatment. If only one drug is given to the patient, the few resistant mutant bacteria may multiply and eventually cause a relapse of the disease. Combined therapy with several drugs to which the organism is sensitive is used in the treatment of tuberculosis, so that each drug kills the few mutants that are resistant to the other. The frequency with which double or triple mutations occur spontaneously in the same cell is so low as to be clinically insignificant.

There are many other examples of chromosomal mutations to antibiotic resistance which have assumed clinical importance. Mutations in the genes controlling the production of chromosomally encoded β-lactamases in Gram-negative bacteria can result in overproduction of these enzymes and consequent resistance to the cephalosporin antibiotics normally regarded as stable to β-lactamase.

Chromosomal mutations leading to antibiotic resistance are in many cases just as important clinically as the types of transferable resistance described in the next section.

Transferable antibiotic resistance

Of the three modes of gene transfer in bacteria, it is plasmid-mediated conjugation which is of greatest significance in terms of drug resistance. Plasmids conferring resistance to one or more unrelated groups of antibiotics (R plasmids) can be rapidly transferred by conjugation throughout the population.

R plasmids were first demonstrated in Japan in 1959 when it was shown that resistance to several antibiotics could be transferred by conjugation between strains of *Shigella* and *Esch. coli*. Many surveys since then in all parts of the world have shown that R plasmids are common and widespread.

The way in which R plasmids are built up in vivo probably varies from case to case, but it is clear that simple transfer factors can pick up resistance genes and combine with non-transmissible resistance plasmids to produce complex transmissible R plasmids that encode resistance to as many as eight or more different antimicrobial drugs. This process of plasmid evolution is considerably accelerated by genetic elements termed *transposons*, which are linear pieces of DNA, often including genes for antibiotic resistance that can migrate between unrelated plasmids and/or the bacterial chromosome independently of the normal bacterial recombination processes. R plasmids can transfer themselves into a wide range of commensal and pathogenic bacteria. Once resistance to antibiotic appears in any one of these species, the process of *transposition* assists the dissemination of the responsible gene between different R plasmids and subsequent distribution to other bacterial species.

As the prevalence of multiple-resistance R plasmids continues to increase, infections caused by a wide range of pathogens become more difficult to treat. For example, the appearance of R plasmids conferring resistance to chloramphenicol (and other antibiotics) in 1972 was followed by epidemics of chloramphenicol-resistant typhoid fever in Mexico and Asia which have proved difficult to control. Similar problems have been encountered with cholera, bacillary dysentery and *Esch. coli* enteritis in infants. Some opportunist pathogens have acquired multiple-resistance R plasmids and these plasmids can also carry genes that confer increased virulence on a bacterial cell. Thus, use of antibiotics may select for bacteria carrying plasmids that confer not only multiple drug resistance but also increased pathogenicity.

Control of antibiotic resistance

The major cause of the spread of genes conferring antibiotic resistance is the selection pressure brought about by the increased, and often indiscriminate, use of antibiotics in man and animals. Plasmid-encoded drug resistance is increased by the widespread use of antibiotics in animal husbandry, where antibiotics are used as animal feed supplements, and whole animal populations may be treated rather than an individual patient as occurs in medical practice. When R plasmids are present, the mass use of antibiotics fails to prevent the spread of resistance and selects R plasmids in the gut flora of the whole population of animals. Such R plasmids, evolved in farm animals, can spread to human commensal *Esch. coli*, followed by transfer to more important human pathogens.

It is important to minimize the use of antibiotics as much as possible and to reduce the chance of cross-infection. Rational use of antibiotics and sensible restriction of their availability in man and animals could prevent further spread of R plasmids and perhaps reduce their incidence. Some R plasmids are unstable and tend to lose resistance genes when the selection pressure is removed. R plasmids are also lost spontaneously from a small proportion of cells in a culture since plasmid replication and segregation are not always precisely synchronous with chromosome replication and segregation. Cells that lose an R plasmid may have a slight metabolic advantage and may slowly outgrow drug-resistant organisms. Moreover, R plasmids that evolve in one species may be unstable in another or may transfer themselves to other organisms much less efficiently. Similarly, organisms that are adapted to the gut of a calf, pig or chicken may not be established readily in man. Such factors may help to contain the spread of R plasmids.

USE OF SPECIFIC GENE PROBES FOR DIAGNOSTIC TESTS

Every properly classified species must, by definition, have somewhere on its chromosome a unique DNA sequence that distinguishes it from every other species. If this sequence can be identified and isolated, a chemical label can then be attached so that the DNA sequence can be used as a probe in hybridization reactions. Hybridization is the process in which two single strands of nucleic acid come together to form a stable double-stranded molecule. As long as the sequence of bases is complementary on each strand, the two strands will bind and stay together. Labelled DNA probes that are specific for particular pathogens can be used to recognize pathogen-specific DNA released from clinical samples. It is not necessary for the infecting pathogen to be initially isolated and DNA probes can conse-

quently be used to detect pathogens that cannot easily be cultured in vitro.

DNA probes have already been used successfully to identify a wide variety of pathogens, from simple RNA-containing polioviruses to pathogenic bacteria and parasites. Probes have also been developed which can recognize specific antibiotic resistance genes, offering the potential for the antimicrobial susceptibility of an infecting organism to be determined directly without primary isolation and growth. Commercial kits incorporating DNA probes for diagnostic use are now becoming available and the future looks increasingly promising for this new technology.

RECOMMENDED READING

Broda P 1979 *Plasmids*. Freeman, San Francisco

Bryan L E (ed) 1984 *Antimicrobial Drug Resistance*. Academic Press, New York

Glass R E 1982 *Gene Function*: E. coli *and its Heritable Elements*. Croom Helm, London

Schleif R 1986 *Genetics and Molecular Biology*. Addison Wesley, Reading, Mass

Stent G S, Calendar R 1978 *Molecular Genetics: An Introductory Narrative*, 2nd edn. Freeman, San Francisco

Stuttard C, Rozee K R (eds) 1980 *Plasmids and Transposons: Environmental Effects and Maintenance Mechanisms*. Academic Press, New York

Tenover F C 1988 Diagnostic deoxyribonucleic acid probes for infectious diseases. *Clinical Microbiology Reviews* 1: 82–101

8

Bacterial pathogenicity

A. Cockayne and J. P. Arbuthnott

Pathogenicity, or the capacity to initiate disease, is a relatively rare quality among microbes. It requires the attributes of *transmissibility* or communicability from one host or reservoir to a fresh host, *infectivity* or the ability to breach the new host's defences, and *virulence*, a variable that is multifactorial and denotes a pathogen's capacity to harm the host. Virulence in the clinical sense is a manifestation of a complex parasite-host relationship in which the capacity of the organism to cause disease is considered in relation to the resistance of the host.

TYPES OF BACTERIAL PATHOGEN

Bacterial pathogens can be classified into two broad groups, *opportunists* and *primary pathogens*.

Opportunistic pathogens

These rarely cause disease in individuals with intact immunological and anatomical defences. Only when such defences are impaired or compromised, as a result of congenital disease or by the use of immunosuppressive therapy or surgical techniques, are these bacteria able to cause disease. Many opportunistic pathogens, e.g. coagulase-negative staphylococci and *Escherichia coli* are part of the normal human flora and are carried on the skin or mucosal surfaces where they cause no harm and may actually have a beneficial effect by preventing colonization by other potential pathogens. However, introduction of these organisms into anatomical sites in which they are not normally found, or removal of competing bacteria by the use of broad-spectrum antibiotics, may allow their localized multiplication and subsequent development of disease.

Primary pathogens

These are capable of establishing infection and causing disease in previously healthy individuals with intact immunological defences. However, these bacteria may more readily cause disease in individuals with impaired defences.

VIRULENCE DETERMINANTS

Both opportunistic and primary pathogens possess *virulence determinants* or *aggressins* that facilitate pathogenesis. Possession of a single virulence determinant is rarely sufficient to allow the initiation of infection and production of pathology. Many bacteria possess several virulence determinants, all of which play some part at various stages of the disease process. In addition, not all strains of a particular bacterial species are equally pathogenic. For example, although six separate serotypes of encapsulated *Haemophilus influenzae* are recognized, serious infection is almost exclusively associated with isolates of serotype b. Moreover, even within serotype b isolates, 80% of serious infections are caused by six out of over 100 clonal types.

Different strains of a pathogenic species may cause distinct types of infection, each associated with possession of a particular complement of virulence determinants. Different strains of *Esch.*

coli, for example, cause several distinct gastro-intestinal diseases, urinary tract infections, septicaemia, meningitis and a range of other minor infections (see Chapter 27).

Expression of virulence determinants in vivo

Many pathogens produce an impressive armoury of virulence determinants in vitro. However, relatively early in the study of pathogenesis, it was appreciated that a knowledge of the behaviour of the pathogen in vivo is crucial to an understanding of virulence.

Comparisons in animal models of the virulence of naturally occurring variants differing in the expression of a particular determinant provided much useful information, but the possibility that observed differences in virulence were due to additional cryptic phenotypic or genotypic variations could not always be excluded. More recently, molecular techniques have been used to construct *isogenic* variants of bacteria that differ only in the particular determinant of interest and these constructs have allowed more detailed analysis of the role of such components in pathogenesis.

Molecular studies have also allowed the genetic basis of virulence and the mechanisms of transmission of virulence determinants to be investigated. Virulence determinants encoded by genomic DNA sequences, plasmids, bacteriophage and transposons have been reported.

Genetic studies have shown that expression of several different virulence determinants in a single bacterium are sometimes regulated in a co-ordinated fashion—possibly in response to environmental stimuli. Such a mechanism is of value to pathogens that can exist outside the mammalian host where expression of virulence determinants is unnecessary and energetically wasteful. Since bacterial pathogens grown in laboratory media express different phenotypes to those grown in animals it is important to study virulence determinants in vivo whenever possible.

Establishment of infection

Potential pathogens may enter the body by a variety of routes including the respiratory, gastro-intestinal, urinary or genital tracts. Alternatively, pathogens may directly enter tissues through insect bites or by accidental or surgical trauma to the skin. Since many opportunistic pathogens are carried as part of the normal human flora, this acts as a ready source of infection in the compromised host. For many primary pathogens, however, transmission to a new host and establishment of infection are more complex processes. Transmission of respiratory pathogens, such as *Bordetella pertussis*, may require direct contact with infectious material since the organism cannot survive for any length of time in the environment. Sexually transmitted pathogens such as *Neisseria gonorrhoeae* and *Treponema pallidum* have evolved further along this route and require direct person-to-person mucosal contact for transmission. Man is the only natural host for these pathogens, which die rapidly in the environment. The source of infection may be individuals with clinical disease or subclinically infected *carriers*, in whom symptoms may be absent or relatively mild either because the disease process is at an early stage or because of partial immunity to the pathogen.

In contrast, for many gastro-intestinal pathogens such as *Salmonella*, *Shigella* and *Campylobacter* species the primary source is environmental and infection follows ingestion of contaminated food or water. Many of these organisms also infect other animals, often without harmful effect, and these act as a *reservoir of infection* and source of environmental contamination.

Once entry into the host is effected, many bacterial pathogens, particularly those that infect mucosal surfaces, attach to host cells. This allows the establishment of a focus of infection that may remain localized or may subsequently spread to other tissues. To survive at these sites the organism must be able to:

1. Multiply by acquisition of nutrients from the host
2. Resist host defence mechanisms designed to combat infection.

Successful multiplication may be accompanied by the secretion of bacterial products that directly or indirectly damage tissues, resulting in the pathology associated with the disease.

Table 8.1 Examples of pili produced by Gram-negative pathogens

Designation	Bacterium	Gene location
Common (type 1)[a]	Enterobacteriaceae Uropathogenic *Escherichia coli*	Chromosome
CFA I, CFA II (CS1, CS2, CS3) E8775 (CS4, CS5, CS6)	Enterotoxigenic *Esch. coli* from humans	Plasmid Unknown
K88 K99 F41	Enterotoxigenic *Esch. coli* from animals	Plasmid Plasmid Unknown
Pap-G, Prs-G P pili X-adhesins (S, M)	Uropathogenic *Esch. coli* Pyelonephritogenic *Esch. coli*	Unknown Chromosome Unknown
N-methylphenylalanine pili	*Pseudomonas, Neisseria, Moraxella, Bacteroides, Vibrio* species	Chromosome

See text for abbreviations and explanation.
[a]Mannose-sensitive pili.

Colonization

For many pathogenic bacteria, the initial interaction with host tissues occurs at a mucosal surface and colonization normally requires *adhesion* to the mucosal cell surface. Adhesion is necessary to avoid innate host defence mechanisms such as peristalsis in the gut and the flushing action of mucus, saliva and urine which remove non-adherent bacteria. For invasive bacteria, adhesion is an essential preliminary to penetration through tissues.

Adhesion involves surface interactions between specific *receptors* on the mammalian cell membrane (usually carbohydrates) and *ligands* (usually proteins) on the bacterial surface. Non-specific surface properties of the bacterium, including surface charge and hydrophobicity, also contribute to the initial stages of the adhesion process. Several different mechanisms of bacterial adherence have evolved, all utilizing specialized cell surface organelles or macromolecules, that help to overcome the natural forces of repulsion that exist between the pathogen and its target cell.

Pili

Examination of the surface of Gram-negative bacteria such as *Esch. coli* by electron microscopy reveals the presence of numerous thin, rigid rod-like structures called *fimbriae* (Latin—fibres or threads) or *pili* (Latin—hairs) that are easily distinguishable from the much thicker bacterial flagella (see Chapter 2). Fimbriae and pili are synonyms and the term pili will be used here.

Pili are involved in mediating attachment of bacteria to mammalian cell surfaces. Different strains or species of bacteria may produce different types of pili which can be identified on the basis of antigenic composition, morphology and receptor specificity (Table 8.1). A broad division can be made between those pili whose adherence in vitro is inhibited by D-mannose (*mannose-sensitive pili*) and those unaffected by this treatment (*mannose-insensitive pili*).

The antigenic composition of pili can be complex. For instance, two pilus antigens called colonization factor antigens (CFA) I and II have been detected in enteropathogenic *Esch. coli* strains. CFA II consists of three distinct pilus antigens designated as coli surface antigens (CS) 1, 2 and 3. Another *Esch. coli* strain, E8775, has been found to produce three other CS antigens, CS4, CS5 and CS6. Pyelonephritogenic *Esch. coli* isolates produce a group of adhesins called X-adhesins; two pili types designated S and M on the basis of receptor specificity have been identified in this group.

The evolutionary significance of such heterogeneity may be that the ability of an individual bacterium to express several different types of pili allows different target receptors to be used at different anatomical sites of the infected host. In vitro, production of pili is influenced by cultural conditions such as incubation temperature and medium composition, which may switch off pilus production or induce a phase change from one pilus type to another.

For some pili the association with infection is clear. Thus the K88 pilus antigen is clearly associated with the ability of *Esch. coli* K88 to cause diarrhoea in pigs; pigs lacking the appropriate intestinal receptors are spared the enterotoxigenic effects of *Esch. coli* strains of this type. In many other instances the association between pilus production and infection remains putative at present. Production of pili is controlled by either chromosomal or plasmid genes (Table 8.1). The structure of one of these pilus types—*type 1* or *common pilus*—has been studied in detail. These consist of aggregates of a structural protein subunit called *pilin* arranged in a regular helical array to produce a rigid rod-like structure of 7 nm diameter, with a central hole running along its length. A highly conserved minor protein, located at both the tip and at intervals along the length of the pilus, is thought to mediate specific adhesion. Type 1 pili bind specifically to D-mannose residues. Their role in vivo remains controversial; however they may be involved in the pathogenesis of urinary tract infections.

Other Gram-negative bacteria, including those of the genera *Pseudomonas*, *Neisseria*, *Bacteroides* and *Vibrio*, produce pili that share some homology, especially in the amino-terminal region of the pilin subunits (the so-called *N-methylphenylalanine pili*). These pili have been shown to act as virulence determinants for *Pseudomonas aeruginosa* and *Neisseria gonorrhoeae*.

Flagella

Flagella may play a role in the virulence of some bacterial pathogens. Bacterial motility is thought to be important in assisting penetration of the intestinal mucus during the initiation of infection by *Vibrio cholerae* and *Campylobacter jejuni*. In these organisms, the flagellum appears to play a double role as an organelle of motility and adhesion.

Non-pilus adhesins

Non-pilus adhesins include the filamentous haemagglutinin of *Bordetella pertussis*, a mannose-resistant haemagglutinin from *Salmonella typhimurium* and a fibrillar haemagglutinin from *Helicobacter pylori*.

Outer membrane proteins are involved in the adherence of *N. gonorrhoeae* and enteropathogenic *Esch. coli* to cell surfaces.

Exopolysaccharides present on the surface of some Gram-positive bacteria are also involved in adhesion. For example, *Streptococcus mutans*, which is involved in the pathogenesis of dental caries, synthesizes a homopolymer of glucose which anchors the bacterium to the tooth surface and contributes to the matrix of dental plaque. Coagulase-negative staphylococci also produce an exopolysaccharide slime which probably mediates adherence of the bacterium to prosthetic devices and catheters.

Binding to fibronectin

Fibronectin is a complex multifunctional glycoprotein found in plasma and associated with mucosal cell surfaces, where it promotes numerous adhesion functions. Many pathogenic bacteria bind fibronectin at the bacterial surface and for some organisms fibronectin has been shown to act as the cell surface receptor for bacterial adhesion. In *Streptococcus pyogenes*, lipoteichoic acid mediates attachment of the bacterium to the amino terminus of the fibronectin molecule. Attachment of *Staphylococcus aureus* to cell surfaces also involves the amino terminus of fibronectin, but the bacterial ligand appears to be protein in this instance. *Treponema pallidum* also binds fibronectin. The significance of the interaction with fibronectin in the pathogenesis of syphilis and many other bacterial diseases needs further clarification. It is likely that the binding to other connective tissue proteins such as collagen and laminin will prove to be an important colonization mechanism.

Invasion

Once attached to a mucosal surface, some bacteria exert their pathogenic effects without penetrating the tissues of the host: toxins or other aggressins mediate tissue damage at local or distant sites. For a number of pathogenic bacteria, however, adherence to the mucosal surface represents but the first stage of the invasion of tissues. Examples of organisms that are able to invade and survive within host cells include mycobacteria and those of the genera *Salmonella*, *Shigella*, *Escherichia*, *Yersinia*, *Legionella* and *Listeria*. Cell invasion confers the ability to avoid humoral host defence mechanisms and potentially provides a niche rich in nutrients and devoid of competition from other bacteria. However, survival of bacteria in professional phagocytes such as macrophages or polymorphonuclear leucocytes, depends on subverting intracellular killing mechanisms that would normally result in microbial destruction (see below).

Heat-shock proteins

In many intracellular bacteria, heat-shock proteins are involved in the infectious process. These are part of a larger family of stress-related proteins synthesized by bacteria in response to adverse environmental stimuli such as heat shock or oxidative stress, and they appear to be involved in the survival of the organism under such conditions. Heat-shock proteins homologous to those detected in bacteria have been found in higher organisms, including man; they may play a role in the induction of auto-immune phenomena such as arthritis following bacterial infections.

Uptake into host cells

The initial phase of cellular invasion involves penetration of the mammalian cell membrane and many intracellular pathogens use normal phagocytic entry mechanisms to gain access.

Shigellae invade colonic mucosal cells but rarely penetrate deeper into the host tissues. Inside the cell, bacteria are surrounded by a membrane-bound vesicle derived from the host cell. Soon after entry, this vesicle is lysed by the action of the plasmid-encoded haemolysin, and the bacterium is released into the cell cytoplasm. *Listeria monocytogenes* produces a heat-shock protein with a similar function termed *listeriolysin*. Once free in the cell cytoplasm, shigellae multiply rapidly with subsequent inhibition of host cell protein synthesis. Several hours later the host cell dies and bacteria spread to adjacent cells where the process of invasion is repeated.

In contrast to shigellae, most salmonellae proceed through the superficial layers of the gut and invade deeper tissues, in particular cells of the reticulo-endothelial system. Salmonellae also occupy a host-derived vesicle but this does not lyse. Instead, several vesicles coalesce to form large intracellular vacuoles. These vacuoles traverse the cytoplasm to reach the opposite side of the cell and initiate spread to adjacent cells and deeper tissues. For both *Salmonella* and *Shigella* species, bacterial protein and RNA synthesis are required for invasion.

Role of cell receptors

The availability of specific receptors defines the type of host cells that are involved. As a result some pathogens can invade a wide range of cell types whilst others have a much more restricted invasive potential. The receptors for some of the invasive pathogens have been identified. For example, *Legionella pneumophila* and *Mycobacterium tuberculosis* adhere to complement receptors on the surface of phagocytic cells. The receptor for *Yersinia pseudotuberculosis* belongs to a family of proteins termed *integrins* that form a network on the surface of host cells to which host proteins such as fibronectin can bind. Mimicry of the amino acid sequence (Arg-Gly-Asp) of fibronectin that mediates attachment to the integrins may represent a common mechanism of effecting intracellular entry.

The ability to utilize integrins may not be restricted to intracellular bacteria. The filamentous haemagglutinin of *Bord. pertussis* may use the fibronectin integrin to mediate attachment in the respiratory tract.

Avoidance of host defence mechanisms

Colonization by bacterial pathogens results in the induction of specific and non-specific humoral and cell-mediated immune responses designed to eradicate the organism from the site of infection. Products of the organism may be chemotactic for phagocytic cells which are attracted to the site. Moreover, complement components may directly damage the bacterium and release peptides chemotactic for phagocytic cells. Other humoral antibacterial factors include lysozyme and the iron chelators transferrin and lactoferrin. Lysozyme is active primarily against Gram-positive bacteria but potentiates the activity of complement against Gram-negative organisms. Transferrin and lactoferrin chelate iron in body fluids, and reduce the amount of free iron to levels below that necessary for bacterial growth.

Pathogenic bacteria have evolved ways of avoiding or neutralizing these highly efficient clearance systems. Since most of the interactions between the bacterium and the immune effectors involve the bacterial surface, resistance to these effects is related to the molecular architecture of the bacterial surface layers.

Capsules

Many bacterial pathogens need to avoid phagocytosis and production of an extracellular capsule is the most common mechanism by which this is achieved. Virtually all the pathogens associated with meningitis and pneumonia, including *H. influenzae*, *Neisseria meningitidis*, *Esch. coli* and *Streptococcus pneumoniae*, have capsules and noncapsulate variants usually exhibit much reduced virulence. Most capsules are polysaccharides composed of sugar monomers that vary among different bacteria. Polysaccharide capsules reduce the efficiency of phagocytosis in a number of ways:

1. In the absence of specific antibody to the bacterium, the hydrophilic nature of the capsule may hinder uptake by phagocytes, a process which occurs more readily at hydrophobic surfaces. This may be overcome if the phagocyte is able to trap the bacterium against a surface—a process referred to as *surface phagocytosis*.

2. Capsules prevent efficient opsonization of the bacterium by complement or specific antibody, events that promote interaction with phagocytic cells. Capsules may either prevent complement deposition completely or cause complement to be deposited at a distance from the bacterial membrane where it is unable to damage the organism.

3. Capsules tend to be weakly immunogenic and may mask more immunogenic surface components and reduce interactions with both complement and antibody.

Streptococcal M protein

The M protein present on the surface of *Str. pyogenes* is not a capsule but functions in a similar manner to prevent complement deposition at the bacterial surface. The M protein binds both fibrinogen and fibrin and deposition of this material on the streptococcal surface hinders the access of complement activated by the alternative pathway.

Resistance to killing by phagocytic cells

Some pathogens are readily ingested by macrophages and other phagocytes but are resistant to the intracellular killing mechanisms of these cells, and may actually multiply intracellularly. Included in this group are the invasive pathogens described above. The normal sequence of events following phagocytosis involves fusion of the *phagosome* in which the bacterium is contained with *lysosomal granules* present in the cell cytoplasm. These granules contain enzymes and cationic peptides involved in oxygen-dependent and oxygen-independent bacterial killing mechanisms (see Chapter 11).

Different organisms use different strategies for survival (Table 8.2). *M. tuberculosis* is thought to resist intracellular killing by preventing phagosome-lysosome fusion; other bacteria are able to resist the action of such lysosomal components following fusion. Some organisms stimulate a normal respiratory burst but are intrinsically resistant to the effects of the potentially toxic oxygen radicals produced. Production of catalase by *Staph. aureus*

Table 8.2 Some strategies adopted by bacteria to avoid intracellular killing

Species	Method
Mycobacterium tuberculosis	Prevents phagosome–lysosome fusion
Salmonella typhi *Yersinia enterocolitica*	Fail to stimulate O_2–dependent killing
Staphylococcus aureus *Neisseria gonorrhoeae*	Produce catalase to negate effect of toxic O_2 radicals
Legionella pneumophila	Inhibits phagolysosome acidification

and *N. gonorrhoeae* is thought to protect these organisms from such toxic products. The smooth lipopolysaccharide of many bacterial pathogens is also thought to contribute to their resistance to the effects of bactericidal cationic peptides present in the phagolysosome.

Antigenic variation

Variation in surface antigen composition during the course of infection provides a mechanism of avoidance of specific immune responses directed at those antigens. This strategy is most highly developed in blood-borne parasitic protozoa, such as trypanosomes, but is also exhibited by bacteria. *N. gonorrhoeae* shows antigenic variation in an outer-membrane protein known as PII and in its pili. Expression of individual PII proteins is controlled by frame shifts in the nucleotide sequence encoding the protein leader sequence, which varies as a result of recombination or mutation during DNA replication. Individual PII genes appear to be independently regulated such that there are many possible combinations of these proteins on a single organism.

Variation in the pilus is controlled by a different mechanism in *N. gonorrhoeae*. Usually only one complete pilin gene is expressed, though several incomplete 'silent' pilin gene sequences are present on the chromosome. Movement of the incomplete gene sequences to an expression locus results in synthesis of a pilin protein that may differ antigenically from that previously expressed. Alternatively, variant pilin gene DNA may be acquired from other gonococci by transformation to allow new pilin genes to be constructed by recombination at the expression site.

The borreliae that cause relapsing fever use a similar strategy to generate antigenic variation. Similar systems may operate in *Borrelia burgdorferi*, the causative agent of Lyme disease.

Group A streptococci produce up to 75 antigenically distinct serotypes of M protein.

The capacity for variation in surface antigens means that antibody produced in response to infection by one strain of a pathogen may not protect against subsequent challenge with a different strain of that bacterium. This makes development of vaccines based on inhibition of attachment or generation of opsonic antibody particularly difficult for these organisms.

IgA proteases

Several species of pathogenic bacteria that cause disease on mucosal surfaces produce a protease that specifically cleaves IgA, the principal antibody type produced at these sites. These proteases are specific for human IgA isotype I. Nearly all the pathogens causing meningitis, with the exception of *N. meningitidis*, possess an IgA protease and a polysaccharide capsule enabling them to persist on the mucosal surface and resist phagocytosis during the invasive phase of the disease.

Serum resistance

To survive in the bloodstream, bacteria must be able to resist lysis as a result of deposition of complement on the bacterial surface. In the Enterobacteriaceae, resistance is due to the composition of the lipopolysaccharide (LPS) present in the bacterial outer membrane. *Smooth* colonial variants which possess polysaccharide 'O' side chains in their LPS are more resistant than *rough* colonial variants that lack such side chains (see below). The side chains sterically hinder deposition of complement components on the bacterial surface. Conversely, however, some O chain polysaccharides activate complement by an alternate pathway leading to lysis of the bacterial cell. In *N. meningitidis* group B and *Esch. coli* K1, sialic acid capsules prevent efficient complement activation and, in *N.*

gonorrhoeae, complement binds but forms an aberrant configuration in the bacterial outer membrane so that it is unable to effect lysis.

Iron acquisition

The concentration of free iron in bodily secretions is extremely low because it is chelated by high-affinity mammalian iron-binding proteins such as transferrin and lactoferrin. In order to multiply in body fluids or on mucous membranes, bacteria must obtain iron and many Gram-negative pathogens have evolved very efficient mechanisms for scavenging iron from mammalian iron-binding proteins. Bacteria such as *Esch. coli* and *Klebsiella aerogenes* produce extracellular iron chelators called siderophores for this purpose. *N. meningitidis*, *Haemophilus parainfluenzae* and *H. influenzae* type b have specific receptors for transferrin and lactoferrin on their surfaces and are able to bind these proteins and their chelated iron directly from body fluids. The exact mechanism by which the iron is then made accessible to the bacterium is as yet poorly understood.

Two other mechanisms of iron acquisition from mammalian iron chelators have been described. Some *Bacteroides* species remove iron by proteolytic cleavage of the chelator. In *List. monocytogenes*, reduction of the Fe^{3+} ion to Fe^{2+} reduces the affinity for the chelator sufficiently for it to be removed by the bacterium.

Toxins

In many bacterial infections the characteristic pathology of the disease is caused by toxins. Toxins may exert their pathogenic effects directly on a target cell or may interact with cells of the immune system resulting in the release of immunological mediators that cause pathophysiological effects. Such effects may not always lead to the death of the target cell but may selectively impair specific functions. Substances that have toxic physiological effects on target cells in vitro do not necessarily exert the same effects in vivo, but a number of toxins have been shown to be responsible for the typical clinical features of bacterial disease.

Two major types of toxin have been described: *endotoxin*, which is a component of the outer membrane of Gram-negative bacteria, and *exotoxins*, which are produced extracellularly by both Gram-negative and Gram-positive bacteria.

Endotoxin

Endotoxin, or lipopolysaccharide (LPS), is a component of the outer membrane of Gram-negative bacteria and is released from the bacterial surface following natural lysis of the bacterium or by disintegration of the organism in vitro. LPS is anchored into the bacterial outer membrane through a unique molecule termed *lipid A* (Fig. 8.1). Covalently linked to lipid A is an eight-carbon sugar, ketodeoxyoctonate (KDO), in turn linked to the oligosaccharides which form the highly variable O antigen structures of Gram-negative bacteria. Bacteria carrying LPS containing O antigen form *smooth* colonies on bacteriological media in contrast to those lacking the O antigen, which form *rough* colonies.

The term *endotoxin* was originally introduced to describe the component of Gram-negative bacteria responsible for the pathophysiology of *endotoxic shock*, a syndrome with high mortality, particularly in immunocompromised or otherwise debilitated individuals. LPS activates complement via the alternative pathway, but most of the biological activity of LPS is attributable to lipid A. Both LPS and lipid A are potent activators of macrophages, resulting in the induction of a range of cytokines which are involved in the regulation of immune and inflammatory responses (see Chapter 11), and which may be partly responsible for many of the pathological changes seen in endotoxic shock.

Exotoxins

Exotoxins, in contrast to endotoxin, are diffusable polypeptides, secreted into the external medium by the pathogen. Some exotoxins can be partially denatured (e.g. by formaldehyde treatment) to generate toxoids which lack toxic activity but still induce protective immunity when used as vaccines. The molecular structure and mechanism of action

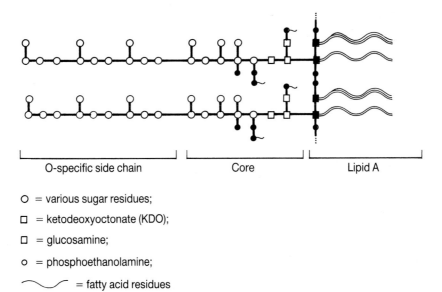

| O-specific side chain | Core | Lipid A |

O = various sugar residues;

□ = ketodeoxyoctonate (KDO);

□ = glucosamine;

o = phosphoethanolamine;

⌒ = fatty acid residues

Fig. 8.1 Diagrammatic representation of the structure of bacterial lipopolysaccharide. (Redrawn from: Reitschel E T, Galanos C, Lüderlitz O 1975 Structure, endotoxicity and immunogenicity of the lipid A component of bacterial lipopolysaccharide. In: Schlessinger D (ed), *Microbiology-1975*. American Society for Microbiology, Washington, pp. 307–314).

of many exotoxins have now been determined. Examples of exotoxins and their effects on target cells are shown in Table 8.3.

Enterotoxins cause symptoms of gastro-intestinal disease, including diarrhoea, dysentery or vomiting. In some cases the disease is caused by ingestion of preformed toxin in food but in the majority of cases colonization of the intestine prior to elaboration of toxin is required.

Cholera toxin and heat labile (LT) toxins of enterotoxigenic *Esch. coli* cause diarrhoea but do not induce inflammatory changes in the intestinal mucosa. These toxins act by perturbing the processes that regulate ion and water exchange across the intestinal epithelium (see Chapters 27 and 31).

In contrast, the enterotoxins of *Clostridium difficile*, *C. perfringens* type A and *Bacillus cereus* cause structural damage to epithelial cells resulting in inflammation. Other gastro-intestinal pathogens such as enteropathogenic *Esch. coli* mediate damage by ill-defined mechanisms, following close contact between the bacterium and the cell surface.

Toxins in respiratory infections

The involvement of exotoxins in the pathogenesis of many bacterial respiratory infections is unclear, but for *Bord. pertussis*—the causative agent of whooping cough—the involvement of toxins is more clear cut. This organism produces a large number of extracellular products, including a tracheal cytotoxin which inhibits the beating of cilia on tracheal epithelial cells, pertussis toxin, which exhibits several systemic effects, and an adenylate cyclase that interferes with phagocyte function (see Chapter 33).

Toxins acting on subepithelial tissues

Another group of toxins cause damage to subepithelial tissues following penetration and multiplication of the pathogen at the site of infection. Many of these toxins also inhibit or interfere with components of the host immune system. Membrane-damaging toxins such as staphylococcal α- and β-toxins, streptolysin O and streptolysin S

Table 8.3 Some effects of bacterial exotoxins

Toxic effect	Examples
Lethal action	
Effect on neuromuscular junction	*Clostridium botulinum* toxin A
Effect on voluntary muscle	Tetanus toxin
Damage to heart, lungs, kidneys, etc.	Diphtheria toxin
Pyrogenic effect	
Increase in body temperature	Exotoxins of *Staphylococcus aureus* and *Streptococcus pyogenes* Staphylococcal toxic shock syndrome toxin-1
Action on gastro-intestinal tract	
Secretion of water and electrolytes	Cholera and *Escherichia coli* enterotoxins
Pseudomembranous colitis	*Clostridium difficile* toxins A and B
Bacillary dysentery	Shigella toxin
Vomiting	*Staph. aureus* enterotoxins A-E
Action on skin	
Necrosis	Clostridial toxins; staphylococcal α-toxin
Erythema	Diphtheria toxin; streptococcal erythrogenic toxin
Permeability of skin capillaries	Cholera enterotoxin; *Esch. coli* heat labile toxin
Nikolsky sign[a]	*Staph. aureus* epidermolytic toxin
Cytolytic effects	
Lysis of blood cells	*Staph. aureus* α-, β- and δ-lysins, leucocidin Streptolysin O and S *Clostridium perfringens* α and θ toxins
Inhibition of metabolic activity	
Protein synthesis	Diphtheria toxin; shiga toxin

[a] Separation of epidermis from dermis.

and *C. perfringens* α *and* θ toxins inhibit leucocyte chemotaxis at subcytolytic concentrations, but cause necrosis and tissue damage at higher concentrations.

Systemic effects of toxins

Some toxins cause damage to internal organs following absorption from the focus of infection. Included in this category are the toxins causing diphtheria, tetanus and botulism and those associated with streptococcal scarlet fever and staphylococcal toxic shock syndrome. The diphtheria toxin, the gene for which is bacteriophage-encoded,

inhibits protein synthesis in mammalian cells. Tetanus toxin, in contrast, exerts its effect by preventing the release of inhibitory neurotransmitters whose function is to prevent overstimulation of motor neurones in the central nervous system, resulting in the convulsive muscle spasm characteristic of tetanus. Diphtheria and tetanus toxins represent the sole determinant of disease and are neutralized by specific antitoxin antibody. As a result, vaccination with diphtheria and tetanus toxoids is highly effective.

Botulism results from the ingestion of preformed toxin produced by *C. botulinum* in food contaminated with this bacterium and is not in reality an infectious disease. The toxic activity is due to a family of serologically distinct polypeptide neuro-toxins. These toxins prevent release of acetylcholine at neuromuscular junctions, resulting in the symptoms of flaccid paralysis.

Other toxins cause disseminated multisystem organ damage. This type of multisystem pathology is seen in staphylococcal *toxic shock syndrome* caused by certain strains of *Staph. aureus* that produce a toxin designated *toxic shock syndrome toxin 1* (TSST-1). This toxin belongs to a group of functionally related proteins collectively referred to as *superantigens*, which includes the staphylococcal enterotoxins, staphylococcal exfoliative toxin and streptococcal pyrogenic exotoxin A. These mole-cules are potent T cell mitogens whose reactivity with lymphocytes induces cytokine release, and may initiate tissue damage by mechanisms similar to those postulated to account for the pathology of Gram-negative endotoxic shock (see Chapter 14).

Other extracellular aggressins

Many bacteria secrete a range of enzymes that may be involved in the pathogenic processes.

Ureases are produced by several pathogenic bacteria. *Proteus* spp. and some other bacteria that cause urinary tract infections break down urea in the urine and the release of ammonia may con-tribute to the pathology. The urease produced by the gastric and duodenal pathogen *Helicobacter pylori* is similarly implicated in the virulence of the organism.

Proteases are produced by many bacteria. For example *L. pneumophila* produces a metalloprotease thought to contribute to the characteristic pathology seen in legionella pneumonia.

Many other degradative enzymes, including *mucinases, phospholipases, collagenases* and *hyaluroni-dases*, are produced by pathogenic bacteria. Many non-pathogenic bacteria also produce such enzymes and their role in pathogenesis requires further clarification.

Understanding of the basic mechanisms of pathogenesis is important for the identification of new or improved vaccines and for the design of appropriate therapies. The body of knowledge gained to date is also invaluable in the analysis of 'new' bacterial pathogens such as *L. pneumophila* and *B. burgdorferi* that are recognized from time to time. However, for a number of bacterial diseases, e.g. syphilis, such approaches have still not defined the mechanisms of pathogenesis or the virulence determinants involved and new strategies employed by such successful pathogens may yet be discovered.

RECOMMENDED READING

Finlay B B and Falkow S 1989 Common themes in microbial pathogenicity. *Microbiological Reviews* 53: 210-230
Inglewski B H and Clark L V (eds) 1990 *The Bacteria. Molecular Basis of Bacterial Pathogenesis.* Academic Press, London, vol XI
Mims C A 1987 *The Pathogenesis of Infectious Disease*, 3rd edn. Academic Press, London
Roth J A (ed) 1988 *Virulence Mechanisms of Bacterial Pathogens.* American Society for Microbiology, Washington, DC
Smith H 1989 The mounting interest in bacterial and viral pathogenicity. *Annual Review of Microbiology* 43: 1-22

9

Virus-cell interactions: antiviral agents

M. Norval

Viruses are totally dependent on the cells they infect to provide the energy, metabolic intermediates and most, if not all, of the enzymes required for their replication. With advances in the techniques of molecular virology, together with the classical methods of electron microscopy, titration and biochemical assay, it has become possible to study virus–cell interactions to a sophisticated level, in at least some instances. The picture that has emerged, and is still emerging, is a fascinating one as viruses affect cells in a variety of ways, some with unexpected consequences. Although an immense diversity of interactions exists, it is possible to make a division into three broad categories:

1. Viruses which infect and replicate within cells causing the cells to lyse when the progeny virions are released. This is called a *cytolytic cycle,* the infection is *productive* and the cell culture shows *cytopathic effects,* which are often characteristic of the infecting virus. The host cells are termed *permissive.* In a few instances viruses are produced from infected cells but the cells are not killed by the process, i.e. the infection is *productive* but *non-cytolytic,* and is termed *persistent.*

2. Viruses which infect cells but which do not complete the replication cycle. Thus the infection is called *abortive.* Abortive infection can be due to a mutation in the virus so that some essential function is lost, or to the production of defective interfering particles, or to the action of interferons. It is possible in some cases to manipulate the conditions to obtain a *steady-state* or *persistent infection* in which infected and uninfected cells coexist and there is some virus production.

3. Viruses which enter cells but are not produced by the infected cell; the virus is maintained within the cell in the form of DNA which replicates in association with the host cell DNA. The host cell is termed *non-permissive* and the infection is *non-productive.* Occasionally this type of interaction can result in the cell being 'transformed' to a malignant phenotype.

Each of the above categories will be considered in turn, and only animal viruses are included in this chapter.

THE LYTIC OR CYTOCIDAL GROWTH CYCLE

While there are large differences in the details of the lytic growth cycle depending on the virus studied and, to some extent, on the host cell, certain features are common and a simplified description will be given first. The quantitative aspects of virion production were determined initially using bacteriophage but have now been ascertained for many animal viruses growing in vitro in cell culture. A one-step growth curve is obtained when samples are removed from an infected cell culture at intervals and assayed for the total content of virus after artificial lysis of the cells (Fig. 9.1).

In the early part of the cycle, virus particles come into contact with the cells and may then

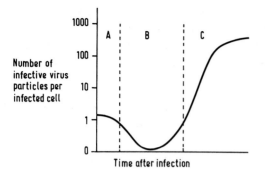

Fig. 9.1 Lytic growth cycle of a virus. Samples are removed from the infected culture at intervals and assayed for the total content of virus. Phase A, adsorption; phase B, eclipse; phase C, assembly and release.

acid replication and the later stages of replication. Viral nucleic acid is then synthesized followed by late mRNA transcription and translation. Most proteins made at this stage are structural ones and will be part of the final virion. There are always antigenic changes at the surface and elsewhere in the cell during these stages. The eclipse phase ends with the *assembly* and *release* of newly formed virus particles. The cycle is shown in diagrammatic form in Fig. 9.2. The whole replication cycle varies from as little as 8 h for some picornaviruses to more than 40 h for cytomegalovirus, a human herpesvirus. Some bacteriophages, in contrast, can go through one replication cycle in only 15 min.

Attachment (adsorption)

There is no known mechanism for bringing together a virus and a susceptible cell; the initial interaction is assumed to be by random collision and depends on the relative concentration of virus particles and susceptible cells. The ionic composition of the culture medium is an important factor as both viruses and cells are negatively charged at neutral pH and would tend to repel each other. The presence of cations, like Mg^{2+}, therefore helps to promote close contact. Adsorp-

attach or *adsorb* to them. This marks the start of the *eclipse phase*. The virion then *penetrates* into the host cell and is partially *uncoated* to reveal the viral genome. *Macromolecular synthesis* of viral components follows. This can often be divided into an *early* and a *late phase* separated by the replication of the viral nucleic acid. Early messenger RNA (mRNA) is first transcribed and translated into proteins. These are often non-structural proteins and enzymes required to undertake nucleic

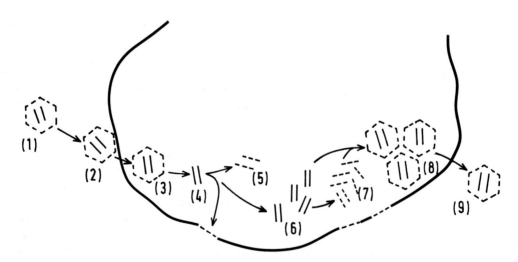

Fig. 9.2 A simplified viral replication cycle showing **1** a hypothetical virus particle, **2** attaching to the surface of a susceptible cell, **3** penetrating into the cell, **4** being uncoated, **5** undergoing early transcription and translation, then **6** replication of the viral nucleic acid, **7** late transcription and translation, and finally **8** assembly of new virus particles and **9** release from the cell.

tion then takes place through a specific binding site on the virus and a receptor on the plasma membrane of the cell. It is largely temperature- and energy-independent.

Viruses vary in the range of cells to which they can adsorb depending on the nature of the site they attach to and how widespread it is amongst cells of different types and from different species. Rabies virus binds to the acetylcholine receptor found on neural cells. Orthomyxo-and paramyxo-viruses have an envelope protein called haemag-glutinin protruding from the surface of the virion, which has a specific binding site for glycoproteins or glycolipids with oligosaccharide side chains terminating in *N*-acetylneuraminic acid (sialic acid). These are found on the membranes of most cells. The haemagglutinin is made up of trimers of two polypeptides, HA_1 and HA_2, and the binding site for sialic acid is located on the globular part of HA_1, which is furthest from the envelope of the virus. Poliovirus infects primate cells only, and only those from the central nervous system or the intestine. The receptor in this case is a lipo- or glycoprotein coded by a gene on chromosome 19 of man. It has been estimated that there are up to 3×10^3 such receptor sites per cell. The attachment is through the VP4 of the virus (see below). Adenoviruses possess fibres at each vertex of the icosahedral capsid which are used for attaching the virus to specific receptors on the cell surface. The adsorption involves non-glyco-sylated polypeptides. Epstein–Barr virus infects B cells of the human leucocyte populations. This selectivity is largely due to the expression in mature B cells of a receptor for one of the complement cleavage fragments to which the virus binds.

Most cellular receptors are glycoproteins and the number expressed on different cell types is an important factor in determining susceptibility, i.e. the capacity of a cell or an animal to become infected with a particular virus. The number per cell is generally several thousand. The expression of these receptors may change if the cells are cultured in vitro. Thus, monkey kidney cells are commonly used for the culture of poliovirus in vitro although poliovirus does not grow in the kidney in infected monkeys.

With some viruses, the requirement for specific receptors on the cell membrane can be bypassed, experimentally at least, by infection with extract-ed viral nucleic acid. Cells which are normally resistant can therefore be infected. For example, chick fibroblasts, resistant to infection by polio-virus, can be infected for one cycle by polio RNA; the virions produced are not infectious for other chick fibroblasts as they still do not possess an appropriate binding site for chick cells.

Penetration (uptake)

Penetration occurs immediately after adsorption and, unlike adsorption, requires energy and does not proceed at $0°C$. Despite much study, it is still not clear how most viruses enter cells and, furthermore, which route of entry leads to a successful infection. There are probably three main mechanisms.

1. Receptor-mediated endocytosis

This method is used by both enveloped and non-enveloped viruses and is essentially the same as the normal uptake of macromolecules like hormones into the cell. Receptors with adsorbed virus particles move together (patch) to pits coated with clathrin, before moving downwards into the cytosol to form small uncoated vesicles which fuse together as endosomes. A proton pump in the endosome lowers the pH to about 5. This change causes a rearrangement of hydrophobic components of some envelope polypeptides leading to fusion of the viral envelope with the endosome membrane. Thus the viral nucleic acid is released into the cytosol. The endosomes combine with lysosomes, which eventually causes degradation of any viral components contained within. This process is outlined in Fig. 9.3. In the case of influenza, a component of the haemag-glutinin (the hydrophobic amino (*N*)-terminal of HA_2) is responsible for the fusion, the fusion sequence being activated by the low pH of the endosome. Herpesviruses also penetrate in a similar way, and several envelope glycoproteins have been identified as taking part in this process.

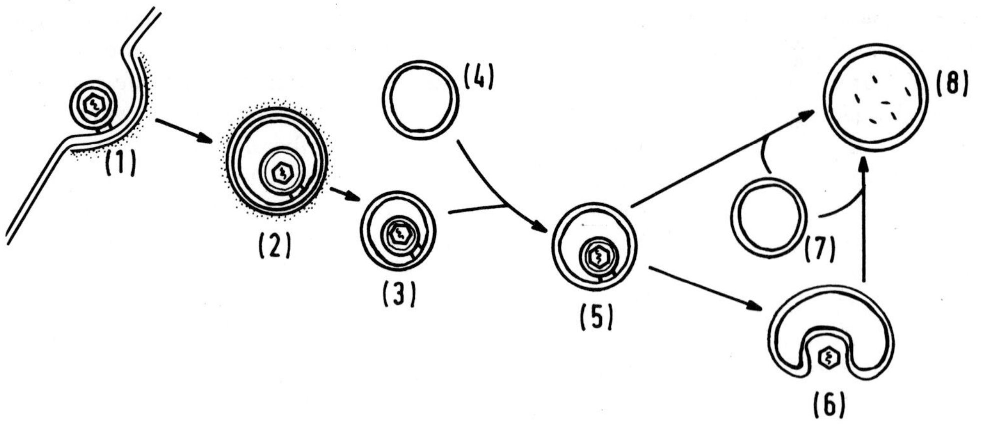

Fig. 9.3 Receptor-mediated endocytosis of an enveloped virus. **1** The virus attaches to specific receptors on the cell membrane, which patch at coated pits before **2** being pinched off to form vesicles. These **3** lose their coat and **4** fuse with other vesicles **5** to form endosomes. **6** At the acid pH of endosomes, fusion of the viral envelope and the endosome membrane occurs releasing the virus into the cytosol. **7** Fusion of the endosome with lysosomes leads to **8** the final degradation of viral components and their return to the surface.

2. Fusion with the plasma membrane

This mechanism is used only by a few enveloped viruses. It requires the presence of a specific viral protein in the envelope which facilitates the fusion between the envelope and the plasma membrane at a physiological pH. Subsequently, there is release of the nucleocapsid into the cytosol. An example of such a protein is the F (fusion) protein of paramyxoviruses.

3. Translocation

Some non-enveloped viruses are able to pass directly across the plasma membrane by an unknown mechanism or mechanisms. From experiments using bacteriophage, it is probable that membrane carrier proteins are involved either in transporting the virus particles or the viral nucleic acid but these have not been identified. Sometimes part of the capsid is left outside, as is the case for adenoviruses which shed their penton capsomeres on entering the cells.

Uncoating

This step in the growth cycle is also not well understood. Some viruses, like polio, undergo conformational changes on attachment which result in the integrity of the particle being lost as it is transported into the cell. Those enveloped viruses entering by receptor-mediated endocytosis may be affected by the action of lysosomal enzymes. For adenoviruses and papovaviruses, it is thought that cellular proteases disaggregate the capsid in the cytosol. Reoviruses never fully uncoat, the viral genome remaining within a recognizable capsid structure. Poxviruses become uncoated in two stages. In the first stage, the outer layers and lateral bodies are removed in endosomal vesicles using host enzymes and the core lies in the cytosol. Poxviruses carry their own DNA-dependent RNA polymerase and this enzyme is used in the second stage to transcribe mRNA which is translated into a special uncoating protein; this enables the final release of viral DNA from the core.

Following uncoating, it is necessary for the viral nucleic acid with, in some instances, viral enzymes or proteins from the capsid, to proceed to the correct place in the cell to commence synthesis of the macromolecules which will comprise the new virus particles. In some cases this happens entirely in the cytosol, e.g. poliovirus, others replicate in the nucleus, e.g. herpesvirus, while a third category has nuclear and cytosol stages, e.g. influenza virus. Again, it is not known how transport is controlled at this stage.

Synthesis of viral components

The nucleic acid in viruses is either single or double stranded, circular or linear, in one piece or segmented. In addition, viruses vary enormously in their complexity, ranging from ones with nucleic acid sufficient to code for only a few proteins like the papovaviruses, up to ones coding for several hundred proteins, like the poxviruses. Although every virus has a unique method of replicating and has a strict temporal control on the synthesis of new components, each must present to the cell functional mRNA, so that new viral polypeptides and nucleic acid can be synthesized using the normal cellular processes. Thus, only viruses which contain DNA and replicate in the nucleus can use cellular enzymes solely for transcription and translation. All other viruses require to synthesize their mRNA by processes other than those found in uninfected cells. Six different classes, first described by Baltimore in 1970, can be distinguished (Fig. 9.4). Conventionally in the scheme, nucleic acid of the same polarity or sense as mRNA is called 'positive' (+), while that of the opposite polarity or anti-sense is called 'negative' (−). Rather than be exhaustive, one illustrative example from each class will now be described.

Class 1. Double-stranded viruses

This comprises a very large group of viruses which contain double-stranded DNA in a linear, e.g. herpesviruses, adenoviruses and poxviruses, or a circular form, e.g. papovaviruses. Herpes simplex virus is used as an example (Fig. 9.5). On uncoating, the viral nucleic acid goes to the nucleus and, using the normal host cell mechanisms of transcription and translation, three groups of viral polypeptides are synthesized in a strict temporal fashion. They are called immediate early (α), early (β) and late (γ). A component in the virus particle induces the transcription of the first set of mRNAs. It is thought that each group of proteins inhibits the synthesis of the one before. Early on, there is inhibition of the host cell protein synthesis and all the metabolic energy of the cell is turned towards the production of new virus particles. Some of the genes coding for the α, β and γ proteins have been mapped on the genome and they are not generally clustered. Amongst the early gene products are thymidine kinase and a virus-specific DNA polymerase. Most of the late proteins are structural proteins. Between β and γ protein synthesis, new viral DNA begins to be made, probably by circularization using a rolling circle model.

Class 2. Single-stranded DNA virus

Parvoviruses, containing single-stranded DNA, are the sole family in this group. They are small viruses with DNA of molecular weight about 2×10^6. Some parvoviruses contain DNA of '−' polarity and grow only in rapidly dividing cells; others contain either '+' or '−' DNA and depend

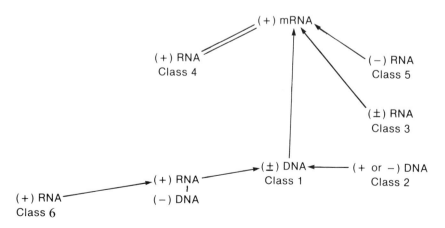

Fig. 9.4 Division of animal viruses into six classes, based on mechanisms of transcription.

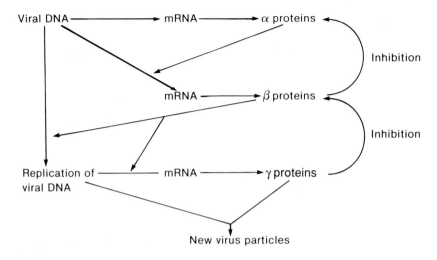

Fig. 9.5   Diagram of macromolecular synthesis during the replication of herpes simplex virus.

on co-infection with a helper virus for their replication. Parvoviruses use the cellular DNA polymerases to make the viral genome double stranded, called the replicative form. Priming is by the viral nucleic acid itself forming a loop at the 3' terminus. This is followed by displacement of the parental DNA strand and synthesis of more DNA complementary to the template strand. Messenger RNAs are made using the appropriate DNA strand as the template and are translated into viral proteins (Fig. 9.6).

Class 3. Double-stranded RNA viruses

In this group are found those viruses with double-stranded RNA, the reoviruses and rotaviruses. All members have segmented genomes and each RNA segment codes for a single polypeptide. Replication of viral nucleic acid, transcription and translation occur solely in the cytosol without nuclear involvement at any stage. The virus carries its own RNA-dependent RNA polymerase, an enzyme unique to some RNA viruses and not found in

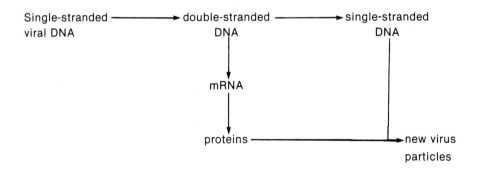

Fig. 9.6   Diagram of parvovirus replication.

own *polymerases,* such as the '–'-strand RNA viruses (RNA-dependent RNA polymerase) and the retro-viruses (reverse transcriptase), it may be possible to inhibit these enzymes without inhibiting the normal cellular mechanisms of transcription.

One of the few successes of antiviral chemo-therapy to date has been in the development of ribonucleoside and deoxyribonucleoside analogues which interfere in the synthesis of the viral genome. One of the first of these was *vidarabine* (adenosine arabinoside, Fig. 9.16c), which is an analogue of the natural nucleoside adenine deoxyriboside and is active against herpesviruses. It is phosphorylated to the monophosphate and triphosphate, the latter then inhibiting viral DNA polymerase selectively without affecting cellular DNA polymerases and also terminating the growing DNA chain. *Acyclovir* (Fig. 9.16d), an acyclic analogue of guanosine, is a later example of the same class of compound. It is effective against most herpesviruses which code for their own thymidine kinase enzyme. The viral thymidine kinase is able to phosphorylate acyclovir to the monophosphate, which is converted to the triphosphate. This is incorporated into the growing DNA strand, which is terminated at that point as there is no group for the next nucleotide triphosphate to be joined on to. Acyclovir also inhibits viral DNA polymerase selectively and has little effect on the cell enzyme. Drug-resistant mutants may emerge after prolonged use of acyclovir. *Zidovudine (azido-thymidine* or AZT, Fig. 9.16e), is a third example presently being used against infections with human immunodeficiency virus. Zidovudine is an analogue of thymidine and is phosphorylated by cellular enzymes to the triphosphate, which inhibits reverse transcriptase and terminates DNA replication when it is incorporated into the growing DNA chain. A similar compound, *tribavirin* (ribavirin, Fig. 9.16f), consists of a triazole attached to ribose and is an analogue of a purine precursor. It is effective against a range of DNA and RNA viruses but has proved particularly useful in infections caused by respiratory syncytial virus. Tribavirin inhibits viral nucleic acid polymerases and may interfere in the capping of viral mRNA. Finally, *phosphonoacetic acid* (Fig. 9.16g) and *foscarnet* (phosphonoformic acid) act by inhibiting DNA polymerases synthesized by herpesviruses, without affecting normal cellular DNA polymerases.

Various other approaches to the production of clinically useful antiviral agents are under investigation and more progress may be anticipated in the future.

RECOMMENDED READING

Barrett A D, Dimmock N J 1986, Defective interfering viruses and infections of animals. *Current Topics in Microbiology and Immunology* 128: 55–84

Bishop J M 1987 The molecular genetics of cancer. *Science* 235: 305–311.

Dimmock N J 1982 Initial stages in infection with animal viruses. *Journal of General Virology* 59: 1–22

Dimmock N J, Primrose S B 1987 *Introduction to Modern Virology,* 3rd edn. Blackwell, Oxford

Fields B N, Knipe D M (eds) 1990 *Virology.* 2nd edn. Raven Press, New York

Kohn A 1985 Membrane effects of cytopathogenic viruses. *Progress in Medical Virology* 31: 107-167

Kozak M 1986 Regulation of protein synthesis in virus-infected animal cells. *Advances in Virus Research* 31: 229–292

Krausslich H-G, Wimmer E 1988 Viral proteinases. *Annual Review of Biochemistry* 57: 701–754

Stephens E B, Compans R W 1988 Assembly of animal viruses at cellular membranes. *Annual Review of Microbiology* 42: 489–516

Strauss E G, Strauss J H 1983 Replication strategies of the single stranded RNA viruses of eukaryotes. *Current Topics in Microbiology and Immunology* 105: 1–98

Streissle G, Paessens A, Dediger H 1985 New antiviral compounds. *Advances in Virus Research* 30: 83–138

PART 2
Infection and immunity

10

Immunological principles: antigens and antigen recognition

J. Stewart and D. M. Weir

ANTIGENS

An antigen is any substance capable of provoking the lymphoid tissues of an animal to respond by generating an immune reaction specifically directed at the inducing substance and not at other unrelated substances. The response is not to the entire molecule but to individual chemical groups that will have a specific three-dimensional shape. The specificity of the response to these *antigenic determinants* or *epitopes* is an important characteristic of immune responses. The reaction of an animal to contact with antigen, called the *acquired immune response*, takes two forms, (1) the *humoral* or *circulating antibody response* and (2) the *cell-mediated response*, and their characteristics are described in Chapter 11. Most of the information available on the specificity of the immune response comes from studies of the interaction of circulating antibody with antigen. An antibody directed against an epitope of a particular molecule will react only with this determinant or other very similar structures. Even minor chemical changes in the conformation of the epitope will markedly reduce the ability of the original antibody to react with the altered material.

The term antigen, referring to substances either acting as stimulants of the immune response or reacting with antibody, is used rather loosely by immunologists. Use is made of the functional classification of antigens into (1) substances which are able to generate an immune response by themselves, which are termed *immunogens*, and

(2) molecules that are able to react with antibodies but are unable to stimulate their production directly. The latter substances are often low molecular-weight chemicals, termed *haptens*, that will react with preformed antibodies but only become immunogenic when attached to large molecules, called *carriers*. The hapten forms an epitope on the carrier molecule that is recognized by the immune system and stimulates the production of antibody. In other words, the ability of a chemical grouping to interact with an antibody is not enough to stimulate an immune response. As we will see later, when discussing the sites on molecules recognized by cells of the immune system, all antigens can be considered to be composed of haptens on larger carrier structures.

General properties of antigens

A substance that acts as an antigen in one species of animal may not do so in another if it is represented in the tissues or fluids of the second species. This underlines the requirement that an antigen must be a foreign substance to elicit an immune response. For example, egg albumin, whilst an excellent antigen in rabbit, fails to induce an antibody response in fowl. The more foreign and evolutionarily distant a substance is to a particular species, the more likely it is to be a powerful antigen.

A widely recognized requirement for a substance to be antigenic in its own right, without having to be attached to a carrier molecule, is that it should have a molecular weight in excess of 5000. It is, however, possible to induce an immune response to substances of lower molecular weight. For example, glucagon (molecular weight of 3800) can stimulate antibody production but only if special measures are taken such as the use of an *adjuvant* which gives an additional stimulus to the immune system. Very large proteins, such as the crustacean respiratory pigment haemocyanin, are very powerful antigens and are widely used in experimental immunology. Polysaccharides vary in antigenicity, e.g. dextran with a molecular weight of 600 000 is a good antigen, whereas dextran with a molecular weight of 100 000 is not.

Some low molecular weight chemical substances appear to contradict the requirement that an antigen be large. Among these are picryl chloride, formaldehyde and drugs such as aspirin, penicillin and sulphonamides. These substances are highly antigenic, particularly if applied to the skin. The reason for this appears to be that such materials form complexes by means of covalent bonds with tissue proteins. The complex of such a substance, acting as a hapten, with a tissue protein acting as a carrier, forms a complete antigen. This phenomenon has important implications in the development of certain types of hypersensitivity (Chapter 11).

Antigenic determinants

The immune system does not recognize an infectious agent or foreign molecule as a whole but reacts to structurally distinct areas — antigenic determinants or epitopes. Thus, exposure to a micro-organism will generate an immune response to many different epitopes. The antiserum produced will contain different antibodies reactive with each determinant. This will ensure that an individual will be protected from the micro-organism by producing a response to at least a few of the possible determinants. If the host only reacted to the organism as a whole then failure to react to this one site would have dire consequences, i.e. it would not be able to eliminate the pathogen. Certain antibodies may react with an epitope composed of residues that can also be part of two other epitopes recognized by different antibodies (Fig. 10.1).

A response to antigen involves the specific interaction of components of the immune system, antibodies and lymphocytes, with epitopes on the antigen. The lymphocytes have receptors on their surface that function as the recognition units — on B lymphocytes surface-bound immunoglobulin is the receptor and on T lymphocytes the recognition unit is known as the T cell receptor. The interaction between an antibody (or cell-bound receptor) and antigen is governed by the complementarity of the electron cloud surrounding the determinants. The overall configuration of the outer electrons, not the chemical nature of the constituent residues, determines the shape of the epitope and its complementary *paratope* (the part of the antibody or T cell receptor that interacts with the epitope). There is no reason why the shape generated by the electron clouds surrounding a group of amino acids should not be identical to that surrounding part of a lipid or polysaccharide. The better the fit between the epitope and the antigen-combining site, or paratope, of the antibody, the stronger the bond formed and consequently the higher the affinity of the interaction.

Antigenic determinants have to be topographical, i.e. composed of structures on the surface of molecules, and can be constructed in two ways. They may be contained within a single segment of primary sequence or assembled from residues far apart in the primary sequence but brought together on the surface by the folding of the molecule into its native conformation. The former are known as *sequential* epitopes and those formed from distant residues are *conformational* epitopes. The antigenic structures seen by antibody depend on the tertiary configuration of the immunogen (conformational), while epitopes seen by T cells are defined by the primary structure (sequential).

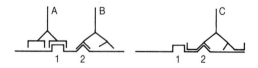

Fig. 10.1 Overlapping epitopes. Two epitopes (1 and 2) on an antigen induce the formation of three antibodies (A, B and C).

Antigenic specificity

Foreignness of a substance to an animal can depend on the presence of chemical groupings that are not normally found in the animal's body. Arsenic acid, for example, can be chemically introduced into a protein molecule and, as a hapten, acts as a determinant of antigenic specificity of the molecule. There are many other examples where antibodies are able to distinguish subtle chemical differences between molecules. Thus, antisera can distinguish between glucose and galactose, which differ only by the interchange of a hydrogen atom and a hydroxyl group on one carbon atom.

The ability of antibody (or T cell receptors) to form a high-affinity interaction with an antigen depends on intermolecular forces which act strongly only when the two molecules come together in a very precise manner. The better the fit, the stronger the bond. An antibody molecule directed against a particularly shaped antigenic determinant might be able to react with another similar but not quite identical determinant, as shown in Fig. 10.2. This type of cross-reaction does occur but the strength of the bond between the two molecules will be diminished in the case of the less well-fitting determinant.

A common source of confusion concerning the specificity of antibodies arises when an antibody to a particular antigen is found to be capable of combining with an apparently unrelated antigen. This raises the need to distinguish clearly between the structural specificity of an antigenic determinant and its distribution specificity. For example, glucose residues are present in many different types of molecule and an antibody that binds to a glucose determinant in antigen X-glucose would be likely to react with the glucose group in antigen Y-glucose provided the two determinants are equally accessible. The antibody directed against

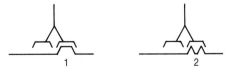

Fig. 10.2 Specificity and cross-reactions. Antibody produced in response to an antigen that contains epitope 1 will also combine with epitope 2.

the glucose determinant is not a non-specific type of antibody but is simply reacting with an identical chemical determinant in another antigen molecule.

In laboratory practice, cross-reactivity is often found between antisera to certain bacterial antigens and antigens present on cells such as erythrocytes. Antigens shared in this way are known as *heterophile antigens*. The best known of the heterophile antigens is the Forssman antigen, which is present on the red cells of many species as well as in bacteria such as pneumococci and salmonellae. Another heterophile antigen is found in *Escherichia coli* and human red cells of blood group B individuals. These cross-reactivities are probably responsible for the generation of antibodies found in individuals of a certain blood group that bind to the red blood cells of individuals of a different blood group. These antibodies are known as *isohaemagglutinins* because they are able to bind the red blood cells and clump them together, i.e. cause agglutination.

IMMUNOGLOBULINS

Towards the end of the 19th century von Behring and Kitasato in Berlin found that the blood serum of an appropriately immunized animal contained specific neutralizing substances or antitoxins. This was the first demonstration of the activity of what are now known as *antibodies* or *immunoglobulins*. Antibodies are glycoproteins, present in the serum and body tissues, that are induced when immunogenic molecules are introduced into the host's lymphoid system. They bind specifically to the antigen that induced their formation.

The liquid collected from blood that has been allowed to clot is known as *serum*. It contains a number of molecules but no cells or clotting factors. If serum is prepared from an animal that has been exposed to an antigen then it is known as an *antiserum* since it will contain antibodies reactive to the inducing antigen. When the components of serum are separated electrophoretically then the heterogeneity of immunoglobulins can be seen, i.e. they appear as broad bands

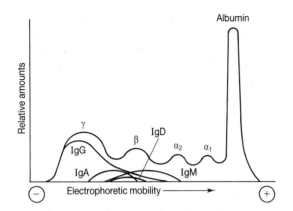

Fig. 10.3 Separation of serum proteins by electrophoresis.

(Fig. 10.3). This technique separates serum components into various fractions, labelled α, β and γ. Most of the antibody molecules are present within the γ fraction and they are sometimes referred to as γ globulins.

There are five distinct *classes* or *isotypes* of immunoglobulins, namely IgG, IgA, IgM, IgD and IgE. They differ from each other in size, charge, carbohydrate content and, of course, amino acid composition (Table 10.1). Within certain classes there are subclasses that show slight differences in structure and function from other members of the class. These classes and subclasses can be separated from each other serologically, i.e. using

antibody. If injected into the correct species they will induce the formation of antibodies that can be used to differentiate between the different isotypes.

Antibody structure

All antibody molecules have the same basic four-chain structure composed of two light chains and two heavy chains (Fig. 10.4). The light chains (molecular weight of 25 000) are one of two types designated κ and λ and only one type is found in one antibody. The heavy chains vary in molecular weight from 50 000 to 70 000 and it is these chains that determine the isotype. They are designated alpha, delta, epsilon, gamma and mu for the respective classes of immunoglobulin (Table 10.1). The individual chains are held together by disulphide bridges and non-covalent interactions.

When individual light chains are studied it is found that they are composed of two distinct areas or *domains* of approximately 110 amino acids. One end of the chain is identical in all members of the same isotype and is termed the constant region of the light chain, C_L. The other end shows considerable sequence variation and is known as the variable region, V_L. The heavy chains are also split into domains of approximately the same size, the number varying between the five types of heavy chain. One of these domains will show considerable sequence variation (V_H) while

Table 10.1 Physicochemical properties of human immunoglobulins. The immunoglobulin serotype is determined by the type of heavy chain present. The different characteristics observed are also controlled by the heavy chain. Variation within a class gives rise to subclasses

Characteristic	Immunoglobulin isotype				
	IgA	IgD	IgE	IgG	IgM[a]
Mean serum concentration (mg/dl)	300	5	0.005	1400	150
Mass (kDa)	160	184	188	160	970
Carbohydrate (%)	7–11	9–14	12	2–3	12
Half-life (days)	6	3	2	21	5
Heavy chain	α alpha	δ delta	ε epsilon	γ gamma	μ mu

[a] Data for IgM as a pentamer.
IgA is also found as a dimer and in secretions IgA is present in dimeric form associated with a protein known as secretory component.

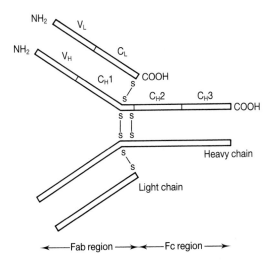

Fig. 10.4 Basic structure of an immunoglobulin molecule. See text for details.

the others (C_H) are similar for the same isotype. The tertiary structure generated by the combination of the V_L and V_H regions determines the shape of the antigen-combining site or paratope. Since the two light and two heavy chains are identical, each antibody unit will have two identical paratopes situated at the amino (N)-terminal end of the molecule that recognize the antigen. The carboxyl (C)-terminal end of the antibody will be the same for all members of the same class or subclass and is involved in the biological activities of the molecule. The area of the heavy chains between the C_H1 and C_H2 domains contains a varying number of interchain disulphide bonds and is known as the *hinge region*. A number of enzymes cleave immunoglobulins at distinct points to generate different peptide fragments. Using these enzymes, antibodies can be divided into a Fab region (fragment antigen binding) containing the paratope and an Fc region (fragment crystallizable) that is similar for all antibodies of the same isotype.

IgG

This is the major immunoglobulin of serum making up 75% of the total and having a molecular weight of 150 000 in man. Four subclasses are

found in man — IgG1, IgG2, IgG3 and IgG4 — that differ in their relative concentrations, amino acid composition, number and position of interchain disulphide bonds and biological function. IgG is the major antibody of the secondary response (see Chapter 11) and is found in both the serum and tissue fluids.

IgA

In man most of the serum IgA occurs as a monomer but in many other mammals it is mostly found as a dimer. The dimer is held together by a J chain, which is produced by the antibody-producing plasma cells. IgA is the predominant antibody class in seromucous secretions such as saliva, tears, colostrum and respiratory, gastro-intestinal and genito-urinary secretions. This secretory IgA (sIgA) is always in the dimeric form and is composed of two basic four-chain units (two light chains and two α heavy chains), a J chain and the secretory component. The secretory component is part of the molecule that transports the dimer produced by a submucosal plasma cell to the mucosal surface (Fig. 10.5). It not only facilitates passage through the epithelial cells but protects the secreted molecule from proteolytic

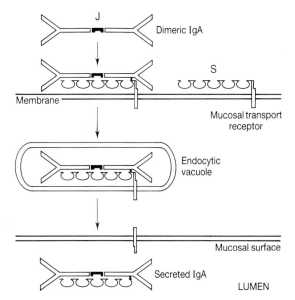

Fig. 10.5 Transport of secretory IgA. J, J chain; S, secretory component.

digestion. There are two subclasses of IgA — IgA1 and IgA2.

IgM

IgM is a pentamer of the basic unit with μ heavy chains and a single J chain. Because of its large size this isotype is mainly confined to the intravascular pool and is the first antibody type to be produced during an immune response.

IgD

Many circulating B cells have IgD present on their surface but it accounts for less than 1% of the circulating antibody. It is composed of the basic unit with δ heavy chains. The protein is very susceptible to proteolytic attack and therefore has a very short half-life.

IgE

The IgE is present in extremely low levels in the serum. However, it is found on the surface of mast cells and basophils, which possess a receptor specific for the Fc part of this molecule.

Despite the differences between the various isotypes, as shown in Table 10.1, all antibody molecules are composed of the same basic unit structure with the Fab portion containing the antigen-recognizing paratope and the Fc region carrying out the activities that protect the host, i.e. effector functions. The diversity seen in the Fc region between the different heavy chains is responsible for the different biological activities of the antibody isotypes.

Antigen binding

The variability in amino acid sequence in the variable domains of light and heavy chains is not found over their entire length but is restricted to short segments. These segments show considerable variation and are termed *hypervariable regions*. Hypervariable regions are now known to contain the residues that make direct contact with the antigen and are sometimes referred to as *complementarity determining regions* (CDRs). Although

the remaining *framework* residues do not come into direct contact with the antigen, they are essential for the formation of the correct tertiary structure of the variable domain and maintenance of the integrity of the binding site. In both light and heavy chains there are three CDRs which, in combination, form the paratope.

The antigen and antibody are held together by various individually weak non-covalent interactions. However, the formation of a large number of hydrogen bonds and electrostatic, van der Waals and hydrophobic interactions leads to a considerable binding energy. These attractive forces are only active over extremely short distances and therefore the epitope and paratope must have complementary structures to enable them to combine. If the electron clouds overlap or residues of similar charge are brought together then repulsive forces will come into play. The balance of attraction against repulsion will dictate the strength of the interaction between an antibody and a particular antigen, i.e. the affinity of the antibody for the antigen.

Antibody diversity

It is now known that an antigen selects from the available antibodies those that can combine with its epitopes. It therefore follows that an individual must have an extremely large number of different antibodies to cope with the vast array of different antigens present in the environment.

Immunoglobulin variability

The paratope is produced by the CDRs of the light and heavy chains generating a specific three-dimensional shape. Any light chain can join with any heavy chain to produce a different paratope. Thus, theoretically, with 10^4 different light chains and 10^4 different heavy chains, 10^8 different specificities could be generated.

The germ-line DNA is the structure of the gene as it is inherited. All cells in the body contain all the inherited genes but different genes become active in different cells at different times. Within B lymphocytes, the cells that differentiate to antibody-producing plasma cells, the functional immunoglobulin genes are formed by gene rearrangements and recombinations. These events give rise to the production of different variable domains in each B lymphocyte. Once a functional gene has been constructed no other rearrangements are allowed to take place within this cell. This dictates that one particular cell will produce only one antigen-combining site and is known as *allelic exclusion*. There is evidence that the gene segments for the variable region of immunoglobulins are particularly susceptible to mutations. This can lead to subtle changes in specificity and/or affinity that are important as an immune response develops (see Chapter 11).

When a B lymphocyte is first stimulated by antigen it will produce IgM. As the immune response develops the class of antibody being produced changes. However, the immunoglobulin produced will have the same variable domain and therefore bind to the same antigen. All that is altered, or *switched*, is the heavy chain constant region. Thus the progeny of a single B cell will produce different immunoglobulin isotypes as the response to a particular antigen develops, but each will have the same paratope.

Secreted and membrane immunoglobulins

At different stages in its development a B cell will produce immunoglobulins that have to be inserted into the membrane or secreted. The membrane-bound immunoglobulin will be used as the antigen receptor of the B cell and a cell that binds antigen through this molecule will then secrete immunoglobulin of the same specificity. The only difference between the two types of antibody is to be found at the C-terminus in that the transcript that will direct the production of the membrane form has an additional part to code for the transmembrane portion.

Antibody function

Knowledge gained from the structural studies discussed above has gone some way towards an understanding of the biological activities of the immunoglobulin molecule. It is now possible to pinpoint areas of the molecule responsible for different activities.

The primary function of an antibody is to bind the antigen that induced its formation. Apart from cases where this results in direct neutralization (e.g. inhibition of toxin activity or of microbial attachment) other effector functions must be generated. The binding of antigen is mediated by the Fab portion and the Fc region controls the biological defence mechanisms. For every antibody the paratope will be different and it will therefore recognize different epitopes. However, for every antibody of the same isotype the heavy chain constant domains will be the same and they will therefore all perform the same functions (Table 10.2).

Neutralization

The fact that antibodies are at least divalent means that they can form a complex with multivalent antigen. Depending on the physical nature of the antigen these *immune complexes* exist in various forms (Fig. 10.6). If the antibody is directed against surface antigens of particulate material such as micro-organisms or erythrocytes then

Table 10.2 Biological properties of human immunoglobulins. These activities are determined by the Fc portion of the molecules

Function	Immunoglubulin isotype							
	IgA	IgD	IgE	IgG1	IgG2	IgG3	IgG4	IgM
Complement fixation	±[a]	−	−	++	+	+++	−	+++
Placental transfer	−	−	−	+	±	+	+	−
Binding to phagocytes	±[b]	−	−	+++	±	+++	+	−
Binding to mast cells	−	−	+++	−	−	−	+	−

[a] IgA will activate the alternative pathway.
[b] Receptors for the Fc portion of IgA have been found on neutrophils and alveolar macrophages.

(a)　　　　　　　(b)

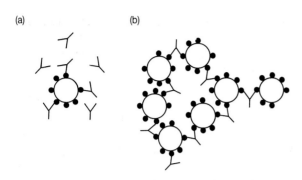

(c)　　　　　　　(d)

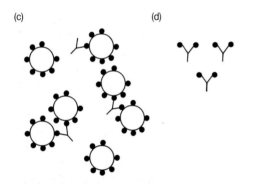

Fig. 10.6 Immune complex formation:
a antibody excess; **b** equivalence; **c** antigen excess;
d monovalent antigen.

agglutination will occur. This is a clump or aggregate that will isolate the potential pathogen, stop its dissemination and stimulate its removal by other mechanisms. If the antigen is soluble then the size of the complex will determine its physical state. Small complexes will remain soluble while large complexes will form *precipitates* .

As might be expected from knowledge of the structure of IgM, its 10 combining sites make it a very efficient agglutinating antibody molecule. Rabbit IgM has been shown to the more than 20 times as active as IgG (molecule for molecule) in bringing about bacterial agglutination. Because of its size, IgM is largely confined to the bloodstream and probably plays an important role in protecting against blood invasion by micro-organisms. Certain sites on micro-organisms are critical to the establishment of an infection. Antibody bound to these sites will interfere with attachment processes and could, therefore, stop infection by the microbe. The binding of an antibody to func-

tionally important residues in a toxin will neutralize their harmful effects.

Complement activation

The activation of the complement system is one of the most important antibody effector mechanisms. The complement cascade is a complex group of serum proteins that mediate inflammatory reactions and cell lysis. It is discussed more fully in Chapter 11. The Fc portion of certain isotypes (Table 10.2), once antigen has been bound, will activate complement; this requires that C1q, a subunit of the first complement component, cross-links two antibody Fc portions. For this to happen the two regions must be in close proximity. It has been calculated that a single IgM molecule is 1000 times more efficient than IgG. This is because two IgG molecules must be close together for complement activation. A large number of IgG molecules would be required for this to occur if the epitopes are spread. Not all isotypes activate complement, presumably because they do not have the required amino acid sequence, and therefore tertiary structure, in the Fc portion. C1q binds to residues in the C_H3 domain of IgM and the C_H2 domain of IgG. Some isotypes when interacting with antigen can activate the alternative pathway of complement that does not use C1 but gives rise to the same biological activities.

Cell binding and opsonization

The Fc portion of certain immunoglobulin isotypes is able to interact with various cell types (Table 10.2). Antibodies specific for particular antigens, such as bacteria, play a valuable role by binding to the surface and making the antigen more susceptible to phagocytosis and subsequent elimination. This process is known as *opsonization* and is again mediated by the Fc portion of the antibody. A specific conformation on the Fc region of certain isotypes is recognized by *Fc receptors* on the surface of the phagocyte. The important residues are in the C_H2 domain near the hinge region. Individually, the interactions are not strong enough to signal the uptake of the antibody molecule, therefore, free immunoglobulin is not internalized. However, when an antigen is coated by many antibody molecules then summation of all the interactions stimulates phagocytosis or other effector mechanisms.

Certain phagocytic cells have receptors for activated complement components, *complement receptors*. If the binding of antibody to the antigen can activate the complement cascade then various complement components will be deposited on the antigen–antibody complex. Phagocytic cells that have receptors for these complement components will then ingest the complexes.

The above-mentioned processes require that the antibody is first complexed with antigen. However, certain cell types will bind free antibody. Mast cells and basophils have Fc receptors that are specific for IgE. These cells perform a protective function but are also involved in hypersensitivity reactions described in Chapter 11. In man, IgG has the ability to cross the placenta and reach the fetal circulation. This is a passive process involving specific Fc receptors. This route is limited to primates whereas, in ruminants, immunoglobulin from colostrum is absorbed through the intestinal epithelium. Another Fc-mediated mechanism, already described, is found for IgA, which is selectively transported into mucosal secretions.

Genetic markers on antibodies

Immunoglobulins are glycoproteins and can behave as antigens if injected into the correct host, i.e. antibodies will be made against epitopes on the immunoglobulin. The parts of the immunoglobulin that the immune system reacts against will depend on the species used to generate the antibody. The type of epitope that these anti-immunoglobulins recognize is given a specific name depending on its position on the molecule (Fig. 10.7).

Antibodies that detect variations between the different classes of immunoglobulin define the *isotype*. The residues that are recognized will be on the constant portions of the heavy and light chains. These anti-isotypic antibodies will be produced by injecting the immunoglobulin of one species into another. Antibodies can also be generated that differentiate between the various subclasses of IgG and IgA.

Allotypes are differences that exist between members of the same species. Allotypic markers are also found on the constant regions of heavy and light chains. The sequences recognized do not appear to influence the activity of the immunoglobulin as marked differences in function between allotypes have not been found.

The variable regions of immunoglobulin molecules exhibit, as described above, immense structural variation. The immune system can recognize these variations and the antibodies generated are known as anti-idiotypic antibodies. Each immunoglobulin contains a number of epitopes that stimulate the production of anti-idiotypic antibodies (Fig. 10.8). Each epitope is known as an *idiotope* and the collection of idiotopes on an immunoglobulin determines its *idiotype*. Thus, each immunoglobulin produced by an individual is capable of stimulating the production

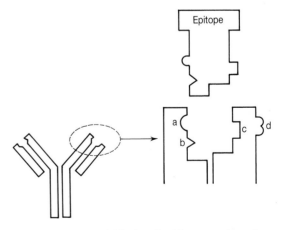

Fig. 10.8 Antibody-variable domains. Idiotopes a, b, and c are located within the paratope (paratope associated) and d is outside the antigen combining site (paratope non-associated).

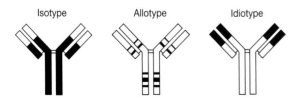

Fig. 10.7 Genetic markers on antibodies. The sites where antibody variants are located are indicated by the shaded areas.

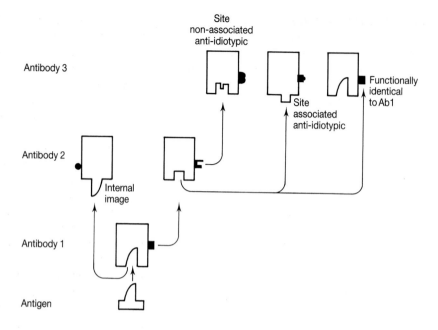

Fig. 10.9 Idiotype network.

of other immunoglobulins, anti-idiotypic antibody, and a network of interaction is generated. This process may have a role in the regulation of immune responses (Chapter 11). Included in the network hypothesis is an important premise that has applications in other areas such as vaccine development. When an antigen is introduced the host will respond by producing specific immunoglobulin. This immunoglobulin will then stimulate the production of anti-idiotypic antibodies and so on. In Fig. 10.9 it can be seen that some of these anti-idiotypic antibodies have a paratope that is similar in shape to the antigen that triggered the process. This antibody is known as the *internal image* and this molecule could be used to vaccinate against agents that are otherwise too difficult or dangerous to obtain.

ANTIGEN RECOGNITION

The immune system has evolved to protect us from potentially harmful material but it must not respond to self molecules. Two separate recognition systems are present: humoral immunity and cell-mediated immunity. Antibody is the recognition molecule of humoral immunity. This glycoprotein is produced by plasma cells and circulates in the blood and other body fluids. Antibody is also present on the surface of B lymphocytes. The interaction of this surface immunoglobulin with its specific antigen is responsible for the differentiation of these cells into plasma cells. Antibody molecules, whether free or on the surface of a B cell, will recognize free native antigen. This contrasts dramatically with the situation in cell-mediated immunity; the T lymphocyte antigen receptor will only bind to fragments of antigen that are associated with products of the *major histocompatibility complex* (MHC). T cell recognition of antigen is said to be *MHC restricted*. These MHC products are present on the surface of cells, therefore T cells only recognize cell-associated antigens. This MHC-restricted recognition mechanism has evolved because of the functions carried out by T lymphocytes. Some T cells produce immunoregulatory molecules, *lymphokines*, some of which influence the activities of host cells and others that directly kill infected or foreign cells. Therefore, it would be inefficient or dangerous to produce these effects in response to either free antigen or antigen sitting idly on some cell membrane. The joint recognition of MHC molecules and antigen ensures that the T cell makes contact with antigen on the surface of the appropriate target cell. Indeed, it is important to remember that immunoglobulins are capable of eliminating free antigens.

B cell receptor

Antibody is found free in body fluids and as a transmembrane protein on the surface of B lymphocytes, i.e. surface immunoglobulin, where it acts as the B cell antigen receptor. The antibody present on the surface of the B cell is exactly the same molecule as will be secreted when the cell develops into a plasma cell except for the extreme C-terminal end as described above. It should be noted that the molecules present on the cell surface are present as monomers even though they are secreted in a polymeric form.

T cell receptor

The complex on T lymphocytes that is involved in antigen recognition is composed of a number of glycoprotein structures. Some of these molecules have been systematically named by CD (cluster of differentiation) nomenclature using antibodies. These generic names shall be used in preference to other symbols sometimes found in the literature since the molecules are designated differently in different species.

The T cell antigen receptor is a heterodimer composed of an α and a β or a γ and a δ chain. The majority of T cells use the α/β heterodimer in antigen recognition. The role of cells that possess the γ/δ molecules is unknown but they may be involved in the immune response to particular types of antigens at specific anatomical sites. The T cell receptor is the molecule that is responsible for the recognition of specific MHC-antigen complexes and will be different for every T cell. Genetic rearrangements of germ-line genes, similar to those seen in B cells, produce functional T cell receptors.

CD3 (T3 in man) is present on all T cells and has a constant structure and is closely associated with the T cell receptor. It is composed of four non-covalently associated polypeptide chains (γ, δ, ε and ζ). (Fig. 10.10). This monomeric complex is thought to be involved in signal transduction when a ligand binds to the T cell receptor.

CD4 and CD8 (T4 and T8 in man) are mutually exclusive molecules. They are present on T cells that are restricted in their recognition of antigen by MHC class II and class I molecules respectively. Due to their almost exclusive correlation with a specific MHC class it is thought that these molecules bind to non-polymorphic determinants on the MHC molecules. This interaction could stabilize the binding of the T cell receptor to the MHC–antigen complex or it may in fact have a co-receptor function. In the former case the CD4 or CD8 molecule could interact with the same MHC molecule as the T cell receptor or with a different one and this interaction does not generate a stimulatory signal, i.e. it solely stabilizes the specific interaction (T cell receptor with antigen – MHC). In the latter case the T cell receptor and CD4 or CD8 bind to the same MHC molecule but at different sites and the joint signal that is generated leads to the stimulation of the T cell.

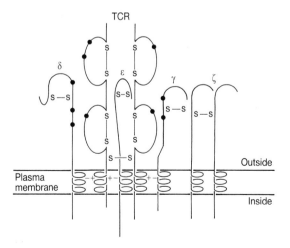

Fig. 10.10 T-cell receptor (TCR)–CD3 complex. Disulphide bonds (S–S) and glycosylation sites (•) are shown.

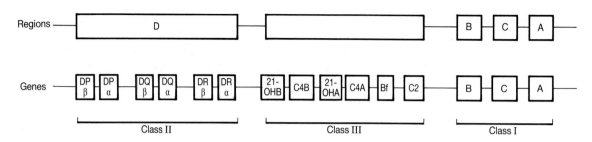

Fig. 10.11 MHC gene map of man.

MAJOR HISTOCOMPATIBILITY COMPLEX

The MHC is part of the genome that codes for molecules that are important in immune recognition — including interactions between lymphoid cells and other cell types. It is also involved in the rejection of allografts. The MHCs of a number of species have been studied but most is known about those of the mouse and man.

The gene complex contains a large number of individual genes that can be grouped into three classes on the basis of structure and function of their products. The products of the genes are usually referred to as *MHC antigens* because they were first defined by serological analysis, i.e. using antibodies.

The MHC of man is known as *human leucocyte group A* (HLA) and in mice it is referred to as *histocompatibility-2* (H-2).

Gene organization

The genes that code for the HLA antigens are found on the short arm of chromosome 6. They are arranged over a region of between 2000 and 4000 kilobases containing enough DNA for over 200 genes. The MHC genes are contained within regions known as A, B, C and D (Fig. 10.11). MHC class I molecules consist of two non-covalently associated polypeptide chains. A single gene that codes for the larger chain is present in the A, B and C regions while the lighter chain, known as β_2-microglobulin, is coded for elsewhere in the genome. The class II molecules are composed of two chains, both of which are coded for within the D region. There are three class II

molecules DP, DQ and DR. The class III genes that code for a number of complement components and other molecules are grouped together in a region between D and B.

Other genes are also present within the MHC, most of which have nothing to do with the immune system. Exceptions to this are the genes for the two types of tumour necrosis factor.

MHC antigen structure and distribution

The MHC class I molecule is a dimer composed of a glycosylated transmembrane peptide, of molecular weight 45 000, coded for within the MHC, linked to a peptide, β_2-microglobulin (Fig. 10.12a). The globular protein formed by these two peptides is

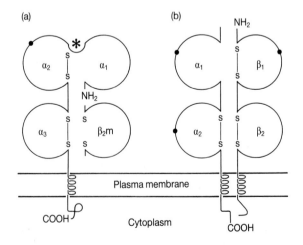

Fig. 10.12 Structure of MHC class I and class II molecules. Schematic representations of **a** class I and **b** class II molecules as found in the plasma membrane. β_2-m, β_2-microglobulin; carbohydrate moieties, •; antigen-binding cleft *.

present on the surface of virtually all nucleated cells in man. β2-Microglobulin is required for the processing and expression of MHC-encoded molecules on the cell membrane. The MHC-encoded class I glycoprotein folds into three globular domains (α_1, α_2 and α_3) held in place by disulphide bonds and non-covalent interactions. These globular domains are found on the outer surface of the cell. There is a short cytoplasmic tail and a transmembrane portion. β2-Microglobulin is non-covalently associated with the α_3 domain.

The MHC class II molecules consist of two polypeptide chains (α and β) held together by non-covalent interactions (Fig. 10.12b). They have a much more limited cellular distribution being limited to the surface of certain cells of the immune system. In man, they are normally found on B lymphocytes, macrophages, monocytes and activated T lymphocytes. The MHC class II molecule consists of two non-covalently associated peptides, α and β. Each chain is composed of two extracellular domains, a transmembrane portion and a cytoplasmic tail.

These two types of molecule are folded into domains of a similar overall structure to immunoglobulin and, along with other molecules of the immune system involved in recognition processes, are thought to have evolved from a common ancestral molecule. A number of members of this *immunoglobulin supergene family* are depicted in Fig. 10.13. MHC class II molecules, some interleukin receptors and Fc receptors are also included in the family.

The MHC antigens of each class have a similar basic structure. However, fine structural differences can be detected in the α_1 and α_2 domains of class I molecules and in α_1 and β_1 domains of class II molecules. These domains form a cleft on the outermost part of the molecules in which antigen fragments are found. The variations found are due to differences in the amino acid sequence and can be detected serologically. The variable residues will give rise to different three-dimensional shapes on the MHC molecules. This will in turn influence the way in which antigen fragments can bind to the MHC molecule.

There are, therefore, many different forms of these molecules that can be identified in a population — they are highly *polymorphic*. Thus, it is highly unlikely that two individuals will have exactly the same MHC antigens. The MHC molecules of a particular individual, their haplotype, can be given a designation using tissue-typing

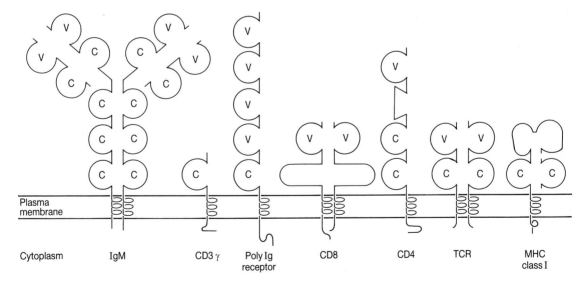

Fig. 10.13 The immunoglobulin supergene family. A number of molecules involved in the immune system display striking similarities in overall structure. Regions similar to immunoglobulin domains are shown as circles; those related to variable and constant domains are designated V and C.

reagents. So, on each chromosome of an individual will be the genes that code for an A, B, C, DP, DQ and DR molecule. As the MHC genes are co-dominant the products of both alleles are expressed on the cell surface. All the nucleated cells in the body will therefore express multiple copies of two HLA-A, two HLA-B and two HLA-C molecules. On certain cell types there will also be HLA-DP, -DQ and -DR molecules that were inherited from both parents.

Function

The MHC antigens are essential for immune recognition by T lymphocytes, which are only able to bind to antigens when they are associated with these molecules. The different classes of MHC antigen are involved in the restriction of different T cell types or subsets. T lymphocytes that have CD4 molecules on their surface recognize antigen in association with MHC class II molecules, while those that have CD8 molecules are restricted by MHC class I molecules.

The T lymphocyte subsets perform different functions, but the division is not absolute. The one thing that they have in common is that they recognize, through their T cell receptor complex (CD3, CD4 or CD8, TCR), antigen fragments in association with MHC molecules (Fig. 10.14). In general terms, CD4 positive (CD4$^+$) cells produce molecules, lymphokines, that stimulate and support the production of immune system cells while the CD8$^+$ fraction are involved in the destruction of virally infected cells.

Viruses replicate within host cells. During this process fragments of viral proteins become associated with MHC class I molecules and these complexes are then transported to the surface of the infected cell. The CD8 T cell recognizes this

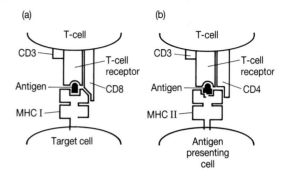

Fig. 10.14 Molecules involved in T cell recognition.
a. Antigen fragments that associate with class I molecules are recognized by T cells that have the CD8 molecule.
b. Antigen fragments that associate with MHC class II are recognized by T cells that have the CD4 molecule on their surface.

complex and destroys the infected cell before it can release progeny virus. If the T cell could bind intact proteins not associated with MHC products, then free virus would also bind, and the elimination of the infected cell and the vast number of viruses it could produce would be inhibited. Thus, MHC-restricted recognition of peptide fragments is responsible for directing the effector cells on to infected targets. These cytotoxic cells are also capable of destroying tissue grafts from MHC-incompatible donors.

The CD4$^+$ cells produce molecules that stimulate growth and differentiation of cells. These molecules are most effective over short distances since they will be more concentrated. This will happen when the two cells involved are actually joined together or in close proximity. The stimulation of CD4$^+$ T cells by antigen fragments on the surface of a responsive cell, or on a cell in the vicinity of a responsive cell, will greatly increase the effectiveness of the messenger molecules produced by the T cell.

RECOMMENDED READING

Paul W E 1989 *Fundamental Immunology* 2nd edn. Raven Press, New York
Roitt I 1989 *Essential Immunology* 6th edn. Blackwell Scientific Publishers, Oxford

Weir D M, Stewart J 1992 *Immunology* 7th edn. Churchill Livingstone, Edinburgh

11

Innate and acquired immunity

J. Stewart and D. M. Weir

The environment contains a vast number of potentially infectious organisms — viruses, bacteria, fungi, protozoa and worms. Any of these can cause damage if they multiply unchecked and many could kill the host. However, the majority of infections in the normal individual are of limited duration and leave very little permanent damage. This fortunate occurrence is due largely to the *immune system.*

The immune system is split into two functional divisions. *Innate immunity* is the first line of defence against infectious agents and most potential pathogens are checked before they establish an overt infection. If these defences are breached the acquired immune system is called into play. *Acquired immunity* produces a specific response to each infectious agent and the effector mechanisms generated normally eradicate the offending material. Furthermore, the adaptive immune system remembers the particular infectious agent and can prevent it causing disease later.

THE IMMUNE SYSTEM

The immune system consists of a number of organs and several different cell types. All the cells of the immune system, tissue cells and white blood cells or *leucocytes,* develop from pluripotent stem cells in the bone marrow. These haemopoietic stem cells also give rise to the red blood cells or *erythrocytes.* The production of leucocytes is through two main pathways of differentiation (Fig. 11.1). The *lymphoid* lineage produces T lymphocytes and B lymphocytes while the *myeloid* pathway gives rise to mononuclear and polymorphonuclear leucocytes as well as platelets and mast cells. Platelets are involved in blood clotting and inflammation while mast cells are similar to basophils but are found in tissues. There is a third population of lymphocytes, also known as null cells or non-T, non-B cells that develop along an unknown pathway.

Lymphoid cells

Lymphocytes make up about 20% of the white blood cells present in the adult circulation. Mature

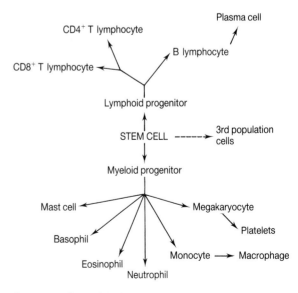

Fig. 11.1   Cells of the immune system.

lymphoid cells are long lived and may survive for many years as memory cells. These mononuclear cells are heterogeneous in size and morphology. The typical small lymphocytes are agranular and comprise the T and B cell populations. The larger cells are referred to as large granular lymphocytes because they contain cytoplasmic granules. Cells within this population are able to kill certain tumour and virally infected cells (natural killing) and destroy cells coated with immunoglobulin (antibody-dependent cell-mediated cytotoxicity).

Morphologically it is quite difficult to distinguish between the different lymphoid cells and impossible to differentiate the subclasses of T cell. Since these cells carry out different processes they possess molecules on their surface unique to that functional requirement. These molecules, referred to as markers, can be used to distinguish between different cell types and also identify cells at different stages of differentiation. The different cell surface molecules have been systematically named by the CD (cluster of differentiation) system and some of those expressed by different T cell populations are shown in Table 11.1. These CD markers are identified using specific monoclonal antibodies. The presence of these specific antibodies on the cell surface is then visualized using labelled antibodies that recognize the first antibody.

Myeloid cells

The second pathway of development gives rise to a variety of cell types of different morphology and function.

Mononuclear phagocytes

The common myeloid progenitor in the bone marrow gives rise to *monocytes* that circulate in the blood and migrate into organs and tissues to become *macrophages*. The human blood monocyte is larger than a lymphocyte and usually has a kidney-shaped nucleus. This actively phagocytic cell has a ruffled membrane and many cytoplasmic granules. These *lysosomes* contain enzymes and molecules that are involved in the killing of

Table 11.1 Major T lymphocyte markers

Marker	Distribution	Proposed function
CD2	All T cells	Adherence to target cell
CD3	All T cells	Part of T cell antigen receptor
CD4	Helper subset (T_H)	MHC class II-restricted recognition
CD5	All T cells	Unknown
CD7	All T cells	Unknown
CD8	Cytotoxic subset (T_C)	MHC class I-restricted recognition

micro-organisms. Mononuclear phagocytes adhere strongly to surfaces and have various cell membrane receptors to aid the binding and ingestion of foreign material. Their activities can be enhanced by molecules produced by T lymphocytes, called *lymphokines*. Macrophages and monocytes are capable of producing various complement components, prostaglandins, interferons and *monokines* such as interleukin-1 and tumour necrosis factor. Lymphokines and monokines are collectively known as *cytokines*.

Polymorphonuclear leucocytes

These cells are sometimes referred to as *granulocytes* and are short-lived cells (2–3 d) compared to macrophages which may survive for months or years. They comprise 60–70% of the leucocytes but also migrate into tissues in response to injury or infection. The mature forms have a multilobed nucleus and many granules. They are classified as *neutrophils*, *eosinophils* and *basophils* on the basis of their histochemical staining.

Neutrophils are the most abundant circulating granulocyte. Their granules contain numerous microbicidal molecules and the cells enter the tissues when a chemotactic factor is produced, as the result of infection or injury.

Eosinophils are also phagocytic cells, although they appear to be less efficient than neutrophils. They are present in low numbers in a healthy, normal individual (1–2% of leucocytes) but their numbers rise in certain allergic conditions. The granule contents can be released by the appropriate signal and the cytotoxic molecules can then kill parasites that are too large to be phagocytosed.

Basophils are found in extremely small numbers in the circulation (<0.2%) and have certain characteristics in common with tissue *mast cells*. Both cell types have receptors on their surface for the Fc portion of IgE and cross-linking of this immunoglobulin by antigen leads to the release of various pharmacological mediators. These molecules stimulate an inflammatory response. There are two types of mast cell; one is found in connective tissue and the other is mucosa associated. Mast cells and basophils are both bone marrow derived but their developmental relationship is not clear.

Platelets

Platelets are also derived from myeloid progenitors. In addition to their role in clotting they are involved in inflammation.

INNATE IMMUNITY

The healthy individual is protected from potentially harmful micro-organisms in the environment by a number of very effective mechanisms, present from birth, that do not depend upon prior exposure to any particular micro-organism. The innate defence mechanisms are non-specific in the sense that they are effective against a wide range of potentially infectious agents. The characteristics and constituents of innate and acquired immunity are shown in Table 11.2.

Determinants of innate immunity

Species and strains

Marked differences exist in the susceptibility of different species to infective agents. The rat is strikingly resistant to diphtheria whilst the guinea-pig and man are highly susceptible. The rabbit is particularly susceptible to myxomatosis and man to syphilis, leprosy and meningococcal meningitis. Susceptibility to an infection does not always imply a lack of resistance to disease caused by the micro-organism. For example, although man is highly susceptible to the common cold he over-comes the infection within a few days. In some diseases, it may be difficult to initiate the infection but once established the disease can progress rapidly — inferring a lack of resistance. For example, rabies occurs in both man and the dog but is not readily established as the virus does not ordinarily penetrate healthy skin. Once infected, however, both species are unable to overcome the disease. Marked variations in resistance to infection have been noted between different strains of mice and it is possible to breed, by selection, rabbits of low, intermediate and high resistance to experimental tuberculosis.

Individual differences and influence of age

The role of heredity in determining resistance to infection is well illustrated by studies on tuberculosis in twins. If one homozygous twin develops tuberculosis, the other twin has a 3 to 1 chance of developing the disease compared with a 1 in 3 chance if the twins are heterozygous. Sometimes genetically controlled abnormalities are an advantage to the individual in resisting infection as, for example, in a hereditary abnormality of the red blood cells (sickling). These red blood cells cannot be parasitized by *Plasmodium falciparum,* thus conferring a degree of resistance to malaria in the affected individuals.

Table 11.2   Characteristics and determinants of innate and acquired immunity

Innate immunity	Acquired immunity
Non-specific	Specific
No change with repeat exposure	Memory
Mechanical barriers Bactericidal substances Natural flora	
HUMORAL	
Acute phase proteins Interferons Lysozyme Complement	Antibody
CELL MEDIATED	
Natural killer cells Phagocytes	T lymphocytes

Infectious diseases are often more severe in early childhood and in young animals; this higher susceptibility of the young appears to be associated with immaturity of the immunological mechanisms affecting the ability of the lymphoid system to deal with and react to foreign antigens. In certain viral infections, e.g. polio and chickenpox, the clinical illness is more severe in adults than in children. This may be due to a more active immune response producing greater tissue damage. In the elderly, besides a general waning of the activities of the immune system, physical abnormalities (e.g. prostatic enlargement leading to stasis of urine) or long-term exposure to environmental factors (e.g. smoking) are common causes of increased susceptibility to infection.

Hormonal influences and sex

There is decreased resistance to infection in diseases such as diabetes mellitus, hypothyroidism and adrenal dysfunction. The reasons for this decrease have not yet been clarified but may be related to enzyme or hormone activities. It is known that glucocorticoids are anti-inflammatory agents, decreasing the ability of phagocytes to ingest material. They also have beneficial effects of interfering in some way with the toxic effects of bacterial products such as endotoxins.

There are no marked differences in susceptibility to infections between the sexes. Although the overall incidence and death rate from infectious disease is greater in the male than in the female, both infectious hepatitis and whooping cough have a higher morbidity and mortality in females.

Nutritional factors

The adverse effects of poor nutrition on susceptibility to certain infectious agents are not now seriously questioned. Experimental evidence in animals has shown repeatedly that inadequate diet may be correlated with increased susceptibility to a variety of bacterial diseases, associated with decreased phagocytic activity and leucopenia. In the case of viruses which are intracellular parasites, malnutrition might have an effect on virus production, but the usual outcome is enhanced disease due to impaired immune responses, especially the cytotoxic responses.

Mechanisms of innate immunity

Mechanical barriers and surface secretions

The intact skin and mucous membranes of the body afford a high degree of protection against pathogens. In conditions where the skin is damaged, such as in burned patients and after traumatic injury or surgery, infections can be a serious problem. The skin is a resistant barrier because of its outer horny layer consisting mainly of keratin, which is indigestible by most micro-organisms, and thus shields the living cells of the epidermis from micro-organisms and their toxins. The relatively dry condition of the skin and the high concentration of salt in drying sweat are inhibitory or lethal to many micro-organisms.

The sebaceous secretions and sweat of the skin contain bactericidal and fungicidal fatty acids and these constitute an effective protective mechanism against many potential pathogens. The protective ability of these secretions varies at different stages of life and some fungal 'ringworm' infections of children disappear at puberty with the marked increase of sebaceous secretions.

The sticky mucus covering the respiratory tract acts as a trapping mechanism for inhaled particles. The action of cilia sweep the secretions, containing the foreign material, towards the oropharynx so that it is swallowed; in the stomach the acidic secretions destroy most of the micro-organisms present. Nasal secretions and saliva contain mucopolysaccharides capable of blocking some viruses and the tears and the mucous secretions of the respiratory, alimentary and genito-urinary tracts contain lysozyme that is particularly active against some Gram-positive bacteria.

The washing action of tears and flushing of urine are effective in stopping invasion by micro-organisms. The commensal micro-organisms that make up the natural bacterial flora covering epithelial surfaces are protective in a number of ways: (1) their very presence uses up a niche that cannot be used by a pathogen; (2) they compete for nutrients and also produce by-products that can inhibit the growth of other organisms. It is important not to disturb the relationship between the host and its indigenous flora.

Commensal organisms from the gut or bacteria normally present on the skin can cause problems if they gain access to an area that they do not normally populate. An example of this is urinary tract infections resulting from the introduction of *Escherichia coli,* a gut commensal, by means of a urinary catheter. Commensal organisms that are provided with the circumstances by which to cause infections are called *opportunistic pathogens.* Infections with these opportunists are quite widespread, often appearing as a result of medical or surgical treatment which breaches the innate defences or reduces the host's ability to respond.

Humoral defence mechanisms

A number of microbicidal substances are present in the tissue and body fluids. Some of these molecules are produced constitutively, e.g. lysozyme, and others are produced in response to infection, e.g. acute-phase proteins and interferon. These molecules all show the characteristics of innate immunity — there is no specific recognition of the micro-organism and the response is not enhanced on re-exposure to the same antigen.

Lysozyme. This is a basic protein of low molecular weight found in relatively high concentrations in neutrophils as well as in most tissue fluids, except cerebrospinal fluid, sweat and urine. It functions as a mucolytic enzyme, splitting sugars off the structural peptidoglycan of the cell wall of many Gram-positive bacteria and thus causing their lysis. It seems likely that lysozyme may also play a role in the intracellular destruction of some Gram-negative bacteria. In many pathogenic bacteria the peptidoglycan of the cell wall appears to be protected from the access of lysozyme by other wall components, e.g. lipopolysaccharide. The action of other enzymes from phagocytes or of complement may be needed to remove this protection and expose the peptidoglycan to the action of lysozyme.

Basic polypeptides. A variety of basic proteins, derived from tissues and blood cells, have some antibacterial properties. This group includes the basic proteins called spermine and spermidine, which can kill tubercle bacilli and some staphylococci. Other toxic compounds are the arginine- and lysine-containing proteins protamine and histone. The bactericidal activity of basic polypeptides probably depends on their ability to react non-specifically with acid polysaccharides at the bacterial cell surface.

Acute-phase proteins. The concentration of acute-phase proteins rises dramatically during an infection. Microbial products such as endotoxin can stimulate macrophages to release endogenous interleukin-1, which stimulates the liver to produce increased amounts of various acute-phase proteins, the concentrations of which can rise over 1000-fold. One of the best-characterized acute-phase proteins is *C-reactive protein,* which binds to phosphorylcholine residues in the cell wall of certain micro-organisms. This complex is very effective at activating the classical complement pathway. Also included in this group of molecules are α_1-antitrypsin, α_2-macroglobulin, fibrinogen and serum amyloid A protein, all of which act to limit the spread of the infectious agent or stimulate the host response.

Interferon. The observation that cell cultures infected with one virus resist infection by a second virus, i.e. viral interference, led to the identification of the family of antiviral agents known as *interferons*. A number of molecules have been identified; α and β interferons are part of innate immunity and γ interferon is produced by T cells as part of the acquired immune response (see Chapter 12).

Complement

The existence of a heat-labile serum component with the ability to lyse red blood cells and destroy Gram-negative bacteria has been known for over 60 years. The chemical complexity of the phenomenon was not appreciated by early workers who ascribed the activity to a single component, called complement. Complement is in fact an extremely complex group of serum proteins present in low concentration in normal serum. These molecules are present in an inactive form but can be activated to form an enzyme cascade, i.e. the product of the first reaction is the catalyst of the next and so on. Complement comprises nine functional components denoted C1 to C9, of which there are further subdivisions.

There are about 20 proteins involved in the complement system, some of which are enzymes, some are control molecules and others are structural proteins with no enzymic activity. A number of the molecules involved are split into two components (a and b fragments) by the product of the previous step. There are two pathways of complement activation, the alternative and classical, that lead to the same physiological consequences — opsonization, cellular activation and lysis — but use different initiation processes. Component C3 forms the connection between the two pathways and the binding of this molecule to a surface is the key process in complement activation.

Classical pathway. The classical pathway of activation leading to the cleavage of C3 is initiated by the binding of two or more of the globular domains of the C1q component of C1 to its ligand–immune complexes containing IgG or IgM and certain micro-organisms and their products. This causes a conformational change in the C1 complex that leads to the auto-activation of C1r. The enzyme C1r then converts C1s into an active serine esterase that acts on the thioester-containing molecule C4 to produce C4a and a reactive C4b (Fig. 11.2). C4a is released and less than 1% of the C4b becomes attached to a surface. The rest is inactivated by reacting with water. C2 binds to the surface-bound C4b, becomes a substrate for the activated C1 complex and is split into C2a and C2b. The C2b is released leaving C4b2a — the classical pathway C3 convertase. This active enzyme then generates C3a and the unstable C3b from C3. A small amount of the C3b generated will bind to the activating surface and act as a focus for further complement activation. The activation of the classical pathway is regulated by C1 inhibitor and by a number of molecules that limit the production of the 'C3 convertase'.

Alternative pathway. Intrinsically, C3 undergoes a low level of hydrolysis of an internal thioester bond to generate C3b. This molecule complexes, in the presence of Mg^{2+} ions, with factor B, which is then acted on by factor D to produce C3bBb. This is a 'C3 convertase' that is capable of splitting more C3 to C3b, some of which will become membrane bound.

The initial binding of C3b generated by either the classical or alternative pathway leads to an amplification loop that results in the binding of many more C3b molecules to the same surface. Factor B binds to the surface-bound C3b to form C3bB, the substrate for factor D — a serine esterase — that is present in very low concentrations in an already active form. The cleavage of factor B results in the formation of the C3 convertase, C3bBb, which dissociates rapidly unless it is stabilized by the binding of properdin (P) — forming the complex C3bBbP. This convertase can cleave many more C3 molecules, some of which become surface bound. This amplification loop is a positive-feedback system that will cycle until all the C3 is used up unless it is regulated carefully.

Regulation. The nature of the surface to which the C3b is bound regulates the outcome. Self cell membranes contain a number of regulatory molecules that promote the binding of factor H rather than factor B to C3b. This results in the inhibition of the activation process. On non-self structures the C3b is protected since regulatory proteins are not present, and factor B has a higher affinity for C3b than factor H at these sites.

Thus the surface of many micro-organisms can stabilize the C3bBb by protecting it from factor H. In addition, another molecule, properdin, stabilizes the complex. The deposition of a few molecules of C3b on to these surfaces is followed by the formation of the relatively stable C3bBbP complex. This C3 convertase will lead to more C3b deposition. Immune complexes composed of certain immunoglobulins, e.g. IgA and IgE, also function as protected sites for C3b and activate complement by the alternative pathway. Poor activation surfaces will be made more susceptible to deposition by the presence of antibody that generates C3b by the classical pathway.

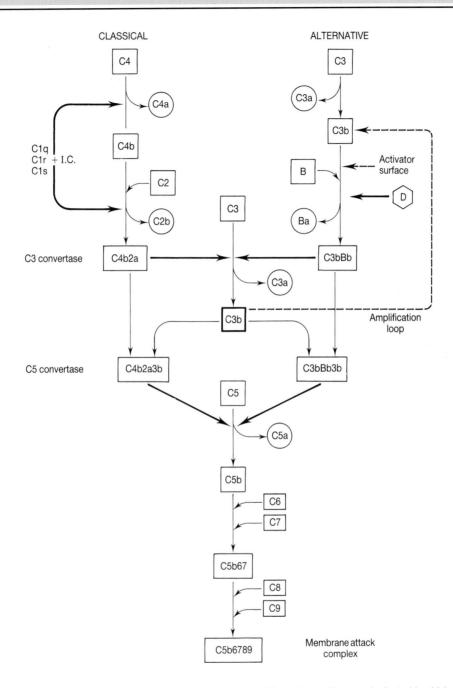

Fig. 11.2 Complement activation: classical and alternative pathways. Enzymic reactions are indicated by thick arrows. I. C., immune complex.

Membrane attack complex. The next step after the formation of C3b is the cleavage of C5 (Fig. 11.3). The 'C5 convertases' are generated from C4b2a of the classical pathway and C3bBb of the alternative pathway by the addition of another C3b molecule. These membrane-bound trimolecular complexes selectively bind C5 and cleave it to give fluid phase C5a and membrane-

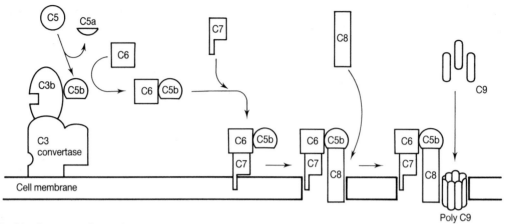

Fig. 11.3 Membrane attack complex.

bound C5b. The formation of the rest of the membrane attack complex is non-enzymic. C6 binds to C5b and this joint complex is released from the C5 convertase. The formation of C5b67 generates a hydrophobic complex that inserts into the lipid bilayer in the vicinity of the initial activation site. Usually this will be on the same cell surface as the initial trigger but occasionally other cells may be involved. Therefore, 'bystander' lysis can take place giving rise to damage to surrounding tissue. There are a number of proteins present in body fluids to limit this potentially dangerous process by binding to fluid phase C5b67. C8 and C9 bind to the membrane-inserted complex in sequence, resulting in the formation of a lytic polymeric complex containing up to 20 C9 monomers. A small amount of lysis can occur when C8 binds to C5b67 but it is the polymerized C9 that causes the most damage.

Functions. The activation of complement by either pathway gives rise to C3b and the generation of a number of factors that can aid in the elimination of foreign material.

The complete insertion of the membrane attack complex into a cell will lead to membrane damage and lysis, probably by osmotic swelling. Some thin-walled pathogens, such as trypanosomes and malaria parasites, are killed by complement-mediated lysis. Some Gram-negative bacteria can be killed by complement in conjunction with lysozyme. However, complement-mediated lysis is of limited importance as a bactericidal mechanism when compared to phagocyte destruction of bacteria. Inherited deficiencies of the terminal components are associated with infection by gonococci and meningococci which can survive inside neutrophils and for which complement-mediated killing is important.

Phagocytic cells have receptors for C3b and iC3b that facilitate the adherence of complement-coated particles. Therefore, complement is an *opsonin* and in certain circumstances this attachment may lead to phagocytosis.

Two of the molecules released during the complement cascade, C3a and C5a, have potent biological activities. These molecules, known as *anaphylatoxins*, trigger mast cells and basophils to release mediators of inflammation (see below). They also stimulate neutrophils to produce reactive oxygen intermediates, while C5a on its own is a chemo-attractant and acts directly on vascular endothelium to cause vasodilation and increased vascular permeability.

Cells

Phagocytes. Micro-organisms entering the tissue fluids or bloodstream are very rapidly engulfed by the *polymorphonuclear leucocytes* or *neutrophils* and the *mononuclear phagocytes*. In the blood the latter are known as *monocytes* while in the tissues they differentiate into *macrophages*. In connective tissue they are known as *histiocytes*, in kidney as *mesangial cells*, in bone as *osteoclasts*, in brain as *microglia* and in the spleen, lymph node and thymus as the *sinus-lining macrophages*.

The three essential features of these cells are that they: (1) are actively phagocytic; (2) contain digestive enzymes to degrade ingested material; and (3) are an important link between the innate and acquired immune mechanisms. Part of their role in regard to acquired immunity is that they can process and present antigens and produce molecules that stimulate lymphocyte differentiation into effector cells.

The role of the phagocyte in innate immunity is to engulf particles (phagocytosis) or soluble material (pinocytosis), and digest them intracellularly within specialized vacuoles. The macrophages present in the walls of capillaries and vascular sinuses in spleen, liver, lungs and bone marrow serve a very important role in clearing the bloodstream of foreign particulate material such as bacteria. So efficient is this process that the finding of a few micro-organisms in the bloodstream usually indicates that there is a continuing release of micro-organisms from an active focus such as an abscess or the heart valve vegetations found in bacterial endocarditis.

The ability of macrophages to ingest and destroy micro-organisms can be impaired or enhanced by depression or stimulation of the phagocyte system. Some micro-organisms such as mycobacteria and brucellae can resist intracellular digestion by normal macrophages, though they may be digested by 'activated' ones.

Chemotaxis. For phagocytic cells to be effective they must be attracted to the site of infection. Once they have passed through the capillary walls they move through the tissues in response to a concentration gradient of molecules that have been produced at the site of damage. These chemotactic factors include products of injured tissue, factors from the blood (C5a), substances produced by neutrophils and mast cells (leukotrienes and histamine) and bacterial products (formyl-methionine peptides). Neutrophils respond first and move faster than monocytes.

Phagocytosis. Phagocytosis involves (1) recognition and binding, (2) ingestion and (3) digestion. It may occur in the absence of antibody, especially on surfaces such as those of the lung alveoli and when inert particles are involved. Cell membranes carry a net negative charge that keeps them apart and stops autophagocytosis. The hydrophilic nature of certain bacterial cell wall components stops them passing through the hydrophobic membrane. To overcome these difficulties the phagocytes have receptors on their surface that mediate the attachment of particles that have been coated with the correct ligand. Phagocytes have receptors for the Fc portion of certain immunoglobulin isotypes and for some components of the complement cascade. The presence of these molecules or *opsonins* on the particle surface markedly enhances the ingestion process and, in some cases, digestion. Whether mediated by specific receptors or not, the foreign particle is surrounded by the cell membrane, which then invaginates and produces an *endosome* or *phagosome* within the cell (Fig. 11.4).

The microbicidal machinery of the phagocyte is contained within organelles known as *lysosomes*. This compartmentalization of potentially toxic molecules is necessary to protect the cell from

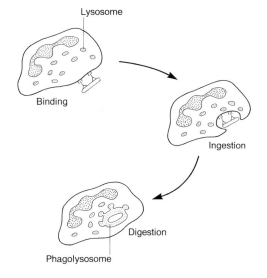

Fig. 11.4 Stages in phagocytosis.

self-destruction and produce an environment where the molecules can function efficiently. The phagosome and lysosome fuse to form a *phagolysosome* in which the ingested material is killed and digested by various enzyme systems.

Ingestion is accompanied by enhanced glycolysis and an increase in the synthesis of proteins and membrane phospholipids. After phagocytosis there is a respiratory burst consisting of a steep rise in oxygen consumption. This is accompanied by an increase in the activity of a number of enzymes and leads to the reduction of molecular oxygen to various highly reactive intermediates, e.g. the superoxide anion (O_2^-.), hydrogen peroxide (H_2O_2), singlet oxygen (O.) and the hydroxyl radical (OH.). All these chemical species have microbicidal activity and are termed oxygen-dependent killing mechanisms. The superoxide anion is a free radical produced by the one-electron reduction of molecular oxygen; it is very reactive and highly damaging to animal cells, as well as to micro-organisms. It is also the substrate for superoxide dismutase that generates hydrogen peroxide for subsequent use in microbial killing. Myeloperoxidase uses hydrogen peroxide and halide ions, such as iodide or chloride, to produce at least two bactericidal systems. In one, halogenation (incorporation of iodine or chlorine) of the bacterial cell wall leads to death of the organism. In the second mechanism, myeloperoxidase and hydrogen peroxide damage the cell wall by converting amino acids into aldehydes that have antimicrobial activity.

A number of oxygen-independent mechanisms are also present within phagocytes that are capable of destroying ingested material. Some of these enzymes can damage membranes. For example, *lysozyme* and *elastase* attack peptidoglycan of the bacterial cell wall and then hydrolases are responsible for the complete digestion of the killed organism. The cationic proteins of lysosomes bind to and damage bacterial cell walls and enveloped viruses, such as herpes simplex virus. The iron-binding protein *lactoferrin* has antimicrobial properties. It complexes with iron, rendering it unavailable to bacteria that require iron for growth. The high acidity within phagolysosomes (pH 3.5–4.0) may have bactericidal effects: it probably results from lactic acid production in glycolysis. In addition, many lysosomal enzymes, such as acid hydrolases, have acid pH optima. There are significant differences between macrophages and neutrophils in the killing of micro-organisms. Although macrophage lysosomes contain a variety of enzymes, including lysozyme, they lack cationic proteins and lactoferrin. Tissue macrophages do not have myeloperoxidase but probably use catalase to generate the hydrogen peroxide system. Normal macrophages are less efficient killers of certain pathogens, such as fungi, than neutrophils. The microbicidal activity of macrophages can, however, be greatly improved after contact with products of lymphocytes, known as lymphokines.

Once killed, most micro-organisms are digested and solubilized by lysosomal enzymes. The degradation products are then released to the exterior.

Natural killer cells. Natural killer cells (NK cells) recognize changes on virus-infected cells and destroy them by an extracellular killing mechanism. After binding to the target cell, by an as yet undefined mechanism, the NK cell produces molecules that damage the membrane of the infected cell, leading to its destruction.

Natural killing can be performed by a number of different cell types. This activity has been shown to be carried out by cells described as large granular lymphocytes and also by cells with T cell markers, macrophage markers and others that do not have the characteristics of any of the main cells of the immune system. Natural killing is present without prior exposure to the infectious agent and shows all the characteristics of an innate defence mechanism. NK cells have also been implicated in host defence against cancers. They are thought to recognize changes in the cell membranes of transformed cells in a mechanism similar to that used to combat virus infection. Natural killing is enhanced by interferons which appear to stimulate the production of NK cells and also increase the rate at which they kill the target cells.

Eosinophils. Eosinophils are polymorphonuclear leucocytes with a characteristic bilobed nucleus and cytoplasmic granules. They are present in the blood of normal individuals at very low levels (<1%) but their numbers increase in patients with parasitic infections and allergies. They are not efficient phagocytic cells but their granules contain molecules that are toxic to parasites. Large parasites such as helminths cannot be internalized by phagocytes and therefore must be killed extracellularly. Eosinophil granules contain an array of enzymes and toxic molecules that are active against parasitic worms. The release of these molecules must be controlled so that tissue damage can be avoided. The eosinophils have specific receptors, including Fc and complement receptors, that bind the labelled target, i.e. antibody or complement-coated parasites. The granule contents are then released into the space between the cell and the parasite, thus targeting the toxic molecules onto the parasite membrane.

Temperature

The temperature dependence of many micro-organisms is well known and it is therefore apparent that temperature is an important factor in determining the innate immunity of an animal to some infectious agents. It seems likely that the pyrexia that follows so many different types of infection can function as a protective response against the infecting micro-organism. The febrile response in many cases is controlled by interleukin-1 produced by macrophages as part of the immune response.

Inflammation

A number of the above factors are responsible for the process of *inflammation*. This is the reaction of the body to injury, such as invasion by an infectious agent, exposure to a noxious chemical or physical trauma. The signs of inflammation are redness, heat, swelling, pain and loss of function. The molecular and cellular events that occur during an inflammatory reaction are: (1) vasodilation, (2) increased vascular permeability and (3) cellular infiltration. These changes are brought about mainly by chemical mediators (Table 11.3) that are widely distributed in a sequestered or inactive form throughout the body and are released or activated locally at the site of inflammation. After release they tend to be rapidly inactivated to ensure control of the inflammatory process.

There is increased blood supply to the affected area due to the action of vaso-active amines such as histamine and 5-hydroxytryptamine and other mediators stored within mast cells. These molecules are released (1) as a consequence of the production of the anaphylatoxins (C3a and C5a) that trigger specific receptors on mast cells and

Table 11.3 Mediators of inflammation

Mediator	Main source	Function
Histamine[a]	Mast cells and basophils	Vasodilation, increased vascular permeability, contraction of smooth muscle
Kinins (e.g. bradykinin)	Plasma	Vasodilation, increased vascular permeability, contraction of smooth muscle, pain
Prostaglandins	Neutrophils, eosinophils, monocytes, platelets	Vasodilation, increased vascular permeability, pain
Leukotrienes	Neutrophils, mast cells, basophils	Vasodilation, increased vascular permeability, contraction of smooth muscle, induce cell adherence and chemotaxis
Complement components (e.g. C3a, C5a)	Plasma	Cause mast cells to release mediator C5a is chemotactic factor
Plasmin	Plasma	Break down fibrin, kinin formation
Cytokines	Lymphocytes, macrophages	Chemotactic factors, colony stimulation factors, macrophage activation

[a] In rodents 5-hydroxytryptamine (serotonin) is present in mast cells and basophils.

(2) following interaction of antigen with IgE on the surface of mast cells or (3) by direct physical damage to the cells. Other mediators, such as bradykinins and prostaglandins, are produced locally or released by platelets. The vasodilation causes increased blood supply to the area, giving rise to redness and heat. The result is an increase in the supply of the molecules and cells that can combat the agent responsible for the initial trigger.

The same molecules, vaso-active amines, prostaglandins and kinins, increase vascular permeability allowing plasma and plasma proteins to traverse the endothelial lining. The plasma proteins will include immunoglobulins and molecules of the clotting and complement cascades. This leaking of fluid will cause swelling (oedema) that will in turn lead to increased tissue tension and pain. Some of the molecules themselves, e.g. prostaglandins and histamine, stimulate the pain responses directly. The inflammatory exudate has several important functions. Bacteria often produce tissue-damaging toxins that will be diluted by the exudate. Clotting factors present result in the deposition of fibrin, creating a physical obstruction to the spread of bacteria. The exudate is continuously drained off by the lymphatic vessels, and antigens, such as bacteria and their toxins, are carried to the draining lymph node where immune responses can be generated.

Chemotactic factors produced, including C5a, histamine, leukotrienes and molecules specific for certain cell types, will attract phagocytic cells to the site. The increased vascular permeability will allow easier access for neutrophils and monocytes and the vasodilation means that more cells are in the vicinity. The neutrophils will arrive first and begin to destroy or remove the offending agent. Most will be successful but a few will die, releasing their tissue-damaging contents to increase the inflammatory process. Mononuclear phagocytes will arrive on the scene to finish off the removal of the residual debris and stimulate tissue repair.

When the swelling is severe there may be loss of function to the affected area. If the offending agent is quickly removed then the tissue will soon be repaired. The inflammatory process continues until the conditions responsible for its initiation are resolved. In most circumstances this occurs fairly rapidly with an acute inflammatory reaction lasting a matter of hours or days. If, however, the causative agent is not easily removed or is reintroduced continuously then chronic inflammation will ensue with the possibility of tissue destruction and complete loss of function.

ACQUIRED IMMUNITY

Micro-organisms that overcome or circumvent the innate non-specific defence mechanisms or are administered deliberately, i.e. active vaccination, come up against the host's second line of defence — *acquired immunity*. To give expression to this acquired form of immunity it is necessary that the antigens of the invading micro-organism should come into contact with cells of the immune system (macrophages and lymphocytes) and so initiate an immune response specific for the foreign material. The cells that respond are precommitted, because of their surface receptors, to respond to a particular epitope on the antigen. This response takes two forms, *humoral and cell mediated*, which usually develop in parallel. The part played by each will depend on a number of factors, including the nature of the antigen, the route of entry and the individual who is infected.

Humoral immunity depends on the appearance in the blood of antibodies produced by plasma cells.

The term 'cell-mediated immunity' was orginally coined to describe localized reactions to organisms mediated by T lymphocytes and phagocytes rather than by antibody. It is now used to describe any response in which antibody plays a subordinate role. Cell-mediated immunity depends mainly on the development of T cells that are specifically responsive to the inducing agent and is generally active against intracellular organisms.

Specific immunity may be acquired in two main ways. (1) It may be induced by overt clinical infection, inapparent clinical infection or deliberate artificial immunization. This is *active acquired immunity* and contrasts with (2) *passive acquired immunity* which is the transfer of preformed antibodies to a non-immune individual by means of blood, serum components or lymphoid cells.

Actively acquired immunity is long-lasting although it may be circumvented by antigenic change in the infecting micro-organism. *Passively acquired immunity* provides only temporary protection. Passive immunity may be transferred to the fetus by the passage of maternal antibodies across the placenta.

Tissues involved in immune reactions

For the generation of an immune response, antigen must interact with and activate a number of different cells. In addition, these cells must interact with each other. The cells involved in immune responses are organized into tissues and organs in order that these complex cellular interactions can occur most effectively. These structures are collectively referred to as the *lymphoid system*, which comprises lymphocytes, epithelial and stromal cells arranged into discrete capsulated organs or accumulations of diffuse lymphoid tissue. Lymphoid organs contain lymphocytes at various stages of development and are classified into primary and secondary lymphoid organs.

The primary lymphoid organs are the major sites of lymphopoiesis. Here, lymphocytes differentiate from lymphoid progenitor cells, proliferate and mature. In mammals, T lymphocytes develop in the thymus and B lymphocytes in the bone marrow (fetal liver). It is in the primary lymphoid organs that the lymphocytes acquire their repertoire of specific antigen receptors in order to cope with the antigenic challenges that the individual receives during its life. The ability to differentiate between self and non-self is also acquired in these tissues.

The secondary lymphoid organs create the environment in which lymphocytes can interact with each other and with antigen and then disseminate the effector cells and molecules generated. Secondary lymphoid organs include lymph nodes, spleen and mucosal-associated lymphoid tissue, e.g. tonsils and Peyer's patches of the gut. These organs have a characteristic structure which relates to the function they carry out, with areas composed mainly of B cells and others of T cells.

Development of the immune system

In man, lymphoid tissue appears first in the thymus at about 8 weeks of gestation. Peyer's patches are distinguishable by the 5th month and immunoglobulin-secreting cells appear in the spleen and lymph nodes at about 20 weeks. From this period onwards, IgM and IgD are synthesized by the fetus (Fig. 11.5). At birth the infant has a blood concentration of IgG comparable to that of the maternal circulation, having received IgG but not IgM via the placenta. The rate of synthesis of IgM in the infant increases rapidly within the first few days of life but does not reach adult levels until about a year. This compares with a much slower rise in IgG and IgA, which do not reach adult levels for some considerable time. Serum IgG does not reach adult levels until after the second year and IgA takes even longer. There is an actual drop in the level of IgG from birth due to the decay of maternal antibody with lowest levels of total IgG at around 3 months of age. This corresponds to an age of marked susceptibility to a number of infections. Cell-mediated

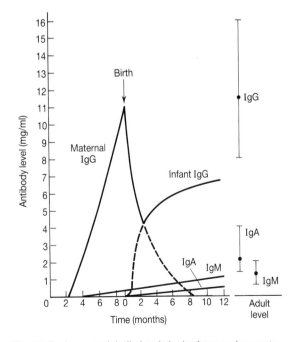

Fig. 11.5 Immunoglobulin levels in the fetus and neonate. The adult levels of the major isotypes are shown as normal ranges with mean serum levels (•).

immunity can be stimulated at birth but these reactions may not be as powerful as in the adult.

Lymphocyte trafficking

Lymphocytes differentiate and mature in the primary lymphoid organs and then enter the blood lymphocyte pool. B cells are produced in the bone marrow and mature there before proceeding via the circulation to the secondary lymphoid organs. T-cell precursors leave the bone marrow and mature in the thymus before migrating to the secondary lymphoid organs. Once in the secondary lymphoid tissues the lymphocytes do not remain there but move from one lymphoid organ to another through the blood and lymphatics (Fig. 11.6). One of the main advantages of this *lymphocyte recirculation* is that during the course of a natural infection the continual trafficking of lymphocytes enables very many different lymphocytes to have access to the antigen. The passage of lymphocytes through an area where antigen has been localized and concentrated on the dendritic processes of macrophages or on the surface of antigen-presenting cells facilitates the induction of an immune response.

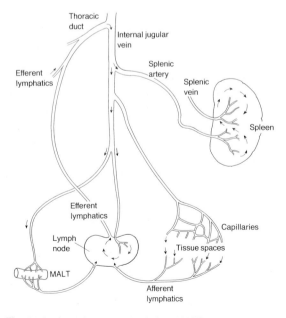

Fig. 11.6 Lymphocyte recirculation. MALT, mucosal-associated lymphoid tissue.

Another possible role of this recirculation process is that it can be used to replenish the lymphoid tissue of, for example, the spleen that might have been depleted by infection or trauma.

There are three main areas where the migration or transfer of lymphocytes from the blood takes place: lymph nodes and Peyer's patches; the spleen; and the peripheral blood vessels. Under normal conditions there is a continuous active flow of lymphocytes through lymph nodes, but when antigen and antigen-reactive cells enter there is a temporary shutdown of the exit. Thus, antigen specific cells are preferentially retained in the node draining the source of the antigen. This is partly responsible for the swollen glands (lymph nodes) that can sometimes be found during an infection.

There is now evidence for non-random migration of lymphocytes to particular lymphoid compartments. For example, lymphocytes that home to the gut are selectively transported across endothelial cells of venules in the intestine. It appears that lymphocytes have specific molecules on their surface that preferentially interact with endothelial cells in different anatomical sites. A lymphocyte that was initially stimulated by antigen in a Peyer's patch will migrate to the draining lymph node, respond and memory cells will be produced. It is important that these memory cells migrate back to the area where the same pathogen might be encountered again. Therefore, they are found preferentially in the mucosal-associated lymphoid tissue.

The flow of lymphocytes from the circulation will be increased if, for example, a local granuloma is formed in response to some foreign agent; then the migration from blood to lymph can be as great as in the lymph nodes themselves.

In the spleen, small lymphocytes seem to enter the peri-arteriolar lymphoid sheath from the blood, passing between the cells rather than through them. The cells later re-enter the blood within the spleen rather than leaving via the lymphatics.

Clonal selection

During their development in the primary lymphoid tissues both T and B lymphocytes acquire specific cell surface receptors that commit them to a single antigenic specificity. For T cells this receptor will remain the same for its life but the surface immunoglobulin on B cells can be modified due to somatic mutations. In the B cell this is mirrored in the modification of the antibody the cell produces on exposure to its specific antigen. The cell is activated when it binds its specific antigen, the lymphocytes then proliferate, differentiate and mature into effector cells.

Each lymphocyte produced has a unique receptor capable of recognizing a particularly shaped epitope. Since the immune system can specifically recognize a very large number of antigens this means that the lymphocytes reactive to any particular antigen are only a small proportion of the total pool. Therefore, antigen binds to the small number of cells that can recognize it and *selects* them to proliferate and mature so that sufficient cells are formed to mount an adequate immune response. A cell that responds to an antigenic trigger and proliferates will give rise to daughter cells with a genetically identical make-up, i.e. *clones*. Therefore, this phenomenon is known as *clonal selection*.

Lymphocyte receptors appear to be created in a random fashion so there is no reason why they should not recognize 'self' molecules. It is obviously an important attribute of the immune system that it is able to discriminate between 'self' and 'non-self'.

Cellular activation

When an individual is exposed to foreign material, those cells with receptors that recognize antigenic determinants are selected to respond. B lymphocytes proliferate and differentiate into antibody-producing plasma cells and memory cells. T lymphocytes are stimulated to become effector cells that can directly eliminate the foreign material or produce molecules that help other cells destroy the pathogen. The type (immunity or tolerance) and magnitude of the response, if generated, will depend on a number of factors, including the nature, dose and route of entry of the antigen and the individual's genetic make-up and previous exposure to the antigen.

The first stage in the production of effector cells and molecules is the activation of the resting cells. This involves various cellular interactions with maturation of the response, leading to a co-ordinated, efficient production of effector T cells, immunoglobulin and memory cells.

B cell activation

Cross-linking of the B cell antigen receptor, surface immunoglobulin, is the initial trigger for activation. When this happens a number of biochemical changes are instigated, including stimulation of phosphatidyl inositol turnover and mobilization of intracellular Ca^{2+} ions. These changes probably act through protein kinases that cause the synthesis of RNA and ultimately immunoglobulin production. In a number of cases this is all that is required to stimulate antibody production. However, for the majority of antigens this initial cross-linking is not enough and molecules produced by T cells are also required.

Thymus-independent antigens. A number of antigens will stimulate specific immunoglobulin production directly. These T independent antigens are of two types: *mitogens* and certain large molecules.

Mitogens (Table 11.4) are substances that cause cells, particularly lymphocytes, to undergo cell division, i.e. proliferation. Certain glycoproteins, called lectins, have mitogenic activity. These molecules have specificity for sugars and bind to the cell surface and will activate all responsive cells. The response to the mitogens will therefore be polyclonal since lymphocytes of many different specificities will be activated. However, at low concentrations these *mitogens* do not cause polyclonal activation but can lead to the stimulation of specific B cells.

Some large molecules with regularly repeating epitopes, e.g. polymers of D-amino acids and simple sugars such as pneumococcal polysaccharide and dextran, can interact directly with the B cell surface immunoglobulin. They may also be held on the surface of specialized macrophages in secondary lymphoid tissues and the B cells interact with them there. The multiple repeats of the epitope interact with a large number

Table 11.4 Lymphocyte mitogens

Mitogen	Sugar specificity	Cell type activated[a]
Phytohaemagglutinin	Oligosaccharides	T lymphocyte
Concanavalin A	α-Methyl-D-mannose	T lymphocyte
Pokeweed mitogen	N-acetyl glucosamine	T and B lymphocytes
Lipopolysaccharide	—	B lymphocytes

[a] Ability to stimulate selectively varies with species and cell source, suggesting that only a subpopulation is capable of responding to mitogens.

of surface immunoglobulin molecules and the signal that is generated is sufficient to stimulate antibody production.

The immune response generated to these antigens tends to be similar on each exposure, i.e. IgM is the main antibody and the response shows little memory. This suggests that class switch and memory production require additional factors.

Thymus-dependent antigens. Many antigens do not stimulate antibody production without the help of T lymphocytes. These antigens first bind to the B cell, which must then be exposed to T cell-derived lymphokines, i.e. helper factors, before antibody can be produced. For the second activation signal, i.e. help, to be effectively targeted at the B cell the T and B cell epitopes must both be physically linked. However, T cells only recognize antigen that has been processed and is presented in association with products of the major histocompatibility complex (MHC). So it is impossible for native antigen to form a bridge between surface immunoglobulin and the T cell receptor. The B cell binds to its epitope on free antigen but there is no site on this molecule that the T cell can bind to since it requires antigen associated with MHC products. The answer to this problem can be seen when the requirements for antigen presentation in T cell recognition are considered.

Antigen processing and presentation

The development of an antibody response to a T-dependent antigen requires that the antigen becomes associated with MHC class II molecules, i.e. *processed*, and expressed on the cell surface, i.e. *presented*, in a form that helper T cells can recognize.

All cells express MHC class I molecules but class II molecules are confined to cells of the immune system — the antigen-presenting cells. These cells present antigen to MHC class II-restricted T cells (CD4 positive (CD4$^+$) population) and therefore play a key role in the induction and development of immune responses. Within lymph nodes, different antigen-presenting cells are found in each of the main areas (Table 11.5).

There are a large number of antigen-presenting cells in the body (Table 11.6), most of which constitutively express MHC class II molecules. Other cells, like T lymphocytes and endothelium, can be induced to express MHC class II molecules by suitable stimuli such as lymphokines. The relative importance of each type depends on whether a primary or secondary response is being stimulated and on the location. The most studied antigen-presenting cells are the macrophages and dendritic cells. However, it is now apparent that in certain situations B cells may be important

Table 11.5 Antigen-presenting cells in the lymph nodes

Area	Antigen-presenting cell	Antigen
Subcapsular marginal sinus	Marginal zone macrophage	T-independent antigens
Follicles and B cell areas	Follicular dendritic cells	Antigen–antibody complexes
Medulla	Classical macrophages	Most antigens
T cell areas	Interdigitating dendritic cells	Most antigens

Table 11.6 Antigen-presenting cells

Group	Type	Location	MHC class II expression
Phagocytic cells	Monocytes	Blood	
	Macrophages	Tissues	
	Marginal zone macrophages	Spleen and lymph node	+
	Kupffer cells	Liver	
	Microglia	Brain	++++
Lymphocytes	B cells	Lymphoid tissue and site of	+ → +++
	T cells	immune responses	0 → ++
Non-phagocytic constitutive presenters	Langerhan's cells	Skin	++
	Interdigitating cells	Lymphoid tissue	++
	Follicular dendritic cells	Lymphoid tissue	0
Facultative presenters	Astrocytes	Brain	
	Follicular cells	Thyroid	0
	Endothelium	Vascular and lymphoid tissue	
	Fibroblasts	Connective tissue	++

Level of MHC class II expression is indicated by number of + signs: 0 = none present. Arrow indicates that MHC class II is inducible.

antigen-presenting cells. The relative importance of B cells becomes greatest during secondary responses, especially if the antigen concentration is low. Here the B cells can specifically engulf antigen via their surface immunoglobulin. In a primary response, specific B cells are at a low frequency and their receptors are of low affinity; in this situation macrophages and dendritic cells are probably most important.

The key feature of all antigen-presenting cells is that they can ingest antigen, degrade it and present it, in the context of MHC class II molecules, to T cells (Fig. 11.7).

Mitogens and T-independent antigens have an inherent ability to drive B cells into division and differentiation. T-dependent responses rely on T cells and their products to control the antibody class, affinity and memory. The first cells to be activated are CD4$^+$ T cells that recognize the antigen in association with MHC class II molecules. These cells respond to the signal of the antigen fragment–MHC complex and produce a variety of lymphokines that act on B cells and other cell types, including macrophages, T cells that mediate cytotoxicity and endothelial cells.

As far as B cell development is concerned, the antigen-stimulated cells develop under the influence of interleukin-4 (previously known as B cell stimulation factor) that is produced by closely adherent T cells or by T cells in the vicinity, i.e. when the antigen-presenting cell is not a B cell. Interleukin-5 and interleukin-6 then bring the cells to a state of full activation with terminal differentiation into an immunoglobulin-producing plasma cell. The characteristics of various inter-

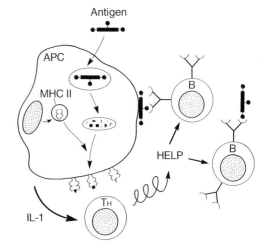

Fig. 11.7 Antigen presentation by mononuclear phagocytes. In this case the antigen has B-cell epitopes (•), equivalent to a hapten, linked to a carrier that contains sequences of amino acids that will generate T cell epitopes after processing and association with MHC molecules. APC, antigen-presenting cell; IL-1, interleukin-1; T$_H$, helper T cell.

leukins are shown in Table 11.7. All these lymphokines are only active at high concentrations, therefore the producing and responding cells must be close together for effective triggering. This will happen within a germinal centre of a lymph node secondary follicle which has evolved to facilitate the necessary cellular and molecular interactions.

T cell activation

As with B cells the activation of resting CD4$^+$ T cells requires two signals. The first is antigen in association with MHC class II molecules and the second is interleukin-1. The generation of the first of these signals has just been discussed, i.e. antigen presentation. There are two related types of interleukin-1 (α and β) that have exactly the same functions. They are produced by a number of cells, most of which can present antigen in response to damage, infection and antigen.

If interleukin-1 binds to its receptor on a T cell when the T cell receptor has been engaged by antigen–MHC, then biochemical changes occur within the cell, leading to RNA and protein synthesis. The responsive cells progress through the cell cycle from the G_o to the G_1 phase. The cells start to express interleukin-2 receptors and produce interleukin-2. Interleukin-2 is a T cell growth factor and causes the expansion of the responsive T cell population. Interleukin-2 was originally thought to be the only T cell growth factor but it is now known that interleukin-4 and interleukin-1 will support T cell growth although they are not as potent. After about 2 d, interleukin-2 synthesis stops while interleukin-2 receptors remain for up to a week if the cell is not re-activated. Therefore, there is a built-in limitation on T cell growth and clonal expansion. When stimulated, T cells secrete interleukin-2, which interacts with interleukin-2 receptors to mediate growth. This can be in an 'autocrine' fashion if the same cell that released the interleukin-2 is stimulated. If the responding cell is in the vicinity of the producer then the stimulation is in a 'paracrine' manner. Interleukin-2 is not present at detectable levels in the blood, therefore there is no 'endocrine' activity involved, i.e. action at a distant site.

The other main type of T lymphocyte is the CD8$^+$ T cell. Antigen recognition by these cells is restricted by MHC class I molecules. Again,

Table 11.7   Interleukins

	Source	Target	Main actions
Interleukin-1 (α and β)	Monocytes Dendritic cells B cells Endothelium Fibroblasts Astrocytes	T lymphocytes B lymphocytes Tissue cells Thymocytes	Lymphocyte activation Inflammatory mediator
Interleukin-2	T lymphocytes NK cells	T lymphocytes B lymphocytes Monocytes	Proliferation Activation
Interleukin-3	T lymphocytes	Stem cells Progenitors	Stimulation of cell production in bone marrow
Interleukin-4	T lymphocytes	B lymphocytes	Division and differentiation
Interleukin-5	T lymphocytes	B lymphocytes Eosinophils	Differentiation
Interleukin-6	T lymphocytes	B lymphocytes Thymocytes	Differentiation
Interleukin-7	Stromal cells	Immature lymphoid cells	Proliferation
Interleukin-8	Monocytes Macrophages Endothelium	Neutrophils T lymphocytes	Chemotactic factors

these cells require two signals to be activated —antigen fragment-MHC is the first and interleukin-2 produced by a helper T (T_H) cell is the other. A cell that 'sees' both these signals responds by clonal expansion and differentiation into a fully active effector T cell.

Therefore, for both B and T cell activation two stimuli are required. The recognition of antigen makes sure that only those cells that will be effective against the foreign material are recruited. The provision of the other signal, T cell help, has evolved to supply growth factors and aid discrimination of 'self' and 'non-self'.

Humoral immunity

Synthesis of antibody

On exposure to antigen, antibody production follows a characteristic pattern (Fig. 11.8). There is a lag phase during which antibody cannot be detected. This is the time taken for the interactions described above to take place and antibody to reach a level that can be measured. Then there is an exponential rise in the antibody level or titre. This log phase is followed by a plateau with a constant level of antibody where the amount produced equals the amount removed. The amount of antibody then declines due to the clearing of antigen–antibody complexes and the natural catabolism of the immunoglobulin.

If the response is to a T-dependent antigen then the B cells can switch to the production of another isotype, e.g. in a primary response IgM

gives way to IgG production. This process is under the control of T cells, since the class of antibody produced will depend on signals from the T cell. At some point, again under the control of T cells, a proportion of the antigen-reactive cells will develop into memory cells. These cells will react if the epitope is encountered again.

There are a number of differences in the reaction profile on second and subsequent exposures to an antigen compared to the primary response (Fig. 11.9). There is a shortened lag and an extended plateau and decline. The level and affinity of antibody produced is much increased and it is mostly of the IgG isotype. Some IgM will be generated but it will follow the same pattern as in the primary response.

When first introduced the antigen selects the cells that can react against it. However, before antibody is produced the B cell must differentiate into a plasma cell, involving the interactions already described. The B cells that are stimulated in the primary response synthesize IgM. With time, class switch will occur in some of the B cells, leading to the production of other isotypes. Somatic mutations will occur giving rise to *affinity maturation* through selection of cells bearing high-affinity receptors as the amount of antigen in the system falls. Memory cells will also be produced. An equilibrium is reached where there is a balance between the amount of antibody synthesized and the amount used. Then various mechanisms come into play to turn off the response when it is no longer needed (see below). The simplest is the removal of the stimulant, i.e. antigen. So the pro-

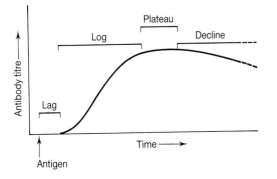

Fig. 11.8 Pattern of antibody production following antigen exposure.

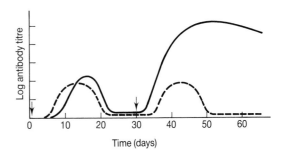

Fig. 11.9 Primary and secondary antibody response. The level of serum IgM (- - -) and IgG (—)detected with time after primary immunization (day 0) and challenge (day 30) with the same antigen.

duction of antibody is stopped and there is a natural decline in antibody levels.

On subsequent exposure the responding cells are at a different level of activation and present at an increased frequency. Therefore, there is a shorter lag before antibody can be detected: the main isotype is IgG. The level of antibody produced is 10 or more times greater than during the primary response. The antibody is present for an extended period and has a higher affinity for antigen due to affinity maturation. As is seen in Fig. 11.9 some IgM is also produced during a secondary response. This immunoglobulin is produced by the activation of B cells that were not present in the lymphocyte pool on the previous exposure but have developed since. The development of these cells follows the characteristics of a primary response and they will give rise to a secondary response if the antigen is encountered again.

Monoclonal antibodies

When an antigen is introduced into the lymphoid system of a mouse all the B cells that recognize epitopes on the antigen will be stimulated to produce antibody. The serum of the immunized animal is known as a polyclonal antiserum since it is the product of many clonally derived B cells. Even if highly purified antigen is used, the antiserum produced will contain a number of antibodies that react to the antigen and others that interact with antigens that the animal encountered naturally during this time. It is extremely difficult to purify the antibodies of interest from this complex mixture but it is possible to fuse single plasma cells with a myeloma (a tumour) cell line to form a hybridoma which secretes monoclonal antibody.

Human monoclonal antibodies are potentially of value in patient treatment. As starting material peripheral blood or secondary lymphoid tissue such as tonsils have been used. It is impossible for ethical reasons to expose human subjects to most of the antigenic material that would be required to induce useful antibodies. Therefore, cells are only available from patients with certain diseases, such as tumours, infections and auto-immune diseases, or from individuals who have received vaccinations.

A preparation of monoclonal antibody molecules will have the same isotype, allotype, idiotype, specificity and affinity, in contrast to the polyclonal antiserum produced by the inoculation of antigen into an experimental animal. In addition, the same antiserum can never be reproduced, not even when using the same animal. Therefore, monoclonal antibodies are defined reagents that can be produced indefinitely and on a large scale. They provide a standard material that can be used in studies ranging from the identification and enumeration of different cell types to blood typing and diagnosis of disease. They are also increasingly used in attempts to treat and prevent disease.

Cell-mediated immunity

Specific cell-mediated responses are mediated by two different types of T lymphocyte. T cells that have the CD8 molecule on their surface recognize antigen fragments in association with MHC class I molecules on a target cell and cause cell lysis. MHC class II-restricted recognition is seen with T cells that have the CD4 marker. These cells secrete lymphokines when stimulated by the antigen–MHC class II complex. CD4$^+$ T cells are involved in two main activities: (1) cell-mediated reactions, as the lymphokines can aid in the elimination of foreign material by recruiting and activating other leucocytes and promoting an inflammatory response; and (2) the generation and control of an immune response, as some of the lymphokines produced are growth and differentiation factors for T and B cells.

The other cell types, NK cells and phagocytes, which can participate in cell-mediated defence mechanisms have been described.

Cell-mediated cytotoxicity

Certain subpopulations of lymphoid and myeloid cells can destroy target cells to which they are closely bound. The stages and processes involved are similar for the different cell types although the molecules that mediate the recognition of the target by the effector differ.

Cytotoxic T lymphocytes. Cytotoxic T cells (T_c cells) are small T lymphocytes that are derived from stem cells in the bone marrow. These cells mature in the thymus. Most cells that mediate MHC-restricted cytotoxicity are $CD8^+$ and, therefore, recognize antigen in association with MHC class I antigens. About 10% are $CD4^+$ and, therefore, MHC class II restricted.

MHC-unrestricted cytotoxic cells. A number of partially overlapping cell populations are able to carry out MHC-unrestricted killing. These include NK cells, lymphokine-activated killer (LAK) cells and killer (K) cells.

Most cells that have the capacity to perform natural killing have the morphology of large granular lymphocytes and have a broad target range. The receptor on the NK cell and the structures that they recognize on the target have not been identified. They have been shown to produce a number of cytokines, including γ-interferon.

Several types of cells are able to destroy foreign material by antibody-dependent cell-mediated cytotoxicity. The cells that carry out this activity have a receptor for the Fc portion of immunoglobulin and are, therefore, able to bind to antibody-coated targets.

Lytic mechanism. Three distinct phases have been described in cell-mediated cytotoxicity: (1) binding to target; (2) rearrangement of cytoplasmic granules and the release of their contents; and (3) target cell death (Fig. 11.10).

Once the effector–target conjugate is formed the cytoplasmic granules appear to become rearranged and concentrated at the side of the cell adjacent to the target. The granule contents are then released into the space between the two cells. There are at least three different types of molecule stored within the granules that can cause cell death. T cells and NK cells contain perforin, which is a monomeric protein related to the complement component C9. In the presence of Ca^{2+} ions the monomers bind to the target cell membrane and polymerize to form a transmembrane pore. This upsets the osmotic balance of the cell and leads to cell death. The granules also contain at least two serine esterases that may play a role in destroying the target cell. A number of

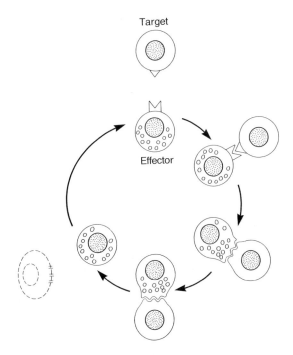

Target

Effector

Fig. 11.10 Mechanism of cell-mediated cytotoxicity. The effector cell has a receptor that is able to bind to a target cell that possess the appropriate ligand (▽).

other toxic molecules are also produced by cytotoxic cells, including tumour necrosis factor (TNFα), lymphotoxin (TNFβ), γ-interferon and NK cytotoxic factor. The process is unidirectional with only the target cell being destroyed. The effector cell can then move on and eliminate another target cell.

Lymphokine production

The other arm of cell-mediated immunity is dependent on the production of lymphokines from antigen-activated T lymphocytes. These molecules produced in an antigen-specific fashion can act in an antigen non-specific manner to recruit, activate and regulate effector cells with the potential to combat infectious agents.

The first documented reference to the production of lymphokines is credited to Robert Koch in 1880. Injection of purified antigen (tuberculin) into the skin of immune individuals produced a reaction that peaked within 24–72 h. The response was characterized by reddening and swelling and was accompanied by the accumulation of lymphocytes, monocytes and basophils. Because of the time course of the reaction this response has become known as *delayed-type hypersensitivity* (DTH) and the cells responsible were called delayed-type hypersensitivity T lymphocytes (T_{DTH} or T_D cells). These cells are identical to the helper T (T_H) cell subset as far as antigen recognition is concerned. CD4+ T cells, usually still referred to as T_H cells, are therefore capable of mediating both helper activities and so-called delayed hypersensitivity reactions by producing lymphokines. Although the term 'delayed hypersensitivity' suggests a disease process the production of lymphokines has a physiological function and only in some situations do pathological consequences occur.

Cytokines are biologically active molecules released by specific cells that elicit a particular response from other cells on which they act. A number of these regulatory molecules produced by lymphocytes (lymphokines) and monocytes (monokines) are shown in Table 11.8. The responses caused by these substances are varied and inter-related. In general, cytokines control growth, mobility and differentiation of lymphocytes but they also exert a similar effect on other leucocytes and some non-immune cells.

The exact signals and mechanisms controlling the activation of T cells and the release of lymphokines are not known. The balance between the different lymphokines produced will determine the response generated. For example, if large amounts of interleukin-4 and interleukin-5 are produced and responsive B cells are present, antibody production will be the main feature of the response. If interleukin-2 is produced then T cell growth will be stimulated while γ-interferon will have multiple effects, including macrophage activation.

Role of macrophages

Macrophages are able to carry out a remarkable array of different functions (Fig. 11.11). They play a key role in several aspects of cell-mediated

Table 11.8 Cytokines of importance in the immune system. Many of the molecules detailed below act synergistically to produce their biological effects

Cytokine	Immune system source	Other source	Target	Effect
Interleukin-1–8[a]				
TNF[b]	Macrophages Lymphocytes	—	Macrophages Granulocytes Tissue cells	Macrophage activation, increased cytotoxic cell activity, cachexia increased adherence of leucocytes to endothelium
IFN[c]	Leucocytes — T lymphocytes NK cells	Fibroblast Epithelium —	Tissue cells Tissue cells Leucocytes and tissue cells	Antiviral effect, induction of MHC class I expression Induction of MHC class I and II, macrophage activation
Macrophage (M–) CSF[d]	Monocytes	Endothelium Fibroblasts	Stem cells	Stimulate division and differentiation
Granulocyte (G–) CSF	Macrophages	Fibroblasts	Stem cells	Stimulate division and differentiation
GM–CSF	T lymphocytes Macrophage	Endothelium Fibroblasts	Stem cells	Stimulate division and differentiation
Migration inhibition factor (MIF)	T lymphocytes	—	Macrophages	Migration inhibition
Chemotactic factors	Lymphocytes Macrophages Granulocytes	Tissue cells and components	Leucocytes	Attract to site of infection or tissue damage

[a] See Table 11.7; [b] tumour necrosis factor; [c] interferon; [d] colony stimulating factor.

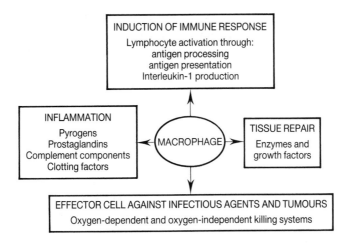

Fig. 11.11   The central role of macrophages.

immunity, being involved at the initiation of the response, as antigen-presenting cells, and as effector cells having microbicidal and tumouricidal activities. They also produce a number of cytokines (or more precisely monokines) that function as regulatory molecules. These monokines contribute to inflammation and fever and affect the functioning of other cells. Macrophages can also produce various enzymes and factors that are involved in reorganization and repair following tissue damage. However, since they contain many important biological molecules they themselves can cause damage if these enzymes and factors are released inappropriately.

Many of these activities are enchanced in macrophages that have been '*activated*' by exposure to lymphokines, such as γ-interferon produced by T cells. Macrophage activation is a complex process which probably occurs in stages with different effector functions being expressed at different stages. Macrophages from different sites in the body show different characteristics, i.e. they are very heterogeneous, and will have different activation requirements.

γ-Interferon is a powerful macrophage-activating molecule which increases the uptake of antigens by an enhanced expression of Fc and complement receptors; the activities of intracellular enzymes involved in killing are also elevated. Since γ-interferon causes an increase in MHC class II expression there will be an enhanced presentation of antigen to CD4+ T cells. This will lead to the production of more lymphokines and more effective elimination of the offending material.

The lymphokines that activate macrophages are secreted by CD4+ T cells. Therefore, the presentation of antigen by an antigen-presenting cell will lead to the production of lymphokines by T cells *specific* for the antigen involved. The lymphokines produced will then activate *any* responsive macrophage in the vicinity of the responding cells. The activation process appears to depend on the presence of a number of lymphokines that act synergistically to induce activation. For example, pure interleukin-2, interleukin-4 or γ-interferon are unable to induce resistance to infection but if γ-interferon is combined with any of the others then resistance is observed.

Macrophages and monocytes themselves are capable of producing a number of important cytokines. These monokines include interleukin-1, interleukin-6, various colony-stimulating factors and tumour necrosis factor (TNF α). Tumour necrosis factor and interleukin-1 acting independently and together have effects on many leucocytes and tissues. Tumour necrosis factor is responsible for the tumouricidal activity of macrophages but is also implicated in the elimination of certain bacteria and parasites. It has a synergistic effect with γ-interferon on resistance to a number of viral infections.

Generation of immune responses

As discussed previously the generation of humoral and cell-mediated responses requires the recognition of antigen, by the responding cell, as the first signal and a second signal, growth and differentiation factors, produced by a T_H cell. T_H cells, as has been emphasized, only recognize antigen fragments in association with MHC class II molecules. The distribution of MHC class II molecules is limited, in normal situations, to certain cells of the immune system — the antigen-presenting cells. In certain circumstances non-lymphoid cells can present antigens if they are induced to express MHC class II molecules. In order to stimulate a T_H cell the antigen must be taken into the cell and re-expressed on the surface in association with MHC class II molecules. Since the T cell antigen receptor recognizes antigen fragments bound to the MHC molecules the antigen-presenting cell must also be able to process the antigen. MHC class I- and class II-restricted recognition by $CD8^+$ and $CD4^+$ T cells requires antigen processing. The pathways that lead to association of an antigen fragment with a particular restriction element are not fully understood.

Immune responses are generated in secondary lymphoid tissues, such as lymph nodes. Since a number of cells and molecules must all interact the architecture of the secondary lymphoid tissue has evolved for the efficient induction of an immune response. In a secondary immune response the cells involved are at a different stage of activation, i.e. they are memory cells having already been exposed to antigen. Therefore, the growth factor signals may not be so critical but antigen in association with MHC class II molecules is still required. In this situation B cells are important as antigen-presenting cells.

$CD8^+$ T cells, as we have seen, recognize antigen fragments associated with MHC class I molecules. All cells have MHC class I molecules on their surface and would therefore be expected to be capable of presenting antigen fragments to cytotoxic T cells that are in the most part MHC class I restricted. The antigen fragments derived from endogenously synthesized molecules, e.g. from a virus, are produced at a site distinct from the endocytotic vesicles where exogenous antigens are processed.

At or around the site of protein synthesis, endogenously produced antigen fragments become associated with the newly produced MHC class I molecules. The MHC class II molecule picks up internalized antigen within a compartment as it moves to the cell surface. In this compartment, probably an endosome, antigen fragments cannot bind to the MHC class I molecules because these structures have already associated with endogenously produced antigenic fragments. Thus the site where the antigen is processed determines whether it will associate with MHC class I or class II molecules. This separation of processing pathways explains why $CD4^+$ and $CD8^+$ T cells are involved in the destruction of exogenous and endogenous antigens, respectively.

If a particular antigen does not become associated with either MHC class I or II molecules then no T-dependent immune response will be directed against that antigen. Since MHC class II molecules are involved in the initiation of immune responses by presenting antigen fragments to T_H cells, they can control whether a response takes place or not. It has been clearly shown that the level of an immune response to a particular antigen is controlled by the MHC class II molecules. The genes that code for these molecules, i.e. MHC class II genes, have therefore been referred to as *immune response genes* (Ir genes).

It should be obvious that if an antigen cannot associate with the MHC class II molecules of an individual then no immune response will be generated. Since the MHC molecules are polymorphic the cells of some individuals will present, and therefore respond to, certain antigen fragments while cells from other individuals will not. Fortunately, more than one antigenic fragment can be generated from each pathogen, otherwise individuals who did not respond to the particular sequence would be vulnerable to that microorganism. In addition, individuals can have six different MHC class II genes and therefore an increased chance that some fragments will bind to at least one of their MHC class II molecules. Variations in the levels and specificity of response will occur in individuals who have different MHC class II molecules and have therefore produced different MHC–antigen complexes on their cells.

Immune response gene effects can also be controlled at the level of the T cell receptor. If an individual does not have a T cell with a receptor that recognizes a particular antigen–MHC complex then no response will be generated. The T cell receptor repertoire is generated in the thymus where the genes of the immature T cells are rearranged to give rise to a functioning receptor. T cells that cross-react too strongly with self molecules are deleted, as are cells whose receptors do not interact with self MHC molecules. Therefore, T cells that interact weakly with MHC molecules are selected to mature and leave the thymus. When these cells later come across antigen–MHC complex the presence of antigen strengthens the weak T cell receptor –MHC interaction leading to a stimulatory signal being transmitted to the T cell. If for some reason T cells that respond to a particular MHC–antigen configuration have been deleted, suppressed or not formed then no immune response will be generated to that antigen. There is what is known as a 'hole' in the T cell repertoire.

Control of immune responses

An antigen can induce two types of response, immunity or tolerance. Tolerance is the acquisition of non-reactivity towards a particular antigen. The generation of immunity or tolerance depends largely on the way the immune system first encounters the antigen. Once the immune system has been stimulated the cells involved proliferate and produce a response that will eliminate the offending agent. It is then important to dampen down the reacting cells and various feedback mechanisms operate to bring this about.

Role of antigen

The primary regulator of an immune response is the antigen itself. This makes sense since it is important to initate a response when antigen enters the host and once it has been eliminated it is wasteful and in some case dangerous to continue to produce effector mechanisms.

Role of antibody

Many biological systems are controlled by the product inhibiting the reaction once a certain level is reached. This type of negative feedback is seen with antibody which may act by blocking the epitopes on the antigen so that it can no longer stimulate the cell through its receptor. In addition, antibody as part of an immune complex may directly inhibit the B cell. In this situation the simultaneous binding of antigen to the surface immunoglobulin and to Fc receptors on the B cell surface leads to a negative signal that switches off antibody production.

As antibody levels rise there is competition between free antibody and the B cell receptor. Consequently, only those B cells that have a receptor with a high affinity for antigen will be stimulated and therefore produce high-affinity antibody. For this reason antibody feedback is thought to be an important driving force in affinity maturation.

Role of immune complexes

As described above, immune complexes can suppress antibody production by interacting with Fc receptors on B cells. Sometimes antibody increases the immune response, especially when antigen is in excess. This process is dependent on the Fc portion of the antibody and is thought to operate by enhancing the uptake of antigen by certain antigen-presenting cells. IgM is most efficient in this context, while IgG is usually suppressive. Thus at the beginning of a response IgM is produced and can stimulate immunoglobulin synthesis whereas, as the response matures, the IgG produced will tend to inhibit antibody production.

Regulatory T cells

T_H cells control the generation of effector cells by producing helper factors. However the factors that stimulate the expansion of B and T cell numbers do not work indefinitely. Maturation factors are also produced that control terminal differentiation into effector cells. Under the influence of these latter lymphokines the action of the proliferation factors is inhibited mainly by making the effector cell unresponsive to its effects.

Other T lymphocytes have been described that provide negative signals to the immune system. Suppressor T cells (T_S cells) limit the development of antibody-producing cells and effector T cells. The activity of suppressor cells can involve both the production of soluble factors and direct cell–cell interactions.

Idiotypes

Antibody can stimulate the production of an anti-antibody, an anti-idiotypic antibody and so on, to form the idiotype network model that can control immune responses. Since these anti-idiotypic antibodies bind to the variable portion of immunoglobulin they can stimulate or inhibit an immune response in the same way as antigen and antigen–antibody complexes.

Tolerance

Two forms of tolerance can be identified — *natural* tolerance and *acquired* tolerance. The non-response to self molecules is due to natural tolerance. If this tolerance breaks down and the body responds to self molecules then an autoimmune disease will develop. Natural tolerance appears during fetal development when the immune system is being formed. In experimental animals the introduction of foreign material at the time of birth leads to tolerance. Acquired tolerance arises when a potential immunogen induces a state of unresponsiveness to itself. This has consequences for host defences since the presence of a tolerogenic epitope on a pathogen may compromise the ability of the body to resist infection.

An antigen can induce different effects on the two arms of the immune system. During an infection the host will be exposed to a variety of antigenic determinants on a micro-organism. These epitopes will be present at differing concentra-tions and possibly at different times during the infection. The epitopes can act as either immunogens or tolerogens. Therefore, it is possible that the antibody response to a particular antigen may be quite pronounced while the cell-mediated response might be lacking, or vice versa. Alternatively, both arms of the immune response may be stimulated or tolerized.

Generally, high doses of antigen tolerize B cells, while minute doses given repeatedly tolerize T cells. A moderate dose of the same antigen might be immunogenic. For acquired tolerance to be maintained the tolerogen must persist or be repeatedly administered. This is probably necessary because of the continuous production of new T and B cells that must be rendered tolerant.

Several mechanisms play a role in the selective lack of response to specific antigens. Since each lymphocyte has a receptor with a single specificity the elimination of a specific cell will render the individual tolerant to the epitope it recognizes and leave the rest of the repertoire untouched. This mechanism relies on self molecules interacting with the receptor and causing their elimination. It is proposed that during lymphocyte development the cell goes through a phase in which contact with antigen leads to death or permanant inactivation. Immature B cells encountering antigen for the first time are particularly susceptible to tolerization in the presence of low doses of antigen. The requirement for two signals in the stimulation of B cells and the generation of effector T cells can give rise to tolerance. Both cell types require stimulation via the antigen receptor and 'help' from a specific T cell. If the helper factors are not produced then the responding cells will be functionally deleted. Therefore, the elimination of self-reactive T cells in the thymus during T cell maturation is an important step in maintaining a state of tolerance. Tolerance can also be induced by active suppression. Some T cells are capable of inducing unresponsiveness by acting directly on B cells or other T cells. These T_S cells can be antigen-specific and probably produce signals that actively suppress cells capable of responding to a particular antigen.

Tolerance to self tissues is fundamental to the functioning of the immune system. It was originally thought that unresponsiveness to self was controlled by the elimination of all self-reactive cells before they matured. This cannot be true since self-reactive B cells are found in normal adult animals. It is thought that these B cells are controlled by a lack of T cell help, i.e. T_H cells have been eliminated. It is thought that T_S cells play a subordinate role acting as a back-up mechanism.

Immunodeficiency

The immunologically competent cells of the lymphoid tissues derived from, renewed by and influenced by the activities of the thymus, bone marrow and other lymphoid tissues, can be the subject of disease processes. The deficiency states seen are due either to defects in one of the components of the system itself, or are secondary to some other disease process affecting the normal functioning of some part of the lymphoid tissues. Deficiency of one or more of the defence mechanisms can be inherited, developmental or acquired. The types of infections and diseases seen in patients with immunodeficiencies relate to the role the affected component plays in the normal situation. An individual whose immune system has been depressed in any of these ways is said to be immunocompromised. The *compromised host* is

prone to infectious diseases that the normal individual would easily eradicate or not succumb to in the first place. A list of predisposing factors is given in Table 11.9.

Defective innate defence mechanisms

Defects in phagocyte function take two forms: (1) where there is a quantitative deficiency of neutrophils which may be congenital (e.g. infantile agranulocytosis) or acquired as a result of replacement of bone marrow by tumour cells or the toxic effects of drugs or chemicals; (2) where there is a qualitative deficiency in the functioning of neutrophils which, while ingesting bacteria normally, fail, because of an enzymic defect, to digest them. Characteristic of these diseases is a susceptibility to bacterial and fungal, but not viral or protozoan, infections. Among the enzyme deficiency disorders are chronic granulomatous disease and Chédiak–Higashi syndrome.

The complement system can also suffer from certain defects in function leading to increased susceptibility to infection. The most severe abnormalities of host defences occur, as would be expected, if there is a defect in the functioning of C3. Severe deficiency or absence of C3 is associated with increased susceptibility to infection,

Table 11.9 The compromised host

Predisposing factor	Effect on immune system	Type of infection
Immunosuppression for transplant or cancer	Diminished cell-mediated and humoral immunity	Lung infections, bacteraemia, fungal infections, urinary tract infections
Viral immunosuppression, e.g. measles, HIV, EB virus[a]	Impaired function of infected cells	Secondary bacterial infections, opportunistic pathogens
Tumour of immune cells	Replacement of cells of the immune system	Bacteraemia, pneumonia, urinary tract infections
Malnutrition	Lymphoid hypoplasia Decreased lymphocytes and phagocyte activity	Measles, tuberculosis, respiratory infections, gastro-intestinal infections
Breakdown of tissue barriers, e.g. surgery, burns, catheterization	Breach innate defence mechanisms	Bacterial infections Opportunistic pathogens
Inhalation of particles due to employment or smoking	Damage to cilia, destruction of alveolar macrophages	Chronic respiratory infections, hypersensitivity reactions

[a] HIV, human immunodeficiency virus; EB virus, Epstein–Barr virus.

particularly septicaemia, pneumonia, meningitis, otitis and pharyngitis.

Defective acquired immune defence mechanisms

Primary immunodeficiencies. Primary deficiencies in immunological function can arise through failure of any of the developmental processes from stem cell to functional end cell. A complete lack of all leucocytes is seen in *reticular dysgenesis* due to a defect in the development of bone marrow stem cells in the fetus. A baby born with this defect usually dies within the first year of life from recurrent, intractable infections. Defects in the development of the common lymphoid stem cell give rise to severe combined immunodeficiency. Both T and B lymphocytes fail to develop but functional phagocytes are present.

There are several types of B cell defect that give rise to hypogammaglobulinaemias, i.e. low levels of γ-globulins (antibodies) in the blood. Deficiency of immunoglobulin synthesis is almost complete in X-linked infantile hypogammaglobulinaemia (*Bruton's disease*). Male infants suffer from severe, chronic bacterial infections after maternal antibody has disappeared. There is an absence, or deficiency, of all five classes of serum immunoglobulins. Therefore, the defect is thought to be caused by the absence of B cell precursors or their arrest at a pre-B cell stage. In these patients cell-mediated immune mechanisms function normally and they seem to be able to handle viral infections relatively well.

Partial defects in immunoglobulin synthesis have been described affecting one or more of the immunoglobulin classes. In *Wiskott–Aldrich syndrome* that is inherited as an X-linked recessive character there are low IgM levels but IgA and IgE levels are elevated. Patients are susceptible to pyogenic infections, along with recurrent bleeding and eczema. The bleeding is due to reduced platelet production (thrombocytopenia) and the allergy-related eczema is linked to the elevated IgE levels. In patients with *dysgammaglobulinaemia* there is a deficiency in only one antibody class. Some patients have reduced levels of IgA

whereas the other isotypes are normal. These patients have an increased incidence of infections in the upper and lower respiratory tracts where IgA is normally protective.

Individuals with T cell defects tend to have more severe and persistent infections than those with antibody deficiencies. A lack of T lymphocytes is often associated with abnormal antibody levels since T_H cells are involved in the generation and control of humoral immunity. Patients with T cell defects suffer from viral, intracellular bacterial, fungal and protozoan infections rather than acute bacterial infections. In *DiGeorge syndrome* (congenital thymic aplasia) the patient is born with little or no thymus. Individuals who survive develop recurrent and chronic infections, including pneumonia, diarrhoea and yeast infections once passive maternal immunity wanes.

Secondary immunodeficiencies. Acquired deficiencies of the immunological mechanisms can occur secondarily to a number of disease states or after exposure to drugs and chemicals.

Deficiency of immunoglobulins can be brought about by excessive loss of protein through diseased kidneys or via the intestine in protein-losing enteropathy. Malnutrition and iron deficiency can lead to depressed immune responsiveness, particularly in cell-mediated immunity. Medical and surgical treatments such as irradiation, cytotoxic drugs and steroids often have undesirable effects on the immune system. Viral infections are often immunosuppressive. For example, measles, human immunodeficiency and other viruses infect cells of the immune system.

In contrast to the deficiency states just described, raised immunoglobulin levels are found in certain disorders of plasma cells due to malignant proliferation of a particular clone or group of plasma cells. In these conditions, such as chronic lymphocytic leukaemia and multiple myeloma, malignant clones will each produce one particular type of antibody. There is usually a decreased synthesis of normal immunoglobulins and an associated deficiency in the immune response to acute bacterial infections. These B-lymphoproliferative disorders contrast to the situation in Hodgkin's disease, a reticular cell neoplasm, where the patients show defective cell-mediated immunity and are susceptible to viruses and intracellular bacteria.

Hypersensitivity

Immunity was first recognized as a resistant state that followed infection. However, some forms of immune reaction, rather than providing exemption or safety, can produce severe and occasionally fatal results. These are known as *hypersensitivity reactions* and result from an excessive or inappropriate response to an antigenic stimulus. The mechanisms underlying these deleterious reactions are those that normally eradicate foreign material but for various reasons the response leads to a disease state. When considering each of the four hypersensitivity states it is important to remember this fact and consider the underlying defence mechanism and how it has given rise to the observed immunopathology.

Various classifications of hypersensitivity reactions have been proposed and probably the most widely accepted is that of Coombs and Gell. This recognizes four types of hypersensitivity that will be considered in turn.

Type 1: anaphylactic

If a guinea-pig is injected with a small dose of an antigen such as egg albumin no adverse effects are noted. If a second injection of the same antigen is given intravenously after an interval of about 2 weeks a condition known as *anaphylactic shock* is likely to develop. The animal becomes restless, starts chewing and rubbing its nose, begins to wheeze and may develop convulsions and die. The initial injection of antigen is termed the sensitizing dose while the second injection causes anaphylactic shock. Such a reaction is seen in humans after a bee sting or injection of penicillin in sensitized individuals. Localized reactions are seen in patients with hay fever and asthma. In all these situations the host responds to the first injection by producing IgE and it is the level of IgE produced to a particular antigen that will determine whether an anaphylactic reaction will occur on re-exposure to the same antigen. Asthma results from a similar response in the respiratory tract.

The biologically active molecules that are responsible for the manifestations of type 1 hypersensitivity are stored within mast cell and basophil granules or are synthesized after cell triggering. The signal for the release or production of these molecules is the cross-linking of surface-bound IgE by antigen. The release of these molecules, vaso-active amines and chemotactic factors, is responsible for the symptoms of type I hypersensitivity. IgE has been implicated in the control of parasitic worms and the importance of this is discussed in Chapter 13.

Type II: cytotoxic

Type II reactions are initiated by the binding of an antibody to an antigenic component on a cell surface. The antibody is directed against an epitope that can be a self molecule or a drug or microbial product passively adsorbed onto a cell surface. The cell that is covered with antibody is then destroyed by the immune system. A variety of infectious diseases due to salmonella organisms and mycobacteria are associated with haemolytic anaemia. There is evidence, particularly in studies in salmonella infections, that the haemolysis is due to an immune reaction against a lipopolysaccharide bacterial endotoxin that becomes coated onto the erythrocytes of the patient.

Type III: immune complex

As discussed previously, when a soluble antigen combines with antibody the size and physical form of the immune complex formed will depend on the relative proportions of the participating molecules and will be affected by the class of antibody. Monocytes and macrophages are very efficient at binding and removing large complexes. These same cell types can also eliminate the smaller complexes made in antibody excess but are relatively inefficient at removing those formed in antigen excess. Type III hypersensitivity reactions appear if there is a defect in the systems, involving phagocytes and complement, that remove immune complexes or if the system is overloaded and the complexes are deposited in tissues. This latter situation occurs when antigens are never completely eliminated, as with persistent infection with an organism, autoimmunity and repeated contact with environmental factors.

The tissue damage that results from the deposition of immune complexes is caused by the activation of complement, platelets and phagocytes, in essence an acute inflammatory response. In general, the degree and site of damage depends on the ratio of antigen to antibody. At equivalence or slight excess of either component the complexes precipitate at the site of antigen injection or production and a mild, local type III hypersensitivity reaction occurs, e.g. Arthus reaction. In contrast, the complexes formed in large antigen excess become soluble and circulate, causing more serious systemic reactions, i.e. serum sickness, or eventually deposit in organs, such as skin, kidneys and joints. The type of disease and its time course will depend on the immune status of the individual.

The local release of antigens from an infectious organism can cause a type III reaction. A number of parasitic worms, although undesirable, cause little or no damage. However, if the worm is killed it can become lodged in the lymphatics and the inflammatory response initiated by antigen –antibody complexes causes a blockage of lymph flow. This leads to the condition of elephantiasis in which enormous swellings can occur. In some cases of tuberculosis, sarcoidosis, leprosy and streptococcal infections, vascular inflammatory lesions are seen mainly in the legs. These are variously referred to as erythema nodosum, nodular vasculitis and erythema induratum and may be due to the deposition of immune complexes and the development of an Arthus reaction.

In systemic disease the clinical manifestations depend upon where the immune complexes form or lodge — skin, joints, kidney and heart being particularly affected.

Drugs such as penicillin and sulphonamides can cause type III reactions. The most susceptible patients will develop rashes (urticarial, morbilliform or scarlatiniform), pyrexia, arthralgia, lymphadenopathy and perhaps nephritis some 8–12 d after being given the drug. It is likely that similar events occur in many bacterial and viral infections (see Chapters 14 and 12).

Type IV: cell-mediated or delayed

This form of hypersensitivity can be defined as a specifically provoked, slowly evolving (24–48 h), mixed cellular reaction involving lymphocytes and macrophages. The reaction is not brought about by circulating antibody but by sensitized lymphoid cells. This type of response is seen in a number of allergic reactions to bacteria, viruses and fungi, in contact dermatitis and in graft rejection. The classical example of this type of reaction is the tuberculin response that is seen following an intradermal injection of a purified protein derivative (PPD) from tubercle bacilli in immune individuals. An indurated inflammatory reaction in the skin appears about 24 h later and persists for a few weeks. In man the injection site is infiltrated with large numbers of mononuclear cells, mainly lymphocytes, with about 10–20% macrophages. Most of these cells are in or around small blood vessels. The type IV hypersensitivity state arises when an inappropriate or exaggerated cell-mediated response occurs.

Cell-mediated hypersensitivity reactions are seen in a number of chronic infectious diseases due to mycobacteria, protozoa and fungi. Because the host is unable to eliminate the micro-organism the antigens persist and give rise to a chronic antigenic stimulus. Thus, continual release of lymphokines from sensitized T cells results in the accumulation of large numbers of activated macrophages that can become epitheloid cells. These cells can fuse together to form giant cells. Macrophages will express antigen fragments on their surface in association with MHC class I and II molecules and will therefore be the targets of cytotoxic T (T_C) cells and stimulate more lymphokine production. This whole process leads to tissue damage with the formation of a chronic granuloma and resultant cell death.

Penicillin sensitization is a common clinical complication following the topical application of the antibiotic in ointments or creams. This and other substances that cause contact sensitivity are not themselves antigenic and only become so in combination with proteins in the skin. The Langerhans' cells of the epidermis are efficient antigen-presenting cells favouring the development of a T cell response. These cells pick up the newly formed antigen in the skin and transport it to the draining lymph node where a T cell response is stimulated. Here, the specific T cells will be stimulated to mature and will then return to the site of entry of the offending material and release their lymphokines. In a normal situation these would help to eliminate a pathogen but in this case the continual or subsequent exposure to the foreign material leads to an inappropriate response. The reaction site is characterized by a mononuclear cell infiltrate peaking at 48 h. The clinical symptoms in these contact dermatitis lesions include redness, swelling, vesicles, scaling and exudation of fluid, i.e. eczema.

Auto-immunity

A fundamental characteristic of the immune system of an animal is that it does not, under normal circumstances, react against its own body constituents. Mechanisms, as we have seen, exist that allow the immune system to tolerate self and destroy non-self. Occasionally these mechanisms break down and auto-antibodies are produced.

Genetic factors appear to play a role in the development of auto-immune diseases and there is a strong association between several auto-immune diseases and particular HLA (human leucocyte group A) specificities suggesting that Ir gene effects may be involved.

There are a number of examples where potential auto-antigenic determinants are present in exogenous material. These preparations may provide a new carrier, i.e. a T cell-stimulating determinant that provokes auto-antibody formation. The encephalitis sometimes seen after rabies vaccination with the older vaccines is thought to result from a response directed against the brain that is stimulated by heterologous brain tissues present in the vaccine.

Micro-organisms are a source of cross-reacting antigens sharing antigenic determinants with tissue components. These may provide an important way of inducing auto-immunity. The group A streptococci, which are closely associated with rheumatic fever, share an antigen with the human heart. Heart lesions are a common finding in

rheumatic fever and anti-heart antibody is found in just over 50% of patients with this condition. Nephritogenic strains of type 12 group A streptococci carry surface antigens similar to those found in human glomeruli and infection by these organisms has been associated with the development of acute nephritis. Some of the immunopathology seen in Chagas' disease has been attributed to a cross-reaction between *Trypanosoma cruzi* and cardiac muscle.

A new helper determinant may appear on a cell during viral infections. These new cell surface antigens (often known as neo-antigens) then promote production of antibodies against other normal molecules. It has been shown that infection of a tumour cell with influenza virus produces a response towards uninfected tumour cells. Infection with *Mycoplasma pneumoniae* is associated with the appearance of cold agglutinins. These IgM antibodies, often directed against blood group I, react with the patient's red cells in the periphery where the temperature is lowest.

Auto-immunity can be induced by bypassing T cells. Self-reactive cells can be directly stimulated by polyclonal activators that directly activate B cells. A number of micro-organisms or their products are potent polyclonal activators; however, the response that is generated tends to be IgM and to wane when the pathogen is eliminated. Bacterial endotoxin, the lipopolysaccharide of Gram-negative bacteria, provides a non-specific inductive signal to B cells, bypassing the need for T cell help. A variety of antibodies are present in infectious mononucleosis, including auto-antibodies, that are caused by the polyclonal activation of B cells by Epstein-Barr virus. Breakdown in the idiotypic network is another way of activating self-reactive cells.

The antibody produced in response to a micro-organism could interact with an idiotope on a self-reactive cell to give a stimulatory signal and an autoreactive response. Alternatively the foreign material might trigger the production of an antibody that has an idiotope that is found on other immunoglobulins or T cell receptors (a cross-reacting idiotope or public idiotope). This cross-reacting idiotope could stimulate autoreactive cells that share this idiotope or are linked through an anti-idiotypic interaction. Micro-organisms use cell surface molecules as attachment sites; therefore, if a response is generated against the microbial structure, an anti-idiotypic antibody to this will be an auto-antibody. The consequences for the host could be quite devastating since a number of micro-organisms use important molecules as their site of attachment and entry.

Undoubtedly, auto-immune diseases have a multifactorial aetiology and a number of the proposed mechanisms may contribute in different combinations to different disorders.

RECOMMENDED READING

Paul W E 1989 *Fundamental Immunology* 2nd edn. Raven Press, New York

Roitt I 1989 *Essential Immunology* 6th edn. Blackwell Scientific Publishers, Oxford

Weir D M, Stewart J 1992 *Immunology* 7th edn. Churchill Livingstone, Edinburgh

12

Immunity in viral infections

J. Stewart and D. M. Weir

The host response to an invading virus will depend upon the characteristics of the infectious agent and where it is encountered. In many cases viral infections are subclinical, i.e. symptomless, but exposure gives rise to protection on re-exposure later in life. What is recognized by the immune system will be dictated by the type of virus and the phase of the infection. A vast array of host defence mechanisms work in a concerted way to protect the individual from viruses and to eliminate them if an infection occurs. In several instances virus-induced immune responses may have immunopathological consequences.

THE RESPONSE TO VIRAL INFECTIONS

Interferons

At the time of their discovery in 1957 the term *interferon* identified a factor produced by cells in response to viral infection that protected other cells of the same species from attack by a wide range of viruses. It is now clear that this activity is mediated by members of a family of regulatory proteins.

In man, as in a number of other species, there are three types of interferon; α-interferon (IFN-α) and β-interferon (IFN-β), produced by peripheral blood mononuclear cells and fibroblasts respectively, and γ-interferon (IFN-γ), a lymphokine produced in response to a specific antigenic signal. There is only one gene for IFN-β and one

for IFN-γ but there are at least 23 different IFN-α genes coding for 15 functional proteins. All the IFN-α genes are closely related and clustered on chromosome 9, close to the IFN-β gene; the IFN-γ gene is on chromosome 12. The production of interferons is under strict inductional control. IFN-α and IFN-β are produced in response to the presence of viruses and certain intracellular bacteria. Double-stranded RNA may be the important inducer. IFN-γ, which has a much more extensive role in the control of immune responses, is produced mainly from antigen-activated T lymphocytes.

To exert their biological effects these molecules must interact with cell surface receptors. IFN-α and IFN-β share a common receptor while IFN-γ binds to its own specific receptor. After binding to the cell surface receptors, interferons act by rapidly and transiently inducing or up-regulating some cellular genes and down-regulating others. The overall effect is to inhibit viral replication and activate host defence mechanisms.

The antiviral activity is mediated by the interferon released from a virus infected cell binding to a neighbouring cell and inducing the synthesis of antiviral proteins (Fig. 12.1). Interferons are extremely potent in this function, acting at femtomolar (10^{-15} M) concentrations. They can inhibit many stages of the virus life cycle — attachment and uncoating, early viral transcription, viral translation, protein synthesis and

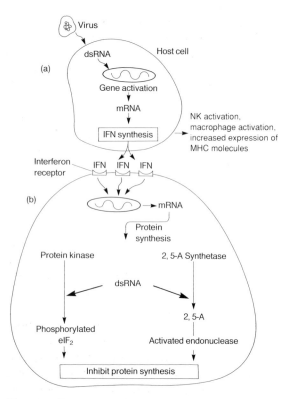

Fig. 12.1 Proposed mechanisms of **a** induction of synthesis of α- and β-interferons and **b** production of resistance to virus infection. dsRNA, double-stranded RNA; mRNA, messenger RNA; 2,5-A, oligoadenylate.

budding. Many new proteins can be detected in cells exposed to interferon, but major roles have been proposed for two enzymes that inhibit protein synthesis: 2',5'-oligoadenylate synthetase (2,5-A synthetase) and a protein kinase. The activity of both these enzymes is dependent on double-stranded RNA provided by viral intermediates in the cell. The protein kinase is responsible for phosphorylation of histones and the protein synthesis initiation factor eIF_2. This leads to the inhibition of protein synthesis within interferon-stimulated cells due to inhibition of ribosome assembly. The 2,5-A synthetase is strongly induced in human cells by all three types of interferon and forms 2',5'-linked oligonucleotides of adenosine from adenosine triphosphate (ATP). These oligonucleotides activate a latent cellular endonuclease that degrades both messenger and ribosomal RNA with a resultant

inhibition of protein synthesis. The requirement for the presence of double-stranded RNA for the full expression of these effects will safeguard uninfected cells from the damaging effects of these enzymes.

Some effects of interferon are viral-specific. The Mx protein induced in mice by IFN-α/β is specifically involved in the resistance to influenza virus infection. There is a related protein in human cells and it is possible that some of the other interferon-induced proteins may confer resistance to specific virus types. Resistance of IFN-γ-treated cells to the parasite *Toxoplasma gondii* is associated with induction of the enzyme indolamine dioxygenase, which catabolizes the essential amino acid tryptophan. However, interferons have effects on host cell growth and differentiation. Interferons, particularly IFN-α and IFN-β, are potent inhibitors of normal and malignant cell growth. A number of clinical trials have shown that IFN-α is active against some human cancers, especially those of haemopoietic origin.

Interferons are able to modify immune responses by (1) altering expression of cell surface molecules, (2) altering the production and secretion of cellular proteins and (3) enhancing or inhibiting effector cell functions. One of the main ways in which interferons control immune responses is by the induction or enhancement of major histocompatibility complex (MHC)-encoded molecules. Class I MHC genes are up-regulated by all types of interferon, as is the production of β_2-microglobulin. IFN-γ induces and increases the expression of MHC class II antigens. In addition, interferons can induce or enhance the expression of Fc receptors and receptors for a number of cytokines. These activities will increase the efficiency of antigen recognition and lead to a more effective immune response.

Interferons have also been implicated in the control of B cell responses. When added in vitro or in vivo they can suppress or enhance primary or secondary antibody responses, depending on the dose and time of addition. The regulatory effects seem to be on the B cells themselves, on increased antigen presentation and through an effect on regulatory T cells.

A number of immune effector cells act by killing infected target cells. The cytotoxicity of macrophages, neutrophils, T cells and natural killer (NK) cells is enhanced by interferons. IFN-γ produced by T lymphocytes is capable of activating macrophages to kill intracellular bacteria. This lymphokine has all the activities of the molecule that used to be known as macrophage-activating factor (MAF). NK cells are able to destroy a range of syngeneic, allogeneic and xenogeneic cells in an MHC-unrestricted fashion (see below). The interaction of NK cells with their target generates the release of IFN-α and IFN-γ. All three types of interferon increase NK cell activity in vitro and in vivo, not only by recruiting pre-NK cells to become actively lytic but also by increasing the spectrum of cells lysed. The mechanisms by which interferons make cells cytotoxic are not clear but it is of interest that interferons can stimulate the production of cytotoxins such as tumour necrosis factor (TNF).

Tumour necrosis factor has also been reported to have several antiviral activities similar to IFN-γ, but working through a different pathway. However, if both tumour necrosis factor and IFN-γ are added together then a synergistic effect is seen. If tumour necrosis factor is added to cells after viral infection, it can lead to their destruction even although the cells are normally resistant to tumour necrosis factor. This effect is also synergistic with IFN-γ. Certain viruses have been shown to trigger the release of tumour necrosis factor from mononuclear cells and it seems likely that this cytokine is an important host response to viral infections.

Certain cell-mediated reactions are also part of the innate defences against viral infections. In natural killing the structures recognized by the effector cells, the NK cells, are not known but changes in the level of expression of a number of surface molecules on the infected cells may be important. One of the most likely candidates is the transferrin receptor. The formation of a close conjugate between the NK cell and the target induces the effector cell to produce toxic molecules that lead to the death of the infected cell. Antibodies that recognize NK cells have been used to deplete these cells in mice. It was found that these treated mice were more susceptible to murine cytomegalovirus than were normal mice. Therefore, natural killing may form a first-line defence against viral attack before the acquired immune response is generated. Natural killing is increased by interferons, both the number of effector cells and their killing potential, and, therefore, these two innate defence mechanisms appear to work together to protect the host from viral infections.

Acquired immunity

The response to viral antigens is almost entirely T cell-dependent. Immunodeficiencies involving T cells are always characterized by markedly enhanced susceptibility to viral infections. However, this tells us little about the effector mechanisms involved as T cells are required for both antibody production and cytotoxic reactions.

The viral epitopes that the immune system responds to have been studied to give an insight into the mechanisms involved in the host response to these pathogens and also to aid in the development of better vaccines. The recognition of viral antigens is similar to that for all foreign material. B cells and immunoglobulin are able to combine with exposed epitopes while processed viral fragments presented in the context of MHC molecules are recognized by T cells. The B cell will recognize a conformationally determined epitope while the T cell epitope is a sequential epitope.

Antigen-specific B cells can act as antigen-presenting cells and therefore support the generation of an immune response by presenting viral antigens in association with MHC class II molecules to helper T(T_H) cells. B cells will present antigen to T cells and in return will be stimulated by growth and differentiation molecules. Intramolecular help may explain hapten–carrier effects. For virus particles the uptake of an intact virion will mean that the B cell will be able to present peptides derived from internal proteins to T cells (Fig. 12.2). Thus, a B cell specific for a surface antigen can receive help from a T cell specific for another molecule as long as it is present within the same particle, i.e. intrastructural help.

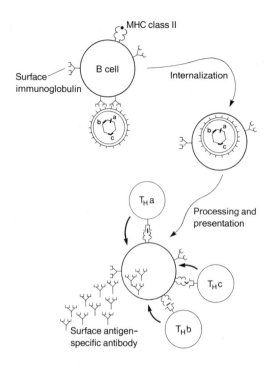

Fig. 12.2   Intrastructural T cell help. A B cell that is specific for a surface component of a virus binds the virus through its receptor, surface immunoglobulin. The virus contains three potential T cell epitopes (a, b and c) within its nucleocapsid. The entire virus can be internalized and all viral polypeptides will be processed and fragments will be re-expressed in association with MHC class II molecules (presentation) on the B cell surface.

In most cases, exogenous virus proteins, i.e. those derived from an extracellular virus and taken into a cell, will be presented in the context of MHC class II molecules and stimulate T_H cells. Cells that are supporting viral replication express virus-derived peptides in association with MHC class I molecules, i.e. the endogenous pathway. The fact that some endogenous viral proteins are presented in the context of MHC class II molecules suggests that the cellular compartment in which they are found is not transected by the MHC class I pathway.

Humoral immunity

There are several ways in which antibody against viral components can protect the host. Antibodies cannot enter cells, and therefore are ineffective against latent viruses and those that spread directly from cell to cell. They will, however, bind to extracellular viral epitopes. These epitopes can be on intact virions or on the surface of infected cells. The binding of antibody to free virus can inhibit a number of processes essential to virus replication. Antibodies to sites that are critical for the binding to the host cell membrane will stop the attachment and penetration processes. IgG and IgM will carry out this important function in serum and body fluids and IgA can neutralize viruses by a similar mechanism on mucosal surfaces. Antibody can also work at stages after penetration. Uncoating with its release of viral nucleic acid into the cytoplasm can be inhibited if the virion is covered by antibody.

Antibody can also cause aggregation of virus particles, thus limiting the spread of the infectious particles and forming a complex that is readily phagocytosed. Complement can aid in the neutralization process by opsonizing the virus or directly lysing enveloped viruses. In certain cases complement alone can inactivate viruses. Some retroviruses have a protein that can act as a receptor for C1q and other viruses have been reported to activate the alternative pathway. In some infections viral proteins remain on the surface of the cell after entry or become associated with the cell membrane during replication. Antibodies against these molecules can cause cell lysis by the classical pathway but an intact alternative pathway is necessary to amplify the initial triggering by the antibody-dependent pathway. In certain situations antibody-mediated reactions are not always of benefit (see below). Antibodies are also capable of modulating or stripping viral antigens from the cell surface, allowing the infected cell to avoid destruction by other effector mechanisms.

Virus infections, particularly those caused by enteroviruses, are frequent and severe when humoral immunity is impaired, as in certain inherited immunodeficiency states. In Bruton-type deficiencies, poliomyelitis may develop after vaccination with the live virus vaccine; meningo-encephalitis caused by echovirus and coxsackie virus may also be seen. In many situations viruses seem to be able to escape the humoral defence mechanisms. Some viruses become latent, e.g. herpesviruses, and are reactivated despite the presence of circulating antibody, as they can pass directly from cell to cell. Other escape mechanisms include antigenic variation in which the antigenic structure of the virus is altered so that antibodies formed to the previous strain are no longer effective.

In virus infections the efficiency of antibody depends largely on whether the virus passes through the bloodstream outside host cells in order to reach its target organ. Poliovirus crosses the intestinal wall, enters the bloodstream to cause a cell-free viraemia and passes to the spinal cord and brain where it replicates. Small amounts of antibody in the blood can neutralize the virus before it reaches its target cells in the nervous system.

In comparison, in viral diseases such as influenza and the common cold, the viruses do not pass through the bloodstream. These infections have a short incubation period, their target organ being at the site of entry into the body, namely the respiratory mucous membranes. In this type of infection a high level of antibody in the blood will be relatively ineffective in comparison with its effect on blood-borne viruses. In this case the antibody must be present in the mucous secretions at the time of infection. There are very low levels of IgG or IgM in secretions but IgA has been shown to be responsible for most of the neutralizing activity present in nasal secretions against rhinoviruses and other respiratory tract viruses.

One consequence of this is that conventional immunization methods using killed virus or viral subunits which produce high levels of circulating antibody are unlikely to be effective against viruses which attack the mucous membranes. Some considerable effort is being directed at developing methods for stimulating local production of IgA in the mucous membranes themselves. Live virus vaccines are effective in this respect and the intranasal administration of a live attenuated influenza virus vaccine is an attempt to overcome this problem. The high degree of immunity provided by the oral polio vaccine is due in part to locally produced antibody in the gut neutralizing the virus before it attaches to cell receptors to cause infection. The presence of IgA against polio has been demonstrated in faeces, in duo-denal fluid and in saliva. Recent evidence suggests that parenteral administration of a killed virus may give rise to a secretory IgA response if the individual has been previously exposed to the virus or has received an oral attenuated vaccine. So there appears to be a link between the systemic immune system and local mucosal immunity.

Humoral immunity does play a major protective role in polio and a number of other viral infections and is probably the predominant form of immunity responsible for protection from re-infection. Passively administered antibody can protect humans against several infections, including measles, hepatitis A and B and chickenpox, if given before or very soon after exposure. Immunity to many viral infections is life-long. This may occur because antibodies are boosted by occasional re-exposure to the virus.

Cell-mediated immunity

The destruction of virus infected cells is an important mechanism in the eradication of virus from the host. Antibody can neutralize free virions but once these agents get into cells other strategies are employed. The destruction of an infected cell before progeny particles are released is an effective way of terminating a viral infection. For this process to occur the immune system must recognize the infected cell and various types of effector cell have evolved to mediate these processes.

Many viruses, such as poliovirus and papilloma virus, replicate and produce fully infectious particles inside the cell. These viruses are liberated from the infected cell as it disintegrates. Other viruses do not wait for the cell to die but are released by a process of budding through the cell membrane. During the replicative process virus-encoded molecules, i.e. viral antigens, are inserted into the host cell membrane and the nucleo-capsid becomes associated with these molecules. The virus particle finally acquires an envelope as it is released. Such viruses include herpesviruses, alphaviruses, flaviviruses, retroviruses, hepadna-viruses and ortho- and paramyxoviruses. Viral antigens often appear on the cell surface very early in the replicative cycle, many hours before progeny virus is liberated. In cells infected with herpes simplex virus as many as five different viral glycoproteins appear on the cell surface. In other virus infections such as those caused by pox viruses and papovaviruses, the viral particles are not released by budding, but viral antigens appear on the cell surface. These molecules, including those which are not incorporated into the released virion, can therefore act as signals indicating the presence of virus within a cell.

Antibody-dependent cell-mediated cytotoxicity is carried out by a number of different cell types all of which have Fc receptors. These killer cells recognize the Fc portion of immunoglobulin bound to viral antigens present on the infected cell surface. This interaction brings the two cells close together and toxic molecules are released onto the target cell membrane causing cell death.

As viral proteins are synthesized within the cell some of these molecules are processed into small peptides. These endogenously produced antigen fragments become associated with MHC class I molecules and this complex is then transported to the cell surface where it acts as the recognition unit for cytotoxic T lymphocytes. Most cytotoxic T cells have a receptor that binds to fragments of the virus sitting in the cleft of an MHC class I molecule. This T cell will also have the CD8 molecule on its surface. Some cytotoxic T cells are restricted in their recognition of antigen by MHC class II molecules and therefore have the CD4 molecule.

$CD4^+$ and $CD8^+$ T cells can produce various lymphokines when stimulated by antigen. These will include molecules that are active in the elimination of virus, e.g. IFN-γ and tumour necrosis factor and others that generally increase the effectiveness of the immune system by attracting cells to the site of infection, stimulating the production of more cells and supporting their growth. Macrophages will be activated and this will lead to enhanced microbicidal activities and the production of monokines.

Induction of an immune response

The precise nature of the acquired immune reactions that are generated in response to infection will depend to a great extent on the site of infection, type of virus, previous exposure to the agent and the genetic make-up of the host. Both humoral and cell-mediated responses will be produced to all infections. The importance of genetic factors is illustrated by the severe X-linked recessive lymphoproliferative syndrome in which fatal infectious mononucleosis results from the unrestricted replication of Epstein–Barr virus as affected males have reduced numbers of normal lymphocytes.

The virus or viral components entering the peripheral tissues or being produced there will be carried to the draining lymph node. Once in the secondary lymphoid tissues the virus is processed by an antigen-presenting cell and viral peptides associate with MHC class II molecules and are transported to the cell surface. When antigen enters the lymph node the outlet is closed so that the antigen-specific cells that enter have a chance to interact with the peptide–MHC complex on the antigen-presenting cells, and the effector cells can respond to the helper factors that will be produced in the node. A T_H cell will bind to the peptide–MHC class II complex and in the presence of interleukin-1 expand clonally and produce helper factors for the growth and differentiation of T and B cells. The proportions of the different lymphokines produced will determine the type and level of the response generated. B cells will enter the node and those that bind antigen through their surface immunoglobulin, or enter the node already having interacted with antigen, will be responsive to the growth factors produced by the T_H cells and will be stimulated into antibody production. Other T cells will enter the lymph node. If these cells have a receptor that interacts with an antigen fragment–MHC class I complex then they will respond to the growth factors present in the node and proliferate and mature into effector T cells. After a period of time the valve on the efferent lymphatic will open and the products of the immune response will leave to circulate round the body and locate at the site of infection. As the response progresses the pathogen will be eliminated, the tissue repaired and memory cells generated. Finally, when all the antigen is eliminated the immune response will be terminated. In some instances virus-induced immune responses may have immunopathological consequences.

IMMUNOPATHOLOGY

Viruses have evolved a multitude of mechanisms for exploiting weaknesses in the host immune system and avoiding, and sometimes actually subverting, immune mechanisms. Some viruses are so successful in avoiding host defences that they persist in the host indefinitely, sometimes in a latent form without producing disease.

One of the most important strategies developed by viruses is to infect cells of the immune system itself. The effect of this is often to disable the normal functioning of the cell type that has been infected. Many common human viruses including rubella, mumps, measles and herpes viruses infect cells of the immune system, as does the human immunodeficiency virus (HIV). The consequences of viral infection of cells of the immune system have been categorized in two ways.

1. Infections that cause temporary immune deficiency to unrelated antigens and sometimes to the antigens of the infecting virus. It is known that infection with influenza, rubella, measles and cytomegalovirus predisposes to bacterial and other infections. This is sometimes associated with depressed immunoglobulin synthesis and interference with the antimicrobial functions of phagocytes.

2. Permanent depression of immunity to unrelated antigens and occasionally to antigens of the infecting virus. The acquired immune deficiency syndrome (AIDS) is an example of such a disease where the patient becomes susceptible to otherwise harmless protozoa, bacteria, viruses and fungi.

Viruses have also developed other mechanisms to avoid the immune system. These include antigenic variation, release of antigens and the production of antigens at sites that are inaccessible to the immune system.

Viruses that cannot enter and replicate within phagocytic cells will be destroyed if they are engulfed by a neutrophil or macrophage. Since neutrophils are short-lived cells they do not usually give rise to progeny virus. On the other hand, monocytes and macrophages are long-lived cells and can be responsible for disseminating a virus throughout the body. Viruses that do replicate within macrophages must escape from the phagosome very rapidly before it fuses with the lysosome. Reovirus infection of macrophages is actually helped by the lysosomal enzymes which initiate 'uncoating' of the virus and therefore enhance viral replication.

A virus will remain relatively safe from immune destruction if it remains within the cell and allows only very low or no viral antigen expression on the infected cell membrane. This is what happens in latent infections where herpes simplex or varicella–zoster virus are present in the dorsal root ganglion.

Antibody can actually remove viral antigens from cell membranes, as cross-linking of antigens on the cell surface can lead to their internalization by capping. Here the antigens complexed with the antibody are drawn to one pole of the cell and are internalized or shed into the surrounding tissue. Capping occurs on brain cells infected with measles virus in subacute sclerosing panencephalitis. Viruses that move from cell to cell without entering the extracellular fluids will also escape the action of antibodies as will those passed from cell to cell by cell division.

A number of infections continually shed virus into external secretions, such as saliva, milk or urine. As long as the infected cell only forms virus on the luminal surface of the mucosa then cells of the immune system and antibody will be unable to destroy the infected cell. IgA present in the secretions may neutralize the virus but this class of antibody does not activate complement efficiently so the cell will not be lysed. A similar situation applies to epidermal infections with wart virus. The infected cell is keratinized and about to be released from the surface of the body before any virus or viral antigens are produced. The infected cell is therefore isolated from the host's immune cells.

During the course of an infection various antibodies will be formed against different epitopes on a virus. These antibodies will be of differing affinities and also stimulate different effector functions. Antibodies against some of the epitopes will neutralize the virus, but other antibodies will be against unimportant epitopes or be of an ineffective isotype, which may fail to neutralize the virus and may actually aid in its infectivity or cause tissue damage through immune complex disease. Soluble antigens liberated from infected cells could 'mop-up' free antibody so that it can no longer interact and destroy extracellular virus. Whether the small particles present in the serum of patients and carriers with hepatitis B virus infections function in this way is not known, although patients in the prodromal phase may suffer from rash, myalgia and arthralgia. Polyarteritis nodosa and glomerulonephritis can also occur, all suggestive of immune complex formation.

Susceptibility to infection is generally greater in the very young and very old because of a weaker immune response. However, the immunopathology tends to be less severe. In the very young, infections can spread rapidly and prove fatal without the clinical and pathological changes seen in adults. Latent infections are kept under control by the immune system and in older people the infections show an increased incidence of activation, e.g. zoster or shingles. Immunological immaturity makes the neonate highly susceptible to many viral infections. Maternal-derived antibody provides passive protection for about 3–6 months, after which time the infant is at risk of infection: respiratory and alimentary tract infections are frequent.

Physical and physiological differences may also contribute to age-related disease susceptibility. Respiratory infections in old age are probably a bigger problem than in young adults because of weaker respiratory muscles and a poorer cough reflex. In the young the airways are narrower and more easily blocked by secretions and exudate. Infants, because of their low body weight, show signs of distress from loss of fluid and electrolytes, so that fever, vomiting and diarrhoea tend to be very serious at this time of life. Often the reasons for the differences between infants and adults are not known. Respiratory syncytial virus causes severe illness in the early months of life with croup, bronchiolitis and bronchopneumonia, despite the presence of maternal IgG. In adults the virus causes an upper respiratory tract infection.

Certain viral infections produce a milder disease in children than in adults, e.g. varicella, mumps, poliomyelitis and Epstein–Barr virus infections. Varicella often causes pneumonia in adults and mumps may involve the testes and ovaries after puberty, giving rise to orchitis and oophoritis. Epstein–Barr virus is excreted in saliva and in developing countries most individuals are infected early in life, usually asymptomatically. In developed countries where the childhood infection is less common, first infection can be delayed to adolescence or early adulthood, when salivary exposure occurs during kissing. In this age group, Epstein–Barr virus infection gives rise to glandular fever. It is not clear why these infections are more severe in adults but it may be linked to the more powerful immune defences giving rise to immunopathological sequelae in adults.

There are also age-related differences in the incidence of infections. It is not surprising that most infections are commonest in childhood when the individual will be exposed to the micro-organisms for the first time.

Antigenic variation

A micro-organism can avoid the acquired immune response by periodically changing the structure of molecules th t are recognized by the host immune system. The immune system will select the variants by not being able to mount an immune response against them before they are shed. The micro-organism will only be able to change a component in a way that does not alter the functioning of the molecule. The molecules involved can be either active enzymes, recognition molecules or structural proteins. HIV shows considerable variation in parts of the envelope glycoprotein within a given individual.

The significance of antigenic variation is well illustrated by influenza viruses. Here changes in the surface glycoproteins are linked to the occurrence of epidemics of infection (see Chapter 50).

With influenza virus the infection is localized to the respiratory tract where the principal protection against reinfection will be secretory IgA. The amount of this antibody produced tends to be low compared to the level of humoral immunity developed against viraemic infections such as poliovirus and measles. The virus-specific IgA still present at the mucosal surface a few years after infection can protect against the original infecting virus but may be insufficient to deal with an antigenic variant despite antigenic overlap. Thus, in effect, IgA levels become a selective pressure which will allow infection by the mutant and antigenic drift occurs. The very short incubation period (1–3 d) is more rapid than the secondary antibody response so that the IgA levels cannot be boosted to abort infection.

Antigenic variation is likely to be an important viral adaptation for overcoming host immunity in long-lived species such as man where there is a need for multiple reinfection of the same individual if the virus is to survive and the virus is unable to become latent. In shorter-lived animals such as mice and rabbits a susceptible population appears quickly enough to maintain the infectious cycle.

Viruses and auto-immunity

Auto-immunity may result from a virus infection in various ways. Epstein–Barr virus can initiate polyclonal B cell activation and some of the resulting antibodies may be directed at self antigens. Alternatively, sequence homology between virus and host components may explain the production of auto-antibodies. Human cytotoxic T (T_C) cells generated in measles infections cross-react with myelin basic protein and can be shown to kill cultured target cells coated with this protein.

Persistence of virus

Certain viruses give rise to a persistent infection which is held in check as long as the immune system remains intact.

Chickenpox is a persistent infection characterized by latency in that there is apparent recovery from the original infection but the virus can reappear later in life when a localized eruption, shingles, results. Other herpesviruses, cytomegalovirus and Epstein–Barr virus, also persist after infection. If the carrier's immune system remains intact, there will be no evidence of disease. However, cytomegalovirus causes many problems in immunosuppressed patients. The polyomavirus, JC, usually causes asymptomatic infections, but, in the immunosuppressed, it has been found in areas of destruction in the central nervous system: the disease is progressive multifocal leukoencephalopathy.

In other persistent infections, the immune system contributes to the pathology of the disease, often over a period of years. Thus, in subacute sclerosing panencephalitis, persistence of measles virus in neurones triggers their destruction by the host's immune system. Similarly the chronic active hepatitis seen in those carriers of hepatitis B who continue to produce virions appears to be triggered by a T_C cell response to the core antigen present in the hepatocyte membrane. In both examples several years may elapse before symptoms appear.

VACCINES

Natural infection with a virus is an extremely effective means of giving life-long immunity from the disease. In most cases, where there is one virus type, this means that second attacks are extremely rare. The memory of the immune system ensures that for these infections a secondary response can be generated before the virus has time to cause the disease. The level of immunity needed to protect an individual will depend on the incubation period of the virus and its life cycle. For viruses with very short incubation periods a high level of protective immunity must be present before exposure to the infective agent. In the case of a virus with a long incubation period (10–20 d) then the immune system has time to generate a protective response.

The amount of antigenic variation that occurs in the virus will also determine the effectiveness of immune protection. If the virus changes its antigen profile between exposures then the individual may not be protected.

It is also important to consider the type of immune response that will be protective against different viruses. If antibody gives protection then steps must be taken to ensure that the material to be used for immunization contains the correct epitopes. A denatured antigen will not generate antibodies that can combine with the native virus. Sometimes the chemical treatment of the antigen may destroy important components. Thus the original killed measles virus vaccine did not contain the fusion protein. As a result, vaccinees suffered enhanced disease when exposed to the virus as viral replication and spread could occur in the presence of antibody to the other viral proteins. If T cell immunity is important then the vaccine must be in a form that will give rise to peptides in the correct compartment of the cell to produce antigen fragments in association with MHC-encoded products. It will have to associate with the MHC class II molecules to generate help and MHC class I molecules to stimulate effector cell formation. For antibody production, T cell help will also be required. Therefore, for an antibody response, a killed vaccine may be sufficient but, when T cell immunity is required, a live attenuated vaccine will be needed.

Vaccination has been responsible for the elimination of smallpox and reducing the incidence of other viral diseases. It should be possible to control many viral diseases but with some the problem is more difficult. New technologies and a better understanding of the immune system are helping with this task.

RECOMMENDED READING

Mims C A 1987 *The Pathogenesis of Infectious Disease* 3rd edn. Academic Press, London

Taussig M J 1984 *Processes in Pathology and Microbiology* 2nd edn. Blackwell Scientific Publishers, Oxford

13

Parasitic infections: pathogenesis and immunity

J. Stewart and D. M. Weir

By convention the term parasitic diseases refers to those caused by protozoa, worms (helminths) and arthropods (insects and arachnids). Such parasites affect many hundreds of millions of people in tropical parts of the world and are responsible for many severe and debilitating diseases (see Chapters 61 and 62).

These infections are associated with a broad spectrum of effects. Some are due to the parasites themselves and others are a consequence of the host response to the invader. The nature and extent of the pathological effects is dependent upon the site and mode of infection and also on the level of the parasite burden.

Development of protective immunity to such parasites is more complicated than to bacteria and viruses because of the complicated life cycles of the parasites involved.

Pathogenic mechanisms

As with other infectious agents the site occupied by a parasite is important. A host will survive with a large number of lung flukes, *Paragonimus* spp., in their usual site in the lungs but a few eggs in the brain may cause far more serious effects. The severity of disease depends not only on the degree of infestation but also on the physiological state of the host. A lowering of general health, due to malnutrition for example, will predispose to more serious consequences following infection by parasites.

Mechanical tissue damage

Physical obstruction of anatomical sites leading to loss of function can be a major component of the diseases caused by parasites. The intestinal lumen can be blocked by worms such as *Ascaris* spp. or tapeworms and filarial parasites (*Wuchereria* and *Brugia* spp.) can obstruct the flow of lymph through lymphatics.

Within tissues the site of a parasite infection can give rise to serious consequences. Intestinal infection with the tapeworm *Taenia solium* is usually of little consequence but the eggs may develop into larvae (cysticerci) in man, causing cysticercosis. The cysticerci can be found in muscle, liver, eye or, most dangerously, in the brain. Hydatid cysts, the larval stage of the dog tapeworm (*Echinococcus granulosus*) in man, may reach volumes of 1–2 litres, and such masses can cause severe damage to any infected organ.

Physiological effects

Large numbers of *Giardia* spp. covering the walls of the small intestine can lead to malabsorption, especially of fats. Competition by parasites for essential nutrients leads to host deprivation. Thus, depletion of vitamin B_{12} by the tapeworm *Diphyllobothrium latum* sometimes leads to pernicious anaemia. Other forms of anaemia result from blood loss, especially in hookworm infection and from red blood cell destruction in malaria.

Some parasites produce metabolites that may have profound effects on the host. *Trypanosoma cruzi* secretes a neurotoxin that affects the autonomic nervous system. Malaria parasites are thought to produce a metabolite with vasoconstrictor activity.

Tissue damage

The presence of parasites can result in the release of proteolytic enzymes that damage host tissues. Ulceration of the intestinal wall occurs in amoebic dysentery and trophozoites (the active, motile forms of a protozoan parasite) can penetrate deep into the wall of the intestine to reach the blood and hence the liver, lungs and brain where secondary amoebic abscesses may occur. The skin damage caused by skin-penetrating helminths, such as *Strongyloides* spp. and hookworms, can also permit entry of other infectious agents.

The host reaction to parasites and their products can evoke immunological reactions that may lead to secondary damage to host tissues. This is seen in schistosomiasis where the host response to parasite eggs in tissues leads to the formation of a granuloma with subsequent tissue destruction through fibrosis. Other types of hypersensitivity reactions can be generated in various parasite infections (see below).

IMMUNE DEFENCE MECHANISMS

The large size of parasites means that they will display more antigens than bacteria or viruses to the immune system. When the parasite has a complicated life cycle some of these antigens may be specific to a particular stage of development. Parasites have evolved to be closely adapted to the host and most parasitic infections are chronic and show a degree of host specificity. For example the malaria parasites of man, birds and rodents are confined to their own particular species. An exception to this is *Trichinella spiralis*, which is able to infect many animal species.

In the natural host there is no one defence mechanism that acts in isolation against a particular parasite. In turn the parasite will have evolved a number of strategies to evade elimination. In general terms, cell-mediated immune mechanisms are more effective against intracellular protozoa while antibody, with the aid of certain effector cells, is involved in the destruction of extracellular targets. Again due to the life cycles of some parasites, either cell-mediated or humoral immunity may be of greater importance at different stages of their development.

Innate defences

Several of the innate or natural defence mechanisms that are active against bacteria and viruses are also effective against parasitic infections. The physical barrier of the skin protects against many parasites but it is ineffective against those that are transmitted by a blood-feeding insect. In addition, other parasites, such as schistosomes, have evolved mechanisms for actively penetrating intact skin. Certain individuals are genetically less susceptible to certain parasites. Thus, individuals with the sickle cell trait have a genetic defect in their haemoglobin that causes a mechanical distortion in their erythrocytes. This somehow leads to the destruction of intracellular malaria parasites. The Duffy blood group antigen is the attachment site for the plasmodium parasite. Individuals who lack this determinant are therefore protected from malaria.

A variety of other non-specific host defence mechanisms are involved in the control of parasitic infections. These include direct cellular responses by monocytes, macrophages and granulocytes, and by natural killer cells. The antiparasitic activity of these cells will be enhanced by products of acquired immune reactions. For example, certain protozoan parasites infect macrophages. In particular, *Leishmania* spp. are obligate parasites of mononuclear phagocytes, and are completely dependent upon macrophages, where they survive in the phagolysosome. The parasite appears to be able to survive within non-stimulated resident macrophages whereas they are destroyed in activated macrophages.

Complement, through activation by the alternative pathway, is active against a number of parasites including adult worms and active larvae of *T. spiralis* and schistosomules of *Schistosoma mansoni*. The spleen is thought to be active in the elimination of intracellular parasites as its filtering of infected erythrocytes is thought to remove intracellular plasmodium.

Acquired immunity

An individual with a parasitic infection will mount a specific response against the invading parasite. These immune reactions will generate antibody and effector T cells directed against specific parasite antigens. Memory B and T cells will also be produced. For a number of reasons described later much of acquired immunity is ineffective in protecting the host against recurrent infection. However, in certain cases, such as amoebiasis and toxoplasmosis, immunity to reinfection is fairly complete. In schistosomiasis, the presence of surviving adult forms protects against further infections. However, this is probably an effect of the parasite and not of the host.

Antibody

The specific immune response to parasites leads to the production of antibody. Infection by protozoan parasites is associated with the production of the immunoglobulins IgG and IgM. With helminths there is in addition the synthesis of substantial amounts of IgE. IgA is produced in response to intestinal protozoa, such as *Entamoeba* and *Giardia* spp.

In addition to these specific T-dependent responses a non-specific hypergammaglobulinaemia is present in many parasitic infections. Much of this non-specific antibody is the result of polyclonal B cell activation by released parasite antigens acting as mitogens. This response is ineffective at counteracting the parasite and can enhance the pathogenicity by causing the production of auto-antibodies and may actually lead to a diminished specific response due to B cell exhaustion. It has also been reported that some parasite molecules are T cell mitogens. This could lead to the generation of autoreactive T cells or activation of suppressor responses.

There are a number of mechanisms by which specific antibody can provide protection against and control parasitic infections (Table 13.1). As with viral infections, antibody is only effective against extracellular parasites and where parasite antigens are displayed on the surface of infected cells. Antibody can neutralize parasites by combining with various surface molecules, blocking or interfering with their proper functioning. The binding of antibody to an attachment site will stop infection of a new host cell. The agglutination of blood parasites by IgM may occur, leading to the prevention of spread, as in the acute phase of infection with *Tryp. cruzi*. Toxins and enzymes produced by certain parasites add to their pathogenicity and antibodies that inhibit these molecules will protect the host from damage and also affect the infection process directly. Intracellular parasites have evolved a number of mechanisms to allow them to survive in this environment. Antibodies against the molecules that aid the parasite in these activities, e.g. to escape from endosomes or inhibit lysosomal fusion, will lead to removal of the intruder by the phagocyte. Parasitic worms are multicellular organisms with defined anatomical features that are responsible for functions such as feeding and reproduction. Antibodies that block particular orifices, e.g. oral and genital, will interfere with critical physiological functions and could cause starvation or curtail reproduction.

Antibodies can bind to the surface of parasites and cause direct damage, or by interacting with complement lead to cell lysis. Antibody also acts as an opsonin and hence increases uptake by phagocytic cells. In this context complement activation will lead to enhanced ingestion due to complement receptors. Macrophage activation leads to the expression of increased Fc and complement receptors, so phagocytosis will be enhanced in the presence of macrophage-activating factors. Phagocytes play an important role in the control of infections by *Plasmodium* spp. and *Tryp. brucei*.

Antibody-dependent cell-mediated cytotoxicity has been shown to play a part in infections caused by a number of parasites, including *Tryp. cruzi*, *T. spiralis*, *S. mansoni* and filarial worms. The effector cells, macrophages, monocytes, neutrophils and eosinophils, bind to the antibody-

Table 13.1 Humoral defence mechanisms against parasite infections

Mechanism	Effect	Parasite
Neutralization	Block attachment to host cell	Protozoa
	Act to inhibit evasion mechanisms of intracellular organisms	Protozoa
	Bind to toxins or enzymes	Protozoa and worms
Physical interference	Obstruct orifices of parasite	Worms
	Agglutinate	Protozoa
Opsonization	Increase clearance by phagocytes	Protozoa
Cytotoxicity	Complement-mediated lysis	Protozoa and worms
	Antibody-dependent cell-mediated cytotoxicity	Protozoa and worms

coated parasites by their Fc and complement receptors. Close apposition of the effector cell and the target are necessary because the toxic molecules produced are non-specific and could damage host cells. Major basic protein from eosinophils damages the tegument of schistosomes and other worms, causing their death. It appears that different cell types and immunoglobulin isotypes are active against different developmental stages of parasites. Eosinophils are more effective at killing newborn larvae of *T. spiralis* than other cells, whereas macrophages are very effective against microfilariae.

T cells

The importance of T cells in counteracting protozoan infections has been shown using nude (athymic) or T cell-depleted mice, which have a reduced capacity to control trypanosomal and malaria infections. The transfer of spleen cells, especially T cells, from immune animals gives protection against most parasitic infections. The type of T cell that is effective depends on the parasite. CD4+ T cells transfer protection against *Leishmania major* and *L. tropica* and may be necessary for the elimination of other parasites. The intracellular parasite of cattle, *Theileria parvum*, is destroyed by cytotoxic T (T$_C$) cells.

CD4+ T cells may act by providing help in antibody production but they also secrete various lymphokines that interact with other effector cells. CD8+ cells may be cytotoxic in certain situations but these cells also produce a variety of lymphokines. Specific T cells respond to antigen stimulation by producing lymphokines. Interleukin-

2 is an important lymphokine that has been shown to be deficient during parasitic infections, such as malaria and trypanosomiasis. Administration of interleukin-2 to mice infected with *Tryp. cruzi* reduces parasitaemia and increases survival.

Colony-stimulating factors, e.g. interleukin-3 and granulocyte/monocyte colony-stimulating factor, are also produced by activated T cells. These molecules act on myeloid progenitors in the bone marrow, causing increased production of neutrophils, eosinophils and monocytes. They also increase the activity of these cells; the monocytosis and splenomegaly in malaria are caused by these T cell-derived molecules. The accumulation of macrophages in the liver as granulomas in schistosomiasis and the eosinophilia that is characteristic of worm infestations are also T cell-dependent phenomena.

In certain cases the production of lymphokines may have adverse effects. Leishmania infect macrophages and the release of molecules that stimulate the production of more host cells may potentiate the infection.

γ-Interferon is secreted by antigen-stimulated T cells and has many effects including the inhibition of proliferation of many mammalian cell types but it does not appear directly to inhibit or kill parasites. Multiplication of the liver stages of the malaria parasite is inhibited by γ-interferon, possibly through the interaction of this lymphokine with its receptor on the surface of hepatocytes. γ-Interferon is a potent macrophage activation factor and is probably involved in the resistance and elimination of intracellular parasites, such as *Toxoplasma gondii* and *Leishmania* spp. Activated macrophages are more effective killers and can destroy intracellular parasites before they establish themselves within the cell.

Macrophages

Macrophages play an important role in the elimination and control of parasitic protozoa and worms. They secrete monokines, such as interleukin-1, tumour necrosis factor and colony-stimulating factors, that influence the inflammatory response. These molecules affect not only T cells and antibody production but also granulocytes. However, other monokines, e.g. prostaglandins, are immunosuppressive. Macrophages are also phagocytic cells and function as such in the elimination of parasites. In the same way as in the eradication of other infectious agents, opsonins will greatly enhance this process. Once internalized, the parasite will be killed, by oxygen-dependent and oxygen-independent mechanisms, and digested. Many of the molecules produced by macrophages are cytotoxic and when produced in close proximity to a parasite will kill it. Specific antibody, IgG and IgE, can mediate the attachment of the macrophage to the surface of parasites that are too large to internalize but are vulnerable to antibody-dependent cell-mediated cytotoxicity. Acting as antigen-presenting cells, they can aid elimination by helping in the initiation of an immune response.

In addition to lymphokines some products of parasites themselves, such as those produced by *Tryp. brucei* and the malaria parasite, can cause macrophage activation. These may be direct effects or result from the production of monokines such as tumour necrosis factor.

In some parasitic infections the immune system is unable to eradicate the offending organism. The body reacts by trying to isolate the parasite within a granuloma. In this situation there is chronic stimulation of those T cells specific for antigens on the parasite. The continual release of lymphokines leads to macrophage accumulation, release of fibrogenic factors, stimulation of granuloma formation and, ultimately, fibrosis. Granuloma formation around schistosome eggs can occur in the liver and this response is thought to benefit the host by isolating host cells from the toxic substances produced by the eggs. It can, however, lead to pathological consequences if the damage to the liver leads to loss of liver function.

Granulocytes

Neutrophils and eosinophils are thought to play a role in the elimination of protozoa and worms. The smaller parasites can be phagocytosed and destroyed by both oxygen-dependent and -independent processes. The phagocytic capacity of neutrophils is superior to that of eosinophils. Both cell types possess receptors for the Fc portion of immunoglobulin and for various complement components, so the presence of opsonins increases phagocytosis. Extracellular destruction of large parasites can occur by antibody-dependent cell-mediated cytotoxicity.

Neutrophils are attracted to sites of inflammation and will clear the offending parasite. They have been reported to be more effective than eosinophils at eliminating several species of nematode, including *T. spiralis*, although the relative importance of the two cell types may depend on the class of antibody present.

Eosinophilia and high levels of IgE are characteristics of many parasitic worm infections. It has been suggested that eosinophils are especially active against helminths, and IgE-dependent degranulation of mast cells has evolved to attract these cells to the site where the parasite is localized. The eosinophilia is T cell-dependent and the lymphokines that induce the production of the cells also cause an increase in their activation state. These effector cells are attracted to the site by chemotactic factors produced by mast cells (see below). Once at the site they degranulate in response to perturbation of their cell membrane induced by antibodies and complement bound to the surface of the parasite. The toxic molecules are therefore released onto the surface of the target and cause its destruction.

Mast cells

The mediators stored and produced by mast cells play an important role in eliminating worm infections. Parasite antigens cause the release of mediators from mast cells; these molecules induce a local inflammatory response. Chemotactic factors are produced and attract eosinophils and neutrophils. Thus the IgE-dependent release of mast cell products helps in the expulsion of the worm. The number of mucosal mast cells rises during a parasitic worm infestation due to a T cell-dependent process.

Platelets

Platelet activation results in the release of molecules that are toxic to various parasites, including schistosomules, *Tox. gondii* and *Tryp. cruzi*. The release process does not require antibody, although IgE-dependent cytotoxicity is possible, but seems to involve acute-phase proteins. The cytotoxic potential of platelets is enhanced by various cytokines, including γ-interferon and tumour necrosis factor.

EVASION MECHANISMS

All animal pathogens, including parasitic protozoa and worms, have evolved effective mechanisms to avoid elimination by the host defence systems (Table 13.2).

Seclusion

Many parasites inhabit cells or anatomical sites that are inaccessible to host defence mechanisms. Those that attempt to survive within cells avoid the effects of antibody but must possess mechanisms to avoid destruction if the cell involved is capable of destroying them. *Plasmodium* spp. inhabit erythrocytes while toxoplasmas are less selective and will infect non-phagocytic cells as well as phagocytes. A number of different ways of avoiding destruction in macrophages have evolved. *Leishmania donovani* amastigotes are able to survive and metabolize in the acidic environment (pH 4–5) found in phagolysosomes while *Tox. gondii* is able to inhibit the fusion of lysosomes with the parasite-containing phagosome.

L. major has a similar escape mechanism by attaching to a phagocyte complement receptor (CR1) that does not trigger the respiratory burst. The activation of the complement system by protozoan parasites seems to be a common mechanism to achieve attachment to target cells. *Tryp. cruzi* trypomastigotes can infect T cells of both the CD4 and CD8 subsets and may be similar to retroviruses in using receptor molecules on the T cell surface for penetration.

The effectiveness of macrophages in the elimination of *Tryp. cruzi* depends upon the stage of development of the parasite. Trypomastigotes are

Table 13.2 Parasite escape mechanisms

Intracellular habitat	Malaria parasites, trypanosomes and *Leishmania* spp.
Encystment	*Toxoplasma gondii* and *Trypanosoma cruzi*
Resistance to microbicidal products of phagocytes	*Leishmania donovani*
Masking of antigens	Schistosomes
Variation of antigen	Trypanosomes and malaria parasites
Suppression of immune response	Most parasites, e.g. malaria parasites, *Trichinella spiralis Schistosoma mansoni*
Interference by antigens Polyclonal activation	Trypanosomes
Sharing of antigens between parasite and host — molecular mimicry	Schistosomes
Continuous turnover and release of surface antigens of parasite	Schistosomes
Exposure to very small numbers of parasites at intervals (trickle infection) so that strong immune response does not develop	

able to escape from the phagocytic vacuole and survive in the cytoplasm whereas epimastigotes do not escape and are killed. Macrophages are also the preferred habitat of *Leishmania* spp., which multiply in the phagolysosome where they are resistant to digestion.

In an immune host these evasion mechanisms are less effective because of the presence of antibody and lymphokines. The ability to resist complement destruction also appears to be important. For example, *L. tropica* is easily killed by complement and causes only a localized self-healing lesion in the skin whereas a disseminating, often fatal, disease is seen with *L. donovani*, which is 10 times more resistant to complement killing. Large parasites such as helminths cannot infect individual cells; however, they can still achieve anatomical seclusion. *T. spiralis* larvae avoid the immune system by encysting in muscle; intestinal nematodes live in the lumen of the intestine.

Evasion

Parasites may avoid recognition by antigenic variation and by acquiring host-derived molecules. African trypanosomes have the capacity to express more than 100 different surface glycoproteins. By producing novel antigens throughout their lives, these parasites continuously evade the immune system. By the time the host has mounted a response against each new antigen the parasite has changed again. Plasmodia pass through several discrete developmental stages, each with its own particular antigens. A similar situation is seen in certain helminths such as *T. spiralis*. As a result, each new stage of the life cycle will be seen by the host as a 'new' infective challenge.

A number of parasites are known to adsorb host-derived molecules onto their surface. This is thought to mask their own antigens and enable them to evade immunological attack.

Parasitic protozoa and worms also use devices to avoid immune destruction. Certain parasites retain a surface coat, or glycocalyx, that blocks direct exposure of its surface antigens.

Immunosuppression

Parasites are not always able to evade detection

and many have evolved mechanisms to suppress or divert immune reactions. Some parasites produce or generate molecules that act against cells of the immune system. Thus, the larvae of *T. spiralis* produce a molecule that is cytotoxic towards lymphocytes, and schistosomes can cleave a peptide from IgG, thereby decreasing its effectiveness. During many parasitic infections a large amount of antigenic material is released into the body fluids and this may inhibit the response to or divert the response away from the parasite. High antigen concentrations can lead to tolerance by clonal exhaustion or clonal deletion. The immune complexes formed can also inhibit antibody production by negative feedback via Fc receptors on plasma cells. Many of these released molecules are polyclonal activators of T and B cells. This leads to the production of non-specific antibody, impairment of B cell function and immunosuppression. It has also been proposed that many parasites can cause unresponsiveness by activating immune suppressor mechanisms.

In many cases the immunosuppression has been attributed to macrophage dysfunction associated with antigen overload or the presence of intracellular parasites. In addition to the non-specific immunosuppression there can be parasite-specific effects. Mice infected by *Leishmania* spp. show antigen-specific depression of lymphokine production. Since this genus inhabits macrophages and is partly controlled by activation of these cells by lymphokines the effect is a diminished response against the pathogen.

Schistosomes have a receptor for part of the antibody molecule. They also release several proteases that cleave antibody molecules and release products that prevent macrophage activation. A schistosome-derived inhibitory factor suppresses T cell activity and is believed to allow other parasites to survive the effects of T cells and may explain the inefficiency of T_C cells in damaging the parasite.

When tested in a lymphocyte proliferation assay, peripheral blood lymphocytes of patients infected with *Plasmodium falciparum* are unresponsive to antigen prepared from the parasite and in nearly 40% of the patients this persists for more than 4 weeks. Patients infected with *P.*

falciparum show a suppression of lymphocyte reactivity which is not related to the degree of parasitaemia or severity of the clinical illness. The depressed lymphocyte reactivity is associated with a loss of both CD4$^+$ and CD8$^+$ lymphocytes from the peripheral blood. Once the parasite is cleared the response returns to normal. An even more sophisticated strategy has been evolved by *L. mexicana* and *L. donovani*, which use interleukin-2 to stimulate their own growth. Mammalian epidermal growth factor has also been shown to stimulate the growth of certain trypanosomes in vitro.

IMMUNOPATHOLOGY

The immune response to parasites is aimed at eliminating the organisms but many of the host reactions have pathological effects.

The IgE produced in parasitic worm infections can have severe effects on the host if it stimulates excessive mast cell degranulation, i.e. type I hypersensitivity. Anaphylactic shock can occur if a cyst ruptures and releases vast amounts of antigenic material into the circulation of a sensitized individual. Asthma-like symptoms occur in *Toxocara canis* infections when larvae of worms migrate through the lungs.

The polyclonal B cell activation seen with many parasitic infections can give rise to auto-antibodies. In trypanosomiasis and malaria antibodies against red blood cells, lymphocytes and DNA have been detected. Host antigens incorporated into the parasite, as an immune evasion mechanism, may stimulate auto-antibody production by giving rise to T cell help and overcoming tolerance. In Chagas' disease about 20% of individuals develop progressive cardiomyopathy and neuropathy of the digestive tract that is believed to be autoimmune in nature. These effects are thought to result from cross-reactivity between antibody or T cells responsive to *Tryp. cruzi* and nerve ganglia.

Immune complex-mediated disease occurs in malaria, trypanosomiasis, schistosomiasis and onchocerciasis. The deposition of immune complexes in the kidney is responsible for the nephrotic syndrome of quartan malaria.

Enlargement of the spleen and liver in malaria, trypanosomiasis and visceral leishmaniasis is associated with increases in the number of macrophages and lymphocytes in these organs. The liver, renal and cardiopulmonary pathology of schistosomiasis is related to cell-mediated responses to the worm eggs. Symptoms similar to those seen in endotoxaemia induced by Gram-negative bacteria are found in the acute stages of malaria.

The non-specific immunosuppression discussed above may explain why individuals with parasite infections are especially susceptible to bacterial and viral infections.

VACCINATION

No effective vaccine, for man, has so far been developed against parasitic protozoa and worms, mainly due to the complex parasite life cycles and their sophisticated adaptive responses. Since protection in many cases depends on both antibody and cell-mediated reactions a vaccine must induce long-lived B and T cell immunity. In addition, since the recognition by T cells is genetically restricted, the vaccine preparation must stimulate T cells from most haplotypes and preferably be without suppressor epitopes. Due to the immunopathology seen in many parasite infections, antigens that induce a potentially damaging response must be avoided.

A much better understanding of the biological mechanisms underlying the natural history of parasitic diseases is required before it will be possible to control these globally important diseases.

RECOMMENDED READING

Mims C A 1987 *The Pathogenesis of Infectious Disease* 3rd edn. Academic Press, London
Taussig M J 1984 *Processes in Pathology and Microbiology* 2nd edn. Blackwell Scientific Publishers, Oxford
Wakelin D 1984 *Immunity to Parasites*. Edward Arnold, London

14

Immunity in bacterial infections

J. Stewart and D. M. Weir

Modern medical science has managed to subdue many of the classical infectious diseases, but has helped to create new ones which result from interference with normal host defence mechanisms — consequent upon medical and surgical procedures such as chemotherapy, catheterization, immunosuppression and irradiation. Infections that develop in this way are known as *iatrogenic* (physician-induced) diseases.

It is important to differentiate infection from disease. A host may be infected with a particular micro-organism and be unaware of its presence. If the microbe reproduces itself to such an extent that toxic products or sheer numbers of organisms begin to harm the host then a disease process has developed. Potentially pathogenic bacteria such as pneumococci, streptococci and salmonellae are found in the nose, throat or bowel; this is known as the carrier state and is a source of infection to other individuals. These bacteria may also cause a disease in the carrier if they enter a vulnerable tissue.

HOST DEFENCES

The immune system has evolved the capacity to respond and react to a large variety of foreign molecules whilst at the same time avoiding self-reactivity. The capacity of the individual to resist infection can be explained in terms of the clonal selection theory of acquired immunity with the production of a specific immune response. The details of the cellular events involved in the control of immune responses and the immune effector mechanisms have been described in Chapters 10 and 11.

Very few organisms can penetrate intact skin and the various other innate defence mechanisms are extremely efficient at keeping bacteria at bay. When bacteria do gain access to the tissues the ability of the host to limit damage and eliminate the microbe will depend on the generation of an effective immune response against microbial antigens. In most cases the host defences will be directed against external components and secreted molecules. Bacteria are surrounded by a cytoplasmic membrane and a peptidoglycan cell wall. Associated with these basic structures there can be a variety of other components such as proteins, capsules, lipopolysaccharide or teichoic acids. There are also structures involved in motility or adherence to the cells of the host (see Chapters 2 and 8). These are some of the components to which the immune system directs its response. In general, peptidoglycan is attacked by lysosomal enzymes and the outer lipid layer of Gram-negative bacteria by cationic proteins and complement. Specific antibodies can bind to flagella or fimbriae, affecting their ability to function properly, and can inactivate various bacterial enzymes and toxins. Antibodies therefore interfere with many important bacterial processes but, ultimately, phagocytes are needed to destroy and remove the bacteria (Fig. 14.1). In some situations cell-mediated responses are required.

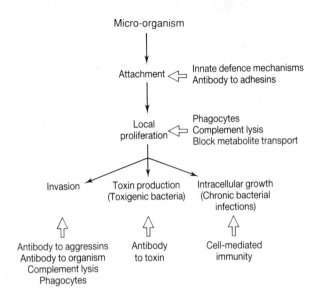

Fig. 14.1 Scheme showing the progress of infection and the immunological defence mechanisms.

Inflammation

Having successfully avoided the innate immune mechanisms that protect the individual (mechanical barriers, antibacterial substances and phagocytosis; described in Chapter 11), a bacterium starts to proliferate in the tissues and its toxic products trigger an inflammatory reaction. The response is initiated by the release of vaso-active amines and other mediators from mast cells. The resulting increase in vascular permeability leads to an exudation of serum proteins, including complement components, antibodies and clotting factors, as well as phagocytic cells. The phagocytes are attracted to the site of inflammation by chemotactic factors released from the mast cells or generated as part of the inflammatory response. Anaphylatoxins generated by complement activation further increase vascular permeability and encourage exudation of fluid and cells at the site of inflammation. Many of these mediators also cause vasodilation, thereby increasing blood flow to the area.

Many types of micro-organisms, e.g. staphylococci and streptococci, are effectively dealt with by the phagocytes. The intensity and duration of the inflammatory process that is stimulated depends on the degree of success with which the micro-organism initially establishes itself. This, in turn, depends on the extent of the injury, the amount of associated tissue damage and the number and type of micro-organisms introduced. A localized abscess may arise at the site of infection.

If bacteria are not eliminated at the site of entry and continue to proliferate, they will pass via the tissue fluids and lymphatics to the draining lymph node where a specific acquired immune response will be generated. The antibody and effector cells generated will leave the node to return to the area of infection to eliminate the bacteria. Some capsulate micro-organisms, such as pneumococci, are able to resist phagocytosis and are not dealt with effectively until large amounts of antibody are made. These 'mop up' the released capsular polysaccharide, and phagocytosis occurs. Other micro-organisms produce exotoxins and damaging effects can occur without the bacteria migrating from their site of entry. Effective immunity to exotoxins requires the development of specific antibodies against the toxin, i.e. *antitoxin*.

The types of infection described above are usually referred to as *acute* infections and contrast with the protracted or *chronic* infections that are usually induced by bacteria that are adapted to survive within the cells of the host. Included amongst these are tuberculosis and leprosy, brucella infections and listeriosis. In these infections cell-mediated immunity plays a predominant part in the final elimination of the micro-organism.

Humoral immunity

The attachment of a micro-organism to an epithelial surface is a prerequisite for the development of an infectious process (see Chapter 8). A first line of attack by antibody could be to inhibit colonization by stopping attachment.

IgA can be detected in many mucous secretions in higher concentrations than those found in serum. IgA-producing plasma cells predominate in the lamina propria of mucosal surfaces and the IgA produced forms a dimer that is specifically transported to the mucosal surface by the poly-immunoglobulin receptor. It is released with the secretory component of the transport molecule still attached. This secretory IgA can stop colonization of the mucosal surface if it interferes with the attachment molecules (*adhesins*) present on the bacterial surface. IgA is thought to be adapted to this role because it survives the presence of proteolytic enzymes of the gastro-intestinal tract better than the other isotypes. In addition, IgA does not activate complement very efficiently; therefore, an inflammatory reaction is not stimulated. Damage to the gut wall during an inflammatory reaction would allow the entry of many potential pathogens into vulnerable tissues.

Many micro-organisms owe their pathogenic abilities to the production of *exotoxins* and are called *toxigenic organisms*. Amongst diseases dependent on this type of mechanism are diphtheria, cholera, tetanus and botulism. Antibodies acquired by either immunization or previous infection or given passively as antiserum are able to *neutralize* bacterial toxins. To give protection, antibodies must either be present in sufficient quantities, as they would after administration of antiserum (*passive immunity*), or be produced by the host (*active immunity*) faster than the toxin is produced by the micro-organisms.

Most bacterial exotoxins are enzymes and protective antibody is able to interfere with the ability of the enzyme to interact with its substrate. The antibody can bind directly to the active site of the enzyme or to adjacent residues and inhibit by steric hindrance. They may also act by stopping activation of a zymogen into an active enzyme, interfere with the interaction between the toxin and its target cell or bind to a site on the molecule, causing a conformational change that destroys the enzymic activity.

The direct binding of antibody to a bacterium can interfere with its normal functioning in numerous ways. Antibody can kill bacteria on its own or in conjunction with host factors and cells. To survive and multiply, bacteria must ingest nutrients and ions mainly by specific transport systems. Antibodies that affect the activity of specific transport systems will deprive the bacteria of its energy supply and other essential chemicals. A number of bacteria are invasive, moving into the tissues aided by enzymes that they produce. Antibodies reactive with these enzymes will stop invasion if they inhibit the activity of the molecules. Invasion can also be inhibited by antibody that attaches to the flagella of the micro-organism in such a way as to affect their motility. Antibodies can agglutinate bacteria, i.e. clump the bacteria together; the formation of the aggregate will impede the spread of the organism. In addition the formation of an immune complex of bacteria and antibody will stimulate phagocytosis and complement activation.

Phagocytic cells have receptors for the Fc portion of IgG (particularly for subclasses IgG1 and IgG3 in man) and for fragments of activated complement (mainly C3b and iC3b). These receptors will interact with the ligand on the surface of the bacteria and cause ingestion. The combination of all the interactions mediated by these opsonins leads to phagocytosis. When a particle is coated with antibody a large number of Fc portions are exposed to the outside. This increases the chance that the particle will be held in contact with the phagocyte long enough to stimulate phagocytosis. The interaction of multiple ligands will increase the overall affinity of the binding and if antibody and complement components are present on the same particle the binding will be even stronger. Phagocytosis is thought to be stimulated by the cross-linking of the cell receptors. This leads to changes in the cytoskeleton and ingestion is initiated.

The bacteria are internalized and attacked by the oxygen-dependent and oxygen-independent killing mechanisms within the phagocyte. Phagocytes are also responsible for the removal and digestion of bacteria that have been killed extracellularly. Bacteria are susceptible to the lytic action of complement, which may be activated by bacterial components. The presence of antibody on the bacterial cell surface will further stimulate the activation of complement. In certain circumstances antibodies in conjunction with other bactericidal molecules lead to more efficient bacterial destruction. Gram-negative organisms are normally resistant to the action of lysozyme, probably due to the lipopolysaccharide component of the cell. The action of antibody and complement is thought to expose the underlying cell wall, which is then attacked by the lysozyme.

Cell-mediated immunity

Ultimately, all bacteria will be engulfed by a phagocyte, either to be killed or removed after extracellular killing. The host defence mechanisms of macrophages and monocytes can be enhanced by various activating stimuli, including such microbial products as muramyl dipeptide and trehalose dimycolate. The chemotactic formyl-methionyl peptides have been shown to increase the activities of various macrophage functions. The linkage of chemotaxis to activation has the advantage that the cell that is being attracted to the site of tissue injury will be better equipped to deal with the insult. Endotoxin present in the cell wall of Gram-negative bacteria and various carbohydrate polymers, such as β-glucans, are also potent macrophage activators.

The immune system is also active in the production of macrophage-activating factors. In particular, lymphokines, produced by T lymphocytes, are often required to potentiate bacterial clearance both by attracting phagocytes to the site of infection and by activating them. The most important activator is γ-interferon although tumour necrosis factor and colony-stimulating factors have also been implicated (see Chapter 11). The production of lymphokines requires a T lymphocyte to bind to processed antigen on the surface of a host cell; the stimulated T cell secretes lymphokines that act non-specifically on any responsive cell in the vicinity. All T lymphocytes produce some lymphokines when stimulated and the balance of the different factors produced dictates the effect on surrounding cells. The overall effect of the lymphokines is to increase the effectiveness of host defence mechanisms, but if these molecules are produced in excess or to an inappropriate signal then a type IV hypersensitivity reaction can occur.

EVASION

Once a micro-organism becomes established in the tissues, having escaped the innate defence mechanisms, it can often make use of a number of evasion strategies that protect it from the immune reactions of the host. Pathogenic bacteria produce a rather ill-defined group of bacterial products called *aggressins* and *impedins*, possession of which is associated with virulence (see Chapter 8). If antibody to such substances is present the pathogenicity of the micro-organism is likely to be reduced.

Intracellular bacteria

Bacteria that can survive and replicate within phagocytic cells are at an advantage as they are protected from host defence mechanisms. Some micro-organisms reside intracellularly only transiently while others spend most, if not all, their life inside cells. An intracellular lifestyle demands potent evasion mechanisms to survive this hostile environment. Some bacteria, like *Mycobacterium leprae*, have become so accustomed to their intracellular environment that they can no longer live in the extracellular space.

Listeria monocytogenes, the causative agent of listeriosis, can survive and multiply in normal macrophages; but it is killed within macrophages activated by lymphokines released from T lymphocytes. Listeriosis is most commonly seen in immunocompromised patients, pregnant women and neonates in whom a lack of adequate T cell-derived macrophage-activating factors is probably the critical factor. *Salmonella* spp. and *Brucella* spp. can also survive intracellularly. Unlike *L. monocytogenes*, they owe their resistance to a glycolipid capsule that is resistant to destruction.

Mycobacteria have a waxy cell wall that is very hydrophobic. This external surface is very resistant to lysosomal enzymes and persists for a long time even when the bacteria have been killed. In addition, these micro-organisms have evolved other strategies to evade destruction. *Mycobacterium tuberculosis* secretes molecules that inhibit lysosome/phagosome fusion, while *M. leprae* can escape from the phagosome and grow in the cytoplasm. The cell wall of both these bacteria contains lipoarabinomannan that blocks the effects of γ-interferon on macrophages.

T lymphocytes represent the major host defence against intracellular pathogens. In many cases the bacteria themselves do not directly harm the host but the pathogenesis is caused by the immune response. After invasion of the host, intracellular bacteria will be taken up by macrophages, evade intracellular killing and multiply. During intracellular replication some microbial molecules will be processed and presented on the surface of the infected cell in association with major histocompatibility complex (MHC) gene products. The exact nature of the microbial molecules and the processing mechanism are not known. The processing appears to produce mainly antigen fragments in association with MHC class II molecules. This complex on the cell surface will be recognized by specific CD4$^+$ T cells, which will be stimulated to release lymphokines. These molecules will in turn activate the macrophage so that the intracellular bacteria are killed.

It has also been proposed that peptides derived from the bacteria can become associated with MHC class I molecules. This complex will lead to the destruction of the infected cell by CD8$^+$ T cells. These cells also produce lymphokines that can aid in the elimination of the infection. The lymphokines produced will attract blood monocytes to the site and activate them. If these newly recruited cells take up the released mycobacteria they will be more likely to destroy them

since they will be in an activated state. The accumulation of macrophages will also cause the formation of a granuloma, which will prevent dissemination of the bacteria to other sites in the body. As conditions for the survival of the pathogens become less suitable they stop replicating and die. Some intracellular bacteria infect cells that are unable to destroy them. In this situation a more aggressive immune response may be needed to remove the pathogen and this can cause pathogenic damage unless kept under control (see below).

IMMUNOPATHOLOGY

The immune response to an organism will lead to some tissue damage through inflammation, lymph node swelling and cell infiltration. Sometimes the damage caused by the immune system is very severe, leading to serious disease and death. Rheumatic fever can follow group A streptococcal infections of the throat and is believed to be due to antibodies formed against a streptococcal cell wall component cross-reacting with cardiac muscle or heart valve. Myocarditis develops a few weeks after the throat infection and can be restimulated if the patient is reinfected with different streptococci.

Immune complex disease (type III hypersensitivity) is frequently associated with bacterial infections. Infective endocarditis due to staphylococci and streptococci is associated with circulating complexes of antibody and bacterial antigen. Detection of these complexes can be helpful in diagnosis, but they can lead to joint and kidney lesions, vasculitis and skin rashes. Immune complexes may play a role in the pathogenesis of leprosy, typhoid fever and gonorrhoea.

Effects of endotoxin

Endotoxin interacts with cells and molecules of inflammation, immunity and haemostasis. Fever is induced by interleukin-1, produced by the liver in response to endotoxin, acting on the temperature-regulating hypothalamus. The action of lipopolysaccharide on platelets and activation of Hageman factor causes disseminating intravascular coagulation with ensuing ischaemic tissue damage to various organs. Septic shock occurs during severe infections with Gram-negative organisms when bacteria or lipopolysaccharide enter the bloodstream. Endotoxin acts on neutrophils, platelets and complement to produce, both directly and through mast cell degranulation, vaso-active amines that cause hypotension. The mortality is very high.

Endotoxin causes macrophages to produce large quantities of potent cytokines such as interleukin-1, tumour necrosis factor and colony-stimulating factors. It also causes polyclonal activation of B cells and can stimulate natural killer cells and other cell types to produce γ-interferon. A substantial part of the pathogenesis of endotoxic shock is probably due to the production of these molecules by cells of the immune system. In small amounts, endotoxin may actually be beneficial to the host but when present in excess the results can be disastrous.

Mycobacterial disease

Activated macrophages secrete a variety of biologically active molecules, including proteases, tumour necrosis factor and reactive oxygen intermediates that are harmful to the surrounding tissue. Hence tissue destruction will be an inevitable side-effect of this important mechanism of resistance. In the acute phase of a response this is likely to be tolerated; but, in the case of resistant organisms such as mycobacteria the process may become chronic and the tissue destruction extensive. Mycobacterial components are still able to stimulate a response after the bacterium has been killed since they persist for a long time, adding to the tissue damage.

Recent evidence suggests that lysis of infected cells may also occur. At first sight this may appear beneficial. Such a direct effect may be particularly relevant in the case of obligate intracellular pathogens like *M. leprae*. Release into the hypoxic centre of a productive granuloma may also be fatal for *M. tuberculosis*, which is highly sensitive to low oxygen pressures. The same cytolytic event may also result in microbial discharge from the granuloma into surrounding capillaries or alveoli and hence facilitate dissemination to other parts of the body or to other individuals. Lysis of infected cells causes tissue destruction, the severity of the effects depending on the importance of the tissue involved. *M leprae* infects a particularly essential cell, the Schwann cell, that is an irreplaceable component of the peripheral nervous system. Although the presence of *M. leprae* does not appear to affect the host cell to any extent, the presence of activated macrophages releasing toxic molecules or direct lysis by cytotoxic cells constitutes a major pathological mechanism in leprosy.

If the leprosy bacillus is released from a lysed non-phagocytic cell to be engulfed by an activated macrophage then the bacterium will be eliminated. Therefore, macrophage activation and target cell lysis can be beneficial as well as detrimental to the host.

The cell-mediated response that has the potential to eliminate these infections will give rise to type IV hypersensitivity reactions if the antigen is not efficiently removed. Chronic production of lymphokines will cause granuloma formation that with time can lead to fibrosis and loss of organ function. This type of response is particularly prevalent in patients with tuberculosis.

RECOMMENDED READING

Mims C A 1987 The Pathogenesis of Infectious Disease 3rd edn. Academic Press, London

Taussig M J 1984 Processes in Pathology and Microbiology 2nd edn. Blackwell Scientific Publishers, Oxford

PART 3

Bacterial pathogens and associated diseases

15

Staphylococcus

Skin and wound infections; abscess; osteomyelitis; food poisoning

J. P. Arbuthnott

The genus *Staphylococcus* consists of cluster-forming Gram-positive cocci. Sir Alexander Ogston, a Scottish surgeon, first showed in 1880 that the organism caused a number of pyogenic diseases in man. He introduced the name 'staphylococcus', which derives from the Greek *staphyle* (bunch of grapes) and *kokkos* (grain or berry). The main pathogen within the genus, *Staphylococcus aureus*, is the cause of a wide range of major and minor infections in man and animals (Table 15.1). Currently there are some 27 different species of staphylococci. These fall into two main groups on the basis of their ability to clot blood plasma by action of the enzyme *coagulase*. *Staph. aureus* is by far the most important coagulase-positive species. The coagulase-negative staphylococci are skin commensals, which are now recognized as

important opportunistic pathogens that can cause infections associated with prostheses, catheters and implants (*Staph. epidermidis*), and urinary tract infections (*Staph. saprophyticus*). It has not been common practice for medical microbiologists to identify coagulase-negative staphylococci to the species level. However, methods are now available that facilitate identification and the importance of other recently recognized coagulase-negative species is being assessed.

Staphylococci, being resistant to dry conditions and high salt concentrations, are well suited to their ecological niche, which is the skin surface of man and animals. Approximately 30% of healthy people are 'carriers' of *Staph. aureus*; an even higher number carry coagulase-negative staphylococci.

Staphylococci are also commonly present on other animals, including farm animals used for milk production, viz., cattle, sheep and goats; mastitis caused by *Staph. aureus* is a common and costly complication of milking. Contamination of food can occur from either human or animal sources; such contamination can result in staphylococcal food poisoning.

Table 15.1 Infections caused by staphylococci

Staph. aureus		Coagulase-negative staphylococci
PYOGENIC INFECTIONS	TOXIN-MEDIATED INFECTIONS	
Boils, carbuncles	Scalded skin	Infected prostheses
Wound infection	syndrome	Infected implants
Abscesses	Pemphigus	Ventriculitis[a]
Impetigo	neonatorum	Peritonitis (CAPD)
Mastitis	Toxic shock	Septicaemia
Septicaemia	syndrome	Endocarditis
Osteomyelitis	Food poisoning	
Pneumonia		

[a] Shunt-associated.
CAPD, continuous ambulatory peritoneal dialysis.

DEFINITION OF THE GENUS

The chief properties characterizing the genus *Staphylococcus* are shown in Table 15.2. Staphylococci resemble members of the genus *Micrococcus* morphologically, but they differ in DNA base composition. Micrococci also differ in having a strictly aerobic metabolism. Members of the genus *Peptococcus* are strictly anaerobic cluster-forming Gram-positive cocci (see Chapter 37). Micrococci and peptococci are usually regarded as harmless commensals.

STAPHYLOCOCCUS AUREUS

DESCRIPTION

Staph. aureus is a Gram-positive coccus about 1 μm in diameter. The cocci are mainly arranged in grape-like clusters (Fig. 15.1); but some, especially when examined in pathological specimens, occur as single cells or pairs of cells. The organisms are non-sporing, non-motile and usually non-capsulate. When grown on nutrient agar, milk agar or blood agar for 24 h at 37°C individual colonies are circular, 2–3 mm in diameter with a smooth, shiny surface; colonies appear opaque and are frequently pigmented (golden-yellow, fawn or cream), though a few strains are unpigmented. Staphylococci are salt-tolerant and can be selectively isolated from materials such as faeces and food by use of media containing 7–10% sodium chloride. The main distinctive diagnostic features of *Staph. aureus* are:

1. Production of an extracellular enzyme, coagulase, that converts fibrinogen in citrated human or rabbit plasma into fibrin, aided by an activator present in plasma. This test is done by adding a drop of fresh young broth culture into a tube containing 0.5 ml citrated plasma diluted 1 in 10. A positive result is seen within a few hours as a distinct clot.

2. Production of thermostable *nucleases* that break down DNA. This activity is detected by the ability of a boiled broth culture to degrade DNA in an agar diffusion test.

Table 15.2 Characteristics of the genus *Staphylococcus*

Gram-positive cocci
Catalase-positive
Divide in more than one plane to form irregular, grape-like clusters
Capable of aerobic and anaerobic metabolism
Occur widely on the surfaces of man and other vertebrate animals

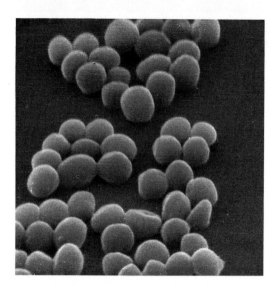

Fig. 15.1 Scanning electron micrograph of *Staph. aureus*.

3. Production of a surface-associated protein known as *clumping factor* or *bound coagulase* that reacts with fibrinogen. Clumping factor is easily detected within a few seconds by adding undiluted plasma to a saline suspension of the organism on a microscope slide.

Various commercial systems based on enzyme production, haemolytic activity and sugar fermentation tests are now available that enable rapid confirmation of the identification of coagulase-positive and coagulase-negative species. Such systems are particularly useful for screening large numbers of strains obtained from environmental and food samples.

PATHOGENESIS

Staph. aureus, which is present in the nose and on the skin of a variable proportion of healthy people, is an opportunistic pathogen in that it causes infection most commonly at sites of lowered host resistance, e.g. damaged skin or mucous membranes or haematomas in the cancellous tissue of a long bone. Staphylococcal pneumonia is a recognized complication of influenza.

Virulence factors

Staph. aureus strains possess a large number of cell-associated and extracellular factors, some of which contribute to the ability of the organism to overcome the body's defences and to invade, survive in and colonize the tissues (Table 15.3).

Though the role of each individual factor is not fully understood, it is likely that they are responsible for establishment of infection, enabling the organism to bind to connective tissue, to resist killing by the bactericidal activities of humoral factors such as complement and to overcome uptake and intracellular killing by phagocytes. Extracellular toxins also play a role.

Animal experiments, with mutants defective in individual virulence factors, support the view that establishment of a focus of staphylococcal infection is multifactorial and that no single virulence factor is pre-eminent in overcoming host resistance. However, particular exotoxins are responsible for the symptoms of certain syndromes.

Staphylococcal toxins

Enterotoxins. Five types of enterotoxin (types A–E) are commonly produced by up to 65% of strains of *Staph. aureus*, sometimes singly and sometimes in combination. These toxic proteins are heat-stable, withstanding exposure to 100°C for several minutes. When ingested as preformed toxins in contaminated food, microgram amounts of toxin can induce nausea, vomiting and diarrhoea (i.e. the symptoms of staphylococcal food poisoning) within a few hours. The serotypes A–E can be detected by a variety of sensitive serological tests (e.g. latex agglutination). Enterotoxins are also potent mitogens which induce the release of mediators such as interleukin-1 from lymphocytes and trigger systemic effects.

Epidermolytic toxins. Two kinds of epidermolytic toxin (types A and B) are commonly produced by strains, mainly belonging to phage group II (see below), that cause blistering diseases. Blistering results from splitting within the plane of the epidermis induced by the toxin. Such blisters range in severity from the trivial to the distended blisters of *pemphigus neonatorum* or the

Table 15.3 Virulence factors of *Staph. aureus*

Virulence factor	Activity
Cell wall polymers	
Peptidoglycan	Inhibitor of inflammatory response
Teichoic acid	Phage adsorption; reservoir of bound divalent cations
Cell surface proteins	
Protein A	Reacts with Fc region of IgG
Clumping factor	Binds to fibrinogen
Fibronectin-binding protein	Binds to fibronectin
Collagen-binding protein	Binds to collagen
Exoproteins	
α-Lysin	
β-Lysin	
γ-Lysin	Impairment of membrane permeability; cytotoxic effects
δ-Lysin	on phagocytic and tissue cells
Panton–Valentine leucocidin	
Epidermolytic toxins	Cause blistering of skin
Toxic shock syndrome toxin	Induces multisystem effects
Enterotoxins	Induce vomiting and diarrhoea
Coagulase	Converts fibrinogen to fibrin in plasma
Hyaluronidase	Degrades hyaluronic acid in connective tissue
Staphylokinase	Degrades lipid
Lipase	Degrades lipid
Phospholipases	Degrade phospholipids
Deoxyribonuclease	Degrades DNA
Proteases	Cause proteolysis

flattened blisters of *impetigo*. Outbreaks of blistering disease are not uncommon in busy nursing units where careful observation of hygiene practice is essential if skin sepsis is to be avoided. The most dramatic manifestation of epidermolytic toxin is the *scalded skin syndrome* in which toxin spreads systemically in individuals that lack neutralizing antitoxin: extensive areas of skin are affected, which, after the development of a painful rash, slough off; the skin surface resembles scalding. Such blistering lesions are seen mainly, but not exclusively, in small children.

Toxic shock syndrome toxin (TSST-1). This was discovered in the early 1980s as a result of epidemiological and microbiological investigations in the USA of an apparently new disease named *toxic shock syndrome*. This multisystem and occasionally fatal condition can occur in any non-immune individual infected with a TSST-1-producing strain. However, the disease reached public notice when large numbers of cases were reported in healthy young menstruating women; an association with highly absorbent tampons was established. Vaginal colonization with toxigenic *Staph. aureus* in the presence of the tampon created conditions favourable to multiplication of the organism and toxin production. The absence of circulating antibodies to TSST-1 was indicative of high risk in such cases.

LABORATORY DIAGNOSIS

One or more of the following specimens may be collected for examination:

1. *Pus* from abscesses, wounds, burns, etc.
2. *Sputum* from cases of lower respiratory tract infections, e.g. influenzal pneumonia
3. *Faeces* or *vomit* from patients with suspected food poisoning; also convenient quantities of the *remains of foods* suspected of causing food poisoning
4. *Blood* from patients with suspected bacteraemia, e.g. in osteomyelitis or endocarditis
5. *Mid-stream urine* from patients with suspected cystitis, pyelonephritis or post-catheterization infection
6. *Anterior nasal* and *perineal swabs* from suspected carriers; the swabs should first be

moistened, if possible, with sterile water or broth, and the nasal swabs should be rubbed in turn over the anterior walls of both nostrils, which are covered by squamous epithelium.

The presence of staphylococci can often be demonstrated by examination of a Gram-stained smear. The organisms can be cultured readily on nutrient, blood or milk agar. Plates are inspected for characteristic golden, cream-coloured or white colonies, and the tube or slide coagulase test is performed to distinguish *Staph. aureus* from coagulase-negative species.

Phage typing

For epidemiological purposes, strains of *Staph. aureus* may be differentiated into different *phage types* by observation of their pattern of susceptibility to lysis by a set of 23 different *Staph. aureus* bacteriophages. The test strain is inoculated confluently over a nutrient agar plate marked out in 23 squares; each of the 23 phage preparations in specially measured dilutions (*routine test dilutions*) is dropped onto the appropriate square before the plate is incubated. Virulent phages cause lysis of staphylococci that they are able to infect, and thus produce a clearing in the lawn of growth (Fig. 15.2). Phage types are designated according to the phages able to cause this effect. Thus, a strain of type 3B/3C/55 is one that is lysed by phage 3B, phage 3C and phage 55 but not by any of the other phages.

Strains isolated from patients, carriers and fomites may be precisely identified ('fingerprinted') by this means and their source and pattern of spread in an outbreak discovered. For example, a group of surgical wound infections may be traced to a surgeon who is a nasal carrier, or to a patient who is shedding staphylococci into the ward, by the demonstration that the strains from all the infected wounds belong to the same phage type as the one isolated from the surgeon or the shedding patient.

In a period of 12 months as many as 100–200 phage types of staphylococci may be isolated from patients and carriers in a maternity unit or a surgical ward, yet only 10–20 types may be found in cases of clinical infection and only two or three types may be responsible for the large majority of the clinical infections.

Strains of *Staph. aureus* can be allocated to three main phage groups, I, II and III, according to their susceptibility to three groups of related phages. Group I contains many hospital epidemic strains, e.g. those of types 80 and 52A/79. Group II contains many of the strains causing minor sepsis outside of hospitals and strains of types 71 and 3B/3C/55 most commonly cause the blistering lesions of impetigo, pemphigus neonatorum and scalded skin syndrome. Group III includes strains of animal origin, many of the antibiotic-resistant hospital strains (e.g. type 47/53/75/77) and most of the enterotoxin-producing strains. The strains of the three groups produce antigenically distinct forms of coagulase. Group IV phages are restricted for typing isolates from animals.

Strains resistant to the typing phages have become common in recent years. Therefore, a number of new typing phages (94, 96), designated

as group V, have been added to the typing set in order to increase typability.

TREATMENT
Sensitivity to antibiotics

Staph. aureus and other staphylococci are inherently sensitive to many antimicrobial agents (Table 15.4). Among the most active is benzylpenicillin, but most strains encountered in patients and carriers outside of hospitals and about 90% of those found in hospitals are now resistant. Resistance to penicillin depends on the ability to produce the enzyme penicillinase, a β-lactamase that opens the β-lactam ring of the penicillin molecule. Penicillinase also inactivates most of the other penicillins, including ampicillin, amoxycillin, carbenicillin, azlocillin and piperacillin, so that penicillin-resistant strains are resistant to other penicillin-type drugs. However, a few compounds have been developed that exhibit stability to

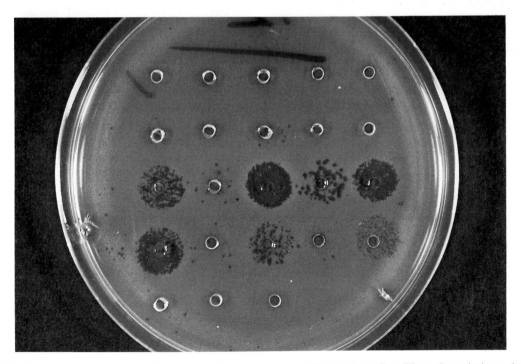

Fig. 15.2 Phage-typing plate showing lysis produced by the International Standard set of 23 different bacteriophages in a lawn of *Staph. aureus*. More than 50 plaques, irrespective of size, in the area surrounding the phage inoculum is scored as a positive result. The *Staph. aureus* strain shown belongs to lytic group III (6/47/53/54/75/83a/85). (Photograph courtesy of George Sharp and Carol Webster.)

Table 15.4 Antibiotics and staphylococci

Agents inherently active against staphylococci	Agents lacking useful antistaphylococcal activity
Penicillins[a]	Mecillinam
Cephalosporins	Temocillin
Aminoglycosides	Monobactams
Tetracyclines	Polymyxins
Macrolides	Nitroimidazoles
Lincosamides	Quinolones[b]
Glycopeptides	
Fluoroquinolones[c]	
Rifampicin	
Fusidic acid	
Trimethoprim	
Chloramphenicol	

[a] Resistance common (see text).
[b] Nalidixic acid, etc.
[c] Ciprofloxacin, etc.

staphylococcal penicillinase; these include methicillin, cloxacillin and flucloxacillin. Cephalosporins and the enzyme inhibitors clavulanic acid and sulbactam also resist penicillinase (see Chapter 6). Resistance to methicillin, cloxacillin and, indeed, virtually all other β-lactam antibiotics may arise by mutation in one of the essential penicillin-binding proteins found in the cell envelope. Such strains may also be resistant to several other antistaphylococcal antibiotics, including gentamicin, erythromycin and tetracycline. These strains (multiresistant *Staph. aureus*; MRSA) are often responsible for hospital cross-infection. Multiresistant hospital staphylococci have probably arisen by a succession of mutations conferring resistance to different drugs and by the acquisition of plasmids that bear genes conferring

antibiotic resistance (Table 15.5). Transposons have also played a part in the transfer of resistance determinants from a plasmid to a chromosomal location (see Chapter 7).

Resistance to vancomycin in *Staph. aureus* is as yet unknown.

Choice of antibiotic for therapy

Since strains of *Staph. aureus* vary in sensitivity to different antibiotics, the choice of antibiotic for use in treatment should be based on the results of sensitivity tests made on a culture of the strain isolated from the patient. Pending receipt of the results, the treatment of severe infections suspected of being staphylococcal should be begun with flucloxacillin. If tests show that the infecting organism is penicillin-sensitive, the drug of choice for further treatment is benzylpenicillin, which is narrow-spectrum and bactericidal. If, as is likely, the strain is found to be penicillin-resistant, flucloxacillin should be continued. If the patient is hypersensitive to penicillin, another antistaphylococcal drug should be used, e.g. gentamicin, clindamycin, fusidic acid or erythromycin. Fusidic acid is not usually used alone in serious infections since mutation to resistance arises readily. If the infecting organism is MRSA, treatment with vancomycin should be initiated immediately. Collections of pus may require surgical drainage if antibiotic treatment is to be successful. Similarly, infection associated with foreign bodies may not be amenable to treatment unless the offending object is removed.

Table 15.5 Common mechanisms of resistance to antistaphylococcal agents

Agent	Mechanism of resistance	Usual genetic location
Penicillins[a]	β-Lactamase	Plasmid
Methicillin[b] Cephalosporins	Altered binding protein	Chromosome
Chloramphenicol	Acetyltransferase	Plasmid
Tetracyclines	Reduced accumulation	Plasmid
Erythromycin	Methylation of ribosome	Plasmid
Streptomycin	Altered ribosomal protein	Chromosome
Other aminoglycosides	Enzymic modification	Plasmid
Fusidic acid	Altered factor G	Chromosome
Rifampicin	Altered RNA polymerase	Chromosome

[a] Except methicillin, nafcillin and isoxazolylpenicillins.
[b] Including nafcillin and isoxazolylpenicillins.

Severe systemic toxin-mediated disease demands urgent appropriate medical treatment as well as antistaphylococcal therapy.

EPIDEMIOLOGY

Sources of infection

Infected lesions

Large numbers of cocci are disseminated in pus and dried exudate discharged from large infected wounds, burns, secondarily infected skin lesions, and in sputum coughed from the lung of a patient with bronchopneumonia. Small discharging lesions, on the hands of doctors and nurses, are a special danger to their patients. Food handlers may similarly introduce enterotoxin-producing food-poisoning strains into food.

Healthy carriers

Staph. aureus grows harmlessly on the moist skin of the nostrils in up to 30–40% of healthy persons; the perineum is also commonly colonized. Organisms are spread from these sites into the environment by the hands, handkerchiefs, clothing, and dust consisting of skin squames and cloth fibres. Some carriers, called *shedders*, disseminate exceptionally large numbers of cocci, comparable to the numbers disseminated by patients with large superficial lesions or lower respiratory tract infections.

During the first day or two of life most babies become colonized by staphylococci acquired from their mother, nurse or environment. In babies born in hospital, the nose, umbilical stump and moist areas of skin are commonly colonized by *Staph. aureus*. Nasal carriage in babies, as in older persons, is usually long-lasting. When a particular strain of *Staph. aureus* has colonized a carrier site in an individual, it can persist in that site for many months or several years. Transmission from babies to nursing mothers, who then develop mastitis, is fairly common.

Animals

Domesticated and some wild species may disseminate *Staph. aureus* from infected lesions or carriage sites and so cause infections in man, e.g. a dairy cow with staphylococcal infection of the udder may give infected milk which can cause staphylococcal food poisoning.

Modes of infection

The mode of acquisition of an infection may be either *exogenous*, i.e. from an external source, or *endogenous*, i.e. from a carriage site, or minor lesion, elsewhere in the patient's own body (see Chapter 67). Staphylococci do not grow outside the body except occasionally in moist nutrient materials such as meat, milk and dirty water. They are, however, very hardy and, though not spore-forming, may remain alive in a dormant state for several months when dried in pus, sputum, bed clothes or dust. They are fairly readily killed by heat (e.g. by moist heat at 65°C for 30 min), by exposure to light and by common disinfectants.

While survival in the environment may be a factor in persistence it is important to remember that the main habitat of *Staph. aureus* is the body surfaces of man and animals.

Cross-infection

Cross-infection is an important method of spread of staphylococcal disease, particularly in closed communities such as hospitals. Direct contact is probably the most important mode of transfer, but air-borne dust and air-borne droplet nuclei may also be involved (see Chapter 67).

COAGULASE-NEGATIVE STAPHYLOCOCCI

Coagulase-negative staphylococci comprise a large group of related species which are commonly found on the surface of healthy persons in whom they are rarely the cause of infection, except in compromised patients.

More than 20 species of coagulase-negative staphylococci are recognized, but only a few are commonly incriminated in human infection. *Staph. epidermidis* accounts for about 75% of all clinical isolates, probably reflecting its preponderance in the normal skin flora; most of the remainder are identified as *Staph. hominis*, *Staph.*

simulans and *Staph. haemolyticus*. One species, *Staph. saprophyticus*, is a common cause of acute cystitis in young women, but is seldom implicated in infections elsewhere.

DESCRIPTION

Coagulase-negative staphylococci are morphologically similar to *Staph. aureus* and the methods for isolation are the same. Colonies are usually non-pigmented (white) and they can be distinguished from *Staph. aureus* not only by their failure to coagulate plasma, but also by their lack of clumping factor and deoxyribonuclease. Various test systems have been devised for the identification of coagulase-negative species of staphylococci but this is seldom worthwhile. Some identification systems are commercially available in kit form.

Because the organisms commonly contaminate clinical specimens and laboratory cultures, care has to be exercised in assessing their significance when isolated, especially from superficial sites that they may be merely colonizing, or from normally sterile specimens such as blood or cerebrospinal fluid.

Coagulase-negative staphylococci are opportunistic pathogens that cause infection in persons with defective resistance, often by colonizing plastic devices. The organisms cause particular problems after cardiac surgery; in patients fitted with ventriculovenous cerebrospinal fluid shunts; in continuous ambulatory peritoneal dialysis (CAPD); and in immunocompromised patients.

The emergence of coagulase-negative staphylococci as major pathogens reflects the increased use of implants such as cerebrospinal fluid shunts, intravascular lines and cannulae, cardiac valves, pacemakers, artificial joints, vascular grafts, and urinary catheters.

PATHOGENESIS

Less is known of the mechanisms of pathogenesis of coagulase-negative staphylococci than of *Staph. aureus*. Unlike *Staph. aureus* they produce few known virulence factors and their major virulence attribute is the ability to form adherent biofilms on the surfaces of polymers used for implants and prosthetic devices. Controversy still rages about the particular surface factor that confers stickiness. Surface slime is widely regarded as important although the precise chemical composition of this slime is not yet known. Surface proteins are also likely candidates in adherence.

TREATMENT

Antibiotic treatment of infections with coagulase-negative staphylococci is complicated because antibiotic sensitivity in this group is generally unpredictable and multiresistant strains are increasingly prevalent. Resistance to penicillin, methicillin, gentamicin, erythromycin and chloramphenicol is common. If such a strain is the cause of systemic infection, then vancomycin or the related drug teicoplanin must be used. A few strains exhibit reduced susceptibility to teicoplanin, but these strains usually retain sensitivity to vancomycin.

It is important to establish, as far as possible, that the organisms are adopting a truly pathogenic role before embarking on therapy. Successful eradication of established infection associated with polymer surfaces usually entails removal of the device involved.

Uncomplicated staphylococcal cystitis ordinarily responds to minimal treatment with trimethoprim, or one of the fluoroquinolones, such as norfloxacin.

RECOMMENDED READING

Easmon C S F, Adlam C 1983 *Staphylococci and Staphylococcal Infections*. Academic Press, London, vols 1 and 2

Elek S D 1959 Staphylococcus pyogenes *and its Relation to Disease*. Livingstone, Edinburgh

Jones D, Board R G, Sussman M 1990 *Staphylococci. Society for Applied Microbiology Symposium Series*, No. 19. Blackwell Scientific, Oxford

Macdonald A, Smith G 1981 *The Staphylococci*. Aberdeen University Press, Aberdeen

Mudd S 1970 In: Mudd S (ed) *Infectious Agents and Host Reactions*. W B Saunders, Philadelphia, ch 5

Pfaller M A, Herwaldt L A 1988 Laboratory, clinical and epidemiological aspects of coagulase-negative staphylococci. *Clinical Microbiology Reviews* 1: 281–299

16

Streptococcus and enterococcus

Sore throat; scarlet fever; impetigo; bacterial endocarditis; rheumatic fever; glomerulonephritis

P. W. Ross

Streptococci form part of the normal flora of man and animals. They inhabit various sites, notably the upper respiratory tract, and usually live harmlessly as commensals. Some species, of which *Streptococcus pyogenes* is the most important, may adopt a more aggressive role. This organism can cause a wide spectrum of diseases, including tonsillitis, erysipelas, impetigo, scarlet fever and septicaemia, which range in severity from the trivial to the life-threatening. *Str. pyogenes* is also involved in the aetiology of rheumatic fever and acute glomerulonephritis. Other pathogenic species include *Str. agalactiae*, an important cause of neonatal infection, and *Str. pneumoniae* (see Chapter 17). Related organisms include: *Peptostreptococcus* spp., which are strictly anaerobic; enterococci, of which *Enterococcus faecalis* is the most important; and certain species that are rarely incriminated in infection, including *Pediococcus* spp. and *Leuconostoc* spp.

The species of streptococci and enterococci that are most commonly encountered in medical laboratory practice are shown in Table 16.1.

CLASSIFICATION OF STREPTOCOCCI

Streptococci are Gram-positive bacteria arranged in chains of varying length (Fig. 16.1); each cell is approximately 1.0 μm in diameter, non-motile, non-sporing and may be capsulate. The majority are facultative anaerobes, but there are species

Table 16.1 Principal types of streptococci and enterococci involved in human infection

Species	Lancefield group	Type of haemolysis on horse blood agar
Str. pyogenes	A	β
Str. agalactiae	B	β
Str. equisimilis	C	β
Str. zooepidemicus	D	β
E. faecalis	D	β or none
E. faecium	D	β or none
Str. bovis	D	α or none
Str. equinus	D	α or none
Str. anginosus[a]	A, C, G or F	α, β or none
Str. pneumoniae	None	α
Str. sanguis	None	α
Str. mitior[b]	None	α
Str. mutans	None	None
Str. salivarius	None	None

[a] Includes strains designated *Str. milleri*, *Str. intermedius* and *Str. constellatus*.
[b] Also known as *Str. mitis*.

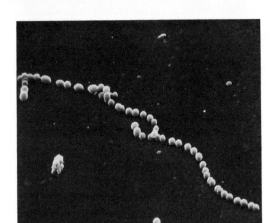

Fig. 16.1 Scanning electron micrograph of *Str. pyogenes* showing typical chain formation.

that are strictly anaerobic. All have an anaerobic type of metabolism and are catalase-negative.

Classification depends traditionally on the type of haemolysis seen on blood agar. Some strains have soluble haemolysins (streptolysins O and S), which produce a clear zone of haemolysis on fresh blood agar media. This is known as β haemolysis, a phenomenon associated with the majority of streptococcal species that cause primary infections in man and animals. These haemolytic streptococci can be further subdivided serologically into a number of broad groups exploiting differences in the group-specific poly-saccharide antigens contained in the cell wall. Lancefield thus identified a number of different groups lettered sequentially A–H and K–V.

Str. pyogenes belongs to Lancefield group A. These strains may be further subdivided by specific sera into Griffith types according to their surface protein antigens (M, T and R). The M protein is the antigen of most importance and it exists in approximately 60 different antigenic forms, each of which is present in a different serotype of *Str. pyogenes* (type 1, type 2, etc.). The determination of the serotype of strains of *Str. pyogenes* isolated from patients and carriers plays a valuable part in the epidemiological investigation of outbreaks of infection in a way compar-

able to the use of phage typing in the study of *Staphylococcus aureus* infection.

Streptococci that do not possess soluble haemolysins are divided into two categories: (1) those that cause a narrow zone of partial clearing and green coloration and are called α-haemolytic streptococci, or viridans streptococci; (2) those that produce no obvious changes around colonies on blood agar and are called non-haemolytic. These are sometimes called γ-haemolytic but this term may be misleading in terms of classification and should not be used. Some oral streptococci such as *Str. mutans* and *Str. salivarius* are usually non-haemolytic.

PATHOGENESIS OF β-HAEMOLYTIC STREPTOCOCCAL INFECTIONS

The most common route of entry of *Str. pyogenes* is the upper respiratory tract where the primary infection is established, usually in the throat, but only a proportion of infected individuals develop tonsillitis or pharyngitis. The others may have mild atypical infections or become symptomless carriers. In tropical climates the skin is a common site of entry. After an acute attack of sore throat the convalescent patient may carry the infecting streptococci in the fauces for some weeks; a few of these convalescent carriers may continue to carry the streptococci in the throat or nose for much longer periods, especially if there is diseased tonsillar tissue or nasal deformity. Nasal carriage is much less common than throat carriage but a nasal carrier sheds far greater numbers of streptococci into the environment than a throat carrier and consequently nasal carriers are more likely sources for the spread of infection than throat carriers.

Several factors are involved in the production of infection by β-haemolytic streptococci — structural components of the organisms and their extracellular products.

Structural components

The virulence of *Str. pyogenes* is closely related to a surface antigen, the M protein, which is the main antiphagocytic factor. M-associated protein antigen, which is not type-specific, is found in M-positive variants. Two other surface proteins, T and R, do not play any part in virulence but are useful in identification of the infecting serotype. Antibodies to M protein are mainly responsible for immunity; they counteract the anti-phagocytic action of the M protein and are effective only against the homologous serotype. Fimbriae on the surface of streptococci enable attachment to epithelial cells and consist of M protein. Hyaluronic acid capsules are produced by streptococci in the early stages of artificial culture and also when spreading in the blood and tissues, but they have only a weak antiphagocytic effect.

Extracellular products

β-Haemolytic streptococci, notably *Str. pyogenes*, possess a formidable battery of diffusible products, but it is not yet possible to link definitively any individual toxin or enzyme, or combination, with any particular syndrome of infection. Not all of these substances are produced by any one strain but most strains can form the majority of them, depending on environmental conditions. These products can also be isolated from some other β-haemolytic streptococci.

Erythrogenic toxins

There are three serologically distinct toxins. The group A streptococci which produce these are infected with temperate bacteriophages. The important activities of the toxins as demonstrated in experimental animals include pyrogenicity, cytotoxicity, suppression of the reticulo-endothelial system, immunosuppression, alteration in permeability of cells of the cerebral cortex and enhancement of susceptibility to endotoxin.

Streptolysin O

Most group A streptococci and some group C and G streptococci produce this haemolysin. Other bacteria also form streptolysin O-like products. Streptolysin O lyses red blood cells by linking to bound cholesterol in the cell membrane, causing holes to form in this structure; it is also cytotoxic

for other cells, including neutrophils, platelets and cardiac tissue. It is inactivated by oxygen.

Streptolysin S

This haemolysin is not inactivated by oxygen and is responsible for the haemolysis produced on the surface of an aerobic blood agar plate. As well as its haemolytic properties it also has a leucocidal action.

Streptokinase (fibrinolysin)

Streptokinase, produced by group A, C and G streptococci, is protein in nature and is antigenic.

The role of streptokinase in streptococcal infections is not clear but because of its action in preventing the formation of an effective fibrin barrier it may well influence the character of the lesions by interfering with the localization of the infection.

Deoxyribonucleases (DNases)

There are at least four of these enzymes, designated A, B, C and D. As with other extracellular products of streptococci, they are found in group C and G as well as in group A streptococci; they are antigenic. DNase B is the most common form in *Str. pyogenes*. They hydrolyse nucleic acids and nucleoproteins, and since the products can be used by streptococci they may have an important nutritional role. Nucleases have been used clinically to liquefy viscous exudates, e.g. empyema.

Hyaluronidase

This antigenic substance is produced by strains of group A, B, C and G streptococci. A characteristic feature of streptococcal infections, whether the portal of entry is the throat, the skin or the genital tract, is the ability of the organisms to spread through the tissues. Cellulitis and erysipelas are classical examples of the spreading lesion, and this may be related to the production of hyaluronidase; however, *Staph. aureus* also produces hyaluronidase, but rarely causes spreading infections in the skin.

Nicotinamide adenine dinucleotidase (NADase)

This is produced by strains of group A, C and G streptococci and is antigenic. There is a close connection between the ability of a streptococcal strain to produce NADase and its leucotoxic effect.

Serum opacity factor (lipoproteinase)

The ability to produce opacity in horse serum is a characteristic of certain M types of group A streptococci. The opacity factor is closely associated with the M protein and is loosely bound to the cell. It is antigenically specific, the specificity corresponding to that of the M antigen.

Other extracellular products that have been isolated from streptococci include bacteriocines, amylase, esterase, proteinase, lipase and β-glucuronidase.

LABORATORY DIAGNOSIS OF β-HAEMOLYTIC STREPTOCOCCAL INFECTIONS

Identification of β-haemolytic streptococci that have been isolated from the patient and examination of patients' sera for a rising titre of antibodies to one or more streptococcal antigens are the means of diagnosis.

Swabs are taken from patients or from suspected carriers. Microscopy is of little help in the diagnosis of streptococcal pharyngitis, though it may reveal other pathogens such as Vincent's organisms. If there is likely to be a delay of more than a few hours before the swab can be despatched to the laboratory or processed, it should be refrigerated. In a search for carriers, as in an institutional outbreak of sore throat or scarlet fever, nasal as well as throat swabs must be taken. Saliva can yield positive results when the throat swab is negative.

Swabs are cultured on blood agar and incubated for 24 h. Anaerobic as well as aerobic incubation should be carried out because group A strains that form only haemolysin O fail to show haemolysis on aerobic culture.

It is unhelpful for a service laboratory to report to the clinician growth of β-haemolytic streptococci from a specimen without grouping the organisms. Grouping of all β-haemolytic streptococci is mandatory for the following reasons: (1) to facilitate epidemiological surveillance of streptococcal infections in hospital and in the wider community; (2) to monitor drug resistance patterns effectively; and (3) because various Lancefield groups are associated with characteristic infections.

For the presumptive identification of β-haemolytic streptococci belonging to group A, bacitracin sensitivity may be tested. Group A organisms are much more sensitive than other groups to bacitracin but the test is not totally reliable as some non-group A strains may also be sensitive. For accurate identification of streptococci, Lancefield's serogrouping must be performed. Commercial kits are used increasingly for streptococcal grouping and are convenient, quick and reliable.

Tests for streptococcal serum antibodies may also be performed, but such tests do not give the clinician an immediate answer during the initial phase of an acute infection. They may be used to identify or confirm primary infections but are more commonly used for the diagnosis of the non-suppurative sequelae of group A streptococcal infection such as rheumatic fever or glomerulonephritis. Single titres are difficult to evaluate as they do not differentiate between past and current infections; a second serum sample must always be tested about 10 d after the first to detect a rise in antibody titre. If the results are equivocal a further sample must be analysed.

Available tests for antibodies to extracellular products are listed in Table 16.2. The antistreptolysin O (ASO) test is most commonly performed and the antideoxyribonuclease B (anti-DNase B) test may also be useful. The other tests are not done by hospital service laboratories.

Table 16.2 Tests for antibodies to extracellular products of haemolytic streptococci

Antistreptolysin O titre (ASO)
Antideoxyribonuclease B (anti-DNase B)
Antinicotinamide adenine dinucleotidase (anti-NADase)
Antihyaluronidase (AH)
Antistreptokinase (ASK)

EPIDEMIOLOGY OF β–HAEMOLYTIC STREPTOCOCCAL INFECTIONS

The severity of streptococcal infections has become steadily and markedly reduced in many countries in the past century. The strongest evidence in support of this statement comes from the mortality rates for scarlet fever, which is a notifiable disease in the UK. Death rates in the UK from this once dreaded disease have fallen from about 1000 per million of the population in the decade 1860–9 to virtually zero at the present time. The remarkable reduction in the severity of scarlet fever was accompanied by a decline in the incidence and mortality of other severe streptococcal infections such as septicaemia, puerperal sepsis, acute endocarditis and rheumatic fever and was apparent before the advent of antibiotics. This general amelioration was probably related to a steady improvement in nutrition and in social and environmental conditions compared with the abject poverty and gross overcrowding of earlier decades when the rapid transfer of *Str. pyogenes* in a highly susceptible population led to an exaltation in the virulence of the pathogen. However, despite the great reduction in severity, there has probably been no corresponding reduction in the incidence of the commonest streptococcal infection, sore throat, and the prevalence of *Str. pyogenes* in the throat has not decreased in recent years.

Besides the acute case of sore throat and the nasal or saliva carrier, other dangerous sources of infection are patients with streptococcal otitis media, vulvovaginitis or infected skin lesions. Although the nasal carrier is important in initiating streptococcal infections, carriage in the throat or saliva is more common. At least 10% of children will be throat carriers at any one time and this proportion increases sharply at times of greater prevalence of clinical infection.

CONTROL OF STREPTOCOCCAL INFECTIONS

Prompt treatment with penicillin of patients with streptococcal infections will quickly reduce the numbers of streptococci. In streptococcal sore throat, complete elimination of the infecting organism can be obtained only if treatment is maintained for the recommended period (see below). A large proportion of children with sore throats will not be seen by a doctor during the acute episode. Such patients will disseminate the infecting organism in the community and be themselves liable to develop septic or non-septic complications.

In outbreaks it is important to search as early as possible for the spreader, most commonly a nasal carrier, but it may be a child who is a heavy salivary carrier or who has an infected skin lesion. Such individuals should be isolated and treated with antimicrobial drugs. Heavy nasal carriers are best treated with systemic rather than local therapy. Treatment of these dangerous carriers is particularly important in children's wards, where young sick patients may develop serious secondary infections. Gross environmental contamination quickly occurs in closed spaces, such as hospital wards, dormitories and barracks.

CHEMOTHERAPY OF STREPTOCOCCAL INFECTIONS

Str. pyogenes is highly sensitive to a wide range of antibacterial drugs, including penicillin and erythromycin, but strains resistant to sulphonamides and tetracyclines are common. Benzylpenicillin (penicillin G) or oral phenoxymethylpenicillin (penicillin V) are the drugs of choice. Others, including flucloxacillin, ampicillin and cephalosporins are less effective and should not be used. Penicillin-resistant strains of *Str. pyogenes* are presently unknown, so that antibiotic sensitivity tests are unnecessary if *Str. pyogenes* is identified as the infecting organism and penicillin is to be used.

Treatment for 3–5 d will limit the effect of severe attacks of streptococcal infection and prevent suppurative complications like otitis media, but studies have shown that only if treatment is continued for 10 d will the streptococci be eliminated from the infected area.

If the use of any other antimicrobial agent is contemplated, as in cases of hypersensitivity to penicillin, antimicrobial sensitivity testing must be done because of dangers of resistance to the drug.

CLINICAL INFECTIONS DUE TO *STR. PYOGENES*

The most common and typical infection caused by *Str. pyogenes* is an acute sore throat. If the infecting streptococcus is capable of producing an erythrogenic toxin and the host has not developed antibodies to this toxin, the sore throat may be accompanied by a generalized punctate erythema or rash. This syndrome is called *scarlet fever*. Local extension of the infection from the throat may result rarely in such complications as peritonsillar abscess (quinsy), sinusitis, otitis media or mastoiditis. Bronchopneumonia may develop as a complication of viral infections of the respiratory tract such as measles and influenza.

Puerperal sepsis or child-bed fever is traditionally associated with infection by *Str. pyogenes*, although other bacteria are now more commonly involved. Besides local inflammation of uterine tissues, infection may spread to the adnexa (pelvic cellulitis or peritonitis). Wounds, burns and chronic skin lesions (eczema, psoriasis) may become infected with *Str. pyogenes*; these superficial infections may extend in the local tissues (cellulitis) or be carried by lymphatics to regional lymph glands (lymphadenitis) or get into the bloodstream and become generalized (septicaemia).

Str. pyogenes can cause two types of primary skin infection, erysipelas and impetigo.

Sore throat

Sore throat — acute tonsillitis and/or pharyngitis — may be caused by non-infective agents such as tobacco smoke and be associated with blood diseases such as leukaemia, but it is caused most commonly by infective agents. It is a feature of the common cold and influenza and with the prodromal stages of infectious diseases such as chickenpox and measles. It accompanies local throat infections such as infectious mononucleosis, candida infection, Vincent's infection and — very rarely now in Western societies — diphtheria. Sore throat is one of the most common ailments seen by family doctors, especially in the winter months. It is uncommon in infants and in the elderly. Boys and girls are equally affected, and its peak incidence is in young schoolchildren who succumb to the cross-infection hazards of the classroom because of a poorly developed level and range of antibodies. It is less common in the older schoolchild, adolescent and young adult.

Acute pharyngitis and acute tonsillitis are caused by both bacteria and viruses. The bacteria are almost exclusively *Str. pyogenes*. Group C and G streptococci may also be involved, but other bacteria such as staphylococci and *Haemophilus* spp. are rarely implicated. For all practical purposes a bacterial sore throat means a streptococcal sore throat. Specific antibodies to the M protein, the virulence antigen of the infecting streptococcus, develop slowly after sore throat or other streptococcal illness but persist for a long time. Consequently, attacks by the same streptococcal serotype are unlikely though specific antibody does not protect against infection with other serotypes. Only 30–40% of cases of sore throat are caused by streptococci. Most of the rest are caused by viruses or, occasionally, *Mycoplasma pneumoniae*. It is not possible to diagnose the aetiology of sore throat on clinical grounds because streptococci and viruses both cause pain on swallowing, tender, enlarged tonsillar lymph nodes, pyrexia, headache and malaise. An exudate over the back of the throat can be produced by both streptococci and viruses. The throat must be swabbed if an accurate diagnosis of the cause of infection is to be established.

Throat swabbing

The technique of swabbing is all important. As large an area of the soft palate as possible should be covered, and rotation of the swab-head is also recommended so that as many bacteria as possible will be gathered on to the swab. A sample of saliva may also be useful as streptococci may be shed into the saliva.

Impetigo

Although *Str. pyogenes* is the predominant infecting agent, impetigo may also be caused by group C and G streptococci and by *Staph. aureus*; the primary skin lesion may be bullous rather than vesicular (bullous impetigo or pemphigus neonatorum).

The streptococci that cause impetigo are derived mainly from skin lesions on other persons. Organisms from these lesions may be found subsequently in the nose and less often in the throat. Spread from the nose or throat to the skin is rare. The lesion is a superficial, discrete, crusted spot that lasts for up to 2 weeks and heals without leaving a scar. Lesions may appear singly or in groups. Young children living under poor hygienic conditions and adults living in institutions are mainly affected. Workers who handle raw meat are also at risk.

In Europe, streptococcal impetigo seldom has serious consequences but in areas of the world with a warm, humid climate it is often followed by acute glomerulonephritis.

Erysipelas

This acute spreading skin lesion is rarer than impetigo. The infected area of the skin shows marked oedema and erythema. In facial erysipelas the attack may be preceded by a streptococcal sore throat and in others an infected abrasion or surgical wound may be associated, but frequently a primary lesion is not identifiable.

Those affected are usually the elderly. An attack confers no protection and some persons suffer many episodes, usually in the same skin area, suggesting that the disease may be a hypersensitivity reaction to streptococcal products.

Scarlet fever

The incidence and severity of scarlet fever have decreased dramatically in the UK in the 20th century. The disease consists of a combination of streptococcal sore throat and a generalized erythema, although occasionally the rash can accompany a streptococcal or staphylococcal wound infection (surgical scarlet fever). The rash is due to an erythrogenic toxin produced by strains of *Str. pyogenes* that have been lysogenized by a temperate bacteriophage. One main eryth-

rogenic toxin and two minor toxins are known to exist; because there are many different serotypes of *Str. pyogenes* an individual may suffer from frequent attacks of streptococcal sore throat although only one attack of scarlet fever.

Many strains of group A and some strains of group G streptococci produce scarlet fever. The incubation period is 2–3 d and the disease occurs most often in children under the age of 10 years. The characteristic rash, consisting of a widespread erythema with punctate spots, varies considerably depending on the severity of the infection. The skin of the face is generally clear and there is frequently circumoral pallor. At the onset of the disease the tongue is often covered by a thick white coat ('white strawberry tongue') and by the 4th day it begins to desquamate. By about the end of a week it is a bright red colour ('red strawberry tongue'). Desquamation of the skin also occurs after about a week.

Although chemotherapy has completely altered the clinical course of the disease by shortening the acute stage and by virtually eliminating suppurative complications, the natural course of the rash is not altered in any way by antibiotics.

NON-SUPPURATIVE COMPLICATIONS OF STREPTOCOCCAL INFECTIONS
Rheumatic fever

An attack of rheumatic fever (RF) is related to antecedent streptococcal throat infection occurring 1–5 weeks earlier. Support for this association is based on clinical, bacteriological, epidemiological serological and chemoprophylactic evidence.

Epidemiology

Altitude, humidity and other physical factors were thought to have a role in the production of RF but it now appears that it can occur anywhere in the world. In general, there is an increased incidence when the streptococcal carriage rate increases and in the UK the age group with the highest incidence of RF (7–9 years) is also that which has the highest incidence of streptococcal sore throat. Social factors such as overcrowding, poor nutrition and clothing are all important.

Diagnosis

RF may be difficult to diagnose clinically and, since throat swabs may or may not yield growth of *Str. pyogenes*, the most important investigations are serological. Two samples of serum must be assayed to check for a rising titre of antibody to *Str. pyogenes*. Titres become detectable in the 2nd week after the onset of infection, are maximal by the 6th week and thereafter decrease.

Many serotypes of *Str. pyogenes* can cause RF, but it does not occur in the absence of immunological evidence of streptococcal infection.

Chemoprophylaxis

Penicillin prophylaxis after a primary attack of RF will reduce substantially the risk of a second attack by preventing further streptococcal infection of the throat. However, prevention of primary attacks is virtually impossible and penicillin treatment of streptococcal sore throat plays little or no part. Moreover, only a few persons with streptococcal throat infection are treated, either because infection is subclinical or because those with a sore throat do not consult their doctor.

Aetiology

There is conclusive evidence of the association between RF and an antecedent streptococcal throat infection, but not with primary streptococcal infections of other tissues. The streptococci are not present in the lesions in the heart and joints. No particular streptococcal serotypes are incriminated, as happens with glomerulonephritis, and it is for this reason that throat infections with different serotypes can cause relapses of RF.

Two main theories have been proposed to explain the occurrence of RF: (1) that the initiation of the chronic lesions in the heart is due to the effect of some of the diffusible products of *Str. pyogenes*, such as streptolysins O and S and proteinase; (2) that immunological phenomena, such as immune complex disease, cross-reactive immunity or delayed hypersensitivity that develop in certain persons who become sensitized to one or more streptococcal products, are responsible for disease in man. An immunological relationship exists between a streptococcal antigen and human myocardial tissue. The antigen responsible for the cross-reactivity is localized in the cell wall and is associated with the M protein. It is probable that several cross-reactive antigen–antibody systems occur between the streptococcus, heart valves and heart muscle. Group-specific polysaccharide antigen of *Str. pyogenes* cross-reacts with the structural glycoprotein of both human and bovine valves.

Specific host factors have not been excluded in the pathogenesis of this disease. Some individuals seem prone to develop the rheumatic syndrome and such individuals are particularly liable to recurrent attacks after further streptococcal sore throats. However, the significance of hereditary predisposition is very difficult to disentangle from predisposing environmental factors, such as overcrowding in families or in communities. Overcrowding is the main reason for the high prevalence of rheumatic heart disease in the cities of many developing countries.

Acute glomerulonephritis

Post-streptococcal glomerulonephritis is a common type of acute nephritis. It is almost always produced by group A streptococci but group C streptococci may also be involved. In comparison with RF, which can be caused by a wide range of serotypes of *Str. pyogenes*, acute glomerulonephritis (AGN) is produced by a much narrower range. Also, whereas the *Str. pyogenes* strains associated with RF are isolated from the upper respiratory tract only, those involved in AGN may be isolated from the upper respiratory tract or from skin lesions such as impetigo (Table 16.3).

Table 16.3 M protein types of *Str. pyogenes* associated with acute glomerulonephritis

Antecedent infection	Common M protein types
Throat infection	12, 1, 25, 4 and 3
Pyoderma	49, 52, 53–55 and 57–61

The role of skin and throat infections in the development of AGN is now firmly established, although there are clear differences in the epidemiology: AGN following streptococcal throat infection occurs at the colder times of the year and mostly in children or young adults. Outbreaks in institutions can occur and there may be epidemic waves in the community. AGN following infected skin lesions occurs in all age groups in hot humid weather, notably in parts of the USA and in the West Indies, where flies of the genus *Hippelates* are important vectors of streptococci. Recurrences of AGN are rare.

Post-streptococcal AGN probably arises because some components of the glomerular basement membrane are immunologically similar to the cell membranes of nephritogenic β-haemolytic streptococci. It is known that some people produce anti-glomerular basement membrane antibody in their urine and plasma from time to time, and this may cause kidney damage. Alternatively, soluble toxic complexes of antigen, antibody and complement may lodge in the glomeruli, from which they are generally removed after a few weeks. According to this theory, the antigen involved is quite unrelated to kidney.

Whichever theory is correct, the events following antigen–antibody combination in the kidney are the same, namely activation of complement and coagulation. This leads to release of histamine and serotonin from neutrophils, causing acute inflammation, deposition of fibrin and tissue destruction in the glomerulus. In most cases the pathological changes are reversible although irreversible scarring may occur.

Laboratory diagnosis

β-Haemolytic streptococci may be isolated from the throat and skin but serological tests are generally more helpful in establishing the diagnosis of AGN. Immune responses vary depending on whether the source of infection is the throat or skin. For example, the ASO estimation is reliable in the throat-associated form but unreliable in pyoderma-associated AGN, whereas the anti-DNase B titre is raised more frequently and to a greater degree in pyoderma-associated AGN.

CLINICAL INFECTIONS DUE TO OTHER STREPTOCOCCI

Group B streptococci

Group B streptococci (*Str. agalactiae*) were known at the end of the last century as a cause of bovine mastitis but it was not until the 1930s that their association with human disease was recognized. Such infections have been reported with increasing frequency, and group B streptococci have now replaced group A streptococci, the scourge of the pre-1940s, as the major streptococcal pathogens in neonates and young infants.

A real change in the incidence and epidemiology of infections has occurred. Improvements in laboratory methods and techniques and a greater awareness of group B infections cannot account for the dramatic increase in the last two decades.

Infections in the neonate

These represent a wide spectrum of clinical disease, some minor, some major.

'Early-onset' infection occurs soon after birth and the 'late-onset' form occurs several days to several weeks after birth. Although these terms are in common use they do not have clear-cut clinical significance, since there is no universally accepted line of demarcation between them.

Early-onset infection. This is a particularly devastating neonatal septicaemic disease. Neonates may be ill at birth or develop acute and fulminating illness a few hours, or a day or two, later. Neonates may be lethargic, cyanosed and apnoeic, and when septicaemia progresses, shock ensues and death will occur if treatment is not quickly instituted. Meningitis and pulmonary infection may be associated.

Early rupture of the membranes, prolonged labour, prematurity, low birth weight and heavy colonization of the mother's genital tract by group B streptococci lead to infection. Group B streptococci may be isolated from many sites in the neonate but diagnosis is sometimes made only after death.

Group B colonization of neonates, with or without infection, is via the mother's genital tract; in almost every case the serotype of group B isolated from the neonate (the anterior nares, external auditory meatus, umbilicus and rectum are the sites from which organisms are most commonly isolated) is similar to that isolated from the cervicovaginal canal, urethra or rectum of the mother. Group B streptococci can be isolated from infants delivered by caesarian section, implying that the organisms can spread directly into the uterus from the genital tract of the mother.

Late-onset infection. Purulent meningitis is the most common group B infection after the immediate newborn period. Signs and symptoms of meningitis relate to the degree of maturity of the infant. There is usually no history of obstetric complications and seldom does the mother have genital tract colonization by group B streptococci. Infection is probably nosocomial, since some studies have shown that a substantial number of ward staff can be group B carriers. Transfer of the organisms to the baby takes place during nursing procedures. Baby-to-baby spread also occurs.

Prevention of group B neonatal infection. Whereas late-onset infection may be prevented or decreased by standard aseptic nursing procedures, early-onset infection is more difficult to prevent. Swabbing the mother's genital tract during pregnancy is not helpful because carriage can be intermittent, and isolation of the organism during pregnancy does not indicate that it will be present during labour. Moreover, administration of antibiotics to women who are positive during pregnancy has little effect on the carriage of group B streptococci. Since the carrier state is difficult to eradicate, the obstetrician and paediatrician should be made aware of mothers who are carriers and be prepared to start immediate antibiotic therapy in any neonate in whom infection is suspected .

Group B streptococci can produce other infections in infants, including septic arthritis, osteomyelitis, conjunctivitis, sinusitis, otitis media, endocarditis, peritonitis and omphalitis.

Localized infections are seen more commonly in older infants.

Infections in the adult

Infections in adults have a bimodal distribution:

1. Abortion, chorioamnionitis, post-partum sepsis (endometritis) and other infections (e.g. pneumonia) in the post-partum period may occur in young, previously healthy women.

2. Meningitis, otitis media, endocarditis, pneumonia, empyema, arthritis, abscesses, infections of wounds and burns, urinary tract infection and osteomyelitis may occur in the elderly and in immunocompromised individuals.

Group C streptococci

These organisms comprise four species, *Str. equi*, *Str. equisimilis*, *Str. dysgalactiae* and *Str. zooepidemicus*. They resemble group A streptococci, although they do not cause as many infections.

Group C streptococci are notably animal pathogens but certain species such as *Str. zooepidemicus* and *Str. equisimilis* can produce disease in humans. They can cause epidemic sore throat, especially in communities such as schools, nurseries and institutions, often associated with unpasteurized milk. Some group C strains have been related to AGN and other infections such as post-partum sepsis, septicaemia, meningitis, pneumonia and skin and wound infections.

Group G streptococci

Although antigenically quite distinct, these streptococci resemble those of groups A and C in their pathogenic properties and in the types of infections produced. They can cause sore throat, sometimes after ingestion of contaminated food, and pneumonia. They are isolated from 3 to 4% of cases of septicaemia and are sometimes associated with underlying malignancy in the patient. Erysipelas and cellulitis may be caused as well as bone and joint infection.

Group D streptococci

Whereas group A, C and G streptococci are commonly linked together because of a number of shared features, group D is a separate entity in terms of its biochemical, serological and pathogenic profiles. Many group D strains are much less sensitive to penicillin than other streptococci. As

laboratories. Methods available include the capsule swelling test (quellung reaction) and the latex agglutination test. Monospecific antisera are used for both these tests.

In the case of pneumococcal meningitis the cerebrospinal fluid is often macroscopically cloudy. The cell count is usually markedly increased and shows a predominance of polymorphonuclear leucocytes. Typical Gram-positive diplococci can commonly be demonstrated, sometimes in enormous numbers, by Gram-stain examination of a CSF deposit. The appearance is often typical and a presumptive diagnosis can be made to allow appropriate therapy to be started before the identity of the organism is confirmed by culture.

Blood cultures are of value in patients with pneumococcal pneumonia, particularly when this is severe, since approximately 15% of patients will be bacteraemic. Blood cultures may also be positive in those with pneumococcal meningitis.

Other body sites which may merit investigation according to the clinical presentation include joint and peritoneal fluids. Tympanocentesis provides the possibility of establishing the microbial cause of otitis media, but since most of these infections settle spontaneously, or with the assistance of a few days' antibiotic treatment, tympanocentesis is not usually necessary.

CHEMOTHERAPY

Str. pneumoniae is sensitive to a wide range of antimicrobial agents. These include the penicillins, cephalosporins, erythromycin, tetracycline, clindamycin, vancomycin, teicoplanin, chloramphenicol and the sulphonamides. Penicillin has had a major impact on the morbidity and mortality of pneumococcal infections. However, mortality rates for pneumococcal infections of the lung and meninges remain at approximately 15 and 20% despite the use of penicillin.

The dose of penicillin necessary to treat pneumococcal infection is largely determined by pharmacological factors at the site of infection. For example, pneumococcal pneumonia will respond to doses of penicillin as low as 0.3 g twice daily, although it is customary to prescribe higher doses; pneumococcal meningitis requires much higher doses, of the order of 7.2 g per day in divided doses. The use of even higher doses is of unproven advantage and runs the risk of inducing convulsions.

Aminopenicillins can also be used to treat pneumococcal infection in the community and amoxycillin is most widely prescribed. This is well absorbed following oral administration and is used to treat many community-acquired infections of the lung, middle ear and the sinuses. In patients unable to tolerate penicillin, erythromycin is the most widely used alternative agent.

Resistance of pneumococci to antibiotics has been recognized for some years and varies geographically. Resistance to erythromycin, tetracycline and chloramphenicol is not uncommon and is often linked to, and reflects the widespread use of, one or more of these agents. For example, tetracycline resistance in the UK occurs in approximately 5–10% of isolates while in France, where erythromycin and other macrolide antibiotics are much more widely used, it can be as high as 30%.

Resistance to penicillin has begun to emerge as a problem world-wide. Strains with reduced susceptibility (minimum inhibitory concentration >0.1 mg benzylpenicillin/l) were first recognized in 1967 in Papua New Guinea. The first strains with reduced susceptibility in the UK were reported in 1976. Although this increase in MIC was a cause of concern it was rarely associated with failure to respond to penicillin. However, high-level penicillin resistance was recognized in 1977 in South Africa where it was responsible for an epidemic of pneumococcal meningitis unresponsive to penicillin. The MIC of penicillin for these isolates was >2 mg/l. The strains were also resistant to several other antibiotics, with the exception of vancomycin and extended-spectrum cephalosporins such as cefotaxime. Since 1977 there has been a world-wide increase in resistance to penicillin in pneumococci and this is quite variable geographically. The highest reported incidence is from Spain, which is a popular destination for many European holidaymakers.

EPIDEMIOLOGY

Str. pneumoniae is second only to *Haemophilus influenzae* as a respiratory tract pathogen. The estimated annual incidence of pneumococcal pneumonia is 68–260 per 100 000 of the population in the USA with a 5% case fatality rate. Comparable data for bacteraemia and meningitis are 7–25 and 1.2–2.8 per 100 000 of the population with fatality rates of 20 and 30% respectively. The annual incidence of pneumococcal pneumonia in the UK is estimated to be between 1–2 per 1000 of the population. Otitis media affects approximately half of all children between the ages of 6 months and 3 years; approximately one-third of cases are caused by *Str. pneumoniae.* Apart from the acute morbidity of otitis media, other complications include mastoiditis and, occasionally, temporal lobe abscess. These complications are reduced significantly by early antibiotic treatment of middle ear disease and are now more common in developing countries.

Mortality from pneumococcal infection is related to age, pre-existing disease and serotype. The highest mortality rates occur in those over 65 years of age with underlying disease and in whom bacteraemia complicates infection. Infections caused by serotype 3 are among the most virulent and bacteraemic pneumococcal pneumonia with this serotype has a mortality rate of up to 50% in the elderly.

IMMUNOPROPHYLAXIS

Before the widespread availability of effective antimicrobial drugs the treatment of pneumococcal infections was based on the use of type-specific antiserum. This reduced mortality in bacteraemic pneumococcal pneumonia, but not to the same extent that penicillin was subsequently shown to achieve. However, it indicated that type-specific antibody had a role in the control of pneumococcal disease and reinforced earlier attempts to produce a vaccine, such as the prototype whole-cell preparation used by Sir Almroth Wright in 1911. In 1945, MacLeod demonstrated the protective efficacy of a quadrivalent polysaccharide vaccine in army recruits and this led to studies by Austrian among novice gold miners in South Africa; this group, although healthy, are known to be at high risk of bacteraemic pneumococcal infection and this was prevented by the use of a polyvalent pneumococcal vaccine.

The vaccine that is currently licensed for use contains a mixture of 23 polysaccharide serotypes chosen according to the prevalence of serotypes responsible for bacteraemic pneumococcal infection. It offers protection against 90% of isolates. Unfortunately, the immunogenicity of this vaccine is inadequate in those below 2 years of age and in those immunosuppressed as a result of malignancy, steroid therapy or other chronic disease. Indications for which the vaccine is licensed in the UK are shown in Table 17.1 In the USA, where the vaccine has been used most widely, it is also recommended for those over 65 years of age, with or without previous ill health, although there have been difficulties in establishing scientifically the efficacy in this group.

Immunization is particularly recommended for those with either functional or anatomical asplenia in whom pneumococcal infection can be fulminant. Such patients include those with congenital or surgical asplenia and those with hereditary haemoglobinopathies such as sickle cell disease. Vaccine efficacy is not complete and many clinicians also prescribe oral phenoxymethyl-penicillin as long-term chemoprophylaxis in this high-risk group.

Table 17.1 Licensed indications for the use of pneumococcal vaccine in the UK

Lack of functioning spleen[a]
Nephrotic syndrome[a]
Sickle cell disease[a]
Leakage of cerebrospinal fluid[a]
Hodgkin's disease
Lymphoma
Alcoholism
Multiple myeloma
Hepatic cirrhosis
Chronic renal failure
Chronic cardiopulmonary disease
Organ transplantation

[a] Licensed for use in children.

RECOMMENDED READING

Applebaum P C 1987 World-wide development of antibiotic resistance in pneumococci. *European Journal of Clinical Microbiology* 6: 367

Gransden W R, Eykyn S J, Phillips I 1985 Pneumococcal bacteraemia: 325 episodes diagnosed at St Thomas's Hospital. *British Medical Journal* 290: 505

LaForce F M, Eickhoff T C 1988 Pneumococcal vaccine: an emerging consensus. *Annals of Internal Medicine* 108: 757

Morbidity and Mortality Weekly Report 1989 Pneumococcal polysaccharide vaccine. 38: 64–8, 73–6

Smart L E, Dougall A J, Girdwood R W A 1987 New 23-valent pneumococcal vaccine in relation to pneumococcal serotypes in systemic and non-systemic disease. *Journal of Infection* 14: 209

18

Coryneform bacteria and listeria

Diphtheria; listeriosis

A. P. MacGowan

The genus *Corynebacterium* includes the diphtheria bacillus but also encompasses many commensals and pathogens of man and animals as well as environmental bacteria. In the medical laboratory '*diphtheroids*' or '*coryneforms*' are defined as pleomorphic Gram-positive rods which stain irregularly, are arranged in V forms or pallisades, are non-motile, catalase-positive, non-acid-fast, non-branching and form acid but not gas from carbohydrates.

Diphtheria is a rare infection in most developed countries but still remains prevalent in many Third World countries. Non-diphtheria coryneforms, mainly *Corynebacterium jeikeium*, may also cause disease, especially in immunocompromised patients.

CORYNEBACTERIUM DIPHTHERIAE

C. diphtheriae is the causative organism of diphtheria, a localized inflammation of the throat with greyish white adherent exudate (*pseudo-membrane*) and a generalized toxaemia due to the secretion and dissemination of a highly potent toxin.

DESCRIPTION

C. diphtheriae has a characteristic appearance in films from growth on suitable culture media. When dividing, the bacilli snap and bend abruptly and appear as angled pairs or parallel rows (*pallisades*), resembling 'Chinese lettering'; the average size is 3.0×0.3 μm but there is considerable pleomorphism with club-shaped, oval and globular forms appearing in older cultures. The rods are Gram-positive, but are easily decolorized. When stained with Neisser or Albert stains the *volutin* (metachromatic) granules stain dark purple in contrast to the brown or green counterstain, giving the rods a beaded appearance. *C. diphtheriae* is non-motile, non-sporing and non-capsulate.

C. diphtheriae is aerobic and facultively anaerobic, growing best at 37°C on a blood- or serum-containing medium. Loeffler's serum slopes allow quick growth and provide characteristic morphology for stained films. On blood or serum tellurite media the bacilli grow more slowly as greyish to black colonies. The shape, size and colour of these colonies enable them to be differentiated into the three main biotypes, called *gravis*, *intermedius* and *mitis* because of a relationship with the clinical severity of the infection (severe, intermediate and mild, respectively). Biochemical tests are important in differentiating *C. diphtheriae* from other coryneforms (Table 18.1)

The demonstration of toxin production is essential to differentiate toxigenic from commensal corynebacteria. Isolates identified as *gravis* or *intermedius* types are usually toxigenic but 10–20% of *mitis* strains isolated from 'sore throats' are non-toxigenic. Toxigenicity is demonstrated by the agar gel precipitation (Elek) test.

EPIDEMIOLOGY

Incidence

Less than 10 cases of diphtheria are reported per

Table 18.1 Biochemical reactions of medically significant corynebacteria

Organism	Catalase	β-haemolysis on blood agar	Urease	Nitrate reduction	Acid production from Glucose	Maltose	Sucrose	Xylose
C. diphtheriae	+	v	−	+	+	+	−	−
C. ulcerans	+	+	+	−	+	+	−	−
C. haemolyticum	−	+	−	−	+	+	v	+
C. pseudotuberculosis	+	+	+	v	+	+	−	−
C. minutissimum	+	−	−	−	+	+	v	−
C. xerosis	+	−	−	+	+	+	+	−
C. pseudodiphtheriticum	+	−	+	+	−	−	−	−
C. jeikeium	+	−	+	−	+	v	−	−
CDC group D-2[a]	+	−	+	−	−	−	−	−

+, 90% or more positive in 4 days; -, 90% or more negative; v, more than 10% and less than 90% positive.
[a] CDC, Centers for Disease Control (Atlanta, USA).

year in the UK; most are imported by visitors returning from the Indian subcontinent or Turkey. No deaths occurred in the UK in the period 1984–91.

Infection is confined to man and usually spreads directly from person to person via nasopharyngeal secretions. Spread is facilitated by intimate contact. Children are susceptible after the age of 3 to 6 months when passive immunity derived from maternal antibodies has disappeared. Incidence is highest among young children, but outbreaks also occur among teenagers and young adults. In the course of immunization programmes directed at pre-school and schoolchildren there may be a shift in distribution of cases to older age groups.

In some tropical countries cutaneous infections with *C. diphtheriae* occur and latent skin infections play an important part in the natural acquisition of immunity.

Transmission

In endemic areas there may be up to 100 healthy carriers for every clinical case. Most clinical infections are probably contracted from carriers rather than symptomatic patients. Nasal carriers are particularly dangerous because they shed large numbers of bacilli. The bacillus is relatively resistant to drying and may survive for many weeks in dust and on dry fomites contaminated with nasal,

oral or pharyngeal secretions. Dust in hospitals and institutions may become heavily infected with dried secretions and may be a source of infection.

PATHOGENESIS

Diphtheria bacilli elicit an inflammatory exudate and cause necrosis of the cells of the faucial mucosa. Infection may spread to the post-nasal cavity or the larynx, causing respiratory obstruction. The serocellular exudate clots and remains adherent to the fauces and attempts to remove the pseudomembrane leave a raw, bleeding surface. The diphtheria bacilli do not as a rule penetrate deeply in the underlying tissues, or the blood, but they produce a very powerful exotoxin which is spread by the bloodstream and has a special affinity for certain tissues, notably heart muscle, nerve endings and the adrenal glands. Diphtheria toxin is a heat-stable polypeptide which is composed of two fragments, denoted A and B. Fragment B is required for transport of fragment A into the cell where it inhibits polypeptide chain elongation at the ribosome. Inhibition of protein synthesis is probably responsible for both the necrotic and neurotoxic effects of the toxin. Death from laryngeal diphtheria may be due to asphyxia because, in the confined space within the larynx, even a small patch of membrane can cause a fatal

Cases of clinical listeriosis fall into two groups: pregnancy and neonatal infection; and infection in non-pregnant adults. Pregnancy and neonatal disease account for between 30 and 45% of cases. In pregnancy-related infection, abortion and stillbirth account for 15–25% of infections, while about 70% are neonatal infections. In about 5% of maternal infections the fetus is not affected.

The incidence of infection increases with age so that with adult infections the mean age is over 55 years. Men are more commonly infected than women over the age of 40 years, and since women are infected in the child-bearing years the overall sex distribution is more or less equal. Most patients with listeriosis live in urban areas and usually have no exposure to animals, although occasional infections occur as a result of direct animal contact, usually in vets or farmers. Immunosuppression is a major risk factor for both the epidemic and sporadic forms of listeriosis and probably accounts for the increasing incidence with age.

The peak incidence of human disease occurs in July, August or September, but in animals it occurs in the spring.

Asymptomatic carriage of listeria in human populations is common; up to 5% of healthy adults are carriers at any one time. The duration of faecal carriage is often short but may exceed a year. About 50% of faecal isolates are *L. monocytogenes* and the remainder are non-pathogenic to man. The high incidence of carriage among humans may reflect the consumption of contaminated foods.

Up to 20% of cheeses imported into the UK are contaminated with listeria, some to high levels. Home-produced cheeses tend to have lower rates of contamination. Soft cheeses are more likely to be affected than hard, but the low pH of cottage cheese prevents the growth of listeria. Listeria are found most commonly on the rinds of cheese, which may suggest contamination during production or may be related to oxygen tension. Epidemiological studies have suggested that pasteurized milk can be a source of listeriosis and listeria can survive some forms of pasteurization within phagocytes.

Cook–chill foods may be contaminated prior to reheating, but microwave ovens are effective in reducing the number of viable bacteria in heavily contaminated food by a factor of 1 million per gram, provided the recommended standing time is observed to ensure even distribution of heat throughout the food. Listeria have been isolated from 15 to 60% of raw and oven-ready chickens and less commonly from other meats. Vegetables, pre-packed salads and chilled main courses have also been shown to be contaminated with listeria.

Although many food products are contaminated with listeria, the number of organisms required to produce infection is unknown and it is difficult to evaluate the importance of these as a source of infection.

Transmission

Various routes of infection have been proposed but the number of infections in which any route can be directly implicated is very small. There is little evidence to support dust or insect spread, but in hospitals neonatal infections have been associated with the contamination of resuscitation equipment in obstetric theatres and also with direct spread between patients.

A small number of pregnancy-associated infections and cases of adult meningitis have been related to consumption of contaminated chickens or cheeses, indicating that food spread is of importance in sporadic listeria infection.

Epidemics of listeriosis usually occur in the community but hospital-associated outbreaks have occurred in renal transplant and in neonatal units. In well-documented community outbreaks in North America, coleslaw, milk and Mexican-style cheese have been implicated.

PATHOGENESIS

The virulence of listeria has not been studied in as much depth as the host response to infection, but the different species within the genus have varying virulence in experimental animals and in man. All strains which are pathogenic to mice produce a haemolysin, listeriolysin O, which is antigenically similar to streptolysin O, suggesting that it may have a potential role in virulence. Listeriolysin O is important for bacterial survival after phagocytosis, and its production is regulated by extracellular iron concentrations. Several other toxins are produced: a factor which promotes bacterial entry into the cells, a cytolysin and enzymes which protect the bacteria from the harmful effects of reactive oxygen radicals such as superoxide dismutase and catalase.

Oral administration of bacteria to germ-free animals causes gut wall infection and occasional spread to the liver and spleen, but colonization of the bowel is inhibited by normal gastro-intestinal flora. In man, gastro-intestinal disease, causing low gastric pH, disrupted bowel flora (perhaps related to antibiotic use) or damaged bowel tissues, may help to establish listeria in the bowel.

Non-specific mechanisms of resistance are important as first lines of defence once the mucous membranes are breached. Lysozyme can lyse some strains of listeria and human neutrophils and non-activated macrophages can phagocytose and kill the bacteria.

In experimental rodent listeriosis, protective immunity depends on T lymphocytes, antibodies playing only a small or no role. T cells confer protection by attracting monocytes to infectious foci and activating them, producing a listeriocidal action which destroys the intracellular bacteria. Granulomata are formed and the listeria are eliminated. It is thought that immunity in man is similar, although little direct evidence exists for this.

CLINICAL ASPECTS OF INFECTION

Infection in pregnancy and the neonate

Listeriosis in pregnancy is classified by fetal gestation at onset, as this correlates best with the clinical features, microbiology and prognosis. Neonatal infection is divided into early (<2 d old), intermediate (3–5 d old) and late (>5 d old).

Maternal listeriosis before 20 weeks of pregnancy is rare. The mother is usually previously well and having a normal pregnancy. Pregnant women often have very mild symptoms and may be asymptomatic until the delivery of an infected infant. Chills, fever, back pain, sore throat and headache are cardinal features of infection, but conjunctivitis, drowsiness and other symptoms are sometimes present. Symptomatic women may have positive blood cultures. High vaginal swabs (HVSs), stool cultures and midstream urines are generally of little help in antepartum diagnosis of listeriosis. With the onset of fever, fetal movements are reduced and premature labour occurs within about 1 week. There may be a transient fever during labour and the amniotic fluid is often discoloured or meconium stained. Culture of the amniotic fluid, placenta or HVS post-delivery usually yields *L. monocytogenes*. Fever resolves soon after birth, and the HVS is usually culture-negative after about 1 month. While the outcome of infection for the mother is usually benign, the outcome for the infant is more variable. Abortion, stillbirth and early-onset neonatal disease are common, depending on the gestation at infection. However, maternal infection without infection of the offspring can occur and even progress to placental infection without ill effects for the fetus.

Repeated pregnancy-associated infections are exceedingly rare and an association between listeria carriage and habitual abortion has not been substantiated.

Early neonatal listeriosis is predominantly a septicaemic illness, contracted in utero. In contrast, late neonatal infection is predominantly meningitic and may be associated with hospital cross-infection. The main characteristics of these two forms of infection are summarized in Table 18.4. Early disease represents a spectrum of mild to severe infection, which can be correlated with the microbiological findings. Those neonates who die of infection usually do so within a few days of birth and have pneumonia, hepatosplenomegaly, petechiae, abscesses in liver or brain, peritonitis and enterocolitis.

Late-onset disease is the third commonest form of meningitis in neonates. The CSF protein content is almost always raised and the glucose level reduced. The total number of white cells is increased but the counts are variable; neutrophils usually predominate, but lymphocytes or monocytes may be the main cell type. In about 50% of Gram films, bacteria are seen which may resemble rods or cocci.

Table 18.4 Characteristics of neonatal infection with *L. monocytogenes*

	Type of infection Early	Late
Onset after delivery	<2 d	>5 d

Maternal factors
  Obstetric problems
  Low birth weight
  Maternal fever
  Abnormal amniotic fluid
	Common	Rare

Source of infection	Maternal	Hospital acquired and (?) maternally acquired
Signs/symptoms	Disseminated infection Cardiopulmonary distress CNS signs Vomiting and diarrhoea Hepatosplenomegaly Skin rash	Meningitis Irritability Poor appetite Fever
Laboratory findings	Leucocytosis or leucopenia Thrombocytopenia Mottling on chest X-ray Increased fibrinogen	Leucocytosis; occasional X-ray changes CSF: total protein and white cell count raised; glucose lowered
Sites of isolation	Commonly, blood, superficial sites and amniotic fluid; less commonly gastric aspirate, CSF and HVS	Commonly CSF Rarely blood
Mortality	30–60%	10–12%

Adult and juvenile infection

Listeriosis in children older than 1 month is very rare, except in children with underlying disease. In adults the main syndromes are CNS infection, septicaemia and endocarditis.

Most cases occur in immunosuppressed patients receiving steroid or cytotoxic therapy or radiotherapy. However, about one-third of patients with meningitis and around 10% with primary bacteraemia have no predisposing factors.

Meningitis

The clinical presentation is the same in all groups, but progression is more rapid in immunocompromised subjects. A peripheral blood leucocytosis occurs and the CSF white blood cells are raised. The CSF glucose is low and the protein is raised; a very high protein may be a poor prognostic indicator. Gram stains of the CSF are often negative, and the clinical features of infection are such that it is not possible to tell listeria meningitis from meningococcal or pneumococcal infection. However, listeria are isolated from blood cultures in most cases.

In the rare cases of encephalitis, cerebritis or abscesses of the CNS the CSF may be normal but often the white blood cell count is mildly raised and the protein slightly elevated with a low glucose concentration. The Gram film and culture are usually negative. Blood cultures are the main source of isolation in many of these patients.

Bacteraemia and endocarditis

Primary bacteraemia is more common in men than in women, and occurs most frequently in patients with haematological malignancy or renal transplants. A small number of patients develop CNS infection, which has a poor prognosis.

Infective endocarditis is twice as common in men as women and the main predisposing factors are prosthetic valves or damaged natural valves. However, some patients belong to other risk groups.

Other infections

Rare manifestations of listeriosis include arthritis and hepatitis. Pneumonia also occurs in renal transplant recipients and other groups of patients.

ANTIMICROBIAL THERAPY

L. monocytogenes is susceptible to a wide range of antibiotics in vitro, including ampicillin, penicillin, tetracyclines, chloramphenicol, aminoglycosides, and co-trimoxazole. There is little agreement as to what is the best treatment, but many patients have been successfully treated with ampicillin or penicillin with or without an aminoglycoside.

Ampicillin and penicillin are probably equivalent agents for the treatment of meningitis. While it is known that aminoglycosides interact synergistically with penicillin or ampicillin in vitro and improve mortality rates in experimental animals, no such evidence exists for human infection. Chloramphenicol has been widely used in the treatment of listeria meningitis but, when used alone, it is probably not as effective as penicillin or ampicillin and may result in relapses. However, the combination of chloramphenicol with penicillin or ampicillin has resulted in increased mortality. Cephalosporins are ineffective in clinical infections.

The antimicrobial treatment of other forms of neonatal and adult listeriosis is probably the same as for meningitis; the combination of ampicillin and an aminoglycoside is used most commonly. Co-trimoxazole has been effective in the small number of patients treated.

Prognosis

The mortality rate in late neonatal disease is about 10%. In contrast, the mortality rate in early disease is 30–60% and approximately 20–40% of survivors will develop sequelae such as lung disease, hydrocephalus or other neurological defects. Early use of appropriate antibiotics in infected mothers may improve neonatal survival.

The mortality in adult infection is about 20–50% in CNS infection; 5–20% in primary bacteraemias; and 50% in infective endocarditis. About 25–75% of patients surviving CNS infection suffer sequelae such as hemiplegias and other neurological defects.

RECOMMENDED READING

Coryneforms

Christie A B 1987 Diphtheria. *Infectious Diseases, 4th edn.* Churchill Livingstone, Edinburgh, vol 2 p 1183–1209

Lipsky B A, Goldberger A C, Tompkins L S, Plorde J J 1982 Infections caused by nondiphtheria corynebacteria. *Reviews of Infectious Diseases.* 4: 1220–1235

Porter I A 1989 Corynebacterium. In: Collee J G, Duguid J P, Fraser A G, Marmion B P (eds) *Mackie and MacCartney. Practical Medical Microbiology*, 13th edn. Churchill Livingstone, Edinburgh, p 374–386

Listeria

Lamont R J, Postlethwaite R, MacGowan A P 1988 *Listeria monocytogenes* and its role in human infections. *Journal of Infection* 13: 187–193

Nieman R E, Lorber B 1980 Listeriosis in adults: a changing pattern. Report of eight cases and review of the literature 1968–1978. *Reviews of Infectious Diseases.* 2:207–227

Porter I A 1989 Listeria: Erysipelothrix. In: Collee J G, Duguid J P, Fraser A G, Marmion B P (eds) *Mackie and MacCartney. Practical Medical Microbiology*, 13th edn. Churchill Livingstone, Edinburgh, p 387–391

Schuchat A, Swaminathan B, Broome CV 1991 Epidemiology of human listeriosis. *Clinical Microbiology Reviews* 4: 169–183

19

Mycobacterium

Tuberculosis; leprosy

J. M. Grange

The mycobacteria, or acid-fast bacilli, are responsible for tuberculosis and leprosy and a number of saprophytic species occasionally cause opportunist disease (see Chapter 20). The name of the genus, *Mycobacterium* (fungus-bacterium), is an allusion to the mould-like pellicles formed when members of this genus are grown in liquid media. This hydrophobic property is due to their possession of thick, complex, lipid-rich, waxy cell walls. A further important characteristic of mycobacteria, also due to their waxy cell walls, is their *acid-fastness*, or resistance to decolorization by a dilute mineral acid (or alcohol) after staining with hot carbol fuchsin or other arylmethane dyes.

There are about 50 species of mycobacteria, which are divisible into two major groups, the slow and rapid growers, although the growth rate of the latter is slow relative to that of most other bacteria. The leprosy bacillus has never convincingly been grown in vitro.

MYCOBACTERIUM TUBERCULOSIS

Tuberculosis is a chronic granulomatous disease affecting man, many other mammals, marsupials, birds, fish, amphibians and reptiles. Mammalian tuberculosis is caused by four very closely related species: *Mycobacterium tuberculosis* (the human tubercle bacillus), *M. bovis* (the bovine tubercle bacillus), *M. microti* (the vole tubercle bacillus) and *M. africanum*.

Most human tuberculosis is caused by *M. tuberculosis* but some cases are due to *M. bovis*, which is the principal cause of tuberculosis in cattle and many other mammals. The name *M. africanum* is given to tubercle bacilli with rather variable properties and which appear to be intermediate in form between the human and bovine types. It causes human tuberculosis and is mainly found in Equatorial Africa. *M. microti* is seldom, if ever, encountered nowadays.

DESCRIPTION

Tubercle bacilli are non-motile, non-sporing, non-capsulate straight or slightly curved rods about $3 \times 0.3\ \mu m$ in size. In sputum and other clinical specimens they may occur singly or in small clumps and in liquid cultures human tubercle bacilli often grow as twisted rope-like colonies termed *serpentine cords* (Fig. 19.1).

Tubercle bacilli are able to grow on a wide range of enriched culture media but Löwenstein–Jensen (LJ) medium is the most widely used in clinical practice. This consists of whole eggs, glycerol, asparagine and some mineral salts and is solidified by heating (inspissation). Malachite green dye is added to the medium to inhibit the growth of some contaminating bacteria and to provide a contrasting colour against which colonies of mycobacteria are easily seen. Agar-based media or broths enriched with bovine serum albumin are also used.

Human tubercle bacilli produce visible growth on LJ medium in about 2 weeks, although on

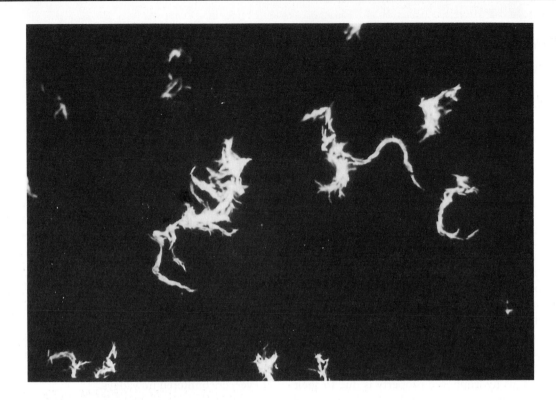

Fig. 19.1 Microcolony of *M. tuberculosis* showing 'serpentine cord' formation.

primary isolation from clinical material colonies may take up to 8 weeks to appear. Colonies are of an off-white (buff) colour and often have a dry breadcrumb-like appearance. Growth is characteristically heaped up and luxuriant or 'eugonic' in contrast to the small, flat 'dysgonic' colonies of bovine tubercle bacilli on this medium. The growth of the latter is much better on media containing sodium pyruvate in place of glycerol, e.g. Stonebrink's medium.

Tubercle bacilli have a rather limited temperature range of growth: their optimal growth temperature is 35–37°C but they fail to grow at 25 or 41°C. Most other mycobacteria grow at one or other, or both, of these temperatures.

Like all mycobacteria, the tubercle bacilli are obligate aerobes but *M. bovis* grows better in conditions of reduced oxygen tension. Thus, when incorporated in soft agar media, *M. tuberculosis* grows on the surface while *M. bovis* grows as a band a few millimetres below the surface. This provides a useful differentiating test. The human tubercle bacillus also differs from the bovine type in its ability to reduce nitrates to nitrites; its production of large amounts of niacin; its sensitivity to pyrazinamide; and, usually, in its resistance to thiophen-2-carboxylic acid hydrazide (TCH), a substance related to the anti-tuberculosis drug isoniazid (Table 19.1).

The tubercle bacilli are obligate pathogens but they survive in milk and in other organic materials and on pasture-land so long as they are not exposed to ultraviolet light, to which they are very sensitive. They are also heat-sensitive and are destroyed in the process of pasteurization. Mycobacteria are susceptible to alcohol, formaldehyde and glutaraldehyde and, to a lesser extent, to hypochlorites and phenolic disinfectants. They are considerably more resistant than other bacteria to acids, alkalis and quaternary ammonium compounds.

Table 19.1 Some differential characteristics of tubercle bacilli causing human disease

Species	Atmospheric preference	Nitratase	TCH	Pyrazinamide
M. tuberculosis	Aerobic	Positive	Resistant[a]	Sensitive
M. bovis	Micro-aerophilic	Negative	Sensitive	Resistant
M. africanum	Micro-aerophilic	Variable	Sensitive	Sensitive

TCH, thiophen-2-carboxylic acid hydrazide.
[a] Strains from south India may be sensitive to TCH.

PATHOGENESIS

The tubercle bacillus owes its virulence to its ability to survive within the macrophage rather than to the production of a toxic substance. The immune response to the bacillus is of the cell-mediated type and the clinical features of tuberculosis are due to the paradox that this ordinarily protective response contributes to the tissue destruction and other pathological characteristics of the disease. As a result of this reactivity, human tuberculosis is divisible into primary and post-primary forms with quite different pathological features.

Primary tuberculosis

The site of the initial infection is usually the lung, following the inhalation of bacilli. These bacilli are engulfed by alveolar macrophages in which they replicate to form the initial lesion or *Ghon focus*. Some bacilli are carried in macrophages to the hilar lymph nodes where additional foci of infection develop. The Ghon focus together with the enlarged hilar lymph nodes form the *primary complex*. In addition, bacilli are seeded by further lymphatic and haematogenous dissemination in many organs and tissues, including other parts of the lung. When the bacilli enter the mouth, as in milk-borne bovine tuberculosis, the primary complexes involve the tonsil and cervical nodes (*scrofula*; Fig. 19.2) or the intestine, often the ileocaecal region, and the mesenteric lymph nodes. Likewise, the primary focus may be in the skin with involvement of the regional lymph nodes. This form of tuberculosis was an occupational disease of anatomists and pathologists and was termed *prosector's wart*.

Within about 10 days of infection, clones of antigen-specific T lymphocytes are produced. These release lymphokines which activate macrophages and cause them to form a compact cluster, or granuloma, around the foci of infection. These activated macrophages are termed *epithelioid cells* from their microscopical resemblance to epithelial cells. Some of them fuse to form multinucleate giant cells. The centre of the granuloma contains a mixture of necrotic tissue and dead macro-

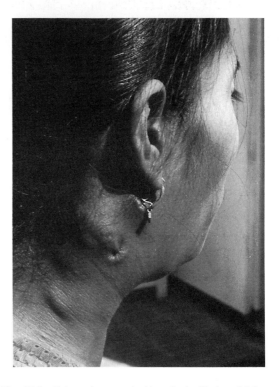

Fig. 19.2 Tuberculous cervical lymphadenitis (scrofula) with sinus formation in an Indonesian lady.

phages which, from its cheese-like appearance and consistency, is referred to as *caseation*.

Activated macrophages inhibit the replication of the tubercle bacillus, but there is no clear experimental evidence that they can actually kill them. Being metabolically very active, the macrophages in the granuloma consume oxygen and the resulting anoxia and acidosis in the centre of the lesion probably kills most of the tubercle bacilli. Granuloma formation is usually sufficient to limit the primary infection: the lesions become quiescent and surrounding fibroblasts produce dense scar tissue which may become calcified. Not all bacilli are destroyed: some remain in a dormant form as persisters which, when reactivated, cause post-primary disease.

In a minority of cases one of the infective foci progresses and gives rise to the serious manifes-tations of primary disease, including progressive primary lesions (particularly in infants; Fig. 19.3), meningitis, pleurisy and disease of the kidneys, spine (*Pott's disease*) and other bones and joints. If a focus ruptures into a blood vessel, bacilli are disseminated throughout the body with the formation of numerous granulomas (Fig. 19.3). This, from the millet seed-like appearance of the lesions, is known as *miliary tuberculosis*. The 'timetable' of events in primary tuberculosis is shown in Table 19.2.

Tuberculin reactivity

About 6 or 8 weeks after the initial infection, the phenomenon of tuberculin conversion occurs. This altered reactivity was discovered by Robert Koch whilst attempting to develop a remedy for

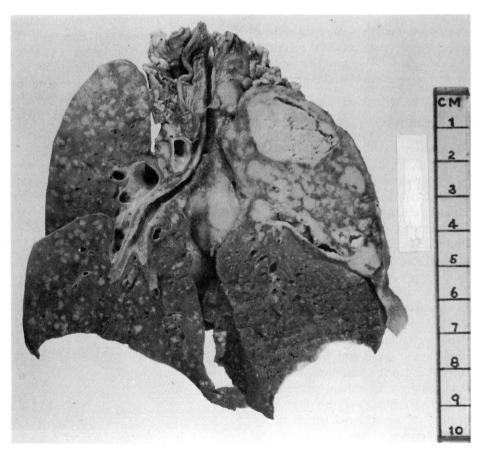

Fig. 19.3 Progressive primary tuberculous lesion in the right upper lobe of the lung and numerous miliary lesions in other parts of the lung in a child aged 6 months.

Table 19.2 Stages of primary tuberculosis in childhood

Stage	Time (from onset)	Characteristics
1	3–8 weeks	Primary complex develops and tuberculin conversion occurs
2	2–6 months	Progressive healing of primary complex Possibility of pleural effusion
3	6–12 months	Possibility of miliary or meningeal tuberculosis
4	1–3 years	Possibility of bone or joint tuberculosis
5	3–5 years or more	Possibility of genito-urinary or chronic skin tuberculosis

Adapted from Miller FJW 1982 Tuberculosis in Children. Churchill Livingstone, Edinburgh.

tuberculosis. When tuberculous guinea-pigs were injected intradermally with living tubercle bacilli, the skin around the injection site became necrotic within a day or two and was sloughed off, together with the bacilli. Koch then found that the same reaction occurred when he injected *old tuberculin*, which was a heat-concentrated filtrate of a broth in which tubercle bacilli had been grown. This reaction became known as the *Koch phenomenon* and its characteristic feature is tissue necrosis.

Injection of old tuberculin, or one of its analogues, into the skin causes an inflammatory reaction with perivascular cuffing and a huge increase in the cellularity of the skin and a compensatory increase in local capillary blood flow. In the more severe tuberculin reactions, the blood flow rate is greatly reduced, leading to an oxygen debt, acidosis, ischaemia and necrosis. This appears to be the result of mediators, including tumour necrosis factor, which are released from lymphocytes and macrophages. It is this necrotic reaction that is largely responsible for the characteristic features of post-primary tuberculosis.

Post-primary tuberculosis

In many individuals, the primary complex resolves and the only evidence of infection is a conversion to tuberculin reactivity. After an interval of months, years or decades, reactivation of dormant foci of tubercle bacilli or exogenous reinfection may lead to post-primary tuberculosis, which differs in several respects from primary disease (Table 19.3). Reactivation may occur spontaneously or after an intercurrent illness or other condition that lowers the host's immune responsiveness (see below). For unknown reasons reactivation or re-infection tuberculosis almost always occurs in the upper lobes of the lungs. The same process of granuloma formation occurs but the necrotic element of the reaction causes tissue destruction and the formation of large areas of caseation termed *tuberculomas*. Proteases liberated by activated macrophages cause softening and liquefaction of the caseous material and an excess of tumour necrosis factor (cachectin) and other immunological mediators cause the wasting and fevers characteristic of the disease.

Table 19.3 Main differences between primary and post-primary tuberculosis

Characteristics	Primary	Post-primary
Local lesion	Small	Large
Lymphatic involvement	Yes	Minimal
Cavity formation	No	Yes
Haematogenous dissemination	Yes	Rare[a]
Tuberculin reactivity	Negative (initially)	Positive
Infectivity	Rare	Usual
Site	Any part of lung	Apical region
Local spread	Rare	Frequent

[a] Except in elderly or in immunosuppressed individuals.

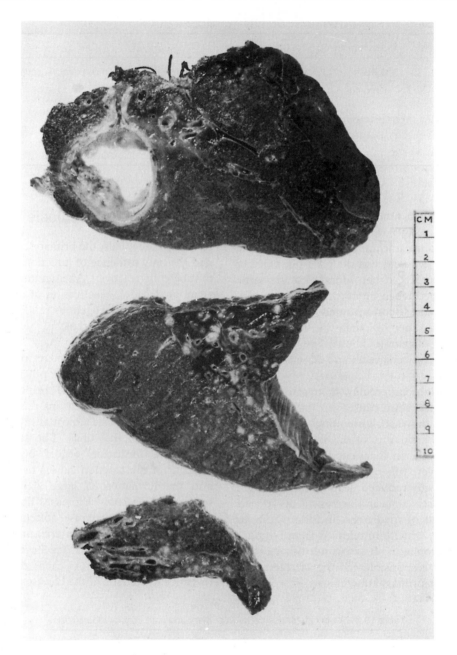

Fig. 19.4 Large tuberculous cavity in the lung of a man aged 24 years. Other parts of the lung show secondary lesions due to endobronchial spread of disease.

The interior of the tuberculoma is acidic and anoxic and contains few viable tubercle bacilli. Eventually, however, the expanding lesion erodes into a bronchus, the liquefied contents are discharged and a well-aerated cavity is formed (Fig. 19.4). The atmosphere of the lung, with a high carbon dioxide level, is ideal for supporting the growth of the bacilli and huge numbers of these are found in the cavity walls. For this reason, closure of the cavities by collapsing the lung, either by artificial pneumothorax or by excising large portions of the chest wall, was a standard treatment for tuberculosis in the pre-chemotherapeutic era.

Once the cavity is formed, large numbers of bacilli gain access to the sputum and the patient becomes an open or infectious case. This is a good example of the transmissibility of a pathogen being dependent upon the host's response to infection. Surprisingly, about 20% of cases of open cavitary tuberculosis resolve without treatment.

In post-primary tuberculosis dissemination of bacilli to lymph nodes and other organs is unusual. Instead, spread of infection occurs through the bronchial tree so that secondary lesions develop in the lower lobes of the lung (Fig. 19.4). Likewise, secondary lesions may occur in the trachea, larynx and mouth and swallowed bacilli cause intestinal lesions; secondary lesions may also develop in the bladder and epididymis in cases of renal tuberculosis. Post-primary cutaneous tuberculosis (*lupus vulgaris*) usually affects the face and neck. Untreated, it is a very chronic condition leading to gross scarring and deformity. Some cases are secondary to sinus formation between tuberculous lymph nodes and the skin (*scrofuloderma*).

Tuberculosis in immunocompromised individuals

Reactivation tuberculosis is particularly likely to occur in immunocompromised individuals, including the elderly, transplant recipients and those who are human immunodeficiency virus (HIV)-positive. In the latter, tuberculosis is usually diagnosed before the other features of acquired immune deficiency syndrome (AIDS) are apparent. Cavity formation is unusual, emphasizing the importance of the immune response in this pathological process. Instead, diffuse infiltrates develop in any part of the lung and non-pulmonary lesions due to lymphatic and haematogenous dissemination are common. Sometimes there are numerous minute lesions teeming with tubercle bacilli throughout the body — a rapidly fatal condition termed *cryptic disseminated tuberculosis*.

The tuberculin test

Although Robert Koch's attempts to use old tuberculin as a remedy for tuberculosis failed, an Austrian physician, Clemens von Pirquet, used the Koch phenomenon in man as an indication of bacterial 'allergy' resulting from previous infection. Individuals with active tuberculosis were usually tuberculin-positive but many of those with widespread and rapidly progressive disease were negative. This led to the widespread but erroneous belief that tuberculin reactivity was an indication of immunity to tuberculosis.

Old tuberculin caused non-specific reactions and it has been replaced by *purified protein derivative* (PPD). This is given by intracutaneous injection (*Mantoux* method) or by means of a spring-loaded gun which fires six prongs into the skin through a drop of PPD (*Heaf* method). In addition, disposable devices with PPD dried onto prongs are available for single tests (*tine tests*).

The biological activity of tuberculins is compared with international standards and their activities are expressed in international units (IU). In the UK, solutions of PPD for Mantoux testing are supplied as dilutions of 1 in 10 000, 1 in 1000 and 1 in 100, which correspond to 1, 10 and 100 IU in the injected dose of 0.1 ml. The standard test dose is 10 IU but those suspected of having tuberculosis, and therefore likely to react strongly, may first be tested with 1 IU. Undiluted PPD is supplied for use with the Heaf gun.

The tuberculin test is widely used as a diagnostic test, although its usefulness is limited by its failure to distinguish active disease from quiescent infections and past BCG (bacille Calmette–Guérin; see later) vaccination. In addition, exposure to various mycobacteria in the environment may induce low levels of tuberculin reactivity. In the USA, more diagnostic reliance is placed on the tuberculin test as BCG is not used in that country. The test is used in epidemiological studies as outlined below.

LABORATORY DIAGNOSIS

The definitive diagnosis of tuberculosis is based on the detection of acid-fast bacilli in clinical specimens by microscopy or cultural techniques. Numerous unsuccessful attempts have been made to develop serological tests for the disease.

Inoculation of guinea-pigs with sputum and other clinical material, once widely used for the diagnosis of tuberculosis, is now obsolete as in-vitro culture methods are equally effective.

Specimens

The most usual specimen is sputum but, if pulmonary tuberculosis is suspected and no sputum is produced, bronchial washings, brushings or biopsies, laryngeal swabs and early-morning gastric aspirates (to harvest any bacilli swallowed overnight) may be examined. Tissue biopsies are homogenized by grinding in Griffith's tubes for microscopy and culture. Cerebrospinal fluid, pleural fluid, urine and other fluids are centrifuged and the deposits are examined.

Microscopy

Use is made of the acid-fast property of mycobacteria to detect them in sputum and other clinical material. In the Ziehl–Neelsen (ZN) staining technique, heat-fixed smears of the specimens are flooded with a solution of carbol fuchsin (a mixture of basic fuchsin and phenol) and heated until steam rises. After washing with water, the slide is flooded with a dilute mineral acid (e.g. 3% hydrochloric acid) and, after further washing, a green or blue counterstain is applied. Red bacilli are seen against the contrasting background colour. In some methods, the acid is diluted in 95% ethanol rather than water. This gives a cleaner background but, contrary to a common belief, it does not enable tubercle bacilli to be distinguished from other species. Fluorescent dyes are also used and there are modifications of the staining techniques for use with tissue sections.

Cultural methods

As sputum and certain other specimens frequently contain many bacteria and fungi that would rapidly overgrow any mycobacteria on the culture media, these must be destroyed. *Decontamination*

methods make use of the relatively high resistance of mycobacteria to acids, alkalis and certain disinfectants. In the widely used *Petroff method*, sputum is mixed well with 4% sodium hydroxide for 15–30 min, neutralized with potassium dihydrogen orthophosphate and centrifuged. The deposit is used to inoculate LJ or similar media. Specimens such as cerebrospinal fluid and tissue biopsies which are unlikely to be contaminated do not require such treament before inoculation on to culture media.

Inoculated media are incubated at 35–37°C and inspected weekly for at least 8 weeks. Cultures of material from skin lesions should also be incubated at 33°C. Any bacterial growth is stained by the ZN method and, if acid-fast, it is subcultured for further identification. A more rapid bacteriological diagnosis is achieved by the radiometric detection of $^{14}CO_2$ released from liquid media containing ^{14}C-labelled palmitic acid.

The first step in identification is to determine whether an isolate is a tubercle bacillus (*M. tuberculosis*, *M. bovis* or *M. africanum*) or one of the other species. Tubercle bacilli grow slowly, do not produce yellow pigment and fail to grow at 25 and 41°C and on egg media containing *p*-nitrobenzoic acid (500 mg/l). Strains differing in any of these properties belong to other species.

Sensitivity testing

Several methods have been described. In the UK there is a preference for the resistance ratio method in which test strains and a number of known sensitive control strains are inoculated on doubling dilutions of drug-containing LJ medium. The results are expressed as the ratio of the drug concentration inhibiting the test strain to that inhibiting the control strains. Sensitive strains have resistance ratios of 1 or 2 while higher ratios indicate resistance (Table 19.4).

TREATMENT

The antituberculosis drugs are divisible into three groups: bactericidal drugs that effectively sterilize tuberculous lesions, bactericidal drugs that only kill tubercle bacilli in certain situations and

20

Environmental ('atypical') mycobacteria

Opportunist disease

J. M. Grange

In addition to the tubercle and leprosy bacilli there are many species of mycobacteria that normally exist as saprophytes of soil and water. Some of these, termed environmental or 'atypical' mycobacteria, occasionally cause opportunist disease in animals and man. Although such opportunist pathogens were described towards the end of the 19th century, their classification remained in a state of chaos for over 50 years and they were often called *anonymous mycobacteria*. Order began to replace chaos in 1959 when a botanist, Ernest Runyon, described four groups of mycobacteria associated with human disease according to their production of yellow or orange pigment and their rate of growth:

Group I   *Photochromogens* — pigmentation on exposure to light
Group II *Scotochromogens* — pigmentation formed in the dark
Group III *Non-chromogens* — no pigmentation
Group IV *Rapid growers*.

All strains in groups I, II and III grow slowly. The photochromogens are colourless when incubated in the dark but if young cultures are exposed to a light source for an hour or more and then re-incubated they develop a bright yellow or orange coloration. The caps of the culture bottles must be loosened during exposure to light as oxygen is essential for pigment formation. Rapid growers, which may be photo-, scoto- or non-chromogens, produce visible growth on Löwenstein–Jensen medium within 1 week on subculture; the appearance of growth on primary culture of clinical material often takes considerably longer.

In 1980 there were 41 approved mycobacterial species and several more have since been described. Identification is usually undertaken by specialist reference laboratories. There is no universally recognized identification scheme for mycobacteria, although reliance is usually placed on cultural characteristics (rate and temperature of growth and pigmentation), various biochemical reactions and resistance to antimicrobial agents. Some centres also use thin-layer chromatography of cell wall lipids or detection of specific antigens by sero-agglutination or immunodiffusion techniques.

ENVIRONMENTAL MYCOBACTERIA OF CLINICAL IMPORTANCE

Species that may be incriminated in human disease are shown in Table 20.1.

Photochromogens

This group contains three species, *M. kansasii*, *M. simiae* and *M. marinum*. The first two grow well at 37°C and are principally isolated from cases of pulmonary disease. *M. marinum*, previously termed the fish tubercle bacillus, is the cause of a warty skin infection known as *swimming pool granuloma*. It grows poorly or not at all at 37°C and cultures from skin lesions should therefore be incubated at 33°C. On microscopy, *M. kansasii*

Table 20.1 Environmental mycobacteria of clinical importance

Runyon group	Species	
I (photochromogens)	M. kansasii M. simiae	M. marinum
II (scotochromogens)	M. scrofulaceum M. szulgai	M. gordonae
III (non-chromogens)	M. avium M. malmoense M. ulcerans	M. intracellulare M. xenopi M. terrae group[a]
IV (rapid growers)	M. chelonei[b]	M. fortuitum

[a] Includes *M. nonchromogenicum* and *M. triviale*.
[b] Also spelt *M. chelonae*.

and *M. marinum* are often elongated with a distinct beaded appearance.

Scotochromogens

The principal pathogen in this group is *M. scrofulaceum* which, as the name suggests, is associated with scrofula or cervical lymphadenitis, although it also causes pulmonary disease. *M. szulgai*, an uncommon cause of pulmonary disease and bursitis, is a scotochromogen when incubated at 37°C but a photochromogen at 25°C. *M. gordonae* (formerly *M. aquae*) is a rare cause of pulmonary disease but is frequently found in water and is a common contaminant of clinical material.

Non-chromogens

The most prevalent and important opportunistic pathogens of man are the avian tubercle bacillus, *M. avium*, and the closely related *M. intracellulare*, formerly known as the *Battey bacillus*. These two species are usually grouped together as the *M. avium-intracellulare* (MAI) complex. Most clinical isolates are smooth, easily emulsifiable and agglutinated by specific antisera, although untypable strains are not uncommon. There are 28 agglutination serotypes in the MAI complex: types 1–3 belong to *M. avium* and types 4–28 to *M. intracellulare*. In man, this complex is responsible for lymphadenitis, pulmonary lesions and disseminated disease, notably in patients with acquired immune deficiency syndrome (AIDS).

M. avium causes tuberculosis in birds and lymphadenitis in pigs as well as occasional disease in wild and domestic animals. The MAI complex is closely related to two animal pathogens: *M. paratuberculosis*, the cause of chronic hypertrophic enteritis or *Johne's disease* of cattle, and *M. lepraemurium*, the cause of a leprosy-like disease of rats, mice and cats.

M. xenopi, first isolated from a xenopus toad, is a thermophile and grows well at 45°C. It is principally responsible for pulmonary lesions and is of limited geographical distribution. Most reported cases have been from London and south-east England and northern France.

M. malmoense is a recently described cause of pulmonary disease and lymphadenitis. It grows very slowly, often taking as long as 10 weeks to appear on primary culture, and is therefore likely to be missed if cultures are not maintained for this length of time.

M. ulcerans, the cause of *Buruli ulcer*, is a very slowly growing species which will only grow in vitro between 31 and 34°C. Colonies are non-pigmented or a pale lemon-yellow colour. Unlike other mycobacterial pathogens, *M. ulcerans* produces a toxin which causes tissue necrosis and which may be involved in the pathogenesis of disease. Inoculation of *M. ulcerans* into the mouse footpad leads to progressive disease with swelling and eventual ulceration or auto-amputation. For unknown reasons, some infected mice develop generalized oedema — the 'fat mouse syndrome'.

Other rare pathogens in this group include *M. terrae* (the radish bacillus), *M. nonchromogenicum* and *M. triviale*, which are sometimes grouped as the *M. terrae* complex. *M. haemophilum*, characterized by its growth requirement for haem or other sources of iron, is a rare cause of granulomatous or ulcerative skin lesions in xenograft recipients and other immunocompromised individuals.

Rapid growers

Only two of the rapidly growing species, *M. chelonei* (*M. chelonae*) and *M. fortuitum*, are well-recognized pathogens of man. These two species were originally identified as the turtle and frog tubercle bacilli, respectively. They occasionally cause pulmonary or disseminated disease but are principally responsible for post-injection abscesses and wound infections including corneal ulcers. Both species are non-chromogenic.

There are many other rapidly growing species of mycobacteria, most of which are pigmented. Disease due to them is exceedingly rare but they frequently contaminate clinical specimens. They are found in the genitalia and gain access to urine samples although, contrary to a common belief, the species *M. smegmatis* is rarely found in this site.

ECOLOGY AND EPIDEMIOLOGY

Mycobacteria are widely distributed in the environment and are particularly abundant in wet soil, marshland, streams, rivers and estuaries. Some species, such as *M. terrae*, are found in soil while others, including *M. marinum* and *M. gordonae*, prefer free water. Some potential pathogens, notably *M. kansasii* and *M. xenopi*, are able to colonize piped-water supplies. Human beings are therefore regularly exposed to mycobacteria as a result of drinking, washing, showering and inhalation of natural aerosols. Such repeated subclinical infection may induce sensitization to tuberculin and other mycobacterial skin-testing reagents. There is also strong evidence that contact with environmental mycobacteria profoundly affects the subsequent ability of BCG (bacille Calmette–Guérin) vaccine to induce protective immunity.

Although man is frequently infected by environmental mycobacteria, they are of low virulence and overt disease due to them is very uncommon. The incidence and type of disease in any region is determined by the species and numbers of mycobacteria in the environment, the opportunities for their transmission to man and the susceptibility of the human population.

Unlike tuberculosis, person-to-person transmission of opportunist mycobacterial disease rarely, if ever, occurs. Thus the incidence of such disease is independent of that of tuberculosis and unaffected by public health measures designed to control the latter. In countries where tuberculosis is now uncommon and declining, the opportunist mycobacterial infections are becoming relatively more common. In south-east England, about 5% of mycobacterial disease is due to environmental species; the proportion is much higher in some parts of the USA. In addition, the absolute incidence is increasing as a result of the growing number of immunocompromised individuals, notably patients with AIDS.

A number of 'epidemics' of falsely diagnosed mycobacterial pulmonary disease and urinary tract infection have resulted from the collection of sputum and urine specimens in containers rinsed out with water from taps colonized by mycobacteria. Likewise, false-positive sputum smear examinations for acid-fast bacilli have occurred when staining reagents were prepared from contaminated water.

DISEASE DUE TO ENVIRONMENTAL MYCOBACTERIA

Four main types of opportunist mycobacterial disease of man have been described: skin lesions following traumatic inoculation of bacteria, localized lymphadenitis, tuberculosis-like pulmonary lesions and disseminated disease (Table 20.2).

Lymphadenitis

This is caused by a number of different species which vary in relative frequency from region to

Table 20.2 Principal types of opportunist mycobacterial disease in man and the usual causative agents

Disease	Usual causative agent
Lymphadenopathy	*M. avium-intracellulare*
	M. scrofulaceum
Skin lesions	
Post-trauma abscesses	*M. chelonei*
	M. fortuitum
Swimming pool granuloma	*M. marinum*
Buruli ulcer	*M. ulcerans*
Pulmonary disease	*M. avium-intracellulare*
	M. kansasii
	M. xenopi
Disseminated disease	
AIDS related	*M. avium-intracellulare*
Non-AIDS related	*M. avium-intracellulare*
	M. chelonei

region. In the USA *M. scrofulaceum* is the usual cause while in Great Britain *M. avium–intracellulare* is the predominant cause. In most cases a single node, usually a tonsillar node, is involved and the majority of patients are children aged less than 5 years. Excision of the node, usually performed for diagnostic purposes, is almost always curative. Lymphadenitis occasionally occurs as part of a more disseminated infection, particularly in individuals with AIDS.

Skin lesions

Three main types have been described: post-injection abscesses, swimming pool granuloma and Buruli ulcer.

Post-injection abscesses

These are usually caused by the rapidly growing pathogens *M. chelonei* and *M. fortuitum*. Abscesses occur sporadically, particularly in the tropics, or in small epidemics when batches of injectable materials are contaminated by these bacteria. Abscesses develop within a week or so or up to a year or more after the injection. They are painful and may become quite large — up to 8 or 10 cm in diameter — and may persist for many months. Treatment is by drainage with curettage or total excision. Chemotherapy is not required unless there is local spread of disease or multiple abscesses, as may occur in insulin-dependent diabetics. Deeper abscesses have developed after more extensive injuries and surgical procedures, including open heart surgery, and corneal infections have followed ocular injuries. Infections by *M. terrae* have occurred in farmers and others who have been injured while working with soil.

Swimming pool granuloma

This is also known as *fish tank granuloma* and *fish fancier's finger* and is caused by *M. marinum*. As suggested by the names, most of those affected are users of swimming pools, keepers of tropical fish and others involved in aquatic hobbies. The bacilli enter scratches and abrasions and cause warty lesions similar to those seen in skin tuber-culosis. The lesions, which usually occur on the knees and elbows of swimmers and on the hands of aquarium keepers, are usually localized but secondary lesions sometimes appear along the line of the dermal lymphatics. This is termed *sporotrichoid spread* as a similar phenomenon occurs in the fungus infection sporotrichosis. The disease is usually self-limiting although chemotherapy with minocycline, co-trimoxazole or rifampicin with ethambutol hastens its resolution.

Buruli ulcer

This disease, caused by *M. ulcerans*, was first described in Australia but the name is derived from the Buruli district of Uganda where a large outbreak of the disease was extensively investigated. Buruli ulcer occurs in several tropical countries, notably Nigeria, Ghana, Zaire, Mexico, Malaysia and Papua New Guinea, and is limited to certain localities which, characteristically, are low-lying marshy areas subject to periodic flooding. Although never isolated from the environment, there is strong evidence that *M. ulcerans* is a free-living species that is introduced into the human dermis by minor injuries, particularly by spiky grasses.

The first manifestation of the disease is a hard cutaneous nodule which is often itchy. This enlarges and develops central softening and fluctuation due to necrosis of the underlying adipose subcutaneous tissues. The overlying skin becomes anoxic and breaks down, the liquefied necrotic contents of the lesion are discharged and one or more ulcers with deeply undermined edges are thereby formed (Fig. 20.1). At this stage the lesion is teeming with acid-fast bacilli, there is no histological evidence of an active cell-mediated immune response and the patient does not react to *burulin*, a skin test reagent prepared from *M. ulcerans*. During this anergic stage the lesion may progressively extend to an enormous size, sometimes involving an entire limb or a major part of the trunk.

For unknown reasons, the anergic phase eventually gives way to an immunoreactive phase when a granulomatous response develops in the lesion, the acid-fast bacilli disappear and the

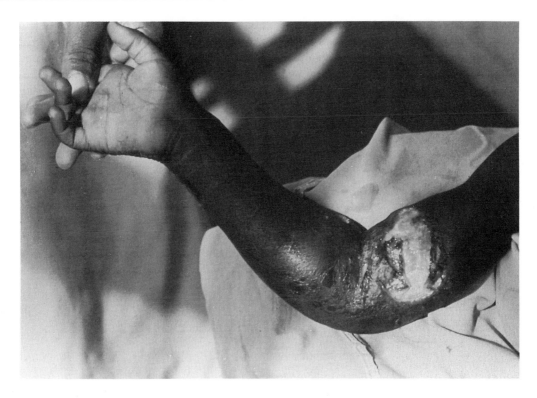

Fig. 20.1 Buruli ulcer. Undermined ulcer overlying the biceps and swelling of the surrounding tissues. (Courtesy of Dr Alan Knell, Wellcome Tropical Institute.)

patient reacts to burulin. Healing then occurs but the patient is often left with considerable disfigurement and disability due to extensive scarring and contractures.

The early, pre-ulcerative, lesions are easily treatable by excision and primary closure by suture. Ulcerated lesions require excision and skin grafting. In the anergic phase, the excision must be extensive enough to remove all disease in order to avoid recurrences. Therapy with rifampicin and clofazimine has been attempted but with unconvincing results.

Pulmonary disease

This is most frequently seen in middle-aged or elderly men with lung damage due to smoking or exposure to industrial dusts. It also occurs in individuals with congenital or acquired immune deficiencies, malignant disease, cystic fibrosis or with no apparent underlying disorder. The disease may be caused by many species but the most frequent are *M. avium-intracellulare* and *M. kansasii*. There are no clinical or radiological characteristics that reliably differentiate opportunist mycobacterial disease from tuberculosis and the diagnosis is made by isolation and identification of the pathogen. Great care must, however, be taken to differentiate true disease from transient colonization or superinfection. As a general rule, a diagnosis of opportunist mycobacterial disease may be made when a heavy growth of the pathogen is repeatedly isolated from the sputum of a patient with compatible clinical and radiological features and in whom other causes of these features have been carefully excluded.

Disseminated disease

Up to a half of all individuals dying of AIDS in the USA have disseminated mycobacterial disease, almost always due to *M. avium-intracellulare*.

Acid-fast bacilli are readily isolated from bone marrow aspirates, intestinal biopsies, blood and faeces. It is not clear to what extent such infection reduces the quality or duration of life and treatment is of limited efficacy. Disseminated disease occasionally occurs in individuals with other congenital or acquired causes of immunosuppression, including renal transplantation. Again, *M. avium-intracellulare* is the usual cause but disseminated *M. chelonei* infections have occurred in recipients of renal transplants and other immunocompromised patients (Fig. 20.2).

TREATMENT OF OPPORTUNIST MYCOBACTERIAL DISEASE

Most environmental mycobacteria are resistant to many antituberculosis drugs in vitro although infections often respond to various combinations of these drugs. Regimens containing five or six antituberculosis drugs have been used for pulmonary disease due to *M. avium-intracellulare*, *M. kansasii* and other slowly growing species, but equal success has been obtained with standard triple therapy — rifampicin, isoniazid and ethambutol — provided that all three drugs are given for up to 18 months. Treatment is, however, unsuccessful in a substantial minority of cases and localized lesions are surgically excised when possible. Pulmonary and non-pulmonary disease due to the rapidly growing species *M. chelonei* and *M. fortuitum* have been treated successfully by various regimens based on one or more of the following drugs: erythromycin, sulphonamides, trimethoprim, amikacin, gentamicin, cephalosporins and fluoroquinolones. Therapy with clofazimine and rifabutin (ansamycin) reduces the bacterial load in AIDS-associated *M. avium-intracellulare* infection but may not totally eliminate the pathogen.

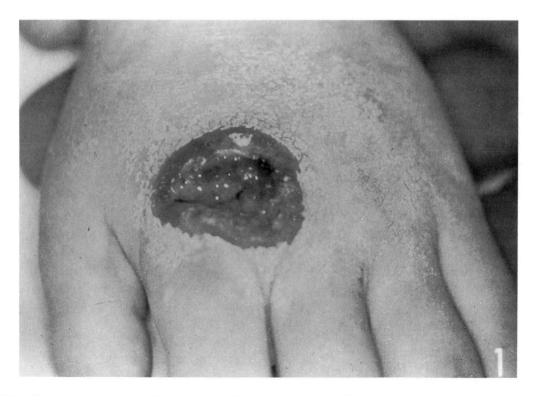

Fig. 20.2 Skin ulcer on the dorsum of the hand due to disseminated *M. chelonei* in an immunocompromised child. (Courtesy of Dr Kurt Schopfer.)

RECOMMENDED READING

Collins C H, Grange J M, Noble W C, Yates M D 1985 *Mycobacterium marinum* infections in man. *Journal of Hygiene* 94: 135–149

Ratledge C, Stanford J L, Grange J M (eds) 1989 *The Biology of the Mycobacteria, Clinical Aspects of Mycobacterial Disease.* Academic Press, London vol 3, ch 3, 10, 11

Stanford J L, Rook G A W 1983 Environmental mycobacteria and immunization with BCG. In: Easmon C S F, Jeljaszewicz J (eds) *Medical Microbiology, Immunization* *Against Bacterial Disease.* Academic Press, London, vol 2, p 43–69

van der Werf T S, van der Graaf W T A, Groothuis D G, Knell A J 1989 *Mycobacterium ulcerans* infection in Ashanti region, Ghana. *Transactions of the Royal Society of Tropical Medicine and Hygiene* 83: 410–413

Wolinsky E 1979 State of the art: non-tuberculous mycobacteria and associated diseases. *American Review of Respiratory Disease* 119: 107–159

21

Actinomyces and nocardia   Actinomycosis; nocardiasis

J. M. Grange

Gram-positive bacteria with branching filaments that sometimes develop into mycelia are included in the rather loosely defined order *Actinomycetales*. Although mostly soil saprophytes, two genera, *Actinomyces* and *Nocardia*, occasionally cause chronic granulomatous infections in animals and man. Another genus, *Streptomyces*, is an extremely rare cause of disease but is the source of several antibiotics. In addition, repeated inhalation of thermophilic actinomycetes, notably *Micropolyspora faeni* and *Thermoactinomyces* species, causes *extrinsic allergic alveolitis (farmer's lung, mushroom worker's lung, bagassosis)* in those who are occupationally exposed to mouldy vegetable matter.

ACTINOMYCES
DESCRIPTION

Actinomyces are branching Gram-positive bacilli. They are facultative anaerobes but they often fail to grow aerobically on primary culture. They grow best under anaerobic or micro-aerophilic conditions with the addition of 5–10% carbon dioxide. Almost all species are commensals of the mouth and have a narrow temperature range of growth around 35–37°C. They are responsible for the disease known as *actinomycosis*, which, in man, is usually caused by *Actinomyces israelii*. A further three species, *A. meyeri*, *A. naeslundii* and *A. odontolyticus*, are very rare causes of actinomycosis and the latter has been isolated from deep caries. *A. meyeri* is sometimes encountered as part of the mixed bacterial flora of brain abscesses. *A. bovis* causes cervicofacial infections in cattle (*lumpy jaw*).

Concomitant bacteria, notably a small Gram-negative rod, *Actinobacillus actinomycetemcomitans*, but also *Haemophilus* species, fusiforms and anaerobic streptococci, are sometimes found in actinomycotic lesions but their contribution to the pathogenesis of the disease, if any, is unknown. *Act. actinomycetemcomitans* is a rare cause of endocarditis.

PATHOGENESIS

Actinomycosis is a very chronic disease characterized by multiple abscesses and granulomas, tissue destruction, extensive fibrosis and the formation of sinuses. Within diseased tissues the actinomycetes form large masses of mycelia embedded in an amorphous protein–polysaccharide matrix and surrounded by a zone of Gram-negative, weakly acid-fast, club-like structures (Fig. 21.1). These clubs were once thought to consist, at least in part, of material derived from host tissue, but it now appears that they are formed entirely from the bacteria. The mycelial masses may be large enough to be visible to the naked eye and, as they are often light yellow in colour, they are called *sulphur granules*. In older lesions the sulphur granules may be dark brown and very hard due to the deposition of calcium phosphate in the matrix.

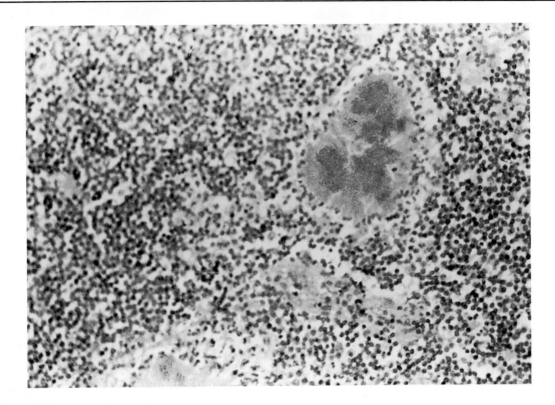

Fig. 21.1 Actinomycotic granule in tissue. (Courtesy of Prof. R. J. Hay.)

In man, about two-thirds of cases of actino-mycosis occur in the cervicofacial region and the jaw is often involved. The disease is endogenous in origin: dental caries is a predisposing factor and infection may follow tooth extractions or other dental procedures. Males are affected more frequently than females and in some regions the disease is more common in rural agricultural workers than in town dwellers, probably due to lower standards of dental care in the former.

Thoracic actinomycosis commences in the lung, probably as a result of aspiration of actino-myces from the mouth. Sinuses often appear on the chest wall and the ribs and spine may be eroded. Abdominal cases commence in the appendix or, less frequently, in colonic diver-ticula. Pelvic actinomycosis occasionally occurs in women fitted with plastic intra-uterine con-traceptive devices. 'Punch actinomycosis' is a rare infection of the hand acquired by injury of the knuckles on an adversary's teeth.

The lymphatics are not usually involved in actinomycosis but haematogenous spread to the liver, brain and other internal organs occasionally occurs.

LABORATORY DIAGNOSIS

Pus from suspected cases is shaken with sterile water in a tube. Sulphur granules settle to the bottom and may be removed with a Pasteur pipette. Granules crushed between two glass slides are used to prepare Gram- and Ziehl-Neelsen-stained films (the latter modified by using 1% sulphuric acid for decoloration), which reveal the Gram-positive mycelia and the zone of radiating acid-fast clubs. Sulphur granules and mycelia in tissue sections are identifiable by use of fluoroscein-conjugated specific antisera. Granules for culture are washed thoroughly in saline in a tube or Petri dish, crushed in a drop of saline with a glass rod and used to inoculate brain–heart infusion agar, blood agar and either glucose broth, enriched thioglycollate broth or commercially available actinomyces broth. Cultures are incubated, both aerobically and anaerobically, with the addition of 5% carbon dioxide for up to 10 d. After incubation for several days, *A. israelii* forms so-called *spider colonies* which resemble molar teeth and its identity may be confirmed by means of biochemical tests or staining with specific fluorescent antisera.

TREATMENT

Actinomyces are sensitive to many antibiotics, but the penetration of drugs into the densely fibrotic diseased tissue is poor. Thus, large doses are required for prolonged periods and recurrence of disease is not uncommon. Surgical debridement reduces scarring and deformity, hastens healing and lowers the incidence of recurrences. Penicillin is frequently used: an injectable penicillin, 0.3–0.6 g or more twice daily, for up to 3 months is usually given but oral phenoxymethylpenicillin, 2 g daily for 6 weeks or more, is often satisfactory for the treatment of cervicofacial disease. Tetracycline is preferred by some physicians, especially if penicillin-resistant bacteria are also present. Erythromycin, fusidic acid, lincomycin and rifampicin have also been used successfully.

NOCARDIA

DESCRIPTION

The nocardiae are branched, strictly aerobic, Gram-positive bacteria which are closely related to the rapidly growing mycobacteria. Like the latter, but unlike actinomyces, they are environmental saprophytes with a broad temperature range of growth. The properties of nocardiae and actinomycetes are compared in Table 21.1. Most species are acid-fast when decolorized with 1% sulphuric acid but a few are not acid-fast and some bacteriologists prefer to place these in the separate genus *Actinomadura*.

Many species of nocardiae are found in the environment but opportunist disease in man is almost always caused by *N. asteroides*, so named because of its star-shaped colonies, *N. brasiliensis*, *N. otitidis-caviarum* (*N. caviae*) and *N. madurae* (*Actinomadura madurae*).

Bovine farcy, a lymphocutaneous disease of cattle in Africa, was thought to be nocardial but the causative agents are now known to be mycobacteria; namely, *M. farcinogenes* and *M. senegalense*.

PATHOGENESIS

Nocardiae, principally *N. asteroides*, are uncommon causes of opportunist pulmonary disease that usually, but not always, occurs in immunocompromised individuals including those receiving corticosteroid therapy and post-transplant immunosuppressive therapy and those with acquired immune deficiency syndrome (AIDS). The infection is exogenous, resulting from inhalation of the bacilli. The clinical and radiological features are very variable and non-specific and diagnosis is not easy. In most cases there are multiple confluent abscesses with little or no surrounding fibrous reaction and local spread may result in empyema. In some cases the disease is very chronic while in others it spreads rapidly through the lungs. Secondary abscesses in the brain and, less frequently, in other organs occur in about one-third of patients with pulmonary nocardiasis.

Nocardiae also cause cutaneous infections with involvement of the lymphatics, mostly in the

Table 21.1 Differences between the genera *Actinomyces* and *Nocardia*

Actinomyces spp.	*Nocardia* spp.
Facultative anaerobes	Strict aerobes
Grow at 35–37°C	Wide temperature range of growth
Oral commensals	Environmental saprophytes
Non-acid-fast mycelia	Usually weakly acid-fast
Endogenous cause of disease	Exogenous cause of disease

USA and the southern hemisphere but very rarely in Europe. The causative agent is *N. brasiliensis* or, less frequently, *N. otitidis-caviarum*. Infections may result in fungating tumour-like masses termed *mycetomas* (Fig. 21.2).

Madura foot is a chronic granulomatous infection of the bones and soft tissues of the foot resulting in mycetoma formation and gross deformity. It occurs in Sudan, north Africa and the west coast of India, principally amongst those who walk barefoot and are therefore prone to contamination of foot injuries by soil-derived organisms. One of the causative organisms is *N. madurae* but it is also caused by other nocardiae and by fungi (see Chapter 60).

LABORATORY DIAGNOSIS

A presumptive diagnosis of pulmonary nocardiasis may be made by a microscopical examination of sputum. In many cases the sputum contains numerous lymphocytes and macrophages, some of which contain pleomorphic Gram-positive and weakly acid-fast bacilli, and occasionally extracellular branching filaments. Nocardiae are not so easily seen in tissue biopsies stained by the Gram or modified Ziehl–Neelsen methods but they may be seen in preparations stained by the Gomori methenamine silver method.

Nocardiae grow on most standard bacteriological media in 2 d to 1 month. Suitable media include brain–heart infusion agar and trypticase–soy agar enriched with blood. In addition, the technique of *paraffin baiting* may be used: a paraffin wax-coated glass rod is placed in inoculated carbon-free broth. Nocardiae grow on the rod at the air–liquid interface and may be subcultured onto agar media.

Colonies of nocardiae are cream, orange or pink coloured and their surfaces may develop a dry, chalky appearance and they adhere firmly to the medium. Identification of species is not easy and is usually undertaken by reference laboratories.

TREATMENT

The therapy of choice for all types of nocardial infections is a sulphonamide, with or without trimethoprim, for an extended period, often 3 months or more. Alternative useful agents are minocycline, amikacin and imipenem, particularly for the treatment of AIDS patients who are unable to tolerate the standard drugs. Mycetomas due to nocardiae are much easier to treat than those due to fungi. Even long-standing cases with extensive mycetoma formation respond well to chemotherapy.

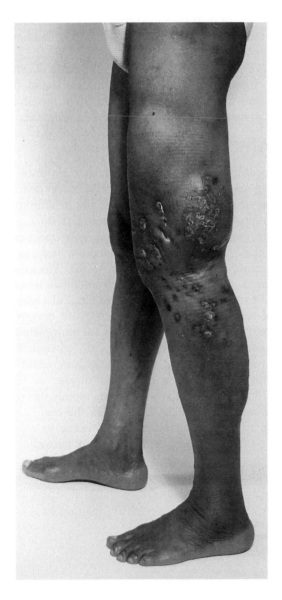

Fig. 21.2 Actinomycotic mycetoma of the thigh, showing multiple fungating nodules and sinuses. (Courtesy of Mr R. D. Rosin.)

RECOMMENDED READING

Bronner M, Bronner M 1971 *Actinomycosis*. John Wright, Bristol

Collins C H, Yates M D, Uttley A H C 1988 Presumptive identification of nocardias in a clinical laboratory. *Journal of Applied cteriology* 65: 55–59

Curry W A 1980 Human nocardosis — a clinical review with selected case reports. *Archives of Internal Medicine*; 140, 818–826

Roberts I F, Karim Q N, Rosin R D 1988 Actinomycotic mycetoma of the thigh. *Journal of the Royal Society of Medicine* 82: 552–553

Stevens D A 1983 Clinical and laboratory aspects of nocardial infection. *Journal of Hygiene* 91: 377–384

Tight R R, Bartlett M S 1981 Actinomycetoma in the United States. *Reviews of Infectious Diseases* 3: 1139–1150

22

Bacillus   Anthrax; food poisoning

R. C. B. Slack

Anthrax is an example of a zoonotic disease primarily recognized in large domesticated animals which infects man accidentally through contact with infected products. *Bacillus anthracis*, the causative organism, is of world-wide distribution and, although rare in the industrialized nations, the very name *anthrax* strikes terror in the public, evoking horrors of 'germ warfare'. It is an important and interesting disease for a number of reasons. It holds a crucial place in the history of medical microbiology because of the work of Robert Koch, who first showed that a causative organism could be isolated from the blood of infected animals, artificially grown in pure culture and then used to reproduce the disease in animals. Koch's work on anthrax led to the development of the present-day methods of isolation and identification of bacteria and to the formulation of *Koch's postulates* (see Chapter 1). Pasteur showed that animals could be actively immunized by infecting them with cultures of *B. anthracis* that had been attenuated by growth at 43°C. Anthrax is a disease in which the infection is transmitted by the spores of the bacillus, which are shed in large numbers in the terminal stages of infection. The disease is therefore unusual in that the infection is spread only from a dying or dead host and that the causative organism may survive for a long time in the environment. More recent work has elucidated the mechanism of virulence of *B. anthracis* and improved protective vaccines.

The genus *Bacillus* originally included all rod-shaped bacteria but now comprises only large, spore-forming Gram-positive bacilli which form chains and will usually grow both aerobically and anaerobically. They are common environmental organisms and are frequently isolated in laboratories as contaminants of media or specimens. *B anthracis* is the most important pathogen of the group. *B. cereus* may contaminate food, especially rice, in large numbers and has been implicated in many episodes of food poisoning. Other species of *Bacillus* are less often incriminated as pathogens, usually in the immunocompromised.

BACILLUS ANTHRACIS

DESCRIPTION

B. anthracis is a non-motile straight, sporing bacillus, rectangular in shape and 4–8 μm by 1–1.5 μm in dimensions, i.e. just smaller in length than the diameter of a red blood corpuscle. The spore is oval, refractile, central in position and of the same diameter as the bacillus. The organism is a strongly Gram-positive aerobe and facultative anaerobe with a temperature range for growth of 12–45°C (optimum, 35°C); it grows on all ordinary media as typical colonies with a wavy margin and small projections, the so-called *medusa head* appearance. Table 22.1 lists some of the differences between *B. anthracis* and other important members of the genus *Bacillus*.

Spores are never found in the tissues but appear when the organism is shed or grown on artificial media; they stain only with special spore-staining

Table 22.1 Distinguishing properties of some important *Bacillus* species

Property	*B. anthracis*	*B. cereus*	*B. subtilis*	*B. stearothermophilus*
Cell Size (μm)	Large (6×1.5)	Large	Small (3×0.6)	Small
Motility	−	+	+	+
Capsule	+	−	−	−
Mouse pathogenicity	+++	+	−	−
Anaerobic growth	+	+	−	+/−
Temperature for optimal growth (°C)	37	30	37	55

procedures. The spores are resistant to chemical disinfectants and heat; the spores of many strains will resist dry heat at 140°C for 1–3 h and boiling or steam at 100°C for 5–10 min. However, autoclaving at 121°C (15 lb/in^2) destroys them in 15 min. The spores are relatively resistant to chemical agents.

PATHOGENESIS

Clinical infection

Man is relatively resistant to infection with *B. anthracis* and anthrax most commonly arises by inoculation through the skin of material from infected animals or their products. The resulting lesion of cutaneous anthrax is often described as a *malignant pustule* because of its characteristic appearance (Fig. 22.1). Coagulation necrosis of the centre of the pustule results in the formation of a dark-coloured *eschar,* which is later surrounded by a ring of vesicles containing serous fluid and an area of oedema and induration which may become extensive. In patients with severe toxic signs and widespread oedema the prognosis is poor.

Inhalation of spores in dust or wool fibres may result in respiratory anthrax: *wool-sorter's disease.* This condition carries a high mortality due to the intense inflammation, haemorrhage and septicaemia which results from the multiplication of organisms in bronchi and spread to the lungs, lymphatics and bloodstream. The production of toxins and the considerable bacterial load which rapidly occurs in the terminal septicaemic phase produce increased vascular permeability and hypotension similar to endotoxic shock.

The intestinal form of anthrax occurs among pastoralists who may be forced through poverty to eat infected animals which have been found dead. An individual may suffer after a day or so from haemorrhagic diarrhoea and dies rapidly from septicaemia. Often these episodes occur as small outbreaks in a family or village. Because some individuals may only suffer cutaneous lesions the recognition of the microbial cuase of the outbreak is easily made clinically.

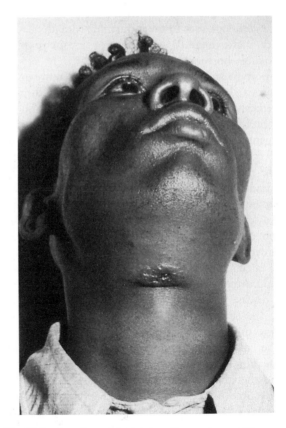

Fig. 22.1 A malignant pustule in a Kenyan farmer. (From Professor I. A. Wamola, University of Nairobi Medical School.)

Animal infection

All mammals are suceptible, though to a varying degree. Guinea-pigs and mice are highly susceptible to experimental inoculation. If a guinea-pig is injected subcutaneously with pathological material containing the bacilli, or with pure cultures, the animals dies, usually within 2–3 d, showing a marked inflammatory lesion at the site of inoculation and extensive gelatinous oedema in the subcutaneous tissues. Large numbers of the bacilli are presented in the local lesion, and are also profusely present in the heart blood and in the capillaries of the internal organs. They are specially numerous in the spleen (Fig. 22.2), which is enlarged and soft, giving rise to the description *splenic fever* in the ox and the German name for the organism — *Milzbrandbazillus* (spleen-destroying bacillus).

The production of anthrax in monkeys and guinea-pigs by inhalation of contaminated aerosols has also been studied experimentally. Spores deposited on the alveolar walls are taken up by phagocytes and carried to the tracheobronchial glands, which become inflamed and enlarged. Infection spreads via the lymphatics to the general circulation. About 20 000 organisms can produce lethal infection if the particle size of the aerosols is less than 5 μm since the smaller particles are more likely to penetrate in the airstream to the alveolar walls, but the lethal dose is much higher if the particles are larger. Much of the work on the aerobiology of infection has been conducted in military establishments and many of the results have not been released in the public domain under the mistaken view that anthrax could be an effective biological weapon.

In natural conditions both wild herbivores and domesticated animals are susceptible. The condition is usually septicaemic following ingestion of contaminated pasture. The spores are ingested with coarse vegetation, which probably predisposes to trauma of the intestinal tract. Infection also occurs by inhalation of dust into the respir-

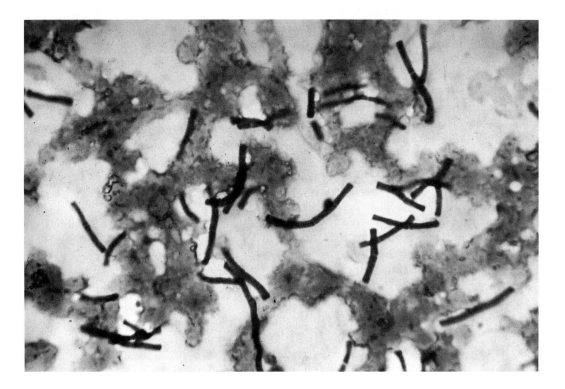

Fig. 22.2 Guinea-pig spleen imprint showing typical anthrax bacilli.

atory tract and, as in human disease, through skin abrasions leading to malignant pustules.

The spores germinate and the vegetative cells produce toxin, leading to the formation of gelatinous oedema and haemorrhage. In susceptible animals the bacilli resist phagocytosis and reach the lymphatics and thence the bloodstream. Before death the bacilli multiply freely in the blood and tissues. In resistant animals there is a more profuse leucocyte response with phagocytosis and decapsulation of the organism.

Virulence determinants

The pathogenicity of *B. anthracis* depends on two properties not found in a saprophytic *Bacillus* spp. The most easily demonstrated is the capsule, which is unusual in being a polypeptide, of D-glutamic acid, which inhibits opsonophagocytosis. The other determinant is the plasmid-encoded toxin complex comprising three proteins, all of which are required for pathogenicity: the *protective antigen* binds the complex to receptors on the macrophage surface; after proteolysis, *oedema factor* and *lethal factor* are released and, after endocytosis, work inside the cell by blocking the adenyl cyclase pathway. The main effect of this toxin complex is to increase vascular permeability which leads to shock. Knowledge of the biochemistry of these determinants has led to the development of protective antigen vaccines to replace the original non-encapsulated avirulent strains.

LABORATORY DIAGNOSIS

Clinical specimens

The fully developed malignant pustule may be dificult to swab and the central necrotic area gives a poor yield. Fluid aspirated from the surrounding vesicles, when present, is more likely to yield anthrax bacilli. Specimens should be taken before antibiotic therapy has been instituted.

In laboratories unfamiliar with the disease additional precautions for staff safety need to be organized. However, the relative ease of clinical diagnosis, given the characteristic appearance and occupational exposure, often makes laboratory confirmation superfluous.

Gram's stain may show typical large Gram-positive bacilli, and culture on blood agar yields the large, flat, greyish colonies with a characterisic swirl (the *medua head*). Staining of films from these colonies will show long chains of Gram-positive bacilli some containing spores. Serological diagnosis by ELISA (enzyme-linked immunosorbent assay) may be of value retrospectively but is seldom used diagnostically.

Confirmatory tests

Animal inoculation was used in the past to confirm that the organism was *B. anthracis*. Guinea-pigs may be inoculated subcutaneously with a suspension of bacilli. Death usually ensues within 2–3 d and post-mortem reveals numerous bacteria on cardiac puncture or impression of splenic cells (Fig. 22.2). These specimens when stained with polychrome methylene blue show large, blue bacilli surrounded by a red granular-stained capsule (*McFadyean's reaction*). This appearance is given only by *B. anthracis*.

Confirmation in vitro is also made by simple biochemical and physiological reactions (Table 22.1). Demonstration of non-motility, gelatin liquefaction, growth in straight chains and enhanced growth aerobically, as seen in the characteristic *inverted fir tree* appearance in a gelatin stab, will generally identify *B. anthracis* completely. Toxin production can be demonstrated by immunological or gene probe methods in reference laboratories.

Environmental samples

It is occasionally necessary to isolate *B. anthracis* from potentially contaminated material such as animal hair, hides or soil. This task is particularly dificult because of the large number of non-pathogenic *Bacillus* spp. found in the environment.

TREATMENT

B. anthracis is susceptible in vitro to a wide range of antimicrobial agents and many have been used successfully in the treatment of anthrax in man. Penicillin remains the drug of choice as β-

precaution must not replace prompt and adequate sugical wound toilet.

CLOSTRIDIUM BOTULINUM

Description

C. botulinum is a strictly anaerobic Gram-positive bacillus (about $5 \times 1\ \mu m$). It is motile with peri-trichous flagella. Its spores are oval and subterminal. It is a widely distributed saprophyte occurring in soil, vegetables, fruits, leaves, silage, manure, the mud of lakes, and sea mud. Its optimum growth temperature is about $35^{\circ}C$, but some strains have been shown to grow and to produce toxin at temperatures as low as $1-5^{\circ}C$.

The widespread occurrence of *C. botulinum* in nature, its ability to produce a potent neurotoxin in food, and the resistance of its spores to inactivation combine to make it a formidable pathogen of man and a range of animals and birds. Spores of some strains withstand boiling in water ($100^{\circ}C$) for several hours. They are usually destroyed by moist heat at $120^{\circ}C$ within 5 min. Spores of type E strains (see below) are usually much less heat-resistant. Insufficient heating in the process of preserving foods is an important factor in the causation of botulism, and great care must be taken in canning factories to ensure that adequate heating is achieved in all parts of the can contents. The resistance of the spores to radiation is of special relevance to food processing.

Toxins of *C. botulinum*

Botulinal toxins are among the most poisonous natural substances known. Seven main types of *C. botulinum* designated A–G produce antigenically distinct toxins with pharmacologically identical actions. Types A, B and E are those most frequently associated with human disease, but all types can cause disease in man. The importance of this point is that, if antitoxin is given to a patient in an emergency, only the type-specific antitoxin will be effective. (The matter is complex and a reference text should be consulted for details of the cross-relationships of some of the toxins within the *C. botulinum* group and the shared antigens with *C. sporogenes* and *C. novyi*.)

Human botulism

Botulism is a severe, often fatal, form of food poisoning characterized by pronounced neuro-toxic effects. The disease has been caused by a wide range of foods, usually preserved hams, large sausages of the German variety, home-preserved meats and vegetables, canned products such as fish, liver paste, and even hazelnut purée. Traditional dishes such as fish or seal's flipper fermented in a barrel buried in the ground cannot be recommended by a bacteriologist. Type E strains are particularly but not invariably associated with a marine source, whereas type A and type B strains are usually associated with soil.

Foods responsible for botulism may not exhibit signs of spoilage. The preformed toxin in the food is absorbed from the intestinal tract. Although it is protein, it is not inactivated by the intestinal proteolytic enzymes. The toxin primarily affects the cholinergic system and seems to block release of acetylcholine, chiefly at points in the peripheral nervous system.

Clinical features

The period between ingestion of the toxin and the appearance of signs and symptoms is usually 1–2 days, but it may be much longer. There may be initial nausea and vomiting. The oculomotor muscles are affected and the patient may have diplopia and drooping eyelids with a squint. There may be vertigo and blurred vision.

There is progressive descending motor loss with flaccid paralysis but with no loss of consciousness or sensation, though weakness and sleepiness are often described. The patient is thirsty, with a dry mouth and tongue. There are difficulties in speech and swallowing, with later problems of breathing and despair. There may be abdominal pain and restlessness. Death is due to respiratory or cardiac failure.

Wound botulism

Rare cases of wound infection with *C. botulinum* resulting in the characteristic signs and symptoms of botulism have been recorded.

Infant botulism

The 'floppy child syndrome' describes a young child, usually less than 6 months old, with flaccid paralysis that is ascribed to the growth of *C. botulinum* in the intestine at a stage in development when the colonization resistance of the gut is poor. There are various grades of the syndrome. Some of the cases recorded in the literature have been attributed to the presence of *C. botulinum* spores in honey; when the honey was given as an encouragement to feed, the spores were ingested and were able to germinate and produce toxin in the infant gut.

Laboratory diagnosis

The organism or its toxin may be detected in the suspected food, and toxin may be demonstrated in the patient's blood by toxin–antitoxin neutralization tests in mice. Samples of faeces or vomit may also yield such evidence. Take care: bear in mind that botulinal toxin is very dangerous — specialist help should be summoned and the laboratory alerted.

Treatment

The priorities are: (1) to remove unabsorbed toxin from the stomach and intestinal tract; (2) to neutralize unfixed toxin by giving polyvalent antitoxin (with due precautions to avoid hypersensitivity reactions to the heterologous antiserum); and (3) to give relevant intensive care and support.

Control

Home canning of foodstuffs should be avoided, and commercial canning must be strictly controlled. The amateur preservation of meat and vegetables, especially beans, peas and root vegetables, is dangerous in inexperienced hands. Acid fruits may be bottled safely in the home with heating at 100°C, since a low pH is inhibitory to the growth of *C. botulinum*.

A prophylactic dose of polyvalent antitoxin should be given intramuscularly to all persons who have eaten food suspected of causing botulism. Active immunity in man can be produced by injecting three doses of mixed toxoid at 2-month intervals, but the very low incidence of the disease under normal conditions does not justify this as a routine. Active immunization should be considered for laboratory staff who might have to handle the organism or who might have to handle specimens containing the organism or its toxin.

CLOSTRIDIUM DIFFICILE

Description

C. difficile is a motile Gram-positive rod with oval spores. It occurs quite commonly in the faeces of neonates, but it is not generally regarded as a normal commensal of adults. The organism produces an enterotoxin (toxin A) and a cytotoxin (toxin B).

Pathogenesis

This organism has a direct relationship with pseudomembranous colitis. There is almost always, but not invariably, a history of prior antibiotic therapy. The lincosamide antibiotics have a special association, but ampicillin is also high in the league table of incriminated drugs and there is virtually no antibiotic that has escaped blame. Evidence often suggests that the organism may be acquired from an exogenous source by a patient whose intestinal colonization resistance has been compromised in some way. The condition is lethal if it is not quickly recognized and treated.

Laboratory diagnosis

C. difficile can be isolated from the faeces by enrichment and selective culture procedures. Toxin can be detected in the patient's faeces by testing extracts against cell monolayers of human embryo fibroblasts or other susceptible cells.

Treatment

It is essential to discontinue the antibiotic that is presumed to have precipitated the disease and to suppress the growth and toxin production of *C. difficile* by giving vancomycin or metronidazole.

Prevention

Clinical awareness is the keynote. If a patient develops unexplained diarrhoea, especially if this is antibiotic associated, the possibility of *C. difficile* and pseudomembranous colitis should be borne in mind. If several cases occur in a hospital unit, the possibility of cross-infection should be considered and the existing antibiotic policy of the unit should be reviewed.

RECOMMENDED READING

Collee J G, van Heyningen S 1991 Systemic toxigenic diseases (tetanus, botulism). In: Duerden B I, Drasar B S (eds) *Anaerobes in Human Disease*. Edward Arnold, London, pp. 372–394

Hobbs B C, Roberts D 1989 *Food Poisoning and Food Hygiene*, 5th edn. Edward Arnold, London

Smith J W G, Collee J G 1990 Tetanus. In: Parker M T, Collier L H (eds) *Topley and Wilson's Principles of Bacteriology, Virology and Immunity. Bacterial Diseases* (Smith G R, Easmon C S F, vol eds), 8th edn. Edward Arnold, London, vol 3, pp. 331–351.

Smith L DS 1977 *Botulism: The Organism, its Toxins, the Disease*. Charles C Thomas, Springfield, Illinois

Willis A T 1969 *Clostridia of Wound Infection*. Butterworths, London

Willis A T, Phillips K D 1983 *Anaerobic Infections. Public Health Laboratory Service Monograph Series 3, 2nd edn.* Her Majesty's Stationery Office, London

24

Neisseria and branhamella

Meningitis; gonorrhoea; respiratory infections

R. J. Fallon and R. C. B. Slack

Neisseriae are Gram-negative diplococci of which the pathogenic members, the meningococcus and the gonococcus, are characteristically found inside the polymorphonuclear pus cells of the inflammatory exudate. Although difficult to differentiate on morphological and cultural characters, these two pathogens are associated with entirely different diseases. *Neisseria meningitidis* is the cause of a range of diseases (Table 24.1), of which acute purulent meningitis (variously called *epidemic cerebrospinal meningitis, cerebrospinal fever* or, because of a purpuric rash which is sometimes present, *spotted fever*) and an acute septicaemic illness with a petechial rash but without meningitis are the commonest. About one-third of cases of meningo-

coccal disease present as septicaemia, most others being of meningitis. The term *meningococcal infection* embraces these and other syndromes associated with the organism.

N. gonorrhoeae is the cause of the sexually transmitted disease *gonorrhoea*. This commonly presents as a purulent infection of the mucous membrane of the urethra and also the cervix uteri in the female; there may be rectal or pharyngeal infection and secondary local and metastatic complications, e.g. epididymitis, salpingitis and arthritis, may occur if the primary infection is not promptly treated. In the newborn the gonococcus may give rise to a purulent conjunctivitis, *ophthalmia neonatorum,* and in young girls a vulvovaginitis. Dis-

Table 24.1 Clinical manifestations of meningococcal infection

Site of infection[a]	Common manifestation	Outcome
Blood	Fulminant septicaemia (Waterhouse–Friderichsen syndrome)	Fatal
Blood	Septicaemia, purpuric rash	Mortality 14–50%
Blood and CSF	Septicaemia, rash and meningitis	
Blood and CSF	Meningitis with no rash	Mortality 2–6%
Blood	Chronic meningococcal septicaemia (rash, arthralgia, metastatic sepsis)	Recover with treatment
Blood and site of sepsis	Arthritis, pericarditis, metastatic sepsis	Recover with treatment
Eye	Conjunctivitis	Recover with treatment
Genital tract	Asymptomatic carriage; rarely vulvovaginitis (children), urethritis, proctitis	Recover with treatment
Chest	Pneumonia	Recover with treatment

[a] In most cases of clinical disease the organism is also carried in the nasopharynx.

seminated gonococcal infection, which is recognized by a rash and evidence of blood spread, may also occur, more commonly in women.

The non-pathogenic or potentially pathogenic members of the genus are common commensals of the upper respiratory tract, which is also the reservoir of the meningococcus. The gonococcus may occasionally be isolated from this site. *N. lactamica* and *N. polysacchareae,* two species of uncertain taxonomic status, have been isolated frequently from the nasopharynx during meningococcal surveys. These organisms have a cultural resemblance to the meningococcus and will grow on selective media, unlike the classical nasopharyngeal commensals. Although similar to the meningococcus in culture, these two neisseriae are of low pathogenicity; *N. lactamica* is occasionally isolated from blood or cerebrospinal fluid (CSF). Nasopharyngeal commensal species include *N. subflava, N. flava* and *N. perflava.*

Branhamella catarrhalis (formerly *N. catarrhalis* and now sometimes called *Moraxella catarrhalis*) is another common commensal of the upper respiratory tract which may give rise to disease, usually as an opportunist pathogen.

DESCRIPTION

The two pathogenic neisseriae, *N. meningitidis* and *N. gonorrhoeae*, are so similar in their morphological and cultural characters that they may be described together. They are Gram-negative, oval cocci occurring in pairs with the apposed surfaces flat or even slightly concave (bean shaped) and with the axis of the pair parallel and not in line as in the pneumococcus. In pus from inflammatory exudates, such as CSF or urethral discharge, many diplococci are found in a small proportion of the polymorphonuclear cells. This is more marked with the gonococcus than with the meningococcus. Extracellular cocci also occur and there may be considerable variation in their size and intensity of staining. In cultures the diplococcal arrangement is less obvious and more coccoid forms may be seen in stained films. Faintly staining involution forms are frequent in older cultures.

Growth requirements

Pathogenic neisseriae are exacting in their growth requirements due, in part, to a susceptibility to inhibitory substances in the culture medium. The addition of heated blood or ascitic fluid, or both, to nutrient agar will ensure a good growth of colonies from infected material, provided incubation is carried out, preferably at 35–36°C, in a moist atmosphere containing 5–10% carbon dioxide. Growth is rather slow (more so with the gonococcus) but, on a good medium, grey, glistening, slightly convex colonies of 0.5–1.0 mm in diameter appear in 8–24 h. Incubation should, however, be continued for another 24 h, when the colonies will be seen to be much larger (2–3 mm) with the gonococcus in particular having a slightly roughened surface and a tendency to crenation of the margins. Gonococci have been divided into four types by Kellogg according to colonial appearance, auto-agglutinability and virulence, as demonstrated by the induction of urethritis in human volunteers. The more virulent strains (Kellogg types T1 and T2) bear numerous pili (fimbriae) and are now designated P^+/P^{++}. The avirulent forms (Kellogg types T3 and T4) are P^-. Both meningococci and gonococci may bear pili. The relationship between these and disease due to the meningococcus is uncertain but gonococcal pili appear to be associated with attachment of the organism to mucosal surfaces and resistance to killing by phagocytic cells.

Colonies of meningococci and gonococci react quickly in the test for cytochrome oxidase; colonies of non-pathogenic neisseriae react more slowly. Species identification depends on carbohydrate utilization reactions: the meningococcus produces acid from glucose and maltose, although strains may be encountered which ferment only one of these sugars; the reactions may be slow and sometimes occur only after several subcultures. The gonococcus produces acid from glucose only and neither species ferments lactose or sucrose. This can easily be remembered by G for gonococcus and M+G for meningococcus.

Most strains of *N. lactamica* can grow on ordinary serum-free culture medium and produce acid from glucose, maltose and, under optimum conditions, lactose but not sucrose or fructose. *N. lactamica* can be differentiated from the pathogenic neisseriae by its positive reaction in the o-nitrophenyl β-galactoside (ONPG) test for β-galactosidase.

Serological classification

Meningococci are divisible into three main serogroups: A, B and C. Group A is, in most countries, the serogroup associated with epidemic cerebrospinal meningitis. The ability to cause epidemics seems to be associated with certain genetically defined clones of the organism. Group C strains have been associated with epidemics but more commonly give rise to local outbreaks, while group B meningococci are seen in both epidemic and outbreak situations. Of other serogroups associated with disease (X, Y, Z, 29E (Z') and W-135), W-135 is isolated most frequently in the UK. A few cases due to serogroups X and Y also occur, but disease due to meningococci of serogroups Z and 29E, which are killed by normal human serum, is rare, and then only in patients with underlying disease. Capsulate meningococci of serogroups H, I, J, K and L have been described but do not appear to cause disease. The serogroup of a meningococcus is determined by its polysaccharide capsular antigen and the serogroup of a culture can be recognized by a slide agglutination test with absorbed group-specific antisera. Meningococci can be typed with antisera directed against outer-membrane proteins. This is useful in epidemiological studies but some serotypes are also found to be associated with more severe disease and, in the case of group B meningococci, with outbreaks. These are so-called *epidemic strains* of group B meningococci which appear to be of a single genotype. Gonococci are antigenically more heterogenous than meningococci so that serogrouping is not practicable.

There is no current serological classification of branhamellae.

MENINGOCOCCAL INFECTION
PATHOGENESIS

The natural habitat of the meningococcus is the human nasopharynx. Surveys of normal popula-tions show that around 5–10% are carriers of meningococci, over half of which are non-capsulate strains. In communities in which outbreaks of cerebrospinal meningitis are occurring, the carrier rate of the epidemic strain (capsulate, as are all pathogenic meningococci) may range from 20% to as high as 90% and some studies have shown that a sharp increase in the carrier rate of group A or other pathogenic groups of meningococci precedes the occurrence of clinical cases. However, this carrier:case ratio is variable in different outbreaks. Smokers appear to carry meningococci more often than non-smokers.

The route of spread of the meningococcus from the nasopharynx to the meninges is controversial: the organism may either spread directly through the cribriform plate to the subarachnoid space by the perineural sheaths of the olfactory nerve; or, much more probably, it passes through the naso-pharyngeal mucosa to enter the bloodstream. In favour of the latter route are the frequent positive blood cultures in the early stages of infection, the purpuric rash in many cases with the isolation of meningococci from the skin lesions, and the occurrence, particularly during epidemics, of meningococcal septicaemia with rash but no clinical meningitis. The problem of main concern in patho-genesis is the occurrence of cerebrospinal meningitis among only a limited proportion of the population at risk. Recent studies have confirmed some early observations that the absence of bactericidal antibody in the blood is the factor most closely related to susceptibility to clinical infection. Evidence in support of this relationship is:

1. The age distribution of meningococcal disease, which has its highest incidence in infants and young children from 3 months to 3 years of age (see Fig. 24.1), amongst whom humoral meningo-coccicidal antibodies are rarely found: the analogy with haemophilus meningitis is obvious.

2. The reciprocal relationship in the appearance of these bactericidal antibodies in older children and adults with the decreasing incidence of cerebrospinal meningitis, except when it occurs in outbreaks among adults brought together for special reasons, e.g. in service training centres and, in earlier days, in ships and gaols.

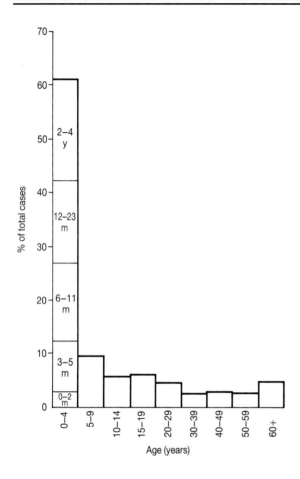

Fig. 24.1 Age distribution of meningococcal infection (Scotland, 1972–82).

3. Prospective studies among military recruits which showed that whereas only 1% of the total population at risk became clinically affected, 38.5% of those lacking specific bactericidal antibody to the meningococcus, and who became infected with the epidemic group C strain, developed meningococcal meningitis.

4. Patients convalescent from meningococcal infection develop typical immunoglobulin and bactericidal antibody to the infecting strains.

It is clear, nevertheless, from the relatively low incidence of meningococcal infections in young children and their absence in the large proportion of adults lacking specific antibody that in most persons the first infection of the nasopharynx with a meningococcus leads to antibody production

without development of clinical disease. It is possible that colonization with *N. lactamica*, which is common in children, may contribute to such antibody production. Group-specific antibody is protective and this is the basis of the success of vaccination against meningococcal disease. Antibodies to outer-membrane proteins may also protect but the range of actual antigens involved in this particular effect and the part non-specific defence mechanisms play in preventing clinical disease is ill-understood. However, the complement system is important as shown by the recurrent attacks of meningococcal infections in complement-deficient subjects.

Apart from serious clinical disease, meningococci are found in purulent conjunctivitis and occasionally in monarticular purulent arthritis without any preceding evidence of septicaemic infection; rarely, a chronic septicaemic form of disease may occur with both joint and skin involvement. Pneumonia, pericarditis and endocarditis are also unusual clinical manifestations.

LABORATORY DIAGNOSIS

In any suspected meningococcal infection, blood culture must be undertaken. If meningitis is suspected, a lumbar puncture must be performed as soon as possible unless signs of raised intracranial pressure render this a dangerous procedure. Lumbar puncture yields more positive cultures than blood culture from patients with meningococcal meningitis.

In meningococcal meningitis, CSF is under pressure and is turbid due to the large number of polymorphonuclear leucocytes present in a typical case. In the very first stages of infection, lumbar puncture may yield unremarkable results due to the fact that the meningeal reaction has not had time to take place, but typically the CSF will contain large numbers of Gram-negative diplococci which can be recognized by microscopical examination of the stained deposit. At a later stage they may be scanty and even apparently absent in films stained by Gram's method. Very scanty organisms may be seen more easily in a film stained with methylene blue. In the early untreated case, Gram-negative diplococci are seen

time and place that regular testing is essential. The use of sulphonamides in the Second World War led to the rapid development of resistance, but the arrival of penicillin at that time solved the problem. Penicillin, especially in slow-release intramuscular forms, such as procaine penicillin, has remained the preferred therapy. Small decreases in susceptibility occurred in the 1950s and 1960s and were overcome by increasing the size of the single dose. The correlation between increasing minimum inhibitory concentration of penicillin for *N. gonorrhoeae* and failure of a single dose of 300 000 units of penicillin to treat acute gonorrhoea in men is shown in Fig. 24.4. This is taken from the pioneering work at the Whitechapel Clinic at the London Hospital by Curtis and Wilkinson and is the clearest example of the relationship between antibiotic susceptibility tests in vitro and the success of a drug in field conditions.

By the 1970s the dose of penicillin required to cure simple acute gonorrhoea in men in some parts of the world had reached an impossibly large injection. In 1976, penicillinase-producing *N. gonorrhoeae* were first found. These strains may carry different plasmids and have arisen in different parts of the world, but all possess the gene coding for the TEM-type β-lactamase commonly found in *Escherichia coli*.

Single-dose therapy appears adequate for the majority of cases of acute genital gonorrhoea in men and women. There are obvious advantages to this approach in obtaining complete compliance and stopping the chain of infection. In disseminated

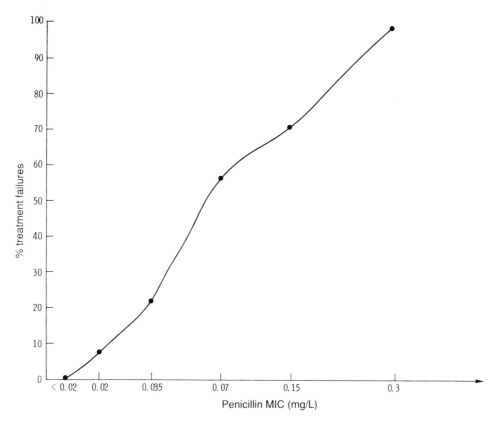

Fig. 24.4 Correlation between minimum inhibitory concentration (MIC) of penicillin for *N. gonorrhoeae* and failure of treatment with a single dose of 300 000 units of penicillin in the treatment of acute gonorrhoea in men. (Data from Curtis F R, Wilkinson A E 1958 *British Journal of Venereal Diseases* 34: 70–82.)

gonococcal disease and any complicated infection treatment for 7–10 d is necessary.

If penicillin is contra-indicated because of allergy or bacterial resistance there are many alternatives; fluoroquinolones have many advocates. Tetracyclines are effective in most places and also treat concomitant chlamydial infection if given in a sufficiently long course of treatment. Tetracycline resistance in gonococci is increasing in some countries. Newer cephalosporins, in particular ceftriaxone, are extremely active, but have to be given by injection and are expensive. Infection with β-lactamase-producing gonococci in a patient not hypersensitive to penicillins responds to co-amoxiclav; this can be given with a large dose of procaine penicillin to overcome intrinsic penicillin resistance which is not reversed by the β-lactamase inhibitor clavulanic acid.

EPIDEMIOLOGY AND CONTROL

There should be little difficulty in the diagnosis and treatment of a typical case of acute gonorrhoea. By extension, one would expect the disease to be limited in distribution and well controlled. This was the case in much of the world until the 1960s. Venereal diseases were seen in small selected populations such as sailors and prostitutes. With the advent of penicillin the number of new cases in countries which had reliable statistics fell rapidly and many felt that venereal disease would be eradicated. The remarkable changes since the 1960s of travel, migration, sexual licence and wide availability of oral contraceptives rapidly reversed this process so that there was an increase in gonorrhoea and non-specific genital infection (mainly caused by chlamydiae) for every year until scares about acquired immune deficiency syndrome (AIDS) in the 1980s. Barrier methods, the condom in particular, greatly reduce the rate of transmission.

BRANHAMELLA CATARRHALIS MORAXELLA CATARRHALIS

PATHOGENESIS

B. catarrhalis is a respiratory tract commensal and it would appear that, as with other members of the upper respiratory tract flora such as the pneumococcus and *H. influenzae,* this organism can gain access to the lower respiratory tract in situations where the host defences are compromised (e.g. in patients with chronic chest disease). *B. catarrhalis* is commonly isolated from sputum, and a pathogenic role is suspected only if the sputum contains large numbers of pus cells and Gram-negative diplococci, and if culture yields a heavy growth of *B. catarrhalis* in the absence of other recognized respiratory pathogens. However, it is much more satisfactory to obtain the organism in pure culture without contamination by upper respiratory secretions so that the true significance of the bacteriological observations may be assessed. This is best done by transtracheal aspiration which, however, is an uncomfortable procedure.

As well as causing chest infection itself, *B. catarrhalis* may also protect other respiratory pathogens from the action of penicillin or ampicillin by producing β-lactamase; such infection only resolves when treated with an antibiotic resistant to β-lactamase.

B. catarrhalis may be associated with conjunctivitis and may be isolated on occasion from blood culture in patients with respiratory tract infection or who are immunocompromised.

LABORATORY DIAGNOSIS

Sputum is examined by Gram film. In true infections large numbers of Gram-negative diplococci may be seen dispersed between the pus cells. Sputum is cultured on media suitable for the isolation of other potential respiratory pathogens (e.g. blood agar and chocolate agar) and incubated in 5% carbon dioxide overnight. In situations in which it is held to be pathogenic, *B. catarrhalis* is predominant in culture.

B. catarrhalis produces rough, circular, convex colonies which can be lifted off intact with a wire loop from agar culture medium. Colonies react positively in the oxidase test. Cultures are examined for their ability to utilize sugars and to produce β-lactamase, which is characteristic of up to 50% of strains. Growth on nutrient agar at

22°C has been suggested as a differential characteristic, but clinically significant isolates of *B. catarrhalis* may not grow in these conditions. Specific tests for deoxyribonuclease (DNase) and for butyrate esterase are positive.

TREATMENT

B. catarrhalis is sensitive to amoxycillin combined with clavulanic acid (co-amoxiclav) and also to cephalosporins, tetracycline and erythromycin.

RECOMMENDED READING

Achtman M 1990 Molecular epidemiology of epidemic bacterial meningitis. *Reviews in Medical Microbiology* 1: 29–38

Broome C V 1986 The carrier state: *Neisseria meningitidis. Journal of Antimicrobial Chemotherapy* 18 (suppl A): 25–34

Cartwright K A V, Jones D M 1989 ACP Broadsheet 121. Investigation of meningococcal disease. *Journal of Clinical Pathology* 42: 634–639

Easmon C S F, Ison C A 1987 *Neisseria gonorrhoeae*: a versatile pathogen. *Journal of Clinical Pathology* 40: 1088–1097

Leading article 1982 *Branhamella catarrhalis*: pathogen or opportunist? *Lancet* i: 1056

McLeod D T, Ahmad F, Power J T, Calder M A, Seaton A 1983 Bronchopulmonary infection due to *Branhamella catarrhalis. British Medical Journal* 287: 1446–1447

Oates J K, Csonka G W 1990 Gonorrhoea. In: Oates J K, Csonka GW (eds) *Sexually Transmitted Diseases.* Baillière Tindall, London, pp. 209–226

25

Salmonella   Food poisoning; enteric fever

M. J. Lewis

Salmonellae are a major cause of food-borne infection world-wide. In the UK and in the USA, reports of salmonella infections have increased steadily since the early 1960s, and this increase has recently accelerated. In the statistics for England and Wales kept by the Public Health Laboratory Service, annual salmonella isolations from humans doubled from 10 251 to 20 532 between 1981 and 1987, and in 1988 exceeded 27 000 isolates (Fig. 25.1). In the USA the figures are double these, and in both countries many, perhaps most, infections go unrecognized. The true incidence of salmonellosis is a matter for guesswork.

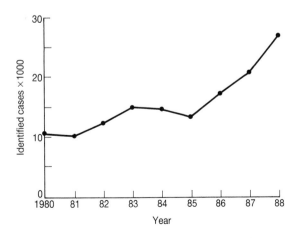

Fig. 25.1 The number of cases of salmonellosis identified in England and Wales during 1980-1988.

DESCRIPTION

Salmonellae are typical members of the Enterobacteriaceae, facultatively anaerobic Gram-negative bacilli able to grow on a wide range of relatively simple media and distinguished from other members of the family by their biochemical characteristics and antigenic structure. Their normal habitat is the animal intestine.

Antigens

Antigenic structure is important, but in day-to-day practice the demonstration of a small number of biochemical characters (Table 25.1) together with the demonstration of some salmonella antigens is sufficient to decide that the organism is a *Salmonella* species. To give the salmonella a name demands a more complete antigenic analysis.

The typical salmonella possesses two sets of antigens which are readily demonstrable by serological reactions in the laboratory. Heat-stable polysaccharides which form part of the cell wall lipopolysaccharide are known as *somatic* or *O antigens*. *Flagellar* or *H antigens* are formed from the structural proteins which make up the flagella that endow the organism with motility. In most salmonellae the flagella exhibit the property of diphasic variation. That is, the flagellar antigens exist in two alternative forms defined by two different sets of genes in the bacterial genome. When one of these sets is expressed the flagella consists of one or more *phase 1* antigens, while when the

Table 25.1 Biochemical tests that help to differentiate salmonellae from common enterobacteria

Organism	Motility	Gas from glucose	Acid from lactose	Urease activity	Citrate utilization	H$_2$S production	Indole production
Salmonella typhi	+	−	−	−	−	+	−
Salmonella spp.	+	+	−	−	+	+	−
Shigella spp.	−	−	−	−	−	−	V
Escherichia coli	+	+	+	−	−	−	+
Citrobacter spp.	+	+	+	−	+	V	V
Klebsiella spp.	−	+	+	+	+	−	V
Proteus spp.	+	V	−	+	V	V	V

V, variable reaction.

other set is operative two or more *phase 2* antigens are synthesized. Some salmonellae also produce a surface polysaccharide, of which the Vi antigen of *Salmonella typhi* is the most important example, which can occasionally make detection of the O antigens difficult. The O antigens have been numbered with Arabic numerals. The flagellar antigens of phase 1 have been labelled with lower-case letters, and of phase 2 with a mixture of lower-case letters and Arabic numerals.

The antigenic structure of any salmonella is expressed as an antigenic formula which has three parts, describing the O antigens, the phase 1 H antigens and the phase 2 H antigens in that order. The three parts are separated by colons and the component antigens in each part by commas. More than 2000 serotypes have so far been described in this way and almost all have been given names. Some of the commoner serotypes are shown in Table 25.2. The Kauffmann–White scheme, which elegantly catalogues this system of description, places the salmonellae into some 30 groups on the basis of shared O antigens, and further subdivides the groups into clusters with H antigens in common. Some salmonellae, such as *S. typhi* (9.12, [Vi]: d: –), express only one flagellar phase. Fortunately, only a small number of salmonellae in the Kauffmann–White scheme regularly cause illness in man.

HOST RANGE AND PATHOGENICITY

Salmonellae are widely distributed in nature. All vertebrates appear capable of harbouring salmonellae in their gut, and salmonellae have also been isolated from a wide range of arthropods such as flies, cockroaches, fleas and ticks. Most animal infections seem to be symptomless, or to cause a self-limiting gastro-enteritis of variable severity. Many serotypes such as *S. typhimurium* show a wide host range, and can be isolated from many different animal species. A small number of strains, the *host-adapted* serotypes, are much more restricted in the species they inhabit, and show a different spectrum of illness.

Table 25.2 The antigenic structure of some representative salmonellae

S. typhi	9, 12, [Vi]	:	d	:	–
S. paratyphi B	1, 4, 5, 12	:	b	:	1, 2
S. typhimurium	1, 4, 5, 12	:	i	:	1, 2
S. enteritidis	1, 9, 12	:	g, m	:	1, 7
S. virchow	6, 7	:	r	:	1, 2
S. kedougou	1, 13, 23	:	i	:	l, w
S. hadar	6, 8	:	z$_{10}$	:	e, n, x
S. heidelberg	1, 4, 5, 12	:	r	:	1, 2
S. infantis	6, 7, 14	:	r	:	1, 5
S. newport	6, 8, 20	:	e, h	:	1, 2
S. panama	1, 9, 12	:	l, v	:	1, 5
S. dublin	1, 9, 12	:	g, p	:	–

Host-adapted serotypes

Among the host-adapted serotypes, *S. typhi* and *S. paratyphi* A, B and C are primarily human pathogens which are rarely, if ever, isolated from animals other than man. *S. paratyphi B*, while essentially a human pathogen, is occasionally isolated from cattle, pigs, poultry and other animals, although cycles of transmission in these hosts have not been demonstrated.

Human infection with these organisms is characterized by a long incubation period of 10–14 d, followed by a septicaemic illness, *enteric fever*, quite unlike the diarrhoea and vomiting that are characteristic of food poisoning.

Other salmonellae adapted to particular animal hosts include *S. cholerae-suis* (pigs), *S. dublin* (cattle), *S. gallinarum-pullorum* (poultry), *S. abortus-equi* (horses) and *S. abortus-ovis* (sheep). These are all responsible for considerable morbidity, mortality and economic loss among domestic animals. Although all are capable of causing illness in man, only *S. cholerae-suis* and *S. dublin* do so with any regularity.

The rest of the 2000 or so serotypes of salmonellae show no apparent host preference. All can potentially cause human infection, but the extent to which any do so is determined by the accident of their prevalence in domestic food animals at any particular time and on the opportunity for the contamination of food in which further multiplication can take place. In developed countries most human infections are caused by a relatively small number of locally prevalent serotypes.

PATHOGENESIS

Salmonella infection is initiated by ingestion of a sufficient number of organisms to overcome the body's defences, in particular gastric acidity, and to colonize the small intestine. The organisms need to be swallowed. Experiments in which volunteers gargled with suspensions of different serotypes without swallowing regularly failed to cause infection.

Infective Dose

The number of salmonellae which must be swallowed in order to set up an infection is still a matter for debate. Whether infection follows exposure to a pathogenic organism is in part a matter of probability. The usual outcome of contact between a pathogenic microbe and a susceptible individual is elimination of the microbe with no discernable effect on the host. Nevertheless, contact with a single organism has a probability, usually very small, that infection will ensue. The more organisms, the greater the likelihood of infection.

The widely accepted dictum that large inocula of salmonellae are required for induction of illness in humans is based largely on volunteer studies. In most of these the median infective dose for most serotypes, including *S. typhi*, has varied from 10^6 to 10^9 organisms. However, investigation of outbreaks suggests that in the naturally occurring situation the infective dose is regularly below 10^3 organisms and sometimes less than a 100 bacteria.

Many factors influence the infective dose. There appears to be considerable strain-to-strain variation in virulence even within a single serotype. Systematic variation in pathogenicity between serotypes is less easy to demonstrate outside the host-adapted strains. The vehicle of ingestion also matters. Organisms in water and other drinks may be carried through the stomach relatively rapidly, and thus escape the effect of the gastric acid. Similarly, the administration of antacids, or the effects of gastric resection, reduce the infective dose. Salmonellosis caused by contaminated endoscopes introduced through the stomach into the small intestine is another example of this effect.

Host Factors

Host factors are also likely to be important, although these again may be difficult to separate from confounding variables. For example, the reported age-specific isolation rates for salmonellae, as for some other gut pathogens, is higher for children less than a year of age than for any other age group, but this reflects the fact that a higher proportion of infections are investigated in this age group. This is often misinterpreted as revealing a greater susceptibility.

Initiation of infection

Once the bacteria enter the lumen of the intestine they are able to multiply. Some of the bacteria attach to the microvilli of the ileal mucosa by means of adhesins on the bacterial surface, which adhere specifically to mannose-containing receptors on the epithelium. Attachment is followed by degeneration of the microvilli to form breaches in the cell membrane through which the salmonellae enter the cell. Further multiplication in these cells and in macrophages of the Peyer's patches follows. Some bacteria penetrate into the submucosa and pass to the local mesenteric lymph nodes. All the clinical manifestations of salmonella infection, including diarrhoea, begin after ileal penetration.

CLINICAL SYNDROMES

Although salmonellae can cause a wide spectrum of clinical illness there are four major syndromes, each with its own diagnostic and therapeutic problems, which are best considered separately. These are enteric fever, gastro-enteritis, bacteraemia with or without metastatic infection, and the asymptomatic carrier state.

Enteric fever

Enteric fever is most usually caused by *S. typhi* or *S. paratyphi* A, B or C, but can be caused by any salmonella serotype. The clinical features tend to be more severe with *S. typhi* (typhoid fever). After penetration of the ileal mucosa the organisms pass via the lymphatics to the mesenteric lymph nodes, whence after a period of multiplication they invade the bloodstream via the thoracic duct. The liver, gallbladder, spleen, kidney and bone marrow become infected during this primary bacteraemic phase in the first 7–10 d of the incubation period. After multiplication in these organs, bacilli pass into the blood, causing a second and heavier bacteraemia, the onset of which approximately coincides with that of the fever and other signs of clinical illness. From the gallbladder a further invasion of the intestine results. Peyer's patches and other gut lymphoid tissues become involved in an inflammatory reaction and infiltration with mononuclear cells, followed by necrosis, sloughing and the formation of characteristic typhoid ulcers occurs.

Onset

The interval between ingestion of the organisms and the onset of illness varies with the size of the infecting dose. It can be as short as 3 d or as long as 50 d, but is usually about 2 weeks. The onset is usually insidious. Early symptoms are often vague: a dry cough and epistaxis associated with anorexia, a dull continuous headache, abdominal tenderness and discomfort are among the most common symptoms. Diarrhoea is not commonly a feature of enteric fever and early in the illness many patients will complain of constipation.

Progression

In the untreated case the temperature shows a step-ladder rise over the 1st week of the illness, remains high for 7–10 d and then falls by lysis during the 3rd or 4th week. Physical signs include a relative bradycardia for the height of the fever, hepatomegaly, splenomegaly and often a rash of *rose spots*. These are 2-4 mm in diameter, slightly raised discrete irregular blanching pink macules most often found on the front of the chest. They appear in crops of up to a dozen at a time and fade after 3 or 4 d, leaving no scar. They are characteristic of, but not specific for, enteric fever.

Relapse

Apparent recovery can be followed by relapse in 5–10% of untreated cases. Relapse is usually shorter and of milder character than the initial illness, but can be severe and may end fatally. Severe intestinal haemorrhage and intestinal perforation are serious complications which can occur at any stage of the illness.

Morbidity and mortality

Classic typhoid fever is a serious and life-threatening infection which, when untreated, has a

26

Shigella   Bacillary dysentery

M. J. Lewis

Dysentery, the bloody flux of biblical times, is a clinical entity characterized by the frequent passage of blood-stained mucopurulent stools. Aetiologically it is divisible into two main categories, amoebic and bacillary. Both forms are endemic in most warm-climate countries. Bacillary dysentery, caused by members of the genus *Shigella*, is also prevalent in many countries with temperate climates.

DESCRIPTION

Shigellae are typical members of the Enterobacteriaceae and are closely related to the genus *Escherichia*. Microscopically, in stained preparations, shigellae are Gram-negative bacilli indistinguishable from other enterobacteria. They are non-motile and non-capsulate. Culturally they are similar to most other enterobacteria except that on MacConkey or desoxycholate-citrate agar (DCA) medium they are non-lactose-fermenting after incubation for 18–24 h. Thus, on such differential media colonies are pale and similar to those of the other common pathogenic genus, *Salmonella*. The main biochemical reactions which differentiate shigellae from the other members of the Enterobacteriaceae are summarized in Table 26.1.

The genus *Shigella* is subdivided on biochemical and serological grounds into four species: *Shigella dysenteriae*, *Sh. flexneri*, *Sh. boydii* and *Sh. sonnei*. One of these, *Sh. dysenteriae*, is unique in being

Table 26.1 Some biochemical reactions of the shigellae and commoner enterobacteria

Organism	Motility	Gas from glucose	Acid from lactose	Urease activity	Citrate utilization	H$_2$S production	Indole production	ONPG test	Acid from mannitol
Shigella dysenteriae 1	–	–	–	–	–	–	–	+	–
Sh. dysenteriae 2–10	–	–	–	–	–	–	V	V	–
Sh. flexneri 1–5	–	–	–	–	–	–	V	–	+
Sh. flexneri 6	–	V	–	–	–	–	–	–	+
Sh. boydii	–	–	–	–	–	–	V	–	+
Sh. sonnei	–	–	(+)	–	–	–	–	+	+
Salmonella typhi	+	–	–	–	–	+	–	–	+
Salmonella (other spp.)	+	+	–	–	+	+	–	–	+
Escherichia coli	+	+	+	–	–	–	+	+	+
Citrobacter spp.	+	+	+	–	+	V	V	+	+
Klebsiella spp.	–	+	+	+	+	–	V	+	+
Proteus spp.	+	V	–	+	V	V	V	–	–

V, variable; (+), positive only after prolonged incubation, ⩾ 48 h.
ONPG, o- nitrophenyl β -galactoside.

unable to ferment mannitol. Another, *Sh. sonnei*, is a late lactose fermenter, and colonies growing on MacConkey or DCA medium for more than 24 h acquire a pink coloration. The antigenic structure of the shigellae is complex. *Sh. dysenteriae* can be subdivided into 10 and *S. boydii* into 15 specific serotypes. A combination of group- and type-specific antigens allows subdivision of *Sh. flexneri* into six serotypes, each of which can be further subdivided. *Sh. sonnei* strains are serologically homogeneous, and a variety of other markers such as the ability to produce specific colicines or the carriage of drug-resistance or other plasmids are used to discriminate between strains for epidemiological purposes.

PATHOGENESIS

Shigellae are pathogens of man and other primates. There are anecdotal reports of infection in dogs, but other animals are immune. Infection occurs by ingestion. The infecting dose is small, between 10 and 100 organisms, and the bacteria seem relatively unaffected by gastric acid or bile.

After reaching the large intestine the shigellae multiply in the gut lumen. Many bacteria adhere to the epithelial cells of the gut mucosa and induce these cells to ingest them. The shigellae multiply within the epithelial cells and spread laterally into adjacent cells and deep into the lamina propria. The infected epithelial cells are killed and the lamina propria and submucosa develop an inflammatory reaction with capillary thrombosis. Patches of necrotic epithelium are sloughed and ulcers form. The cellular response is mainly by polymorphonuclear leucocytes, which can be seen readily on microscopical examination of the stool, together with red cells and sloughed epithelium. Dysentery bacilli rarely invade other tissues. Transient bacteraemia can occur but septicaemia with metastatic infection is rare.

Although the main determinant of pathogenicity in shigella infection is invasion of the wall of the large bowel, with its consequent inflammatory reaction, many strains have been shown to produce an exotoxin able to cause secretion of water and electrolytes by cells of the small bowel by a mechanism similar to that of cholera and *Escherichia coli* toxins. This toxin may be responsible for the brief episode of watery diarrhoea which often precedes the onset of the severe bloody flux of classical dysentery.

CLINICAL FEATURES

The incubation period is usually between 2 and 3 d, but may be as short as 12 h. The onset of symptoms is usually sudden and frequently the initial symptom is abdominal colic. This is followed by the onset of watery diarrhoea, and in all but the mildest cases this is accompanied by fever and malaise. Many episodes resolve at this point, but others progress to abdominal cramps, tenesmus and the frequent passage of small volumes of stool, predominantly consisting of bloody mucus. In a typical case of dysentery the symptoms last about 4 d but, exceptionally, may continue for 10 d or more.

The severity of the clinical illness is to some extent associated with the particular species involved. Infection with *Sh. dysenteriae* is usually associated with a severe illness in which prostration is marked and in young children may be accompanied by febrile convulsions. The special virulence of *Sh. dysenteriae* has been ascribed to its ability to produce a potent exotoxin; this was formerly described as a neurotoxin because of the neurological effects resulting from vascular endothelial damage produced by the toxin when injected intravenously in experimental animals. However, this toxin, which also has a fluid transuding effect on the intestinal mucosa, is elaborated by many other strains of shigellae and its role in the pathogenesis of dysentery is uncertain.

Sh. dysenteriae type I has also been responsible for many cases of the haemolytic uraemic syndrome accompanying outbreaks of dysentery in several countries. The condition, with its triad of haemolytic anaemia, thrombocytopenia and acute renal failure, can be caused by many pathogens (in particular, *Esch. coli* O157). It is associated with complement activation and disseminated intravascular coagulation and in some parts of the world is one of the commonest forms of acute renal failure in children.

The illness caused by members of the *Sh. flexneri* and *Sh. boydii* groups may be as prostrating as that caused by *Sh. dysenteriae*. At the other end of the clinical spectrum of bacillary dysentery, the illness associated with *Sh. sonnei* in an otherwise healthy person may be confined to the passage of a few loose stools with vague abdominal discomfort and the patient often continues at school or work. Death from bacillary dysentery is uncommon; it occurs mostly at the extremes of life or in individuals who are suffering from some other disease or debilitating condition.

LABORATORY DIAGNOSIS

A specimen of faeces is always preferable to a rectal swab. Rectal swabs do not allow adequate macroscopic and microscopic examination of the stool and unless properly taken and bearing obvious faecal material may be no more than a swab of peri-anal skin. Moreover, because of drying of the swab, pathogenic species die off quite rapidly, and may not survive transport to the laboratory.

Fresh unstained suspensions of faeces should be examined microscopically for the presence of protozoa that may be responsible for the diarrhoea (see Chapter 61) and also to note the character of the cellular exudate.

The faeces are inoculated on DCA or MacConkey agar. Mucus, if present in the specimen, may be used as the inoculum. Suitable cultures should also be set up to detect other possible bacterial pathogens such as *Salmonella* (Chapter 25) or *Campylobacter* (Chapter 30) species.

After incubation at 37°C for 18–24 h pale non-lactose-fermenting colonies from DCA or MacConkey agar are tested for urease production (negative for shigellae), motility (negative) and for the ability to utilize certain sugar substrates. Colonies that give the characteristic reactions must have their identity confirmed by serological investigation with species-specific sera and then with type-specific sera unless the strain is *Sh. sonnei*. It is rarely necessary to take strain identification any further except when investigating major outbreaks in endemic areas. With *Sh.*

sonnei, plasmid pattern analysis and colicine typing may help elucidate patterns of spread.

Tests for specific antibodies in the patient's serum are of little value since in an endemic area the patient's serum rarely shows any increased level of specific antibody compared with sera from healthy people.

TREATMENT

Most cases of shigella dysentery, especially those due to *Sh. sonnei*, are mild and do not require antibiotic therapy. Symptomatic treatment with the maintenance of hydration by use of oral rehydration salt solution (see Chapter 31, Table 31.2) is all that is required. As with salmonella infections, drugs which impair gut motility should be avoided. Treatment with a suitable antibiotic is necessary in the very young, the aged or the debilitated, and in severe infections. Ampicillin, co-trimoxazole, tetracycline or ciprofloxacin are appropriate choices, provided they are shown to be active in vitro; each may be administered orally. There is no evidence that antibiotics reduce the period of excretion of the organisms, and they should not be used in the asymptomatic person either prophylactically or in attempts to hasten clearance after recovery.

EPIDEMIOLOGY

Over the past half century there has been a steady and remarkable change in the relative frequency of the different shigella species in the UK and other European countries. Infections due to *Sh. dysenteriae*, common before the First World War, are now rare. Between 1920 and 1930 both *Sh. flexneri* and *Sh. sonnei* were endemic and approximately equal in incidence, but by 1940 *Sh. sonnei* had become dominant, increasing in incidence annually to a peak of over 49 000 notifications (99% of all shigellae notified) in 1956. The incidence of Sonne dysentery has declined steadily since then (Fig. 26.1) to its present annual average of about 3000 notified cases, but shows little sign of falling further. Infections due to the other shigellae, usually imported, have also remained fairly constant at about 800–900 a year for the past decade.

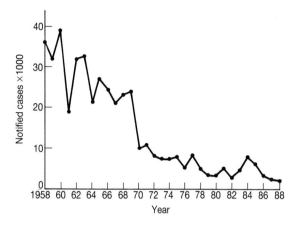

Fig. 26.1 The number of cases of Sonne dysentery notified annually in England and Wales during 1958–88.

Similar changes have taken place in the USA although more slowly. Up to 1968 *Sh. flexneri* and *Sh. sonnei* were equally common, but *Sh. sonnei* now accounts for 65% of cases and *Sh. flexneri* for about 30%. Over the past several decades the other two shigella species have been responsible for less than 5% of notifications, but there has been a recent increase in cases imported from Asia and South America.

Sources and spread

Bacillary dysentery is usually spread faecal–orally by fingers. The case or carrier, after contaminating his or her hands while cleansing at toilet touches and thus contaminates the lavatory flush handle, door knobs, washbasin taps, hand towels and other objects which, when handled by another individual, allow transfer of dysentery bacilli to the recipient's hands and thence to the mouth. Such spread is facilitated by separating the wash-basin from the lavatory compartment so that the handle of the intervening door acts as an efficient vehicle of infection. The carrier may also handle and thus infect food that is eaten, or eating utensils that are used by another person, who is thereby infected. Dysentery bacilli are also liberated into the air in an aerosol when an infected loose stool is flushed from the toilet and after settling on the surfaces of toilet seats, furniture and surroundings may survive for some days in a moist atmosphere.

An important feature of the epidemiology of bacillary dysentery in the UK and other countries with good environmental sanitation is that the main patient group involved is school age children and particularly primary school children. Here, unwitting neglect of toilet hygiene by children at school undoubtedly plays a part. The disease is often endemic among adults living in residential institutions where for one reason or another high standards of hygiene are difficult to maintain, and has in the past been a scourge in gaols and in armies in the field. The seasonal distribution of bacillary dysentery in the UK is bimodal, with the highest incidence in spring and a second peak in October and November. Incidence is at its lowest in summer, when schoolchildren are on holiday. Since this is the period when flying insects are most abundant, this suggests that in this country insects play little if any part in trans-mission. However, in communities without satis-factory methods of sewage disposal insects can gain access to infected human excreta and transfer shigellae mechanically to foodstuffs. Foods may also be contaminated directly by human cases or carriers.

Occasional epidemics of bacillary dysentery have been traced to water supplies when chlori-nation of the supply has not been instituted or has been defective. Such water-borne epidemics are usually spectacular in the large number of people simultaneously infected and in the speed with which they can be terminated when the water supply is adequately treated. Epidemic infection may also follow the contamination of milk or ice-cream.

Control

The mild and often fleeting nature of the clinical illness associated with *Sh. sonnei* infection means that frequently the case of bacillary dysentery remains ambulant and follows his or her daily labour and leisure pursuits, remaining in circulation as a disperser of the causal organism. The pressure on toilet facilities, particularly in schools, allows hand-to-mouth spread of the bacilli. The provision of washbasins in the same compartment as the toilet pedestal would allow some reduction in spread, especially if flushing mechanisms and washbasin taps could be operated by foot instead of by hand. However, hand washing, although very important, cannot be guaranteed to remove all the dysentery bacilli from the hands. During diarrhoea, faecal soiling of the fingers can be heavy, and hand washing will at best only reduce the numbers of bacteria present. The normal disinfecting effect of the skin fatty acids and competing skin organisms may take up to half an hour to destroy the rest. For this reason it is important that people with symptoms such that they need to go to stool during a normal working shift should stay off work and as far as possible out of circulation until the symptoms have subsided, especially when their work involves preparation of food or direct contact with other people. Asymptomatic carriers are far less important in the spread of this disease, and seldom if ever need to be excluded from any employment.

Control of an outbreak

Outbreaks of dysentery in schools and other institutions are notoriously difficult to control. In nursery school outbreaks infection is usually widespread before the first cases are notified, with considerable environmental contamination. Some children will be incubating the infection; others will have recovered from the diarrhoea but still be excreting the organisms. In this situation the acute case is far more important in the spread of infection than the symptomless excreter. There is

little to be gained by trying to ascertain bacteriologically who is infected and who is not, once the cause of the outbreak has been established, since there is little reason to exclude an asymptomatic carrier and it is pointless to seek confirmation of a clearly symptomatic case. The practical course is usually to exclude acute cases but to allow children without symptoms to remain at or return to school.

Having determined the exclusion policy it is important to try to stop hand-to-hand spread among those who remain at school. Supervision of children using the lavatory, supervised hand washing before meals, frequent disinfection of water closets, including seats, lavatory chain and door handles, and the general use of paper towels all play a part. No single measure alone will be sufficient. Staff need support as morale can flag, and they themselves are vulnerable to infection. Outbreaks can persist for weeks despite all measures, and then subside abruptly for little apparent reason.

Similar principles can be applied to other outbreak situations, e.g. in residential institutions or a hospital ward. The most important single factor in all these situations is the need for adequate communication. Teachers, nurses, parents and all who are involved in trying to control the outbreak need to have explained to them exactly how the infection spreads, and the reasons for the measures taken or not taken. Finally, the temptation to use antibiotics prophylactically in an attempt to limit the spread must be resisted.

RECOMMENDED READING

Bennish M L, Harris J R, Wojtyniak B J, Struelens M 1990 Death in shigellosis: incidence and risk factors in hospitalized patients. *Journal of Infectious Diseases* 161: 500–506

Christie A B 1987 *Infectious Diseases: Epidemiology and Clinical Practice*, 4th edn. Churchill Livingstone, Edinburgh, ch 6

Keusch G T 1979 Shigella infections. In Lambert H P (ed) *Clinics in Gastro-enterology, Infections of the GI Tract*, W B Saunders, London, vol 8 (3), pp 645–662

Maurelli A T, Sansonetti P J 1988 Genetic determinants of shigella pathogenicity. *Annual Review of Microbiology* 42: 127–150

27

Escherichia

Urinary tract infection; travellers' diarrhoea; haemorrhagic colitis; haemolytic uraemic syndrome

R. J. Gross

Strains of *Escherichia coli* and related Gram-negative 'coliform' bacteria predominate among the aerobic commensal flora present in the gut of man and animals. Individuals have a rich flora in the lower ileum and, more especially, in the colon, which includes *Esch. coli*. It is acquired by ingestion of the organisms during the first few days after birth. The species *Esch. coli* encompasses a great variety of strains that include purely commensal organisms as well as those possessing combinations of virulence determinants that enable them to act as specific pathogens of the gut and of extra-intestinal sites, especially the urinary tract.

DESCRIPTION

Esch. coli is the type species of the genus but several other species have been described. Strains of *Esch. coli* are usually motile and some strains, especially those from extra-intestinal infections, produce a polysaccharide capsule. They grow well on non-selective media, forming smooth, colourless colonies 2–3 mm in diameter in 18 h on nutrient agar, and large, red colonies on MacConkey agar; there may be haemolysis on blood agar. They grow over a wide range of temperature (15–45°C). Some strains are more heat-resistant than other members of the Enterobacteriaceae and will survive 60°C for 15 min or 55°C for 60 min.

The characteristic biochemical reactions of *Esch. coli* are given in Table 27.1 where they are compared with those of the other *Escherichia* species. Although most strains ferment lactose with the production of acid and gas within 24–48 h, some do so only after extended incubation or are non-lactose fermenters. Many characteristic biochemical reactions, such as indole production and the formation of acid and gas from lactose and other carbohydrates, take place at 44°C as well as at 37°C.

Studies of DNA–DNA recombination show that *Esch. coli* and *Shigella* organisms form a single genetic species and it is therefore to be expected that intermediate strains will occur. Certain of these, which are non-motile and anaerogenic, and often ferment lactose late or not at all, have caused difficulties in classification. They were at one time included in the so-called 'Alkalescens-Dispar' group but these strains are now considered to be atypical *Esch. coli*. Some workers believe that an intermediate group between *Escherichia* and *Shigella* should be established and that an important criterion for inclusion in it should be the ability to cause dysentery-like disease.

Antigenic structure

The diagnostic serotyping scheme is based on the distribution of O, H and K antigens, as detected by the reactions obtained in agglutination tests.

Over 160 different somatic or O antigens have been described. Agglutination tests must be carried out on boiled or autoclaved cultures to overcome inagglutinability caused by K antigens. Numerous cross-reactions occur between individual *Esch. coli* O antigens, and between these and the O

Table 27.1 Biochemical test reactions of *Escherichia* species

Property	Esch. blattae	Esch. coli	Esch. fergusonii	Esch. hermanii	Esch. vulneris
Motility	−	+	+	+	+
Christensen's citrate	V	+	+	V	−
Growth in KCN medium	−	−	−	+	−
Malonate fermentation	+	−	−	−	+
β-Galactosidase	−	+	+	+	+
Arginine dihydrolase	−	V	V	−	+
Ornithine decarboxylase	+	V	+	+	−
Adonitol: acid production	−	−	+	−	−
Cellobiose: acid production	−	−	+	+	+
Dulcitol: acid production	−	V	−	+	−
Glycerol: acid production	+	+	−	−	−
Mannitol: acid production	−	+	+	+	+
Raffinose: acid production	−	V	−	−	+
Salicin: acid production	−	V	+	V	+
Sorbitol: acid production	−	+	−	−	−
Indole production	−	+	V	+	−

+, Most strains positive; −, most strains negative; V, some strains positive, others negative.

antigens of organisms belonging to the genera *Citrobacter, Providencia, Salmonella, Shigella* and *Yersinia*. In some instances the antigens appearing in the different genera are identical serologically and structurally. In contrast to *Salmonella* and *Klebsiella* species, which produce only neutral O-specific polysaccharide, that produced by *Esch. coli* strains may be neutral or acidic. In most cases the acidic components are hexuronic acids.

Over 50 H (flagella) antigens are known, all of them are usually monophasic but rare diphasic strains have been reported. There are only a few significant cross-reactions between them and with the H antigens of other members of the Enterobacteriaceae. Before use for H antigen determination it is often necessary to grow cultures in semi-solid agar.

The term 'K antigen' was first used collectively for surface or capsular antigens that cause 'O inagglutinability'. In the past these antigens were divided into three classes (L, A and B) according to the effect of heat on the agglutinability, antigenicity and antibody-binding power of bacterial strains that carry them.

In modern usage the term 'K antigen' refers to the acidic polysaccharide capsular antigens and those of *Esch. coli* may be divided into two groups (groups I and II; see Table 27.2) that largely correspond to the old A and L antigens.

Antisera for serotyping purposes are not readily available except for enteropathogenic O groups (EPEC).

Many of the Enterobacteriaceae possess fimbriae. There is a distinction between common fimbriae, which are chromosomally determined and do not have an essential role in bacterial conjugation, and sex pili, which are determined by conjugative plasmids, and appear to be organs of conjugation. Strains may carry both common fimbriae and sex pili, as well as more than one type of common fimbriae. Within a culture, there are individual cells with many common fimbriae and others with none, and there is reversible variation between the fimbriate and the non-fimbriate phase.

Little is known about the function of the common fimbriae. Type 1 fimbriae are able to mediate adhesion to a wide range of human and animal cells that contain mannose residues. Such adhesion might favour pathogenicity and there are some examples of this. The possible role of type 1 fimbriae in urinary tract infection remains controversial.

More recently, a number of filamentous protein structures resembling fimbriae have been described in *Esch. coli*. These cause a mannose-resistant haemagglutination, and there is good evidence that they play an important part in the pathogenesis of diarrhoeal disease and in urinary tract infection. They include the K88 antigen found in

Table 27.2 K antigens of *Esch. coli*

Properties	Group I	Group II
Molecular weight	>100 000	<50 000
Acidic component	Hexuronic acid, pyruvate	Glucuronic acid, phosphate, KDO, NeuNAc
Heat stability (100°C, pH 6)	All stable	Mostly labile
O groups	08, 09	Many
Chromosome site	*his*	*serA*
Expressed at 17–20°C	Yes	No
Electrophoretic mobility	Low	High

KDO, ketodeoxyoctonate; NeuNAc, *N*-acetylneuraminic acid.

strains causing enteritis of pigs, the K99 antigen found in strains causing enteritis of calves and lambs, and the colonization factor antigens (CFAs) found in enterotoxigenic *Esch. coli* of human origin. Fimbriae that are of importance in urinary tract infection and cause mannose-resistant haemagglutination are distinguished according to their receptor specificities. These include the P fimbriae that bind specifically to receptors present on the P blood group antigens of human erythrocytes and uroepithelial cells (see Chapter 8).

PATHOGENESIS

Esch. coli is a widespread intestinal parasite of mammals and birds and, although present wherever there is faecal contamination, appears not to lead an independent existence outside the animal body. Certain strains are pathogens in man and animals and cause both septic infection and diarrhoea.

Urinary tract and septic infections

Esch. coli is commonly implicated in infections of the urinary tract and is by far the most common cause of acute, uncomplicated urinary tract infection outside hospitals. *Esch. coli* also causes neonatal meningitis and septicaemia as well as sepsis in operation wounds and abscesses in a variety of organs.

Strains of *Esch. coli* possess a battery of virulence determinants. The polysaccharides of the O and K antigens protect the organism from the bactericidal effect of complement and phagocytes in the absence of specific antibodies. However, in the presence of antibody to K antigens alone, or to both O and K antigens, phagocytosis is successful. In a capsulate strain the presence of K antigens exerts only a partial protection against the effect of antibody to O antigens alone. As many as 80% of *Esch. coli* strains causing neonatal meningitis and 40% of those isolated from infants with septicaemia but without meningitis possess the K1 antigen. Strains possessing the KI or the K5 antigen may have greater virulence than those with other K antigens since they are very poorly immunogenic because of their structural identity with host components.

Many strains of *Esch. coli* form a haemolysin and a much higher proportion of *Esch. coli* isolated from human extra-intestinal infections are haemolytic than are those from human faeces. Furthermore, haemolytic strains have been found to be more virulent than non-haemolytic ones in animal experiments. It is likely that haemolytic strains of *Esch. coli* obtain iron from the lysed erythrocytes of the host. Its cytotoxic activity may also be important in some infections.

Some strains possess the Col V plasmid which carries the genetic determinants for an aerobactin-mediated iron uptake system and this may be responsible for enhanced virulence. Expression of the aerobactin-mediated iron uptake system occurs more frequently in strains from septicaemia, pyelonephritis and lower urinary tract infection than among human faecal isolates.

Esch. coli that cause urinary tract infection often originate in the gut of the patient and the infection is thought to occur in an ascending manner. There is evidence that the ability of

Esch. coli to infect the urinary tract is associated with fimbriae that specifically mediate adherence to the uroepithelial cells. The receptor is part of the P blood group antigen and the fimbriae have therefore been termed P fimbriae. Some authorities doubt the importance of P fimbriae because bacteria freshly shed in the urine of infected patients do not adhere to epithelial cells. On the other hand, this may simply reflect the fact that a culture may contain a mixture of fimbriate and non-fimbriate cells; in this case it would not be too surprising if the non-fimbriate cells were shed in the urine.

Epidemiology

Urinary tract infection is much commoner in females than in males since the shorter, wider female urethra appears to be less effective in preventing access of the bacteria to the bladder. Sexual intercourse is a predisposing factor. The high incidence in pregnant women can be attributed to impairment of urine flow due partly to hormonal changes and partly to pressure on the urinary tract. Other causes of urinary stagnation that may predispose to urinary tract infection include urethral obstruction, urinary stones, congenital malformations and neurological disorders, all of which occur in both sexes. In men, prostatic enlargement is the most common predisposing factor. Catheterization and cystoscopy may introduce bacteria into the bladder and therefore carry a risk of infection.

Since most urinary tract infections are thought to be caused by organisms originating from the patient's own bowel, each infection is generally regarded as sporadic. However, the prevalence of various serotypes of *Esch. coli* in urinary tract infections varies with geographical location and this fits well with the view that *Esch. coli* that cause such infections are specific pathogens for the urinary tract. Pathogenic strains, possibly transmitted in contaminated foods, are able to colonize the bowel and individuals with predisposing factors may acquire a urinary tract infection. The prevalence of infections due to a particular strain may therefore increase for a time in a locality.

Laboratory diagnosis

Clinical specimens may be stained by Gram's method for microscopical examination and are cultured on suitable media so that the organism may be isolated for identification and sensitivity testing. In the case of suspected urinary tract infection, culture is semiquantitative and in acute *Esch. coli* infections the organism is generally present in virtually pure culture at a count of 10^5 or higher per ml of urine (see Chapter 64).

Treatment and control

Esch. coli is naturally sensitive to many antibiotics; although moderately resistant to benzylpenicillin, it is sensitive to ampicillin and the cephalosporins, and usually to tetracycline, streptomycin, chloramphenicol, kanamycin, gentamicin, trimethoprim, sulphonamides and the polymyxins. Many strains, however, have acquired plasmids conferring resistance to one or more of these drugs. Strains resistant to ampicillin, streptomycin, sulphonamides and tetracyclines are particularly common and strains resistant to chloramphenicol, trimethoprim and cephalexin are no longer rare; the resistances are usually transferable.

Extra-intestinal *Esch. coli* infections are treated with specific antimicrobial therapy, preferably guided by the results of laboratory tests for sensitivity. In particular, bacterial meningitis is a medical emergency and vigorous early treatment is required. Urinary catheterization and cystoscopy require rigorous aseptic technique to minimize the introduction of bacteria into the bladder. Bladder irrigation and systemic treatment with antimicrobial agents has been used in catheter-associated infections but such treatment is seldom more than palliative and encourages infections with resistant organisms.

Diarrhoea

Esch. coli may cause: acute enteritis of young animals, including human infants, piglets, calves and lambs; acute enteritis in human subjects of all ages occurring mainly in the tropics and including travellers' diarrhoea; a dysentery-like disease affecting man at all ages; and haemorrhagic colitis or 'bloody diarrhoea'.

Strains that cause diarrhoea fall into four groups with different pathogenic mechanisms (Table 27.3):

1. *Enteropathogenic Esch. coli (EPEC)*. EPEC were first discovered by serotyping in epidemiological studies. They cause infantile enteritis, especially in tropical countries; outbreaks often occur in hospitals and may have a high mortality, but such outbreaks have become uncommon in industrialized countries.

2. *Enterotoxigenic Esch. coli (ETEC)*. These strains produce a heat-stable enterotoxin (ST) or a heat-labile enterotoxin (LT) or both. In addition, they possess colonization factors that are specific for the host animal species and which enable the organisms to adhere to the epithelium of the small intestine.

3. *Entero-invasive Esch. coli (EIEC)*. EIEC cause an illness identical to shigella dysentery in patients of all ages.

4. *Vero cytotoxin-producing Esch. coli (VTEC)*. *Esch. coli* O157 is by far the most common serogroup found in human VTEC infections. VTEC produce one or both of two Vero cytotoxins (VT1 and VT2). VT1 is closely related to the so-called Shiga toxin produced by strains of *Shigella dysenteriae* 1 and is sometimes called Shiga-like toxin. VTEC cause a range of symptoms from mild, watery diarrhoea to a severe diarrhoea with large amounts of fresh blood in the stool (*haemorrhagic colitis*). An important complication, especially in children, is the *haemolytic uraemic syndrome*.

Enteropathogenic Esch. coli *(EPEC)*

Pathogenesis. The ability of EPEC strains to cause diarrhoea has been confirmed by oral administration of the organisms to babies and adults, but the mechanism by which they do so is incompletely understood. Most strains do not produce ST, LT or VT and are non-invasive.

Colonization of the upper part of the small intestine occurs in infantile enteritis associated with EPEC but the adhesive mechanism is less well understood than that of ETEC. In many patients EPEC are seen by electron microscopy to be intimately associated with the mucosal surface and to be partially surrounded by cup-like projections ('pedestals') of the enterocyte surface and in areas of EPEC attachment the brush border microvilli are lost. Such strains of *Esch. coli* have been termed attaching, effacing *Esch. coli* or entero-adherent *Esch. coli* (EAEC).

It is clear that there is considerable diversity among the strains previously designated EPEC. A few are enterotoxigenic and are best regarded as ETEC while some produce VT and are best regarded as VTEC. The term EPEC is best reserved for strains that do not produce ST, LT or VT. Many of these are strongly adhesive to intestinal epithelial cells and this represents an important pathogenic mechanism. Nevertheless, some EPEC strains associated with human diarrhoea possess none of these characters and their pathogenic mechanism is still unclear.

Epidemiology. Since 1971 few epidemics of EPEC enteritis have been reported in the UK or the USA, but a satisfactory explanation for this has not been put forward. Strains isolated recently from sporadic cases in the UK possess the same virulence determinants as those that caused outbreaks in the 1960s and early 1970s. In the absence of epidemics, the incidence of sporadic cases of infantile enteritis in the UK shows a peak in the summer months.

Table 27.3 The major groups of diarrhoea-causing *Esch. coli*

Pathogenic group	Common serogroups
1. Enteropathogenic *Esch. coli* (EPEC)	O26, O55, O86, O111, O114, O119, O125, O126, O127, O128, O142
2. Enterotoxigenic *Esch. coli* (ETEC)	O6, O8, O15, O25, O27, O63, O78, O115, O148, O153, O159, O167
3. Entero-invasive *Esch. coli* (EIEC)	O28ac, O112ac, O124, O136, O143, O144, O152, O164
4. Vero cytotoxin-producing *Esch. coli* (VTEC)	O157[a]

[a] VTEC have been found in many other serogroups but these are far less common than O157 in human disease.

Although EPEC enteritis now appears to be of little importance in areas with good standards of hygiene, it is still common in communities with poor hygiene. In these countries sporadic cases and outbreaks occur very frequently in the general community as well as in institutions.

The importance of EPEC as a cause of enteritis in adults is difficult to evaluate since few laboratories look for these organisms in patients over 3 years of age. However, a few outbreaks have been described.

Laboratory diagnosis of EPEC. Stool specimens are plated on non-selective media such as MacConkey agar and several colonies are examined by slide agglutination with polyvalent antisera for the EPEC serogroups. Those giving positive reactions are subcultured and again tested by slide agglutination with monovalent antisera; identification is finally confirmed by tube agglutination tests. Strains provisionally serogrouped in this way should also be identified as *Esch. coli* because there is widespread sharing of antigens among the Enterobacteriaceae.

Tests for adhesion to HEp-2 cells and DNA probes for the detection of the EPEC adherence factor are available in some laboratories.

Enterotoxigenic Esch. coli *(ETEC)*

Pathogenesis. *Heat-labile enterotoxin* (LT). LT is closely related to the toxin produced by strains of *Vibrio cholerae*. Both are protein complexes consisting of one polypeptide A subunit and five polypeptide B subunits with molecular weights of about 25 000 and 11 500 respectively. The B subunits are responsible for binding of the toxin to the epithelial cells. After translocation across the membrane of intestinal epithelial cells, subunit A catalyses the nicotinamide adenine dinuleotide (NAD)-dependent activation of adenylate cyclase to cause an increase in the concentration of cyclic adenosine 5'-monophosphate (cAMP). In the intestinal villus cells. cAMP inhibits the absorption of sodium and therefore of chloride and water while in the crypt cells cAMP increases sodium secretion and causes loss of chloride and water leading to profuse watery diarrhoea.

LT has been shown to be plasmid encoded in many strains of human and animal origin and the organization of the operon encoding the A and B subunits is known in detail.

Occasional *Esch. coli* strains produce a heat-labile toxin (LT-II) which has similar biological activity to LT but which does not react with antiserum in neutralization or immunodiffusion tests. The structural genes for LT-II appear to be chromosomal although few strains have been studied.

Heat-stable enterotoxin (ST). In contrast to LT, the STs of *Esch. coli* have a low molecular weight and are poorly immunogenic. Two major classes of *Esch. coli* STs have been recognized and are designated ST_A and ST_B (or ST-I and ST-II). ST_A is detected by an infant mouse test in which secretion occurs in the intestine within 4 h following intragastric administration. This toxin activates guanylate cyclase activity resulting in an increase in the level of cyclic guanosine monophosphate (cGMP). The activity of ST_A is rapid, whereas LT acts after a lag period. The mechanism of secretion caused by ST_A, via cGMP, is not known but calcium may play a role.

ST_A has been shown to be plasmid encoded and these plasmids may also carry genes for LT, adhesive factors or antibiotic resistance.

ST_B is distinguished from ST_A by its biological activity and by its insolubility in methanol. ST_B stimulates fluid accumulation in ligated intestinal loops of piglets but not in the infant mouse test. The mechanism of action of ST_B is not known but it appears not to act via cAMP or cGMP.

Adhesive factors. Enterotoxin is not sufficient to enable an *Esch. coli* strain to cause diarrhoea. The organism must also be able to adhere to the mucosal surface of the epithelial cells of the small intestine. This adhesion is usually mediated by fimbriae which bind to specific receptors in the cell membrane. Adhesive or *colonization factors* are antigenic and can be recognized by means of agglutination or immunodiffusion tests. Their presence can also be demonstrated by haemagglutination, by experimental colonization of animal intestines or by tissue or organ culture methods. In contrast to the haemagglutination due to type 1 pili of *Esch. coli*, that due to colonization factors associated with diarrhoeal disease is not inhibited by mannose. Plasmids that simultaneously carry genes for both a colonization factor and enterotoxin production have been described.

The first colonization factor in *Esch. coli*, initially recognized as a surface antigen (K88), is controlled by a transferable plasmid and is fimbrial in nature. Its importance in the pathogenesis of piglet enteritis was demonstrated in experiments in which it was shown that the loss of the K88 plasmid from a strain of *Esch. coli* O141 was accompanied by the loss of its capacity to cause diarrhoea when given orally to piglets. This was restored by introducing a K88 plasmid from another strain of *Esch. coli*. There is a gene in pigs which is inherited in a simple Mendelian manner and which determines the presence of receptors for K88 in the pig intestinal epithelium; pigs lacking this receptor are resistant to colonization of the small intestine by *Esch. coli* strains with the K88 antigen.

Several colonization factors have subsequently been discovered in human strains of ETEC and, no doubt, others remain to be discovered. The properties of some of the more important colonization factors are shown in Table 27.4.

Epidemiology. ETEC are uncommon in geographical regions where hygiene and nutrition are good, but occasional outbreaks of diarrhoea and sporadic cases have been reported. In the developing countries, diarrhoeal diseases are a major cause of death in children under 5 years of age and ETEC cause a large proportion of these. In its most severe form ETEC infection resembles cholera.

ETEC are the commonest cause of travellers' diarrhoea. This is a world-wide illness, usually of brief duration, often beginning with the rapid onset of loose stools and accompanied by variable symptoms, including nausea, vomiting and abdominal cramps. It occurs most frequently among those travelling from areas of good hygiene and temperate climate to areas with lower standards, particularly in warmer countries.

There have been several studies of travellers' diarrhoea in Mexico where 'turista' has an attack rate of 29–48%; for example, among students and Peace Corps volunteers, ETEC have been found in 45–72% of sufferers in different surveys. Similarly, in African countries ETEC have been found in 31–75% of Peace Corps volunteers with diarrhoea.

Table 27.4 Properties of some important human colonization factors

Colonization factor	Components	MRHA			Fimbrial type	Associated toxin	Associated serogroups
		Human	Bovine	Guinea-pig			
CFA I		+	+	−	Rod-like	ST or ST/LT	O4, O7, O15, O20, O25, O63, O78, O90, O104, O110, O126, O128, O136, O153, O159
CFA II	CS1	(+)	+	−	Rod-like	ST/LT	O6, O139
	CS2	−	+	−	Rod-like	ST/LT	O6
	CS3	−	+	−	Fibrillar	ST/LT	O8, O78, O80, O85, O115, O128, O139, O168
CFA III		−	−	−	Rod-like	LT	O25
CFA IV	CS4	+	+	−	Rod-like	ST/LT	O25
	CS5	+	+	+	Helical	ST	O6, O29, O92, O114, O115, O167, O25, O27, O79, O89, O92, O148, O153, O159, O169
	CS6	−	−	−	No fimbriae detected	ST or LT	

MRHA, mannose-resistant haemagglutinin; ST, heat-stable toxin; LT, heat-labile toxin; CS, coli surface antigen.

The sources and modes of spread of ETEC infection in warm-climate countries are not well understood but it seems likely that water contaminated by human or animal sewage plays an important part in the spread of infection.

Laboratory diagnosis of ETEC. *Detection of LT.* Tests in tissue cultures of Y1 mouse adrenal cells and Chinese hamster ovary (CHO) cells are accepted as standard methods for the detection of LT, but other cell lines, including Vero monkey kidney cells, are also sensitive to the toxin. Exposure of the cells to culture supernates containing LT or cholera toxin leads to a morphological response which can be seen by microscopy. The response can be regarded as stimulatory or 'cytotonic' in contrast to the cytotoxic effect of VTEC supernates on Vero cells.

A wide range of immunological techniques is available for the detection of LT, including an enzyme-linked immunosorbent assay (ELISA) and a solid-phase radio-immunoassay (RIA). These tests are performed in microtitration trays or in tubes and the results can be read spectrophotometrically. A precipitin test (the *Biken test*) performed directly on bacterial colonies growing on a special agar medium has been evaluated and may be suitable for use in field laboratories. Additionally, a staphylococcal coagglutination test and a latex particle agglutination test have been described; the latter is available commercially and may prove to be valuable as a simple screening test.

Detection of ST. Many enterotoxigenic strains of *Esch. coli* produce only ST and it is essential to include tests for ST production in any survey of enterotoxigenicity. Unfortunately the usual tests are cumbersome and time consuming.

Injection of enterotoxin preparations, both LT and ST, into ligated ileal loops of rabbits leads to the accumulation of fluid. The action of ST can be distinguished from that of LT both by its relative stability to heat and by the rapidity of its action. So far it has proved impossible to devise tissue culture tests for ST and the most widely used method for detecting ST_A is the infant mouse test. The intestines are removed after the injection of culture supernates and the ratio of gut weight to remaining body weight is used as an objective measure of fluid accumulation.

The non-antigenic nature of ST at first prevented the development of immunological tests. This problem was overcome by preparing antiserum from toxin coupled to a bovine serum albumin carrier and using the antiserum in an RIA. Subsequently, ELISA tests with monoclonal antibody specific for ST became available.

Genetic probes for the detection of ST and LT. Radiolabelled or biotin-labelled gene probes have been developed for the detection of ST or LT in stool, food or water samples containing ETEC.

Enteroinvasive Esch. coli (EIEC)

Epidemiology. The epidemiology and ecology of EIEC is poorly studied but there is no evidence of an animal or environmental reservoir. Surveys suggest that they cause about 5% of all diarrhoeas in areas of poor hygiene. In the UK and USA outbreaks are occasionally described, especially in schools and hospitals for the mentally handicapped. Infections are usually foodborne but there is also evidence of cross-infection. The most common serogroup is O124.

Pathogenesis. Shigellae and EIEC cause bacillary dysentery by an invasive mechanism in which the organisms penetrate the epithelial cells of the large intestine and multiply intracellularly. In order to survive their passage through the upper intestine they must resist the effects of gastric acidity, bile salts and pancreatic enzymes. They are assisted in this by the possession of a complete, 'smooth' lipopolysaccharide capsule. The invasive mechanism depends on the presence of certain outer-membrane proteins that are cleaved by pancreatic enzymes during passage through the small intestine, rendering the organisms temporarily non-invasive; it is assumed that these proteins are restored in the colon. Once they arrive in the colonic lumen the organisms encounter a reducing environment in which they must compete with the resident flora for available carbon sources. These environmental factors have probably provided selective pressure for the maintenance of the invasive phenotype which enables shigellae and EIEC to escape the lumen and to occupy an intracellular niche in which an endless source of carbon is available in the form of the host blood glucose.

In the course of the invasive process the organisms first penetrate the mucus layer with the help of glycosidases produced by the normal flora. They then attach to the cell surface where they appear to induce an endocytic process that does not rupture the plasma membrane. The intracellular organisms are briefly contained within an endocytic vacuole. The ability to lyse these vacuoles is an important virulence attribute as organisms that are unable to do this are unable to spread to neighbouring cells.

Following endocytosis there is an inhibition of host cell protein synthesis. Glucose and amino acid transport continue but these nutrients are used to support bacterial multiplication. There is tissue destruction and a consequent inflammation that is the underlying cause of the symptoms of bacillary dysentery.

Virulence in shigellae and EIEC depends on both chromosomal and plasmid genes. A large plasmid (120 MDa in *Sh. sonnei* and 140 MDa in other shigellae and in EIEC) carries genes for the expression of outer-membrane proteins that are required for invasion as well as genes that may be necessary for the insertion of these proteins into the cell membrane. Plasmid genes are also required for the ability to escape from the endocytic vacuole and to invade contiguous host cells. Chromosomal virulence genes include those required for the expression of a smooth lipopolysaccharide and genes for an aerobactin iron-binding system.

Laboratory diagnosis of EIEC. The original test for entero-invasive potential is the guinea-pig eye or *Sereny test*. The organism is instilled into the conjunctival sac of the guinea-pig and the animal is examined for up to 7 d for signs of conjunctivitis. Tissue culture methods are also available in which monolayers of HEp-2 or HeLa cells are exposed to suspensions of the organism under test. After an appropriate infection period the cells are washed with a solution containing gentamicin and lysozyme to remove extracellular organisms. After a further period to allow intracellular growth the cells are examined microscopically for the presence of intracellular organisms.

Vero cytotoxigenic Esch. coli *(VTEC)*

The importance of VTEC in human disease has only become clear since the association was established between VTEC and two diseases of previously unknown aetiology: *haemorrhagic colitis* and *haemolytic uraemic syndrome* (HUS).

Haemorrhagic colitis is a grossly bloody diarrhoea, usually in the absence of pyrexia. It is usually preceded by abdominal pain and watery diarrhoea. Outbreaks were recognized in the USA in 1982 and, since then, outbreaks and sporadic cases have been reported in several other countries.

HUS is characterized by acute renal failure, micro-angiopathic haemolytic anaemia and thrombocytopenia. HUS occurs in all age groups but is more common in infants and young children and is a major cause of renal failure in childhood. HUS may be classified into two principal subgroups; 'typical' HUS is associated with a prodromal bloody diarrhoea while an 'atypical' form occurs without a diarrhoeal phase. *Esch. coli* O157 is associated with the typical form of HUS.

VTEC infection in man can be associated with a range of clinical symptoms from mild, non-bloody diarrhoea to severe manifestions such as HUS and a wide spectrum of illness can occur even within a single outbreak. VTEC infection may also be accompanied by thrombotic thrombocytopenic purpura in which the clinical features of HUS are further complicated by neurological involvement and fever.

VTEC have also been implicated as a cause of disease in animals, particularly calves and pigs.

Pathogenesis. *Nature and mode of action of VT.* When VT was first described it was found to be very similar to Shiga toxin, produced by strains of *Sh. dysenteriae* type 1, in terms of biological properties, physical characteristics and antigenicity. The term 'Shiga-like toxin' (SLT) was therefore used to describe the toxin produced by *Esch. coli* strains and both terms, VT and SLT, are widely used. VT that is neutralized by anti-Shiga toxin is now designated VTI and a second VT, first shown in strains of serogroup O157 and not neutralized by anti-Shiga toxin, is termed VT2. VT1 and VT2 are also known as SLT-I and SLT-II.

Like Shiga toxin, VTI and VT2 are made up of A and B subunits. For both toxins the A subunit possesses the biological activities of the toxin while the B subunits are thought to mediate specific binding and receptor-mediated uptake of the toxin. VTI and VT2 have the same biological activities as Shiga toxin: cytotoxicity for Vero and HeLa cells, enterotoxicity in ligated rabbit gut loops and mouse paralytic lethality.

The genes controlling production of VT are phage encoded in several *Esch. coli* strains. VT genes have been cloned in *Esch. coli* K12 from phages originating in strains of serogroups O26 and O157 and probes for the VT genes have been developed.

Human umbilical cord endothelial cells have been used in studies of the action of VT1. There is a direct, dose-dependent cytotoxic effect on these cells in culture and actively dividing cells are the most sensitive. Since a micro-angiopathy of the capillaries is a characteristic renal lesion in HUS the results with this model support the hypothesis that vascular endothelial cells are a primary target for VT.

A plasmid in VTEC of serogroup O157 is necessary for the expression of fimbriae that determine the attachment of small numbers of bacteria in tissue culture. However, surface structures other than fimbriae may also mediate attachment. A DNA probe derived from this plasmid has been evaluated for the detection of VTEC.

Epidemiology. VTEC outbreaks have occurred in the community, in nursing homes for the elderly and in day care centres for young children. The most severe clinical manifestations are usually seen in the paediatric and geriatric populations.

Food is an important source of VTEC infection. In several outbreaks of haemorrhagic colitis due to *Esch. coli* O157 in the USA and Canada the causative organism has been isolated from hamburger meat and unpasteurized milk. *Esch. coli* O157.H7 was also isolated from healthy heifers on the farms associated with the milk-borne incidents and it seems likely that cattle are a reservoir of *Esch. coli* O157.H7.

Laboratory diagnosis. The proportion of VTEC in the faecal flora may be low, often less than 1%, so that picking and testing of individual colonies from culture plates may not always detect the presence of VTEC. DNA probes for the VTI and VT2 genes have been developed and by using these probes in colony hybridization tests several hundred colonies from each faecal specimen can be examined giving a considerable increase in sensitivity.

While 95% of *Esch. coli* are sorbitol fermenters, O157 VTEC do not ferment sorbitol in 24 h and this characteristic has been used as the basis of tests to detect them, e.g. using sorbitol–MacConkey agar for primary culture followed by agglutination with an O157 antiserum. VT production is confirmed by testing strains for a cytotoxic effect on Vero cells.

Evidence for VTEC infection has also been obtained by observing rising levels of VT-neutralizing antibodies or of antibody directed against the O157 lipopolysaccharide in patients' sera.

Prevention and treatment of Esch. coli enteritis

General measures. The early correction of fluid and electrolyte imbalance is the most important single factor in preventing the death of the patient in severe infections.

The most effective means of preventing infection is to avoid exposure to the infecting agent. Contaminated food and water are probably the most important vehicles of ETEC infection in developing countries. The provision of safe supplies of water together with education in hygienic practice in the handling and production of food, particularly that given to young children, are essential. Travellers to countries with poor hygiene, especially in the tropics, should select eating places with care and if possible should consume only hot food and drinks, or bottled water. Self-peeled fruits are probably safe, but salads should be avoided. Unheated milk should always be considered unsafe.

The spread of infantile enteritis in hospitals and nurseries is mainly from patient to patient — generally on the hands of attendants — or from contaminated infant feeds. It can be prevented only by very strict hygiene. Infected patients, and recently admitted patients suspected of being infected, must be isolated by barrier nursing techniques to prevent faecal spread. In some cases outbreaks can be terminated only by closing the ward or nursery and cleaning thoroughly before reopening.

It is likely that VTEC infections are acquired most frequently from meat and from unpasteurized milk. Such infections should be avoided by normal food hygiene with particular attention to the thorough cooking of raw meats, especially if minced.

Vaccination. The most extensive studies of the use of vaccines have so far been in the veterinary field. Recently, a potential vaccine for human use has been prepared by cross-linking a synthetically produced ST with the non-toxic B subunit of LT. Tests in the rat showed that the vaccine protects against subsequent challenge with ST or LT or with organisms that produce them. In human volunteers oral administration causes an increase in antitoxin levels in serum samples and jejunal aspirates.

Inhibition of enterotoxin activity. A number of substances such as activated charcoal, bismuth subsalicylate and non-steroidal anti-inflammatory drugs inhibit or reverse the secretory effects of enterotoxins in experimental animals and may be of value in the prevention or treatment of diarrhoea. Clinical trials have shown some benefit from such substances but more work needs to be done to establish the optimum conditions for their use.

Antimicrobial prophylaxis. A number of antimicrobial drugs reduce the incidence of diarrhoea in travellers to tropical areas. These include phthalylsulphathiazole, neomycin, doxycycline, trimethoprim, norfloxacin and other fluoroquinolones. However, the widespread use of antibiotic prophylaxis has been criticized both on the grounds of drug toxicity and because of the possibility that the development and spread of drug resistance might be encouraged among a variety of enteropathogenic organisms.

OTHER PROPOSED ESCHERICHIA SPECIES

Esch. blattae was first described among bacteria isolated from the gut of the cockroach. It differs from *Esch. coli* both in oxidizing gluconate and fermenting malonate, as well as in failing to form indole, acidify mannitol or sorbitol, or produce β-galactosidase. It would probably be better placed in another genus. The species has not been reported from human clinical specimens but its characters are given along with those of the other *Escherichia* species in Table 27.1, for completeness. *Esch. fergusonii* has been recovered from various clinical specimens, especially faeces, but its clinical significance is as yet unknown. Similarly, the pathogenic potential of *Esch. hermanii* and *Esch. vulneris* is also largely unknown but they are particularly associated with wound colonization.

RECOMMENDED READING

Gross R J, Rowe B 1985 *Escherichia coli* diarrhoea. *Journal of Hygiene* 95: 531–550

Gross R J 1991 The Pathogenesis of *Escherichia coli* diarrhoea. *Reviews in Medical Microbiology* 2: 37–44

Hale T L, Formal S B 1987 Pathogenesis of shigella infections. *Pathology and Immunopathology Research* 6: 117–127

Johnson JR 1991 Virulence factors in *Escherichia coli* urinary tract infection *Clinical Microbiology Reviews* 3: 80–128

Levine M M 1987 *Escherichia coli* that cause diarrhoea: enterotoxigenic, enteropathogenic, enteroinvasive,

enterohemorrhagic, and enteroadherent. *Journal of Infectious Diseases* 155: 377–389

Ørskov I, Ørskov F 1985 *Escherichia coli* in extra-intestinal infections. *Journal of Hygiene* 95: 551–575

Schoolnik G K 1989 How *Escherichia coli* infects the urinary tract. *New England Journal of Medicine* 12: 804–805

Scotland S M 1988 Toxins. *Journal of Applied Bacteriology Symposium* suppl: 109S–129S

Smith H R, Scotland S M 1988 Vero cytotoxin-producing strains of *Escherichia coli*. *Journal of Medical Microbiology* 26: 77–85

28

Klebsiella, enterobacter, proteus and other enterobacteria

Pneumonia; urinary tract infection; opportunistic infection

R. J. Gross

The genera described in this chapter conform to the general definition of the Enterobacteriaceae in that they are aerobic or facultatively anaerobic, ferment glucose, and give a positive catalase and a negative oxidase reaction. Together with organisms of the genera *Salmonella* (Chapter 25), *Shigella* (Chapter 26), *Escherichia* (Chapter 27) and *Yersinia* (Chapter 36), they are commonly referred to as *coliform* bacteria.

The generic and specific names of organisms of clinical interest are listed alphabetically in Table 28.1, along with a few of their common synonyms. Numerous tests are used to differentiate the various species of coliform bacteria; a highly simplified scheme that allows presumptive identification to the genus level is shown in Table 28.2.

KLEBSIELLA

CLASSIFICATION

The classification of the genus *Klebsiella* has a complex history that must be considered briefly to avoid the confusion that might be caused by changes in the nomenclature. In the past the name *Klebsiella aerogenes* was used for the non-motile, capsulate, gas-producing strains commonly found in human faeces and in water. These probably corresponded to strains described in the 19th century as *Bakterium lactis aerogenes*, referred to later as *Bact. aerogenes*, and subsequently transferred to the genus *Klebsiella*. Unfortunately, the term '*Bact. aerogenes*' (later *Aerobacter aerogenes*)

was also used by water bacteriologists to refer to organisms that were subsequently shown to be motile and are now classified as *Enterobacter* species. In an attempt to resolve the resultant confusion, some taxonomists adopted *pneumoniae* as the species name for the non-motile *aerogenes*-like organisms, although it had earlier been used to designate certain biochemically atypical *Klebsiella* strains isolated from the respiratory tract of man and animals. This view has now been accepted formally and the name *K. pneumoniae* appears in the Approved Lists of Bacterial Names while *K. aerogenes* is omitted. In this chapter the name *K. pneumoniae* is therefore used for the species as a whole, but the most frequently encountered, biochemically typical form of it is referred to as *K. pneumoniae* ssp. *aerogenes*. The atypical respiratory strains are included in the subspecies *ozaenae*, *pneumoniae* and *rhinoscleromatis*. A further species, *K. oxytoca*, is occasionally encountered in clinical specimens.

DESCRIPTION

Members of the genus *Klebsiella* tend to be slightly shorter and thicker than the other enterobacteria and are straight rods about 1–2 μm long and 0.5–0.8 μm wide. The capsule is often pronounced and can be demonstrated even by Gram's stain. Capsular material is produced in greater amounts in media rich in carbohydrate. In these conditions the growth on agar is luxuriant, greyish white and extremely mucoid (Fig. 28.1). The

Table 28.1 The principal genera and species of Enterobacteriaceae of clinical interest

Genus	Species	Synonyms
Citrobacter	*C. amalonaticus*	*Levinea amalonatica*
	C. freundii	
	C. koseri	*C. diversus, L. amalonatica*
Edwardsiella	*E. tarda*	*E. anguillimortifera*
Enterobacter	*Ent. aerogenes*	*K. mobilis*
	Ent. cloacae	
Erwinia	*Erw. herbicola*	*Ent. agglomerans*
Escherichia[a]		
Hafnia	*H. alvei*	*Ent. alvei, Ent. hafniae*
Klebsiella	*K. oxytoca*	
	K. pneumoniae	
	ssp. *aerogenes*	*K. aerogenes*
	ssp. *ozaenae*	*K. ozaenae*
	ssp. *pneumoniae*	*K. pneumoniae*
	ssp. *rhinoscleromatis*	*K. rhinoscleromatis*
Morganella	*M. morganii*	*Pr. morganii*
Proteus	*Pr. mirabilis*	
	Pr. vulgaris	
Providencia	*Prov. alcalifaciens*	
	Prov. rettgeri	*Pr. rettgeri*
	Prov. stuartii	
Salmonella[a]		
Serratia	*S. liquefaciens*	*Ent. liquefaciens*
	S. marcescens	
	S. odorifera	
Shigella[a]		
Yersinia[a]		

[a] See appropriate Chapter.

Table 28.2 Simplified scheme for the presumptive identification of the most important genera of enterobacteria

Test	*Escherichia*	*Salmonella*	*Shigella*	*Klebsiella*	*Enterobacter*[a]	*Proteus*	*Providencia*	*Citrobacter*	*Yersinia*
PPA test[b]	–	–	–	–	–	+	+	–	–
Gluconate oxidation	–	–	–	+	+	–	–	–	–
Citrate utilization	–	+	–	+	+	V	+	+	–
Lysine decarboxylase	+	+	–	+	V	–	–	–	–
ONPG test[c]	+	–	V	+	+	–	–	+	+
Urease production	–	–	–	V	–	+	–	–	+
Indole formation	+	–	V	V	–	V	+	V	–
Motility	+	+	–	–	+	+	+	+	V

+, most strains positive; – most strains negative; V, variable.
[a] Including the genus *Serratia*.
[b] Deamination of phenylalanine to phenylpyruvic acid.
[c] ONPG, *o*-nitrophenyl β-galactosidase. This is a test for β-galactosidase activity.

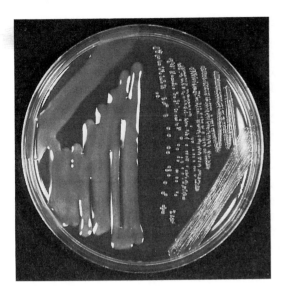

Fig. 28.1 Mucoid (left) and non-mucoid (right) variants of *Klebsiella* species on carbohydrate-rich medium. (Photograph courtesy of George Sharp and Richard Edwards.)

polysaccharides of the different capsular types are all complex acid polysaccharides, which usually contain glucuronic acid and pyruvic acid. They resemble the K antigens of *Escherichia coli* (see pp. 323–325).

Klebsiellae are non-motile but most strains are fimbriate. The organisms grow between 12–43°C (optimum, 37°C) and are killed by moist heat at 55°C in 30 min. They may survive drying for months and, when kept at room temperature, cultures remain viable for many weeks. They are facultatively anaerobic but growth under strictly anaerobic conditions is poor. There is no haemolysis of horse or sheep red cells.

Members of the genus can be differentiated by simple biochemical tests (Table 28.3). A useful character of practically all strains of *K. pneumoniae*, spp. *aerogenes* and *pneumoniae*, and practically no other members of the Enterobacteriaceae, is the ability to form gas within 4 d from starch.

Antibiotic susceptibility

Clinical isolates of *Klebsiella* are generally resistant to a wider range of antibiotics than most *Esch. coli* strains. They are nearly always naturally resistant to ampicillin and amoxycillin, but usually sensitive to cephalosporins, especially the newer derivatives such as cefuroxime and cefotaxime. Resistance to chloramphenicol and tetracycline varies from strain to strain; they are often sensitive to gentamicin but transferable enzymic resistance to gentamicin and various cephalosporins has become common in strains found in some hospitals.

Antigenic structure

About 80 capsular (K) antigens are presently recognized. Among current UK isolates types K2, K3 and K21 predominate and the prevalence of these types limits the usefulness of capsular serotyping as an epidemiological tool.

In addition to the capsular antigens, five different somatic or O antigens occur in various combinations with the capsular antigens. Four of the five *Klebsiella* O antigens are identical with or

Table 28.3 Some differential biochemical reactions of medically important *Klebsiella* species

| Property | *K. oxytoca* | *K. pneumoniae* ssp. | | | |
		aerogenes	*ozaenae*	*pneumoniae*	*rhinoscleromatis*
Gas from glucose	+	+	V	+	−
Indole formation	+	−	−	−	−
Growth in KCN medium	+	+	+	−	+
Malonate fermentation	+	+	−	+	+
Methyl red test	V	−	+	+	+
Urease formation	+	+	−	+	−

+, most strains positive; −, most strains negative; V, variable.

related to *Esch. coli* O antigens. It is therefore possible to divide *Klebsiella* strains into a small number of groups which may be further subdivided into capsular types, but this is of little practical value in the classification of the capsulate members of the genus.

There is some association between antigenic structure, biochemical activities and habitat. Members of capsular types 1–6 occur most frequently in the human respiratory tract.

Considerable overlap occurs between *Klebsiella* antigens and those of unrelated organisms. Capsular type 2, for example, is immunologically similar to the type 2 pneumococcus. Capsular antigens are usually detected by means of the capsular 'swelling' reaction, but agglutination, complement fixation, indirect immunofluorescence and countercurrent immuno-electrophoresis may also be employed.

Other typing methods

Many *Klebsiella* strains produce bacteriocines, which appear to be distinct from colicines because they have no action on *Esch. coli*. They have a narrow range of activity on other klebsiellae and epidemiological analysis may be improved by the use of bacteriocines as an adjunct to capsular serotyping. Phage typing has also been used and biotyping has been recommended instead of serotyping for use in less well-equipped laboratories.

PATHOGENESIS

Klebsiellae are a fairly common cause of urinary tract infection and occasionally give rise to cases of severe bronchopneumonia, sometimes with chronic destructive lesions and multiple abscess formation in the lungs (*Friedländer's pneumonia*). Cases are sporadic and usually occur in members of the general population rather than in hospital patients. In many cases there is also bacteraemia and mortality is high. This condition is usually but not always associated with members of capsular types 1–5, which are often biochemically atypical. However, the main importance of klebsiellae as human pathogens is in causing infections in hospital patients; the strains respon-

sible are nearly always biochemically typical members of *K. pneumoniae* ssp. *aerogenes,* most of which belong to higher-numbered capsular types. Clinical sepsis develops in surgical wounds and in the urinary tract; a number of patients have bacteraemic infections and some of them die. Colonization of the respiratory tract is very common in hospitalized patients receiving antibiotics, but its clinical significance is often difficult to assess. Some debilitated patients develop bronchopneumonia in which klebsiella appears to be the primary infecting agent. In the early days of antibiotic usage, klebsiellae were naturally resistant to the available antibiotics and with the passage of time they acquired resistance to the newly developed ones. The emergence of klebsiella as an important cause of infection in hospitals is undoubtedly related to the use of antibiotics.

The *ozaenae* and *rhinoscleromatis* subspecies of *K. pneumoniae* take their names from the diseases with which they are associated. Rhinoscleroma is a chronic upper respiratory tract disease that occurs in a number of countries in eastern Europe and other parts of the world where it is associated with prolonged exposure to crowded and unhygienic conditions. The lesions occur in the nose, larynx, throat and, to a lesser extent, in the trachea and consist of granulomatous infiltrations of the submucosa. Ozaena is an uncommon, chronic disease in which there is atrophy of the nasal mucosa in which *K. pneumoniae* ssp. *ozaenae* is of doubtful significance.

Virulence determinants

Bacterial pathogens must multiply in order to establish an infection and in order to multiply they need to acquire iron. *Klebsiella* strains possess two high-affinity iron uptake systems, one employing *aerobactin,* the other *enterochelin.* Production of aerobactin can be correlated with virulence and the genes encoding aerobactin are located on a plasmid.

Klebsiella strains show resistance to complement-mediated serum killing and phagocytosis if both K and O antigens are present; resistance to the former seems related to the O antigens and the latter to the K antigens. The virulence of *K.*

pneumoniae in animal models varies considerably and does not appear to depend on capsule formation.

TREATMENT

Klebsiella infection of the urine often responds to trimethoprim, nitrofurantoin, co-amoxiclav or oral cephalosporins. Pneumonia and other serious infections require vigorous treatment with an aminoglycoside or a cephalosporin such as cefotaxime.

ENTEROBACTER
DESCRIPTION

Enterobacter (formerly *Aerobacter*) species have many features in common with those of the genus *Klebsiella*, but are readily distinguished by their motility. Several species are now recognized; *Enterobacter aerogenes* and *Ent. cloacae* are much the most important clinically.

Although motility is the main distinguishing character between *Enterobacter* and *Klebsiella* species, a few strains that in all other respects resemble *Ent. cloacae* are non-motile. The colonies of *Enterobacter* strains may be slightly mucoid.

In general, the fermentative activity of *Enterobacter* strains is more limited than that of typical *Klebsiella* strains. *Ent. aerogenes* and *Ent. cloacae* can be distinguished according to decarboxylase activity: *Ent. aerogenes* is usually able to decarboxylate lysine, but not arginine, whereas *Ent. cloacae* decarboxylates arginine, but not lysine.

Antibiotic susceptibility

Enterobacter strains are nearly always highly resistant to penicillins and to the earlier cephalosporins because they produce a chromosomal β-lactamase with cephalosporinase activity. Many are also resistant to tetracycline, chloramphenicol and to streptomycin, although most are sensitive to other aminoglycosides including gentamicin. Most strains of *Ent. cloacae* appear susceptible to cefotaxime on primary testing, but they often possess an inducible chromosomal cephalosporinase which allows the rapid development of

resistance during therapy. *Enterobacter* strains differ from *Serratia* strains in being sensitive to the polymyxins.

PATHOGENESIS

The normal habitat of *Enterobacter* species is probably soil and water, but the organisms are occasionally found in the faeces and the respiratory tract of man. In recent years, infection of hospital patients with *Ent. cloacae* and *Ent. aerogenes* has been reported more frequently, but *Enterobacter* species are a much less important cause of hospital infection than *Klebsiella* species. Most infections are of the urinary tract, although members of the genus are an important cause of bacteraemia in some hospitals.

TREATMENT

Cephalosporins are contra-indicated because of the risk of treatment failure due to inducible β-lactamases. Aminoglycosides are often effective.

HAFNIA
DESCRIPTION

In the past this organism was placed in the genus *Enterobacter* under the names *Ent. alvei* and *Ent. hafniae* but DNA–DNA hybridization studies show that the organism deserves separate generic status. Three DNA-related groups have been recognized among *Hafnia alvei* strains but these are not given separate species names and, at present, the genus *Hafnia* contains only one species.

Strains grow well on ordinary media, producing greyish convex colonies 1.0–2.0 mm in diameter on nutrient agar at 37°C after incubation for 24 h. *H. alvei* ferments a much narrower range of sugars than members of the genus *Enterobacter*. It is not capsulate and does not liquefy gelatin. All *H. alvei* strains are lysed by a single phage, which is without action on any other members of the Enterobacteriaceae. There is an antigenic scheme that includes 197 serotypes.

PATHOGENESIS

Strains are isolated from the faeces of man and other animals and are also found in sewage, soil, water and dairy products. They are occasionally encountered as opportunist pathogens.

SERRATIA

DESCRIPTION

Although numerous species of the genus *Serratia* have been described, until about 10 years ago only *Serratia marcescens* was generally recognized. Since then, several others have been added, including *S. liquefaciens* (formerly known as *Ent. liquefaciens*) and *S. odorifera*.

S. *marcescens* is the species most commonly encountered in clinical specimens. It is smaller than the average coliform bacterium but its size is subject to considerable variation. Even on the same type of medium a single strain may at one time give rise to coccobacilli and at another to rods indistinguishable from other coliform bacteria. Capsules are not normally formed, but capsular material has been shown to be formed on a well-aerated medium poor in nitrogen and phosphate. Most *Serratia* strains are motile.

Colonies of *S. marcescens* on agar are usually homogeneous for the first day or two, and then may become differentiated into a convex, pigmented and relatively opaque centre and an effuse, colourless, almost transparent periphery with an irregular crenated edge. Pigment is formed only in the presence of oxygen and at a suitable temperature, which is not necessarily the same as that for optimal growth. Thus, many strains grow best at 30–37°C but form little or no pigment whereas at lower temperatures growth is poorer and pigment formation is abundant.

The red pigment *prodigiosin* is soluble in absolute alcohol and other organic solvents but is insoluble in water. It has been separated into three red fractions and one blue fraction with different absorption spectra. Prodigiosin is also formed by certain organisms unrelated to *S. marcescens*, including an actinomycete, and certain Gram-negative rods from sea water.

Antibiotic susceptibility

Serratia strains, like *Enterobacter* strains, are commonly resistant to cephalosporins. Resistance to ampicillin and gentamicin is variable from strain to strain, but many strains destroy these antibiotics enzymically.

PATHOGENESIS

S. *marcescens* is widely distributed in nature but faecal carriage is uncommon in the general population. Pigmented strains may cause concern by giving rise to red colours in various foods or by simulating the appearance of blood in the sputum or faeces. Pigmented and non-pigmented strains are found occasionally in the human respiratory tract and in faeces. Accounts of human disease due to *S. marcescens* have become increasingly frequent in recent years. Most of the infections occur in hospital patients; they include infections of the urinary and respiratory tracts, meningitis, and wound infections. Septicaemia is common, and endotoxic shock and endocarditis have been reported. Some strains become endemically established in hospitals and outbreaks of infection are also frequently reported. *Serratia* strains are able to multiply at ambient temperatures in fluids containing minimal nutrients and outbreaks have followed the introduction of the organisms directly into the bloodstream in contaminated transfusion fluids. Only a small proportion of the strains responsible for infection are pigmented.

The other *Serratia* species also occur commonly in the natural environment, especially in water, but *S. liquefaciens* and *S. odorifera* are not uncommon in human clinical specimens.

TREATMENT

An aminoglycoside, such as gentamicin, is usually the most reliable first-line choice.

PROTEUS, PROVIDENCIA AND MORGANELLA

CLASSIFICATION

The history of these genera is inextricably linked and they are best considered together. The organism first isolated by Morgan early this century was formerly included in the genus *Proteus* but genetic evidence and enzyme studies show that a separate genus is justified with a single species — *Morganella morganii*. There has been similar debate over the taxonomy of the remaining species in this group with successive proposals to combine and separate the genera *Proteus* and *Providencia*. The organisms once known as biotypes A and B of *Proteus inconstans* are now regarded as separate species of the genus *Providencia: Providencia alcalifaciens* and *Prov. stuartii*. As a result of genetic studies *Proteus rettgeri* has also been transferred to the genus *Providencia* as *Prov. rettgeri*, even though it resembles *Proteus* species rather than other organisms of the genus *Providencia* in producing urease. This leaves only *Pr. vulgaris* and *Pr. mirabilis* in the genus *Proteus*.

DESCRIPTION

Morphological and cultural characters

There is considerable morphological variation but in agar cultures after 24 h the microscopical appearance is much like that of other coliform bacteria with rods $1–3 \times 0.6\ \mu m$. The flagella vary more in shape than most enterobacteria with both normal and 'curly' forms occurring in the same organism.

All these organisms grow well on ordinary nutrient media. A notable property of *Pr. vulgaris* and *Pr. mirabilis* strains is the ability to *swarm* on solid media: the bacterial growth spreads progressively from the edge of the colony and eventually covers the whole surface of the medium. This swarming characteristically takes place in a discontinuous manner with each period of outward progress followed by a stationary period (Fig. 28.2). A number of methods have been devised to inhibit swarming, mainly to avoid interference with the isolation of clinically more important organisms.

Biochemical activities

M. morganii and *Proteus* and *Providencia* species have the almost unique ability to oxidatively de-

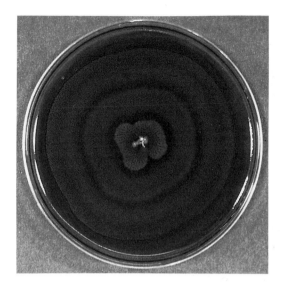

Fig. 28.2 Swarming growth of *Pr. mirabilis* inoculated centrally onto a blood agar plate and incubated overnight at 37°C. (Photograph courtesy of George Sharp and Richard Edwards.)

aminate amino acids, which is tested for by growing the organism in a medium containing phenylalanine, from which phenylpyruvic acid is formed (the PPA test). Some other differential characteristics are shown in Table 28.4.

Typing methods

Phage-, bacteriocin- and serotyping schemes have been developed for *Proteus* and *Providencia* species. Swarming *Proteus* strains exhibit the *Dienes phenomenon* (the mutual inhibition of swarming) and this forms the basis for a precise method of differentiation among such strains. Test organisms are inoculated onto the surface of an agar plate and those that show no line of demarcation in areas where the swarming growths meet are regarded as identical.

Antibiotic susceptibility

Most strains of *Pr. mirabilis* do not produce β-lactamase; they are consequently moderately sensitive to benzylpenicillin and fully sensitive to ampicillin, and most other β-lactam antibiotics. *Pr. vulgaris* strains are usually resistant to peni-

Table 28.4   Some differential biochemical reactions of *Proteus, Providencia* and *Morganella* species

Test	Pr. mirabilis	Pr. vulgaris	Prov. alcalifaciens	Prov. rettgeri	Prov. stuartii	M. morganii
Ornithine decarboxylase	+	−	−	−	−	+
Gas from glucose	+	+	V	−	−	+
H$_2$S production	+	V	−	−	−	−
Indole formation	−	+	+	+	+	+
Urease formation	+	+	−	+	−	+

+, most strains positive; −, most strains negative; V, variable.

cillins and early cephalosporins such as cephaloridine, although they may be sensitive to newer derivatives such as cefotaxime. All strains are resistant to polymyxins while susceptibility to chloramphenicol and tetracycline varies. *Proteus* and *Providencia* strains are inherently sensitive to aminoglycosides but resistance, which may be due to enzymic or non-enzymic mechanisms, is now common.

PATHOGENESIS

Strains of *Pr. mirabilis* are a prominent cause of urinary tract infection in children and in domiciliary practice. Indole-positive *Proteus* and *Providencia* strains are usually seen in hospital patients, especially in elderly males following surgery or instrumentation. Septicaemia generally occurs only in patients with serious underlying conditions or as a complication of urinary tract surgery, but outbreaks of septicaemia, often with meningitis, may occur among the newborn in hospitals. A variety of other infections, usually of surgical wounds or bedsores, occur in hospitals and are usually considered to originate from the gut flora. Urease-producing organisms such as those of the genus *Proteus* may provoke the formation of *calculi* (stones) in the urinary tract.

M. morganii is uncommon in human disease but occasionally causes infections in hospital patients.

TREATMENT

Pr. mirabilis urinary tract infections usually respond to ampicillin or trimethoprim but nitrofurantoin is not effective. Treatment of infection associated with renal stones is often unsuccessful. Serious infection with other *Proteus, Providencia* or *Morganella* strains can often be treated with an aminoglycoside or one of the newer cephalosporins such as cefotaxime. However, susceptibility is unpredictable and treatment should be guided by laboratory findings.

CITROBACTER
DESCRIPTION

The genus *Citrobacter* was first proposed for a group of lactose-negative or late lactose-fermenting coliform bacteria that share certain somatic antigens with salmonellae and were also known as the *Ballerup–Bethesda* group. These organisms are now known as *Citrobacter freundii*. Other species included in the genus are *C. koseri* (known as *C. diversus* in the USA) and *C. amalonaticus* (formerly *Levinea amalonatica*).

Morphological and culture characters

Citrobacter strains grow well on ordinary media, producing smooth, convex colonies 2–4 mm in diameter on nutrient agar. They are not pigmented. Rough or mucoid forms sometimes occur.

Antibiotic susceptibility

C. freundii is usually sensitive to aminoglycosides and chloramphenicol while sensitivity to ampicillin, tetracycline and cephalosporins varies. *C. freundii* strains are commonly resistant to cephaloridine whereas most *C. koseri* strains are sensitive. Resistance to aminoglycosides occurs frequently among *C. koseri* strains.

PATHOGENESIS

Members of the genus *Citrobacter* are often found in the faeces of man and may be isolated from a variety of clinical specimens. They do not often give rise to serious infections. *C. koseri* occasionally causes neonatal meningitis; in this condition there is a high mortality and the formation of cerebral abscesses is common.

OTHER GENERA

ERWINIA HERBICOLA

This anaerogenic, yellow-pigmented organism, known as *Ent. agglomerans* in the USA, is not uncommon in the human upper respiratory tract and in swabs from superficial lesions. It resembles closely organisms that are frequently isolated from plants and soil, some of which are plant pathogens.

This organism is an occasional pathogen in predisposed human patients and may be isolated from upper respiratory tract and urinary tract infections. It has also caused bacteraemia when administered in contaminated intravenous fluids.

EDWARDSIELLA TARDA

E. tarda was first described under the name *Asakusa* to include a group of enterobacteria that appeared to be quite distinct from all others. It grows well on ordinary media but produces only small colonies of 0.5–1 mm diameter after 24 h.

Edwardsiella strains are frequently isolated from healthy cold-blooded animals and their environment. They are pathogenic for eels, catfish and other animals, sometimes causing economic losses. *E. tarda* is an occasional pathogen of man; wound infection is the most common source but meningitis and septicaemia have also been reported. *E. tarda* is rarely found in the faeces of healthy people, but a higher isolation rate has been found in patients with diarrhoea, and the role of the species in the aetiology of diarrhoea requires further study. Human infections with *E. tarda* probably originate from contact with cold-blooded animals.

RECOMMENDED READING

Ewing W H 1986 *Edwards and Ewing's Identification of Enterobacteriaceae*, 4th edn. Elsevier, New York

Farmer J J, Wells H G, Griffin P M, Wachsmuth K I 1987 Enterobacteriaceae infections. In: Wentworth BB (ed), *Diagnostic Procedures for Bacterial Infections*, 7th edn. American Public Health Association, Washington, pp. 233-296

Lund B M, Sussman M, Jones D, Stringer M R (eds) 1988 *Enterobacteriaceae in the Environment and as Pathogens*. Society of Applied Bacteriology Symposium Series No. 17. Blackwell Scientific Publications, Oxford. (Published as a supplement to *Journal of Applied Bacteriology* 65.)

Williams P, Tomas J M 1990 The pathogenicity of *Klebsiella pneumoniae*. *Reviews in Medical Microbiology* 1: 196-204

29

Pseudomonas and non-fermenters

Opportunistic infection; cystic fibrosis; melioidosis

J. R. W. Govan

The genus *Pseudomonas* comprises more than 200 species, mostly saprophytes found widely in soil, water and other moist environments. A few species are pathogenic for plants, insects and animals. *Pseudomonas aeruginosa* is the species most commonly associated with human disease but *Ps. mallei* and *Ps. pseudomallei* are also important pathogens in some parts of the world. Several other species of pseudomonas and a number of other glucose non-fermenters are occasionally isolated from human clinical specimens as opportunistic pathogens. The reasons for the pre-eminent status of *Ps. aeruginosa* as an opportunistic pathogen lie in its adaptability, its innate resistance to many antibiotics and disinfectants, its varied armoury of putative virulence factors, and in an increasing supply of patients compromised by age, underlying disease or immunosuppressive therapy.

PSEUDOMONAS AERUGINOSA

DESCRIPTION

Ps. aeruginosa is a Gram-negative bacillus, non-sporing, non-capsulate, and usually motile by virtue of one or two polar flagella (Fig. 29.1). It is a strict aerobe but can grow anaerobically if nitrate is available. The organism grows readily on a wide variety of culture media over a wide temperature range and emits a sweet grape-like odour that is easily recognized. Most strains of *Ps. aeruginosa* produce diffusible pigments; typically, the colony and surrounding medium is greenish blue due to production of a soluble blue phenazine pigment, *pyocyanin*, and the yellow-green fluorescent pigment *pyoverdin*, which acts as the major siderophore; additional pigments include *pyorubrin* (red) and *melanin* (brown). Some 10–15% of *Ps. aeruginosa* strains readily produce pigment only when grown on pigment-enhancing media. Individual colonies of *Ps. aeruginosa* can occur as five distinct types ranging from dwarf colonies to large mucoid colonies; the most common colonial

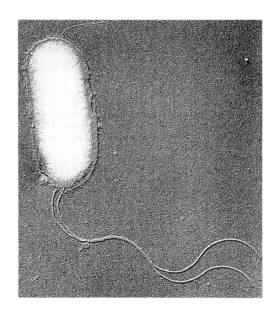

Fig. 29.1 Shadowed electron micrograph of *Ps. aeruginosa* showing two polar flagella and a single polar pilus.

form is relatively large, low-convex with an irregular surface, an edge that is translucent and an oblong shape with the long axis parallel to the line of inoculum.

Ps. aeruginosa differs from members of the Enterobacteriaceae by deriving energy from carbohydrates by an oxidative rather than a fermentative metabolism. In carbohydrate fermentation tests, *Ps. aeruginosa* appears inactive and only glucose is utilized. However, all strains give a positive oxidase reaction and this is a useful preliminary test for non-pigmented strains. Although a few Gram-negative bacilli are also oxidase-positive, none reacts as swiftly as *Ps. aeruginosa*, which gives a positive reaction within 30 s.

For epidemiological purposes, or to confirm the clonal relationship between isolates, *Ps. aeruginosa* can be characterized on the basis of: O and H antigens; sensitivity to sets of bacteriophages; bacteriocin typing; and DNA probes prepared from fragments of the exotoxin A or pilin genes. At present, serotyping and pyocin typing are generally accepted as the most readily usable and reliable methods. Seventeen serotypes based on heat-stable somatic (O) antigens are recognized but, in practice, four or five serotypes account for the majority of strains. Pyocin typing depends on the production of pyocins (bacteriocines) by the strain under investigation; pyocin types of *Ps. aeruginosa* are designated on the basis of the inhibition patterns observed when tested against 13 indicator strains and on the size of the inhibition zones. In this manner at least 105 pyocin types of *Ps. aeruginosa* are recognized.

PATHOGENESIS

Ps. aeruginosa can infect almost any external site or organ. In the community, infections caused by *Ps. aeruginosa* are mostly mild and superficial, e.g. otitis externa and varicose ulcers; such conditions are often chronic, but not disabling. Recreational and occupational conditions associated with susceptibility to pseudomonas infections include Jacuzzi or whirlpool rash (an acute self-limiting folliculitis) and industrial eye injuries, which may lead to panophthalmitis.

In hospitalized patients, pseudomonas infections are more common, more severe and more varied. Infection is usually localized, as in catheter-related urinary tract infection, in infected ulcers, bed sores or burns, and in eye infections. In patients compromised by age, or immuno-suppressing diseases such as leukaemia, and in those treated with immunosuppressive drugs or corticosteroids, pseudomonas infections frequently become generalized and the organism may be cultured from the blood or from many organs of the body post-mortem. *Ps. aeruginosa* is not a major cause of Gram-negative septicaemia or necrotizing pneumonia but is associated with high mortality in these conditions. The lungs of children with cystic fibrosis are very susceptible to infection with *Ps. aeruginosa*. In these patients, asymptomatic pulmonary colonization with typical non-mucoid forms of *Ps. aeruginosa* eventually leads to the emergence of mucoid variants (Fig. 29.2); debilitating episodes of pulmonary exacerbation due to mucoid *Ps. aeruginosa* are the major cause of morbidity and mortality in cystic fibrosis.

Most strains of *Ps. aeruginosa* produce two exotoxins, exotoxin A and exo-enzyme S, and a variety of cytotoxic substances including proteases, phospholipase, pyocyanin and rhamnolipids; an alginate-like exopolysaccharide is responsible for the mucoid phenotype (Fig. 29.3). The importance of these putative virulence factors depends upon the site and nature of infection: proteases play a key role in corneal ulceration; exotoxin and proteases are important in burn infection; and phospholipases, proteases and alginate are associated with chronic pulmonary colonization.

LABORATORY DIAGNOSIS

Ps. aeruginosa grows on most common culture media. If specific investigation for *Ps. aeruginosa* is desired, material should be cultured on a medium such as *Pseudomonas* isolation agar (Difco), which is both selective and enhances the production of the characteristic blue-green pigment pyocyanin. If *Ps. aeruginosa* is sought in aqueous environments or soil, then enrichment media containing acetamide as the sole carbon and nitrogen source

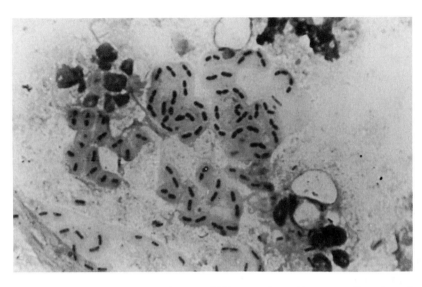

Fig. 29.2 Gram-stained sputum from patient harbouring mucoid *Ps. aeruginosa*. Note spawn-like microcolony and adjacent phagocytes.

may be used before culture on *Pseudomonas* isolation agar. Resultant colonies are usually easily identified. About 10% of *Ps. aeruginosa* isolates do not produce readily detectable pigment even on suitable media; in such cases an oxidase test should be performed and, if positive, further identification should be carried out with an appropriate multitest system. If the result is equivocal, production of pyocins is a useful confirmation of identity. Except in patients with chronic obstructive airway diseases, tests for serum antibodies have no place in diagnosis.

TREATMENT

Strains of *Ps. aeruginosa* are normally intrinsically resistant to most commonly employed antimicrobial agents. Before the introduction of the first antipseudomonal β-lactam agent, carbenicillin, in the 1960s, pseudomonas infections were usually treated with polymyxins, agents that exhibit considerable toxicity. With the development of more potent β-lactam compounds, such as ticarcillin and azlocillin, and the discovery of antipseudomonal aminoglycosides like gentamicin and tobramycin, treatment with a combination of an aminoglycoside and a penicillin was commonly adopted. Such a combination possesses the potential advantage of antibacterial synergy, although there is no convincing clinical evidence of the superiority of combined therapy, and the newer, broad-spectrum β-lactam agents such as ceftazidime and imipenem are often used alone.

Each of the agents mentioned so far has to be administered parenterally, but the fluoroquinolones of the ciprofloxacin type can also be given by mouth and this may be an advantage if therapy has to be prolonged. Ciprofloxacin exhibits good activity against *Ps. aeruginosa* and penetrates well into most tissues. It has been successfully used in pseudomonas infection, but resistance sometimes emerges during therapy.

Passive vaccination may be useful for the treatment of septicaemia and burn infections due to *Ps. aeruginosa* which are associated with high mortality; active vaccination to prevent pulmonary colonization would be highly desirable for patients with cystic fibrosis and a polysaccharide-based vaccine is under clinical trial at the time of writing.

Ps. aeruginosa is resistant to, and may multiply in, many of the disinfectants and antiseptics commonly used in hospitals. It can be a troublesome contaminant in pharmaceutical preparations and may cause ophthalmitis following the faulty chemical 'sterilization' of contact lenses.

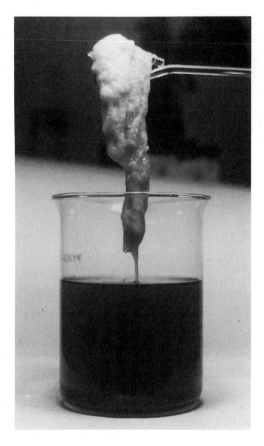

Fig. 29.3 Alcohol extraction of alginate from mucoid *Ps. aeruginosa.*

EPIDEMIOLOGY

Ps. aeruginosa can be isolated from a wide variety of environmental sources and is a competent and hardy saprophyte. The ability of the species to persist and multiply, particularly in moist environments, and on moist equipment (e.g. humidifiers) in hospital wards, bathrooms and kitchens, is of particular importance in cross-infection control. Consumption of salad vegetables contaminated with pseudomonas is a potential risk for immunocompromised patients in intensive care units.

Most hospital-acquired infections with *Ps. aeruginosa* originate from exogenous sources but some patients suffer endogenous infection, particularly of the urinary tract. Healthy carriers of *Ps. aeruginosa* usually harbour strains in the gastro-intestinal tract, but in the open community the carriage rate seldom exceeds 10%. In contrast, acquisition of *Ps. aeruginosa* in a hospital is rapid and up to 30% of patients may excrete the organisms within 2 days of admission.

Epidemics of pseudomonas infection in newborn and young infants in maternity units and paediatric wards are not uncommon. The ability of *Ps. aeruginosa* to survive, and occasionally to flourish, in many supposedly antiseptic or disinfectant solutions explains the method of spread in some of these episodes. In one large maternity unit 71 cases of infection, including gastroenteritis and eye infections, suddenly occurred among infants in a period of 5 weeks. Only babies that were artificially fed were affected and *Ps. aeruginosa* was cultured from milk feeds immediately before use. Investigation showed that although the milk and the bottles had been adequately sterilized, rubber bungs used to close the bottles had been stored in a solution of antiseptic. The epidemic strain of *Ps. aeruginosa* was isolated from the stored bungs. Heat sterilization of the fully prepared and treated milk feeds terminated the epidemic.

Burned patients are another category especially at risk from *Ps. aeruginosa*; the presence of the organism in ward air, dust and in eschar shed from the burns suggests that infection can be airborne. However, contact spread has been demonstrated and is probably now more important than the airborne route with the use of effective topical agents for prophylaxis and treatment of burn and wound infection. Transmission may occur directly via the hands of medical staff, or indirectly via contaminated apparatus. Severely burned patients and those with chest injuries who require artificial ventilation are very susceptible to *Ps. aeruginosa*; pulmonary infection not infrequently precedes septicaemia, which is associated with high mortality. Modern intensive care equipment can be difficult to clean and there is little doubt that infection can be spread by this source.

Eye infection may result from contaminated contact lenses, or from installation of pseudomonas-contaminated medicament during ophthalmic procedures. Similarly, in the early days of North Sea oil exploration, diving operations had occasionally to be aborted because of outbreaks of troublesome ear infection due to *Ps. aeruginosa*. The organism thrives in the conditions of high humidity and poor sanitation associated with prolonged saturation diving, even in the helium-rich atmosphere of the diving bell. Moreover, the low-level pain normally associated with otitis externa is particularly intense under conditions of saturation diving and is exacerbated by the need for lengthy periods of decompression. The warm, moist and aerated conditions under which *Ps. aeruginosa* thrives are ideally met in poorly maintained whirlpools or Jacuzzis. An irritating folliculitis known as *Jacuzzi rash* is a typical example of an opportunistic pseudomonas infection that may be acquired from such a source.

CONTROL

Prevention is easier than cure; once *Ps. aeruginosa* has gained access to the hospital environment, or has established infection, it is notoriously difficult to eradicate. Four guide-lines to control infection are offered in the knowledge that it is not always easy to put them into practice:

1. Patients at a high risk of acquiring infection with *Ps. aeruginosa* (e.g. a patient being evaluated for renal or heart–lung transplantation) should not be admitted to a ward where cases of pseudomonas infection are present.
2. A patient infected with *Ps. aeruginosa* should, if at all possible, be isolated until the infection has been eradicated.
3. Strict infection control measures should be followed by all medical and nursing staff handling patients. All instruments and apparatus, dressings, etc. must be not only clean but sterile. Antimicrobial and other therapeutic substances and solutions must be free from bacteria; a particular danger exists when multidose ointments, creams or eye drops are used to treat several individuals over a period. Initially, the preparation may be sterile but contamination can easily occur between uses, and *Ps. aeruginosa* can multiply readily at a range of temperatures in many medicaments.
4. In hospital units, episodes of cross-infection due to a single strain of *Ps. aeruginosa* may occur as sporadic infections in individual patients over

a considerable period of months or years. For this reason, if facilities are available, it is advantageous to monitor all clinically relevant isolates of *Ps. aeruginosa* by a suitable typing system to identify epidemic strains.

PSEUDOMONAS MALLEI AND PS. PSEUDOMALLEI

These organisms were previously assigned to various genera, including *Bacillus* and *Loefflerella*, but are now considered to belong to the genus *Pseudomonas*. *Ps. mallei* is an animal parasite occasionally transmitted to man whereas *Ps. pseudomallei* is a free-living organism that can infect an animal or human host. Laboratory-acquired infection with these organisms is a hazard; both species are categorized as category A pathogens and must be handled with great care and under strictly designated conditions.

Both species are easily cultured. *Ps. pseudomallei* produces a characteristic wrinkled colonial appearance after several days of growth on nutrient agar; fresh cultures emit a characteristic pungent odour of putrefaction. Both organisms are oxidase-positive but neither species produces diffusible pigment. *Ps. mallei* is invariably non-motile.

GLANDERS

Glanders is a disease of horses caused by *Ps. mallei*. It is nowadays restricted to Asia, Africa and the Middle East. Guinea-pigs are highly susceptible to infection; if an inoculation is made intraperitoneally into a male guinea-pig, the tunica vaginalis is rapidly invaded by the bacilli and swelling of the testes results (*Straus reaction*). The infected animals die within a few days of inoculation and generalized lesions can be seen at necropsy.

Glanders, in the natural host, is associated with a profuse catarrhal discharge from the nose, and the nasal septum shows nodule formation; later in the disease the nodules break down with the production of irregular ulcers. When infection occurs in superficial lymph vessels and nodes following infection through the skin — e.g. via abrasions caused by a rubbing harness — the clinical term *farcy* is used to describe the infection. The lymph vessels show irregular thickening, become corded and are termed *farcy pipes*. Humans may become infected via skin abrasions or wounds which come into contact with the discharges of a sick animal.

MELIOIDOSIS

Melioidosis is a tropical disease of animals and humans that is endemic in South-East Asia and northern Australia. The causative organism, *Ps. pseudomallei*, is found in soil and surface water in rice paddies and monsoon drains; the isolation rates are highest during the rainy season and in still rather than flowing water. Human infection is mainly acquired cutaneously through skin abrasions or by inhalation of contaminated particles. In humans the clinical manifestations range from a subclinical infection, diagnosed by the presence of specific antibodies, to a benign pulmonary infection that may resemble tuberculosis, or to a fulminating septicaemia with a mortality rate of 80–90%. Virtually every organ can be affected and hence melioidosis has been called the 'great imitator' of every infectious disease. Melioidosis commonly presents as pyrexia and, in endemic areas, serological testing for *Ps. pseudomallei* is important in the evaluation of pyrexia of unknown origin. *Ps. pseudomallei* can survive intracellularly within elements of the reticuloendothelial system and this ability may account for latency and the emergence of symptoms many years after exposure. Suppurative parotitis is a characteristic presentation of melioidosis in children.

Early diagnosis and appropriate antibiotic therapy are key factors in the successful management of melioidosis. The organism may be observed, usually in very small numbers, as small, bipolarstained Gram-negative bacilli in exudates and may be isolated from sputum, urine, pus or blood. Enzyme-linked immunosorbent assay (ELISA) for the detection of specific IgG and IgM antibody to *Ps. pseudomallei*, as well as an indirect haemagglutination test for serum immunoglobulin antibody, are useful serological screening tests in the investigation of subclinical melioidosis. Combinations of antimicrobial agents such as tetra-cycline and chloramphenicol have been standard therapy in the treatment of melioidosis; prolonged treatment is necessary to avoid relapse. The ability of *Ps. pseudomallei* to survive and multiply in phagocytes may be the cause of the difficulty of treating melioidosis in spite of the fact that antibiotics are effective against the organism in vitro and the frequent recurrences when the duration of treatment is not long enough. Of the newer agents, ceftazidime is especially effective in vitro.

GLUCOSE NON-FERMENTERS

A small but increasing percentage of clinically relevant Gram-negative bacilli belong to pseudomonas species other than those already discussed. This group includes *Ps. cepacia*, *Ps. maltophilia* (*Xanthomonas maltophilia*), *Ps. putida*, *Ps. fluorescens* and *Ps. stutzeri*. In addition, there is a group of bacteria that are commonly referred to as glucose-non-fermenters that are taxonomically distinct from the carbohydrate-fermenting Enterobacteriaceae and the oxidative members of the genus *Pseudomonas*. The clinical relevance of non-fermenters is based on their role as opportunistic pathogens in hospital-acquired infections and their intrinsic resistance to many antimicrobial agents. Glucose non-fermenters comprise a heterogeneous group of species and none requires specific cultural conditions. Unequivocal identification may be difficult as most species are relatively inert in the biochemical tests used in identification of Gram-negative bacteria. Tests for motility and oxidase production are useful and identification is assisted by computer-based probabilistic methods or multi-test identification systems.

SPECIES OTHER THAN *PSEUDOMONAS*

Eikenella corrodens is a commensal of mucosal surfaces which may cause a range of infections, in particular endocarditis, meningitis, pneumonia and infections of wounds and various soft tissues.

Flavobacterium meningosepticum is a saprophyte whose natural habitat is soil and moist environments, including nebulizers; it may cause opportunistic nosocomial infections, particularly in infants. As the name suggests, this species is associated with meningitis and has been responsible for high mortality in epidemic outbreaks.

Moraxella lacunata and *M. phenylpyruvica* are commensals of mucosal membranes but may give rise to opportunistic infections.

Acinetobacter calcoaceticus is a saprophytic species found in soil and aquatic environments, including sewage, and occasionally as a commensal of moist areas of human skin. The most important hospital-acquired infections associated with the two subspecies *A. calcoaceticus* ssp. *anitratus* and *A.* *calcoaceticus* ssp. *lwoffi* include pneumonia and other infections of the upper respiratory tract.

Two other genera of Gram-negative bacteria, *Alcaligenes* and *Achromobacter*, are often included among non-fermenters. They may be confused with *Pseudomonas* species. Like other non-fermenters, they are saprophytes found in moist environments in nature and in the hospital environment, and are associated with a range of hospital-acquired opportunistic infections, including septicaemia and ear discharges.

RECOMMENDED READING

Dance D A B 1991 Melioidosis: the tip of the iceberg? *Clinical Microbiology Reviews* 4: 52–60

Govan J R W 1988 Alginate biosynthesis and other unusual characteristics associated with the pathogenesis of *Pseudomonas aeruginosa* in cystic fibrosis. In: Donachie W, Griffiths E, Stephen J (eds) *Bacterial Infections of Respiratory and Gastrointestinal Mucosae*. IRL Press, Oxford, pp 67–96

Holmes B, Pinning C A, Dawson C A 1986 A probability matrix for the identification of Gram-negative aerobic, nonfermentative bacteria that grow on nutrient agar.

Journal of General Microbiology 132: 1827–1842

Leelarasemee A, Bovornkitti S 1989 Melioidosis: review and update. *Reviews of Infectious Diseases* 11: 413–415

Vasil M L 1986 *Pseudomonas aeruginosa*: biology, mechanisms of virulence, epidemiology. *Journal of Pediatrics* 105: 800–805

von Graevenitz A 1978 Clinical role of infrequently encountered nonfermenters. In: Gilardi G L (ed) *Glucose Nonfermenting Gram-negative Bacteria in Clinical Microbiology*. CRC Press, Boca Raton, pp 119–153

chickens are almost certainly the most important single source of human infection in developed countries. However, as there would have to be gross undercooking for campylobacters to survive as far as the dinner plate, most infections are probably acquired from other foods, such as bread and salads, that become cross-contaminated from the raw bird in the kitchen. Other raw meats and offal may also be a source of campylobacters in the kitchen, but to a lesser extent than poultry.

Outbreaks

Fortunately, the fastidious nature of campylobacters ensures that they do not multiply in food standing at room temperature, so large outbreaks of food poisoning do not occur. On the other hand, the distribution of untreated water and raw milk have given rise to major outbreaks of campylobacter enteritis affecting several thousand people.

Figure 30.3 portrays the principal sources and routes of transmission of campylobacters to man.

CONTROL

The wide distribution of campylobacters in nature precludes any possibility of reducing the reservoir of infection. To interrupt transmission the proper purification of water and heat treatment of milk are obvious and basic measures. The control of infection in broiler chickens is also highly desirable, though not yet possible; gamma irradiation of broiler carcasses is another possibility. Public education on basic hygiene in food handling, particularly the need to wash hands and utensils

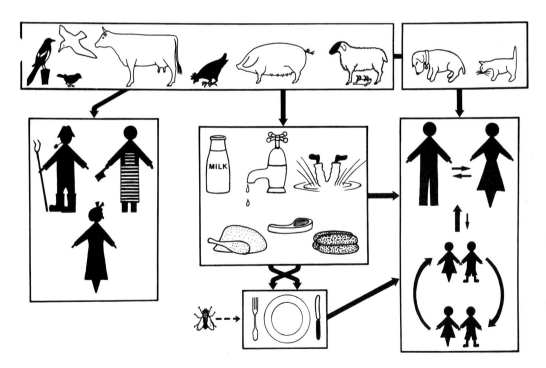

Fig. 30.3 Sources and transmission of *C. jejuni* and *C. coli*. Top boxes: animal reservoirs and sources of infection (the sheep has just given birth to a dead campylobacter-infected lamb). Left-hand box: transmission by direct contact — occupational (farmer, butcher, poultry processor). Right-hand box: transmission by direct contact — domestic (puppy or kitten with campylobacter diarrhoea; person-to-person spread under conditions of poor hygiene). Central box: indirect transmission through consumption of untreated water, raw milk, raw/undercooked meat and poultry, food cross-contaminated from raw meats and poultry; transmission by flies unproven. (Reproduced by permission of the World Health Organization.)

between handling raw meats and other foods, should be promulgated energetically.

HELICOBACTER

The discovery in 1983 of *H. pylori* (formerly *C. pylori* or *C. pyloridis*) overturned several traditionally held beliefs about gastric physiology and pathology. The human stomach was not supposed to have a resident bacterial flora, yet *H. pylori* colonizes the gastric mucosa of at least one in four of the adult population and appears to be an important, perhaps essential, factor in the pathogenesis of peptic ulceration. Moreover, gastric urease, which was thought to be intrinsic, is now known to be produced by *H. pylori*.

DESCRIPTION

H. pylori is a Gram-negative spirally shaped bacterium, 0.5–1.0 μm wide by about 3 μm long. Like the campylobacters, it is strictly microaerophilic and it requires carbon dioxide for growth, but it has a tuft of sheathed polar flagella, unlike the single unsheathed polar flagellum of campylobacters (Fig. 30.1). It is biochemically inactive in most conventional tests, but it produces an exceptionally powerful urease, almost 100 times more active than that of *Proteus vulgaris*. It undergoes coccal transformation even more rapidly than *C. jejuni* when exposed to adverse conditions.

The antimicrobial sensitivities of *H. pylori* are similar to those of campylobacters, notably resistance to trimethoprim and sensitivity to nitroimidazoles. *H. pylori* is sensitive to penicillin, most other β-lactam antibiotics, and bismuth compounds, which are valuable for the treatment of infection (see below).

H. mustelae is a closely related species that colonizes the stomach of ferrets.

PATHOGENESIS

H. pylori is a highly adapted organism that lives only on gastric mucosa. Most infections are symptomless, and endoscopic appearances of the stomach are usually normal, but colonization is associated with histological gastritis of the type known as chronic active or type B gastritis (not to be confused with type A atrophic auto-immune gastritis of pernicious anaemia). There is some evidence that the gastritis can cause non-ulcer dyspepsia, but the more important issue is whether it predisposes to peptic ulceration.

The course of infection

Little is known of the early stages of infection, but it seems that after an incubation period of a few days, patients suffer a mild attack of acute achlorhydric gastritis with symptoms of abdominal pain, nausea, flatulence and bad breath. This may resolve spontaneously, with simultaneous disappearance of the organism, but in many patients infection persists, usually with chronic active gastritis. Such patients may remain hypochlorhydric for as long as 12 months, but gastric acidity eventually returns to normal. It is not known whether infection is permanent, burns itself out to leave atrophic gastritis, or eventually resolves spontaneously.

Site of infection

The gastric antrum is the site most favoured by *H. pylori* but any part of the stomach may be colonized. The bacteria are present in large numbers in the mucus overlying the mucosa where the pH is about 7.0 (they are not acid-tolerant). Colonization often extends into gastric glands, but they do not invade the mucosa (Fig. 30.4). Colonization ceases abruptly where gastric mucosa ends, e.g. in areas of intestinal metaplasia in the stomach. Conversely, areas of gastric metaplasia elsewhere in the gut, notably the duodenum, may become colonized with *H. pylori*.

The mucosa underlying areas of colonization may be normal, but more often than not foveolar cells are damaged and there is gastritis. The presence of polymorphonuclear leucocytes is characteristic of the gastritis, hence the description chronic *active* gastritis. There is little doubt that *H. pylori* causes the gastritis. Its association with the lesions is close, its elimination by antibiotics results in resolution of the gastritis, and experimental infection reproduced the lesions in two volunteers.

Peptic ulceration

Type B gastritis of the stomach antrum and *H. pylori* are present in virtually all patients with duodenal ulceration and most with gastric ulceration. There is good evidence that colonization with *H. pylori* is a prerequisite for the primary development of duodenal ulceration. However, as only a small minority of colonized patients develop ulceration, other factors must also operate. The most telling evidence of the importance of *H. pylori* in the pathogenesis of peptic ulceration is that healed ulcers are less likely to recur in patients who have been cleared of *H. pylori* by antimicrobial therapy.

There are several reasons why *H. pylori* might predispose to ulceration. One theory is that the ammonia produced by the metabolism of urea by its powerful urease causes ionic changes in the mucus layer, which in turn cause back-diffusion of hydrogen ions in the mucosa. A mucus-degrading protease produced by the organism may also play a part in pathogenesis.

LABORATORY DIAGNOSIS
Microscopy

H. pylori was seen in histological sections long before it was cultured, and microscopy remains as sensitive a method as any in experienced hands. Warthin–Starry silver staining, as used for legionella bacteria, shows the organisms most clearly (Fig. 30.4), but many less complex staining methods are satisfactory. The bacteria are barely visible in haemotoxylin and eosin-stained sections. They can be seen in freshly made smears of biopsy material examined either wet by dark-ground or phase-contrast microscopy, or dried and stained with Gram's stain.

Culture

Biopsy specimens of gastric mucosa, preferably from the antrum, are needed for successful cul-

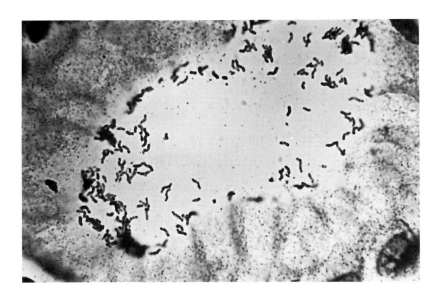

Fig. 30.4   Section of gastric mucosa showing colonization with *H. pylori*. × 1400. Warthin–Starry silver stain. (Photomicrograph by Mr G.H. Green, Worcester Royal Infirmary.)

ture. Specimens must be kept moist and must not be more than 2 h old. Most strains of *H. pylori* will grow on Skirrow's campylobacter-selective agar, which is best used in conjunction with a non-selective medium. Plates are incubated at 37°C in the same atmosphere as used for campylobacters. High humidity is essential, so it is best not to dry plates before inoculating them. They should be left undisturbed for 3 d and incubated for a week before being discarded as negative. *H. pylori* forms discrete domed colonies unlike the effuse colonies of *C. jejuni* and *C. coli*.

Biopsy urease test

H. pylori produces such abundant urease that it is detectable in biopsy material without having to grow the organism. Biopsy tissue is put into a small quantity of urea solution with an indicator; if *H. pylori* is present the pH changes, within a few minutes to 2 h, from acid to alkaline because of the formation of ammonia. The test can be done in the clinic while the patient is still in attendance.

Urea breath test

This test has the merit of being non-invasive. Urea containing an isotope of carbon (carbon-14 or -13) is fed to the patient and the emission of the isotope as carbon dioxide in the breath is measured. Patients infected with *H. pylori* give high readings of the isotope because of the breakdown of urea to carbon dioxide (and ammonia) through the action of the urease. The disadvantages of the test are that carbon-14 is radioactive, and carbon-13, though not radioactive, can be measured only with a mass spectrometer, which is too costly for general use.

Serology

An ELISA can be used to detect antibodies to *H. pylori* or its urease. Their presence correlates well with colonization; titres fall over several months if infection is eradicated.

TREATMENT

The treatment of *H. pylori* infection is relevant only in relation to peptic ulceration, and some gastro-enterologists question even this. Healed ulcers are less likely to recur in patients in whom *H. pylori* has been eradicated, but there is no simple and effective treatment that will guarantee eradication.

The mainstay of treatment is colloidal bismuth in the form of the subcitrate or subsalicylate, which exerts a direct contact action on the bacteria. Used alone it causes temporary disappearance of the organism, but relapse is common. *H. pylori* is sensitive in vitro to a number of antibiotics, but only those that are acid-stable and can penetrate gastric mucus have any effect in vivo. Best results so far have been obtained with a combination of colloidal bismuth, amoxycillin and metronidazole.

EPIDEMIOLOGY

H. pylori infection rates increase with age. In developed countries infection is rare in childhood but by the age of 60 years at least half the population is colonized. In developing countries infection arises early in childhood and many children are infected by the time they reach puberty. People living in close contact with one another have especially high rates of infection.

This pattern suggests that infection is spread by personal contact, though the route is unknown. Although *H. pylori*-like organisms are found in other animals, typical strains have been found only in human beings and other primates. Clearly, nothing can be done to control infection until we know how infection is spread.

GASTROSPIRILLUM HOMINIS

Gastrospirillum hominis was first described in 1989 in patients with chronic active gastritis. It is much less common than *H. pylori* and its clinical significance is unknown. It is more tightly spiralled than *H. pylori* and it has bipolar tufts of up to 12 sheathed flagella. Although it has not been cultured in vitro, it produces sufficient urease to give a positive biopsy urease test. Similar bacteria are common in the stomachs of cats and other animals.

raw shellfish. It is thought that the organisms enter the bloodstream by way of the portal vein or the intestinal lymph system. Elderly males with liver function defects due to alcohol abuse are particularly susceptible but any deficiency in the immune system may also be a contributing factor.

2. A rapidly progressing cellulitis following contamination of a wound sustained during exposure to a saline aquatic environment. Infections of this kind occur in otherwise healthy persons as well as in the debilitated and are characterized by wound oedema, erythema and necrosis which only occasionally progresses to septicaemia. The infection can be rapidly fatal.

3. Acute diarrhoea following the consumption of shellfish. This is less common; victims generally have mildly debilitating underlying conditions. Mortality is rare.

There have also been rare reports of meningitis and pulmonary infection.

Virulence is closely associated with the presence of a polysaccharide capsule that probably contributes to the ability to resist phagocytosis and the killing effects of human serum. Virulent strains are able to use transferrin-bound iron, but not at the level of transferrin saturation normally found in man. This may explain the association of infection with pre-existing liver or other disorders that may result in elevated serum iron levels.

Strains of *V. vulnificus* produce several toxins that may contribute to tissue damage. They include a collagenase and cytolytic and proteolytic substances. A vascular permeability factor has also been described.

VIBRIO ALGINOLYTICUS

Description

Strains of *V. alginolyticus* were previously regarded as biotype 2 of *V. parahaemolyticus*. The organism is halophilic; it fails to grow on CLED agar but grows in the presence of 10% sodium chloride. It grows well on TCBS, forming large, yellow (sucrose-fermenting) colonies. There is pronounced swarming on non-selective solid media.

Pathogenesis

V. alginolyticus is only weakly pathogenic. Most infections are of wounds and are opportunistic and self-limiting. Clinical features include mild cellulitis and a seropurulent exudate. The pathogenic mechanism is unknown.

Epidemiology

This organism is widely distributed in sea-water and seafood and is probably the most common vibrio found in these sources in the UK. It occurs in large numbers throughout the year. Infections are invariably associated with exposure to saline aquatic environments.

OTHER VIBRIOS

V. damsela is a recently described halophilic, aerogenic marine vibrio found in tropical and semi-tropical aquatic environments. It is associated with severe infections of wounds acquired in warm coastal areas.

Strains of *V. fluvialis* were previously known as group F vibrios or as EF-6. Strains of one of the two biotypes are now regarded as a separate species, *V. furnissii*. Both species are easily confused with *Aeromonas hydrophila* because of their superficial phenotypic similarities.

V. fluvialis was first recognized as a cause of diarrhoeal disease in the late 1970s and a significant outbreak was reported in Bangladesh in 1980. Patients experienced diarrhoea, abdominal pain, fever and dehydration. *V. fluvialis* can be isolated in low numbers from fish and shellfish, and from seawater in areas where this is warm. Epidemiological studies are few but it seems likely that infection is from contaminated seafood.

V. hollisae has been associated with bacteraemia and diarrhoea, especially in the USA in areas where the sea water is warm, such as the Gulf of Mexico. Infections are strongly associated with the consumption of raw seafood. *V. hollisae* is unique in possessing gene sequences homologous with those encoding the thermostable direct haemolysin of *V. parahaemolyticus*.

V. mimicus occurs in similar environments to *V. cholerae* and has been isolated from a variety of infections. Most isolates are from the stools of patients who develop gastro-enteritis after consumption of raw oysters, although a few ear infections have also been reported.

Other aquatic organisms that are probably related to vibrios include *Aeromonas* spp. and *Plesiomonas shigelloides*. *Aeromonas* spp., notably *A. hydrophila*, have been debatably implicated in diarrhoea and occasionally cause more serious infection in compromised individuals. *A. salmonicida* is an economically important pathogen of fish. *P. shigelloides* is an organism of uncertain taxonomic status that sometimes causes water-borne outbreaks of diarrhoea in warm countries.

MOBILUNCUS

The name *Mobiluncus* was first proposed for a group of curved, motile, Gram-variable, anaerobic bacteria isolated from the vagina of women with bacterial vaginosis. Although the genus was first placed tentatively in the family *Bacteroidaceae* its taxonomic position is uncertain. Recent studies of 16S RNA suggest that the genus *Mobiluncus* belongs to the order *Actinomycetales* in which it is most closely related to the genus *Actinomyces*.

Description

There are two species, *M. curtisii* and *M. mulieris*. The former is short (mean length 1.5 µm, range 0.8–2.5 µm) and Gram-variable while the latter is long (mean length 3.0 µm, range 1.9–4.2 µm) and Gram-negative. Both species have multiple flagella originating from the concave aspect of the cells. Cell wall studies show that there is no outer membrane and, although the cell wall is thinner than that of most Gram-positive organisms, it is generally considered that both species are Gram-positive. Two subspecies have been proposed for *M. curtisii*, spp. *curtisii* and *holmesii*. The differential characteristics of these species and subspecies are shown in Table 31.3.

Epidemiology, pathogenesis and treatment

The clinical condition previously known as non-specific vaginitis and more recently described as bacterial vaginosis is characterized by the presence of a thin, homogeneous vaginal discharge with a characteristic 'rotten fish' smell. This becomes more pronounced on alkalization, and can be evoked by placing a drop of potassium hydroxide solution on the fresh exudate on a slide or the speculum used for the vaginal examination. In addition, 'clue cells' (epithelial cells covered with bacteria) can be seen in fresh unstained smears and there is a raised vaginal pH (>4.5). The characteristic smell is ascribed to amines which are assumed to be produced by one or more of the bacterial species that form the complex microbial flora of the vagina.

The microbiology of bacterial vaginosis is complex. For some time it was believed that *Gardnerella vaginalis* (formerly *Corynebacterium vaginale*

Table 31.3 Differential characteristics of *Mobiluncus* species

Characteristic	*M. curtisii* ssp *curtisii*	*M. curtisii* ssp *holmesii*	*M. mulieris*
Mean cell length (µm)	1.5	1.5	3.0
Gram stain reaction	V	V	–
NH_4^+ from arginine	+	+	–
Hippurate hydrolysis	+	+	–
CAMP reaction	W	W	S
Produces >1 mEq acetate per 100 ml	–	–	+
Acid (pH<5.5) from glycogen	–	–	+
Acid (pH<6.0) from melibiose	+(–)	–(+)	–
Nitrate reduction	–	+	–(+)
Migration through soft agar	+	–	V
Susceptibility to metronidazole	Resistant	Resistant	sensitive

+ (–), usually positive; – (+), usually negative; V, variable; S, strong; W, weak.

or *Haemophilus vaginalis*) was the only aetiological agent. This is a micro-aerophilic, pleomorphic, Gram-variable rod of uncertain taxonomic status. More recent evidence suggests a polymicrobial cause for vaginosis with certain organisms playing a key role, especially when they overgrow the lactobacilli of the normal flora. In most studies *Mobiluncus* species have been isolated from only 10–50% of women with bacterial vaginosis, but this almost certainly underestimates the prevalence of these fastidious and slow-growing organisms. By use of DNA probes, *Mobiluncus* species have been found in the vaginal secretions of over 80% of women with vaginosis but are demonstrated only rarely in women without vaginosis. *Mobiluncus* are frequently found in association with *G. vaginalis* and with other organisms that may also be of aetiological importance. It appears that both the combination of species and their relative numbers are of importance in the development of the syndrome.

Although *Mobiluncus* species do not appear to be particularly invasive there are several reports of their isolation from extra-genital sites, especially from breast abscesses.

Both *Mobiluncus* species are susceptible to most antimicrobial agents, including benzylpenicillin, clindamycin, erythromycin and gentamicin. *M. mulieris* is more susceptible than *M. curtisii*, to metronidazole, but treatment with metronidazole appears to eliminate *Mobiluncus* species in patients with vaginosis, suggesting that other anaerobic species that are susceptible to metronidazole may be important for the multiplication of *Mobiluncus* species. Penicillins are appropriate drugs for the treatment of infection by *Mobiluncus* species.

'SPIRILLUM MINUS'

The organism commonly known as *Spirillum minus*, one of the causes of rat-bite fever in man, is of uncertain taxonomic position. It was once regarded as a spirochaete but was later placed in the genus *Spirillum*. According to the 8th edition of Bergey's Manual it does not belong to the genera *Spirillum*, *Oceanospirillum* or *Aquaspirillum* and it is therefore regarded as a *species incertae sedis*.

Description

S. minus is a short, spiral, Gram-negative organism about 2–5 μm in length and 0.2 μm in diameter. Longer forms up to 10 μm may be observed. The regular short coils have a wavelength of 0.8–1.0 μm. The organisms are very actively motile, showing darting movements like those of a vibrio. The movement is due to polar flagella which vary in number from one to seven at each pole. The organisms can be demonstrated in fresh specimens by dark-ground illumination or by staining with Leishman's or other stains. Although there have been many unconfirmed claims the organism has not been cultivated on artificial media and many of its properties are therefore unknown.

Laboratory diagnosis

In rat-bite fever *S. minus* may be demonstrated in the local lesion, the regional lymph glands, or in the blood, either by direct microscopical methods or by animal inoculation. Guinea-pigs, white rats and mice are susceptible to infection and the organism may be detected by microscopy in the peripheral blood following intraperitoneal challenge.

Epidemiology, pathogenesis and treatment

S. minus occurs naturally in wild rats and other rodents, causing bacteraemia. The clinical syndrome of rat-bite fever begins with an acute onset of fever and chills 1–4 weeks after the animal bite. The rodent bite usually heals before the onset of symptoms but it often re-ulcerates. Local lymphadenopathy and lymphangitis develop with the onset of fever and systemic disease. A generalized rash with large brown to purple macules is usually observed, but some patients present with urticarial lesions. A roseolar rash may spread from the area of the original bite. Fever usually declines within 1 week before returning again after a few days; the fever may then recur in an episodic fashion for months or even years. Endocarditis, meningitis, hepatitis, nephritis and myocarditis are rare complications. In most untreated cases, symptoms resolve within 2 months after six to eight episodes of fever, although up to 6.5% of untreated cases may be fatal. This form of rat-bite fever occurs mainly in Japan and the Far East and is known as *sodoku*. Cases have been diagnosed, however, in other parts of Asia and in Europe and the USA.

S. minus infections respond to treatment with antibiotics, including penicillin and tetracyclines. In the rare case of endocarditis the addition of an aminoglycoside may be of value.

RECOMMENDED READING

Hammann R 1989 Newly recovered and delineated microbial species of the human genital tract. *Infection* 17: 188–193

Janda J M, Powers C, Bryant R G, Abbott S L 1988 Current perspectives on the epidemiology and pathogenesis of clinically significant Vibrio spp. *Clinical Microbiology Reviews* 1: 245–267

Jenkins S G 1988 Rat-bite fever. *Clinical Microbiology Newsletter* 10: 57–59

Lassnig C, Dorsch M, Wolters J et al 1989 Phylogenetic evidence of the relationship between the genera Mobiluncus and Actinomyces. *FEMS Microbiology Letters* 65: 17–21

Sturm A W 1989 Mobiluncus species and other anaerobic bacteria in non-puerperal breast abscesses. *European Journal of Clinical Microbiology and Infectious Diseases* 8: 789–792

Tison D L, Kelly M T 1984 Vibrio species of medical importance. *Diagnostic Microbiology and Infectious Disease* 2: 263–276

32

Haemophilus

Respiratory infections; meningitis; chancroid

A. J. Howard

The major pathogen in this group of organisms is *Haemophilus influenzae*, which is associated with a variety of invasive infections such as meningitis, epiglottitis, pneumonia and septic arthritis and localized disease of the respiratory tract such as bronchitis and otitis media. Other haemophili of medical importance include *H. aegyptius*, a cause of epidemic conjunctivitis, *H. ducreyi*, the causative organism of chancroid, and *H. parainfluenzae*, *H. aphrophilus* and *H. paraphrophilus*, three organisms which are occasionally encountered in patients with infective endocarditis and a variety of other miscellaneous conditions, including dental infections, lung abscess and brain abscess. The generic name relates to the inability of this group of organisms to grow on culture media without the presence of whole blood or certain of its constituents.

The first recorded observation of haemophili is thought to have been made by Robert Koch who described the microscopical appearance of a profusion of minute rods in pus from patients with conjunctivitis while engaged on cholera research in Egypt. A few years later, during the influenza pandemic of 1889–92, Pfeiffer noted the constant presence of large numbers of small bacilli in the sputum of patients affected with the disease. He had established these organisms in stable subculture by 1892, and in 1893 published a complete account of his work on influenza arguing that the bacillus he had isolated was the causative agent of the disease.

In the succeeding years considerable controversy surrounded this issue. It was observed that the influenza bacillus was sometimes absent in the localized outbreaks of infection which followed the pandemic and that the organism could be isolated from the respiratory tract of healthy individuals and from others with diseases in which clinical influenza was absent. The matter was resolved in 1933 when Smith, Andrewes and Laidlaw confirmed that the true aetiological agent was a virus. It still remains a possibility that secondary infection with *H. influenzae* contributed to the high mortality seen in the 1889–92 and 1918–19 pandemics.

DESCRIPTION

Morphology

Haemophili are pleomorphic Gram-negative rods. In clinical specimens *H. influenzae* is most commonly seen as a small, uniform coccobacillus. In some cultures, and occasionally in clinical material, longer, filamentous forms may be seen, often in association with large, spherical or fusiform bodies.

Encapsulation

Some strains of *H. influenzae* produce a capsule

which is demonstrable by capsule stains and a *Quellung reaction* (swelling of the capsule) with type-specific antisera. The capsules are polysaccharide in composition and represent six distinct antigenic types, designated a–f. The most important of these is type b, which is a polymer of ribosyl ribitol phosphate. Strains possessing this capsule are associated with most invasive infections seen with this species.

Growth factors

The dependence on blood for growth on laboratory culture media is based on a requirement for two factors, termed *X* and *V*. X factor — haemin — is required for the synthesis of the iron-containing respiratory enzymes cytochrome C, cytochrome oxidase, catalase and peroxidase. Unlike most bacteria, haemin-dependent haemophili have an inability to synthesize protoporphyrin from aminolaevulinic acid. V factor is nicotinamide adenine dinucleotide (NAD) or phosphate (NADP) or certain unidentified precursors of these compounds. It is essential for the oxidation–reduction processes in cell metabolism. The differential requirements for X and V factors are important criteria for defining *Haemophilus* species (Table 32.1): *H. influenzae* and *H. aegyptius* require both; *H. parainfluenzae*, V factor only; and *H. aphrophilus* and *H. ducreyi*, X factor only.

Growth on laboratory media

Ordinary blood agar contains X and V factors, but growth of *H. influenzae* on this medium is poor. The major growth restriction is lack of availability of V factor and enhancement of growth is obtained if the medium is supplemented with NAD. Streaking an organism which excretes an excess of this substance (e.g. *Staphylococcus aureus*) across the surface of the agar will produce growth stimulation in its vicinity (*satellitism*). Utilization of V factor in blood agar is also limited by the presence of serum nicotinamide adenine dinucleotidase (NADase). This can be inactivated by heating blood agar for a few minutes at 80–90°C until it turns brown (*chocolate agar*). This process also liberates extra X and V factor into the medium. X factor is heat-stable, but heating of media at 120°C for several minutes will destroy the heat-labile V factor. Good growth is also obtained on certain transparent media containing blood extracts (e.g. Levinthal agar or Fildes' peptic digest agar). The latter are useful for demonstrating capsulate strains, colonies of which are iridescent when viewed obliquely with transmitted light.

Metabolism

Haemophilus species are aerobic but facultatively anaerobic. Anaerobic growth considerably reduces the haemin requirement of X-dependent species. There is a variable requirement for carbon dioxide within the genus (Table 32.1). *H. influenzae* does not require a carbon dioxide-enriched atmosphere for growth but will often exhibit growth enhancement in such conditions.

Biochemical reactions

Haemophili are catalase-positive, oxidase-positive and ferment glucose and galactose. *H. influenzae* can be divided into eight biotypes on the basis of indole production, urease activity and ornithine decarboxylase reactions (Table 32.2). Biotypes

Table 32.1 Some characters of *Haemophilus* species associated with disease in man

Character	H. influenzae	H. aegyptius	H. parainfluenzae	H. aphrophilus	H. ducreyi
X requirement	+	+	−	+[b]	+
V requirement	+	+	+	−	−
CO_2 (5%) requirement	−	−	−	+[b]	−
Haemagglutination[a]	−	+	−	−	−

[a] Reaction with human or guinea-pig cells at 4°C.
[b] These characters may be lost on subculture.

Table 32.2 Differentiation of biotypes of *H. influenzae*

Reaction	Biotype							
	I	II	III	IV	V	VI	VII	VIII
Indole	+	+	−	−	+	−	+	−
Urease	+	+	+	+	−	−	−	−
Ornithine decarboxylase	+	−	−	+	+	+	−	−

I–III are the most common and the majority of invasive, type b, organisms are biotype I.

PATHOGENESIS

Normal carriage

H. influenzae is exclusively a human parasite which resides principally in the upper respiratory tract. Non-capsulate organisms are present in the nasopharynx or throat of between 25 and 80% of healthy people and capsulate strains in 5–10%, of which capsular type b strains are found in 1–5%.

Invasive infections

Invasive infections, usually caused by strains possessing the type b polysaccharide capsule, are quite distinct from the local (mostly respiratory) infections seen with non-typable *H. influenzae* and the other five serotypes. Meningitis is the most common invasive disease, followed by epiglottitis, bacteraemia without a clearly defined focus of infection (though often associated with pharyngitis), septic arthritis, pneumonia and cellulitis (Table 32.3).

These infections are unusual in the first 2 months of life, but are otherwise mainly seen in early childhood. Most cases occur in children under 2 years of age, but acute epiglottitis tends to present in slightly older children, having a peak incidence between 2 and 4 years of age.

The polysaccharide capsule is the major virulence factor for type b *H. influenzae*. The rarity of infections in the first 2 months of life correlates with the presence of maternal antibodies to this substance and the occurrence of infection in early infancy with the absence of antibodies having such specificity. As the prevalence and mean level of capsular antibodies in the population rises, *H. influenzae* type b infections become less common (Fig. 32.1).

What determines whether acquisition of type b organisms in a susceptible host will lead to asymptomatic carriage and the stimulation of protective antibodies, or to the induction of invasive disease, is unclear. However, animal experiments suggest that when invasion occurs, the organism penetrates the submucosa of the nasopharynx

Table 32.3 The clinical presentation of 126 cases of invasive, *H. influenzae* type b infections (data from Wales 1988–89)

Disease	Number of cases (%)	%
Meningitis	74	59
Epiglottitis	18	14
Bacteraemia	11	9
Pneumonia	8	6
Septic arthritis	8	6
Cellulitis	7	6

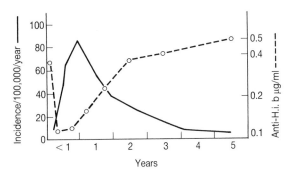

Fig. 32.1 The incidence of *H. influenzae* meningitis (continuous line) during the first 5 years of life and the corresponding mean level of anti-*H. influenzae* type b capsular polysaccharide antibodies (broken line). (Reproduced with permission from Peltoler H, Käyhty H, Sivonen A, Mäkelä H 1977 *Haemophilus influenzae* type b capsular polysaccharide vaccine in children: a double blind field study of 100 000 vaccinees 3 months to 5 years of age in Finland. *Pediatrics* 60: 730–737.)

and establishes systemic infection by haemato-genous spread. This is facilitated by a number of bacterial factors. Principal among these is the type b capsular polysaccharide, which has been shown to facilitate all phases of the invasion process. Other virulence factors which may be involved include: pili (fimbriae), which assist attachment to epithelial cells; IgA proteases, which are also involved in colonization; and outer-membrane components, which may contribute to invasion at several stages. It is possible that the initiation of invasive infection is potentiated by intercurrent viral infection. Genetic factors and immunosuppression may also play a role. It is unclear whether it is exposure to type b *H. influenzae*, or some other organism (e.g. *Escherichia coli* K100) possessing cross-reacting antigens which usually stimulates protective antibody production.

Occasionally, non-capsulate *H. influenzae* may also be responsible for invasive disease. These are usually associated with some predisposing factor such as cranial trauma or surgery, pre-existing joint disease and general conditions, including malignancy, diabetes, alcoholism or immuno-globulin defects. Meningitis and septicaemia due to non-capsulate *H. influenzae* is sometimes seen in the neonate.

Non-invasive disease

H. influenzae also produces a variety of local infections which are usually associated with some underlying physiological or anatomical abnormality. The commonest infections affect the respiratory tract and consist of otitis media, sinusitis and purulent episodes in patients with exacerbations of chronic obstructive airway disease.

Acute sinusitis and otitis media are usually initiated by viral infections. These predispose to secondary infection with potentially pathogenic components of the local resident microbial flora through mechanisms which may involve obstruction to the outflow of respiratory secretions, decreased clearance of micro-organisms via the normal mucociliary mechanism and depression of local immunity. It is usually non-capsulate strains that are responsible when *H. influenzae* is involved.

A similar aetiology probably accounts for the bacterial infections seen in association with chronic obstructive airway disease and again it is the non-capsulate strains of *H. influenzae* that are chiefly responsible. Acute exacerbations of this disease are usually, like acute otitis media and sinusitis, initiated by acute viral infections. These further compromise an already impaired mucociliary clearance mechanism in patients with chronic lung disease and further potentiate bacterial colonization of the lower respiratory tract. In this situation *H. influenzae* can establish purulent infection which further compromises pulmonary function and has been shown to have direct toxic effects on cilia.

LABORATORY DIAGNOSIS
Direct examination

Gram-stained smears of clinical material such as cerebrospinal fluid, pus, sputum or aspirates from joints, middle ears or sinuses can be useful in providing a rapid, presumptive identification. Haemophili tend to stain poorly and dilute carbol fuchsin is a better counterstain than neutral red or safranin.

General considerations

The viability of *H. influenzae* in clinical specimens declines with time, particularly at 4°C. For optimal yield, specimens should be transported to the laboratory and seeded onto appropriate culture media without delay. Chocolate agar represents a good, general purpose medium and can be used without further supplementation for specimens obtained from sites that would normally be expected to be sterile. Plates should be incubated in an aerobic atmosphere enriched with 5–10% carbon dioxide.

Sputum

Specimens of sputum collected by expectoration will inevitably become contaminated by upper respiratory flora. This will commonly include *H. influenzae* and the finding of the organism in such specimens cannot be automatically taken to imply involvement in a pathological process. Support for the significance of *H. influenzae* is provided if, in a purulent sample, the organism is present as the predominant isolate, or in a viable count of $>10^6$ colony-forming units per ml. Addition of bacitracin (10 IU/ml) facilitates the selective isolation of *H. influenzae* from mixed cultures of respiratory organisms. Obtaining bronchial secretions by transtracheal aspiration or via protected channel bronchoscopy will reduce the problem of contamination with commensal organisms.

Throat swabs

Throat swabs in patients with suspected acute epiglottitis should not be attempted since attempts to obtain the sample may precipitate complete airway obstruction. Blood cultures are usually positive in this condition.

Blood culture

Blood should be drawn for culture from patients with suspected invasive disease. Any good blood culture medium is satisfactory. Visual examination of the bottles cannot be relied upon to indicate positive growth. Bottles must be routinely subcultured onto solid medium, or some other detection system (e.g. release of radiolabelled carbon dioxide) used.

Antigen detection

The detection of type b polysaccharide antigen in body fluids or pus can be a useful and rapid diagnostic aid, particularly in patients who have received antibiotics before specimens are obtained. Techniques available include: countercurrent immuno-electrophoresis; agglutination of latex particles coated with rabbit antibody to type b antigen; and co-agglutination of *Staph. aureus* coated with anti-type b antibody.

In the absence of confirmatory cultures, the results should be regarded with caution as some serotypes of *Streptoccoccus pneumoniae* and *Esch. coli* may share similar antigens.

Antibiotic sensitivity tests

Because of the fastidious nature of the organism, accurate determination of the antibiotic susceptibility of *H. influenzae* requires careful standardization of the methodology. Disc tests have proved less reliable for detecting enzyme-mediated ampicillin and chloramphenicol resistance than microbiological or biochemical techniques that demonstrate antibiotic inactivation.

TREATMENT

H. influenzae is sensitive to a wide range of antibiotics and is usually inhibited by low concentrations of ampicillin, chloramphenicol, tetracycline, sulphonamide and trimethoprim. Early cephalosporins were relatively ineffective against this species, but later compounds such as cefuroxime, cefotaxime and ceftazidime are highly active. Other antibiotics active against *H. influenzae* include ciprofloxacin, aztreonam and co-amoxiclav.

Chloramphenicol has long been considered the antibiotic of first choice for the treatment of meningitis. It is bactericidal for *H. influenzae*, achieves good concentrations in the meninges and cerebral tissues and has proved highly effective in clinical practice. Resistance may be encountered; however, in most parts of the world this remains uncommon. Ampicillin is also effective and for a time enjoyed popularity for the primary treatment of bacterial meningitis as it appeared to cover all the pathogens likely to be responsible and avoided the potential toxicity of chloramphenicol. However, resistance to the drug is now encountered in up to 25% of type b strains in the UK. In view of this level of resistance, ampicillin should no longer be used as a single agent in meningitis if *H. influenzae* is a possibility and the results of sensitivity tests are not available. Resistance to ampicillin is due to the production of a β-lactamase, which was probably originally derived from Enterobacteriaceae (so-called TEM–1 enzyme). Cefotaxime and related cephalosporins exhibit high activity against *H. influenzae*, and are effective for the treatment of this condition.

Antibiotic therapy is only a component of the clinical management of patients with haemophilus meningitis and full supportive care is required to achieve the most favourable outcome. Skilled medical and nursing care is also vital in the management of acute epiglottitis where maintenance of a patent airway is crucial. Chloramphenicol or cefotaxime are the antibiotics of choice.

For the treatment of less serious respiratory infections such as otitis media, sinusitis and acute exacerbations of chronic bronchitis, oral antibiotics such as ampicillin, cefaclor, tetracycline and co-trimoxazole are all effective. β-Lactamase-mediated ampicillin resistance is less common in non-capsulate strains than in type b strains. It is seen in about 10% of isolates in the UK.

EPIDEMIOLOGY OF INVASIVE DISEASE

H. influenzae is an important cause of serious systemic bacterial disease in children throughout the world. In the USA infections have become more common since the Second World War and for several decades *H. influenzae* has been the leading cause of bacterial meningitis in that country, accounting for some 12 000 cases annually. In the UK *Neisseria meningitidis* remained the commonest cause of bacterial meningitis until 1980, but on several occasions in the 1980s the annual incidence of haemophilus meningitis exceeded that due to the meningococcus. The incidence reported recently from several locations in England and Wales has approached more closely the situation in the USA than estimates made previously.

Meningitis is more common in winter months, in families of low socio-economic status and in household contacts of a case. The disease is usually seen in the youngest member of a family and uncommonly in children who have no siblings. Outbreaks of infection have been described in close communities, such as nursery schools. Very high rates have been reported in several distinct populations, e.g. Navajo and Apache Indians and Alaskan eskimos. It is possible that socio-economic considerations are important in determining such racial differences but genetic factors may also play a role. Immunosuppression, whether iatrogenic or associated with malignancies (especially Hodgkin's disease), asplenia or agammaglobulinaemia also predispose to invasive disease.

The mortality associated with *H. influenzae* meningitis is around 5%. Neurological sequelae, especially hearing loss, may be present in 10–30% of survivors.

CONTROL

Active immunization

A purified capsular polysaccharide vaccine has been prepared and used extensively in several parts of the world. Unfortunately, it produces a poor response in children less than 2 years of age and in patients with immunodeficiency. New vaccines have been developed in which the polysaccharide is covalently coupled to various proteins such as *N. meningitidis* outer-membrane protein, diphtheria toxoid, tetanus toxoid and a non-toxic variant of diphtheria toxin. These produce a lasting anamnestic response which is not age related, and may also be effective in high-risk patients who give a poor response to polysaccharide vaccine alone.

Antibiotic prophylaxis

Data from the USA have shown that household contacts of patients with invasive disease have an increased risk of acquiring infection if they are under 5 years of age. The attack rate has been calculated to be 4% in the 30 d following presentation of the index case for children under 2 years, 2% for children of 2–3 years, and 0.1% for children of 4–5 years of age. The risk for children under 2 years of age is 600–800-fold higher than the age-adjusted risk for the general population. Contact with a case in the setting of a day care centre or nursery has also been associated with increased attack rates in children under 2 years of age although the calculated risk is lower than that seen in household contacts.

Rifampicin in a dosage of 20 mg/kg (up to a maximum of 600 mg) given orally once daily for 4 d is effective in eradicating carriage of *H. influenzae* and has been used in attempts to prevent secondary infection in both household and nursery contacts. Conclusive data regarding its efficacy are not available.

HAEMOPHILI OTHER THAN *H. INFLUENZAE*

H. ducreyi

This organism is responsible for a sexually-transmitted disease, *chancroid*, which is most prevalent in tropical regions, particularly Africa and south-east Asia. Patients present with painful penile ulcers (*soft sore* or *soft chancre*) and inguinal lymphadenitis. Typical small Gram-negative bacilli can be seen in material from the ulcers or in pus from lymph node aspirate. It is likely that the lesions of chancroid have facilitated the transmission of human immunodeficiency virus (HIV) in some tropical countries.

Chancroid has traditionally been treated with sulphonamides (alone or in combination with streptomycin), tetracyclines or erythromycin, but resistant strains occur. Newer drugs, including co-trimoxazole, co-amoxiclav, cefotaxime and ciprofloxacin have also been shown to be effective.

An unrelated Gram-negative rod, *Calymmatobacterium granulomatis* causes a somewhat similar sexually-transmitted disease, *granuloma inguinale*, in parts of the tropics. Intracellular organisms, known as *Donovan bodies* (not to be confused with the Leishman–Donovan bodies of leishmaniasis) can be demonstrated in the stained smears from the lesions. Tetracyclines are usually used in treatment.

H. aegyptius

This organism, formerly known as the *Koch–Weeks bacillus* is probably a biotype of *H. influenzae*. It causes a purulent conjunctivitis and appears to be responsible for *Brazilian purpuric fever*, a clinical syndrome that was first recognized in Brazil in 1984, in which conjunctivitis leads to an overwhelming septicaemia resembling fulminating meningococcal infection. Ampicillin in combination with chloramphenicol has been successful when treatment has been started sufficiently early.

Other haemophili

Various other species of *Haemophilus*, notably *H. parainfluenzae*, *H. aphrophilus*, *H. paraphrophilus* and *H. haemolyticus* are occasionally implicated in human disease, especially bacterial endocarditis. A combination of ampicillin and gentamicin has been successfully used to treat such cases.

RECOMMENDED READING

Brazilian Purpuric Fever Study Group 1987. Haemophilus aegyptius bacteraemia in Brazilian purpuric fever. *Lancet* ii: 761–763

Kilian M 1976 A Taxonomic study of the genus Haemophilus and the proposal of a new species. *Journal of General Microbiology* 93: 9–62

Morse S A 1989 Chancroid and *Haemophilus ducreyi*. *Clinical Microbiology Reviews* 2: 137–157

Sell S H, Wright P F 1982 Haemophilus influenzae. *Epidemiology, Immunology, and Prevention of Disease.* Elsevier, New York

Shapiro E D 1990 New vaccines against *Haemophilus influenzae* type b. *Pediatric Clinics of North America* 37: 567–583

Turk D C 1984 The Pathogenicity of *Haemophilus influenzae*. *Journal of Medical Microbiology* 18: 1–16

33

Bordetella

Whooping cough

N. W. Preston

The genus *Bordetella* constitutes one of the groups of very small ovoid or rod-shaped Gram-negative bacilli, often described as parvobacteria. The genus contains two human pathogens, *Bordetella pertussis* and *B. parapertussis*, which cause one of the most frequent and serious bacterial respiratory infections of childhood in communities not protected effectively by vaccination.

The pertussis syndrome

Pertussis has been recognized as a clinical entity for several centuries. Typically, the child suffers many bouts of paroxysmal coughing each day; during these the tongue is protruded fully, fluids stream from the eyes, nose and mouth, and the face becomes cyanotic; when death seems imminent, a final cough appears to clear the secretions and, with a massive inspiratory effort, air is sucked through the narrowed glottis, producing a long high-pitched whoop — hence the term *whooping cough*. Such attacks often terminate with vomiting. Between them the patient does not usually appear ill.

If a characteristic attack is witnessed, there may be little hesitation in making a clinical diagnosis of pertussis. However, the illness is often mild and atypical, especially in older children and adults, in younger children who have been in-completely immunized, and in very young infants partially protected by maternal antibody.

In these cases, the laboratory has a vital role in diagnosis, because similar coughing may be caused by a variety of viruses, and such illness is generally mild and of short duration. Here, the term *pseudo-whooping cough* has been applied aptly. False diagnosis may create a popular impression of pertussis as a trivial disease; and it has been recommended that, in the absence of positive bacterial culture, whooping cough should not be diagnosed for an illness of less than 3 weeks of duration. With genuine pertussis, the cough is likely to persist for months rather than weeks. Furthermore, because pertussis vaccine cannot be expected to protect against viral infection, estimates of vaccine efficacy require an accurate diagnosis. Thus, a study in the UK by the Public Health Laboratory Service found an efficacy of 93% against pertussis confirmed by bacterial culture, compared with only 82% for cases diagnosed solely on clinical criteria.

DESCRIPTION

Bordetellae used to be classified in the genus *Haemophilus*. However, growth is not dependent on either of the nutritional factors X and V and *B. parapertussis* and *B. bronchiseptica* do not require blood for their growth. The three species resemble each other in being small Gram-negative bacilli, in causing infection of the respiratory tract, and in sharing some common surface antigens.

Bordetella pertussis

This is the most fastidious of the bordetellae. It produces toxic products which must be absorbed by a constituent of the culture medium, such as charcoal, starch or a high concentration of blood, as in the original Bordet–Gengou medium. Because agglutination forms an important part of identification, a smooth growth is essential, and this is best provided by charcoal–blood agar: *B. pertussis* is a strict aerobe, with an optimal growth temperature of 35–36°C. Even under these conditions it usually takes 3 d before colonies are visible to the naked eye.

Typical colonies are shiny, greyish white, convex, and with a butyrous consistency. By slide agglutination, they can be shown to react strongly with homologous (pertussis) antiserum, and weakly or not at all with parapertussis antiserum, depending on the specificity of the reagent. Subculture reveals no growth on nutrient agar.

The organism produces three major agglutinogens (1, 2 and 3) which can be detected by the use of absorbed, single-agglutinin sera. Factor 1 is common to all strains; the three serotypes pathogenic to man (type 1,2, type 1,3, type 1,2,3) also possess factor 2 or factor 3 or both factors, and these type-specific agglutinogens have a role in immunity to infection.

Bordetella parapertussis

This organism is readily distinguished from *B. pertussis* by its ability to grow on nutrient agar, with the production of a brown diffusible pigment after 2 days (Table 33.1). It also grows more rapidly than *B. pertussis* on charcoal–blood agar, and is agglutinated more strongly by parapertussis than by pertussis antiserum.

It causes less severe illness than *B. pertussis*, and is uncommon in most countries, though occasionally it has been responsible for outbreaks of whooping cough.

Bordetella bronchiseptica

Colonies of this species are visible on nutrient agar after overnight incubation; it differs from the other species by also being motile and by producing an obvious alkaline reaction in litmus milk and in the Hugh and Leifson medium that is used to differentiate oxidative from fermentative action on sugars. For this reason it is placed by some taxonomists in the genus *Alcaligenes*; however, it is readily distinguished from the intestinal commensal *Alcaligenes faecalis* by its rapid hydrolysis of urea.

Although it is rarely encountered in human infection, *B. bronchiseptica* is a common respiratory pathogen of animals, especially laboratory stocks of rodents. Because it shares antigens with other bordetellae, it is important that animals be checked for freedom from bordetella antibody before they are used in the preparation of specific antisera. For this reason, sheep or donkeys have sometimes been used in preference to rodents.

PATHOGENESIS

Whooping cough is a non-invasive infection of the respiratory mucosa, with man as the only natural host. In a typical case, there is an incuba-

Table 33.1 Differential properties of *B. pertussis* and *B. parapertussis*

Property	B. pertussis	B. parapertussis
Duration of incubation to yield visible colonies	3 d	2 d
Growth on nutrient agar	None	Good
Pigment diffusing in medium	None	Brown
Slide-agglutination with		
Pertussis antiserum	Strong	Weak
Parapertussis antiserum	Weak	Strong

tion period of 1–2 weeks, followed by a 'catarrhal' phase with a simple cough but no distinctive features. Within about a week, this leads gradually into the 'paroxysmal' phase, with increasing severity and frequency of paroxysmal cough, which may last for many weeks and be followed by an equally prolonged 'convalescent' phase.

In the initial preventable stage of the infection there is heavy colonization of the ciliated epithelium of the bronchi and trachea with vast numbers of bacteria whose agglutinogens play a vital and type-specific role in attachment. Once established, *B. pertussis* produces a tracheal cytotoxin which paralyses the cilia, and leads to paroxysms of cough as an alternative means of removing the increased mucus. Another bacterial product, called pertussis toxin (PT), is responsible for the characteristic lymphocytosis in uncomplicated whooping cough. Subsequent increase in neutrophils, together with fever, suggests bronchopneumonia or other secondary infection, maybe with pyogenic cocci. Blockage of airways may lead to areas of lung collapse, and anoxia may lead to convulsions, though with modern intensive care the disease is rarely fatal.

In developing countries, whooping cough is still a major cause of death; but, in developed countries, concern is focused on a very prolonged and frightening illness with possible respiratory and neurological sequelae, on the anxiety and exhaustion of parents, and on the heavy use of hospital and community medical resources.

Experimental infection in animals

Some, though not all, of the features of human disease have been produced in animals. Thus, marmosets and rabbits develop catarrh during prolonged colonization of the respiratory tract; they produce a similar range of agglutinin response to vaccination, and this immunity shows evidence of serotype specificity.

However, the mouse, which has long been used in the evaluation of pertussis vaccine potency, does not show these features. It can be infected and even killed by degraded organisms of serotype 1, which have lost the type-specific agglutinogens (2 and 3) that are necessary for human infection.

It also reveals additional properties of PT that are not seen in man: histamine sensitization, and islets activation (inducing hyperinsulinaemia and hypoglycaemia). Furthermore, PT and another component of the organism (filamentous haemagglutinin, FHA) are virulence factors in the mouse; but their role in human infection is uncertain. It is therefore necessary to interpret with caution experimental evidence from mice, or from other small rodents whose suitability as models of human pertussis infection is not known.

LABORATORY DIAGNOSIS
Bacterial culture

Because atypical clinical cases frequently occur, laboratory confirmation of the diagnosis is often essential. Bacterial culture has the highest specificity of the tests available for confirmation of the clinical diagnosis. In the absence of any really effective therapy, accuracy in the diagnosis is more important than speed. Bacterial culture has the additional advantage that the isolate can be serotyped and thus provide valuable epidemiological information.

So rarely has a positive culture been obtained from a healthy person, other than one incubating the disease, that a false-positive result can be discounted. Moreover, with good technique of swabbing and culture, the organism can be recovered up to 3 months from the onset of illness when coughing persists. This casts doubt on the widespread belief that the bacterium is eliminated in a few weeks, and has implications for the transmission of infection.

Though the main disease is in the lower respiratory tract, the organism can be recovered readily from the nasopharynx. 'Cough plates' and post-nasal swabs are unsatisfactory because of overgrowth by commensal bacteria. A pernasal swab acquires fewer commensals, and these can be suppressed by penicillin (0.25 unit/ml = 0.15 mg/l) or cephalexin (30 mg/l) in the charcoal–blood agar plate; higher concentrations may suppress bordetellae. Pernasal swabs on flexible wire are available commercially; the tip is directed downwards and towards the mid-line, passing gently along the floor of the nose for about 5 cm (depending on the patient's age) until stopped by the posterior wall of the nasopharynx. Practice in swabbing is necessary, initially with a co-operative adult! If old enough, patients should be warned to expect a tickling sensation but no pain; and a child's head should be held steady. Whenever possible a segment of the culture plate should be inoculated immediately after withdrawal of the swab. The use of transport medium reduces the isolation rate. A single swab may yield a negative culture, but isolation rates of up to 80% may be achieved by taking specimens on several successive days.

In the laboratory, the inoculum is spread to give separate colonies, and the plate is incubated for at least 7 d before being discarded as negative. Because of the prolonged incubation, the medium should have a depth of 6–7 mm (40 ml in a 9 cm dish); and a bowl of water may be placed in the incubator, to reduce drying of the culture. Cephalexin tends to give 'rough' growth which may have to be subcultured on cephalexin-free medium for reliable serological identification.

Detection of bacterial antigens

Bordetella antigens may be detected in serum and urine in tests with specific antiserum. Alternatively, bacteria in nasopharyngeal secretions are labelled with fluorescein-conjugated antiserum and examined by ultraviolet microscopy. This method has the theoretical advantage, compared with culture, of detecting dead bordetellae. However, false-negative results are likely unless the patient's own antibody is removed from the bacteria by enzyme, before application of the fluorescent reagent. Moreover, false-positive results may occur because of serological cross-reactions with organisms such as staphylococci, yeasts, haemophili and moraxellae, some of which resemble bordetellae microscopically. Bordetella antiserum should be absorbed with these organisms, but appropriate reagents are not readily available. Reports on the high specificity of this test lack conviction, in the absence of reliable evidence on the true diagnosis.

Detection of bordetella antibody

Sera and nasopharyngeal secretions can be examined for antibody. However, a negative result does not exclude pertussis because the serological response is often slow and weak, especially in very young children. More importantly, a positive result is ambiguous because antigens are shared with other organisms (see above). Even with insensitive tests, such as agglutination, pertussis antibodies are readily detected in the sera of healthy persons. More sensitive techniques, such as enzyme-linked immunosorbent assay (ELISA), are liable to increase the number of false-positive results, and thereby give spurious respectability to a diagnosis that should rightly be 'pseudo-whooping cough'. The need at present in serological diagnosis is not for greater sensitivity but for greater specificity.

Differential blood count

Although lymphocytosis is a characteristic response to pertussis infection, many cases of true pertussis do not develop a significant increase in circulating lymphocytes; conversely, there are so many other causes of lymphocytosis that a positive result lacks diagnostic specificity.

TREATMENT
Antimicrobial drugs

Most antibiotics have little or no clinical effect when the infection is well established, even though the organism may be sensitive in vitro.

The drug of choice is erythromycin, which may reduce the severity of the illness if given before the paroxysmal stage. If given for at least 14 d it sometimes eliminates the organism and so reduces the exposure of contacts. However, positive cultures are frequently obtained after short periods of erythromycin therapy.

Erythromycin may also be given to protect non-vaccinated infants, though it seems unrealistic to expect this treatment to be maintained throughout the several months that the older sibling (or adult) may remain infectious.

Appropriate antibiotics should, of course, be administered to patients who show signs of secondary bacterial infection.

Other measures

Cough suppressants and corticosteroids may control the paroxysms, but may be harmful by encouraging retention of secretions. Cyanosis and anoxia can be reduced by avoiding sudden noises, excitement or excessive medical examination, which tend to precipitate paroxysms; but mucus and vomit should be removed to prevent their inhalation.

Treatment with pertussis immunoglobulin has been tried, but without success — probably because such materials have never been checked for the presence of all three agglutinins.

Because of the dearth of effective therapy for whooping cough, the widespread use of pertussis vaccine is of supreme importance (see below).

EPIDEMIOLOGY

Source and transmission of infection

Most new cases arise from patients (usually children, sometimes adults) with typical symptoms, presumably because the paroxysmal cough provides an efficient means of droplet dissemination. Atypical cases have only a minor role in transmission; long-term asymptomatic carriage is unknown. The degree of contact is important: 80–90% of non-immune siblings exposed in the household become infected, compared with less than 50% of non-immune child contacts at school.

Antibiotic therapy may reduce transmission, but is not completely effective.

Incidence and mortality

Pertussis infection occurs world-wide, affects all ages and is a major cause of death in malnourished populations. In the developed countries, mortality has gradually declined with a combination of improved socio-economic conditions, availability of intensive care in hospitals, and antibiotic therapy to combat secondary infection. However, the latter constitute an unnecessary use of medical resources on a disease that is eminently preventable by vaccination.

The disease is most severe, and the morbidity rate highest, in the first 2 years of life; most fatal cases are in infants under 1 year old. Even very young babies are not immune: maternal antibody does pass to the fetus, but it rarely contains all three agglutinins, and protection is incomplete.

Although one attack usually confers long-lasting immunity, infection with a different serotype of the organism can subsequently occur.

The disease occurs in epidemic waves at about 4 year intervals, reflecting the time necessary to build up a new susceptible population after the 'herd' immunity produced by an epidemic. Figure 33.1 illustrates the pattern, for England and Wales, where whooping cough has been a notifiable disease since 1940. The maintenance of a 4

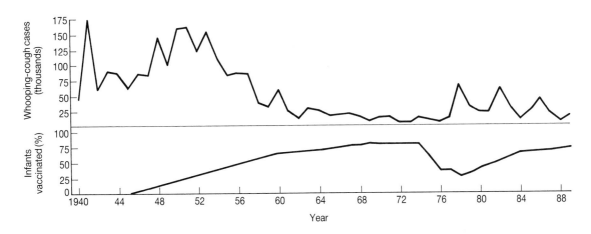

Fig. 33.1 Whooping cough in England and Wales since 1940.

year cycle presumably results from the interaction of various factors, such as the degree of artificial immunity produced by high vaccination rates, and the levels of natural immunity that follow either large epidemics or a high background incidence of endemic pertussis in interepidemic intervals.

Figure 33.1 also illustrates how variations in the rates of uptake of pertussis vaccine have affected the incidence of whooping cough more than the steady improvement in the general health of the population that continued throughout the period. After the gradual introduction of pertussis vaccination during the 1950s, there was a steady reduction in the size of epidemics until the 1970s. Unfounded fear of brain damage caused a loss of faith in the vaccine and three large epidemics occurred before the slow restoration of confidence in the vaccine began to take effect.

Prevalence of serotypes

The three serotypes of *B. pertussis* pathogenic for man are liable to spontaneous reversible variation, as shown by the arrows in Table 33.2. Fimbriae are readily demonstrable on strains possessing agglutinogen 2, aiding colonization of the respiratory mucosa; serotypes 1,2 and 1,2,3 predominate amongst the strains isolated from patients in non-vaccinated communities.

In the 1960s, many countries used type 1,2 vaccine and these two serotypes were suppressed. However, type 1,3 organisms, which have a weak factor 1 component, became predominant in these countries, and caused infection even in vaccinated children before the vaccine was modified in the late 1960s by addition of agglutinogen 3. Similarly, countries which used a vaccine deficient in agglutinogen 2, or both agglutinogens 2 and 3, saw a predominance of type 1,2 infection, even in vaccinated children.

To be effective, a vaccine must contain all three agglutinogens, as recommended by the World Health Organizaton. However, because the agglutinin 3 response is usually the weakest (when type 1,2,3 vaccine is used), type 1,3 organisms are the last to be eliminated from a community with an effective vaccination programme.

CONTROL

Treatment and quarantine

Neither the antibiotics nor the immunoglobulins currently available are very effective in influencing the course of the illness, even if given during the incubation period or the catarrhal phase. They are equally unreliable for the prophylaxis of contacts.

Because patients typically disseminate the organism for many weeks or months, and because children are infectious even before the most characteristic symptoms develop, control of the disease by quarantine is unrealistic.

Vaccination

Vaccination is safe and more than 90% effective and is strongly recommended.

Table 33.2 Occurrence of serotypes of *B. pertussis* in different communities

	Serotypes of *B. pertussis* which cause whooping cough	
	1,2 ↔[a] 1,2,3 ↔[a] (1),3[b]	
Prevalence in non-vaccinated communities	High	Low
Prevalence in communities vaccinated with type 1,2	Low	High[c]
Prevalence in communities vaccinated with type 1,3 or type 1	High[c]	Low
Relative incidence in communities vaccinated with type 1,2,3 (prior to complete elimination)	Lower	Higher

[a] The arrows indicate spontaneous reversible variation of serotype.
[b] The parentheses (1) indicate a weak factor 1 component, so that type 1,3 does not protect against type 1,2 infection, and vice versa.
[c] Infection occurs even in vaccinated children.

The vaccines currently in use are suspensions of whole bacterial cells, killed by heat or chemicals, which are administered by deep intramuscular injection. Adsorption of the bacteria onto an adjuvant, such as aluminium hydroxide, enhances the immune response (particularly important with factor 3) and also causes fewer adverse reactions (Table 33.3).

Three items are essential for good protection:

1. Presence of all three agglutinogens in the vaccine
2. Use of adsorbed vaccine (i.e. with adjuvant)
3. Minimum of three doses, at monthly intervals from 3 months of age.

Moreover, since there is little passive protection from the mother, and since effective active immunity cannot be achieved until after the third injection of vaccine, it is important that immunization schedules are strictly adhered to. These and other aspects of vaccination are dealt with in Chapter 68.

Safety of pertussis vaccine

Minor adverse reactions occur in up to one-third of vaccinated children, and can be considered as part of the normal immune response. Parents should therefore be warned to expect possible erythema and local swelling, slight feverishness, and crying. Of much more concern are possible neurological sequelae. In 1981, the National Childhood Encephalopathy Study reported that persistent neurological disorder, commencing within 7 d of vaccination, may have resulted from 1 in 310 000 vaccinations. However, this low figure includes disorders that would have occurred in those children within 1 month in the absence of vaccination. Pertussis vaccination thus seems merely to advance the appearance of neurological disorders that would occur in any case and there is no firm evidence that the vaccine causes serious long-term adverse side-effects.

Contra-indications to pertussis vaccination

Severe adverse reaction to a previous dose is probably the only firm contra-indication. A current feverish illness (not merely snuffles) is cause for postponement until the child is well. Parental concern over a possible neurological contra-indication is due reason for consultation with a paediatrician. Allergy is not a contra-indication; neither is age — children who missed vaccination in infancy may receive the normal three-dose course. Vaccination is also sometimes advised for adults, e.g. nurses and doctors in appropriate hospitals.

Acellular pertussis vaccine

Although doubts about the efficacy and safety of whole-cell pertussis vaccine have largely passed, the urge to identify the essential protective components persists. An efficacy trial of acellular PT–FHA vaccine in Swedish children showed poor protection and a lack of correlation between protection and the antibody response to either component. An extract containing the type-specific agglutinogens might be better, but trials in millions of children would be necessary to show that it was as effective and safe as whole-cell vaccine. Furthermore, a satisfactory acellular vaccine may be too expensive, especially for developing countries where the need is greatest.

Eradication

Vaccination aims at a herd immunity, which breaks the cycle of transmission because the organism dies before finding a new susceptible host (see Chapter 68).

In the UK, good vaccine is readily available. Eradication is possible, but, even if high levels of vaccination of infants are maintained, it will be some years before adequate herd immunity is achieved within the child population.

Table 33.3 Plain and adsorbed pertussis vaccine

Vaccine	Immune response	Adverse reactions
Plain	Weaker	More
Adsorbed (onto adjuvant)	Stronger	Less

RECOMMENDED READING

Bass J W 1985 Erythromycin for pertussis: probable reasons for past failures. *Lancet* ii: 147

Baxter D N, Gibbs A C C 1987 How are the sub-unit pertussis vaccines to be evaluated? *Epidemiology and Infection* 99: 477–484

Bowie C 1990 Lessons from the pertussis vaccine court trial. *Lancet* 335: 397–399

Cherry J D, Brunell P A, Golden G S, Karzon D T 1988 Report of the Task Force on pertussis and pertussis immunization — 1988. *Pediatrics* 81: 939–984

Preston N W 1987 Eradication of pertussis by vaccination. *Lancet* i: 1312

Smith M H 1988 National Childhood Vaccine Injury Compensation Act. *Pediatrics* 82: 264–269

Thomas M G, Lambert H P 1987 From whom do children catch pertussis? *British Medical Journal* 295: 751–752

Wardlaw A C, Parton R (eds) 1988 *Pathogenesis and Immunity in Pertussis*. Wiley, Chichester

34

Legionella Legionnaires' disease; Pontiac fever

R. J. Fallon

The Legionellaceae are Gram-negative rods whose natural habitat is water. Man is accidentally infected and the disease is not transmissible from person to person. There are 36 genetically defined species of *Legionella*, much the most important of which is *Legionella pneumophila*. This species can be subdivided on the basis of DNA relationships into three subspecies: *L. pneumophila* ssp. *pneumophila* and *L. pneumophila* ssp. *fraseri*, which have been described in human disease; and *L. pneumophila* ssp. *pascullei*, which has so far been isolated only from the environment. A total of 15 *Legionella* species have been associated with human disease (Table 34.1) but most infections are caused by

just one of the many serogroups of *L. pneumophila*, serogroup 1 (SG1).

Legionellae give rise to two main clinical syndromes:

1. *Legionnaires' disease*, a pneumonia which may progress rapidly unless treated with appropriate antibiotic therapy, and extend to involve two or more lobes of the lung. The incubation period is 2–10 d and the illness is characterized by high fever and symptoms such as respiratory distress, cough, confusion and focal neurological signs. In previously healthy subjects the mortality is about 10%, but in nosocomial infection the rate may be much higher.

2. *Pontiac fever*. In contrast to Legionnaires' disease, which develops in only a small proportion of the total population exposed to an identified source of infection, Pontiac fever has a high attack rate with no mortality. It is a brief febrile influenza-like illness which may sometimes be slow to resolve fully.

Legionellae have rarely been associated with other infections such as prosthetic valve endocarditis or wound infection but these are usually nosocomial infections. Legionellae are not normally carried by man.

Table 34.1 *Legionella* species associated with human disease

Species	Number of serogroups	Autofluorescence under ultraviolet light
L. anisa	1	+
L. birminghamensis	1	−
L. bozemanii	2	−
L. cincinnatiensis	1	−
L. dumoffii	1	+
L. feeleii	2	−
L. gormanii	1	+
L. hackeliae	2	−
L. jordanis	1	−
L. longbeachae	2	−
L. maceachernii	1	−
L. micdadei	1	−
L. pneumophila	>14	−
L. tucsonensis	1	+
L. wadsworthii	1	−

+, blue-white fluorescence; −, no autofluorescence.

DESCRIPTION

In biological material (e.g. sputum, lung or in water deposits) legionellae are short rods or cocco-bacilli but in culture they become longer and sometimes filamentous. Although they are weakly Gram-negative, they are difficult to visualize in biological material by Gram's stain, but may be stained non-specifically using a silver impregnation method. Specific fluorescent antibody stains are used diagnostically. The organisms may be numerous, particularly in patients who are infected in hospital or who are immunosuppressed, but are often present only in very small numbers in the scanty sputum, which is characteristic of Legionnaires' disease. They have not been demonstrated in patients with Pontiac fever. Legionellae are exacting in their growth requirements and grow best on buffered charcoal–yeast extract agar (BCYE) which contains iron plus cysteine as an essential growth factor. Some legionellae grow better in the presence of 2.5–5% carbon dioxide at 35–36°C. Colonies do not appear until after incubation for 48 h. Usually they will appear by 5 d but species other than *L. pneumophila* may take up to 10 d. Colonies have a classical 'cut-glass' appearance on examination under the plate microscope. Colonies of some *Legionella* species show autofluorescence on illumination with long-wave ultraviolet light (Table 34.1). Species and serogroups within species have specific heat-stable lipopolysaccharide antigens and further identification depends on serological examination, usually by the fluorescent antibody test or by slide agglutination with specific antisera. Species may be differentiated further, on the basis of serology, into serotypes within serogroups but this applies, at the present time, almost entirely to *L. pneumophila* SG1. Subtyping is usually by the use of monoclonal antibodies in an immuno-fluorescence test. Similarities or differences between strains of the same serogroup may be revealed by genetic studies.

PATHOGENESIS

Legionella infection arises as the result of inhalation of an aerosol of fine water droplets containing the organism. Such aerosols are usually generated from warm water sources, typically:

1. The ponds in cooling towers of refrigeration plants in air-conditioning systems

2. Domestic hot water systems in hotels and hospitals

3. Warm water in nebulizers and oxygen line humidifiers

4. Whirlpool spa baths and showers.

It has been shown that legionellae may be engulfed by, and survive within, free-living amoebae and it may well be that the bacteria are protected from drying and disinfectants if they are present in the cysts formed by such amoebae. There is presently no evidence that ingestion plays a part in the pathogenesis of legionella infection, although the demonstration of *L. pneumophila* in bowel contents raises this as a possibility.

Animal models have given some insight as to the train of events when legionellae reach the lungs. Guinea-pigs infected by inhalation of an aerosol containing legionellae develop a lobular pneumonia which rapidly becomes confluent. It has been shown that instillation of a protease produced by *L. pneumophila* into the lungs of guinea-pigs will produce a pneumonia which appears to be the same in nature as that caused by inhalation of intact bacteria.

Once infection is established in man the patient develops pneumonic consolidation with an outpouring of proteinaceous fibrinous exudate, containing macrophages and polymorphs, into the alveoli. Despite the outpouring of cells, patients usually produce little sputum. Apart from the pneumonic consolidation there are distant toxic effects of the infection on the nervous system with confusion, hallucinations and, occasionally, focal neurological signs; renal impairment leading to renal failure may occur. The mechanism of these toxic changes is unknown. The patient develops high fever and the disease may range from a rapidly progressing fatal pneumonia to a relatively mild pneumonic illness.

At the cellular level, legionellae are engulfed by monocytes and can survive therein as intracellular parasites. The duration of intracellular parasitization is unknown but the persistent excretion of group-specific legionella antigen in the urine of some patients, as opposed to its more transient appearance in the majority of cases of legionella pneumonia, points to the possibility that in some patients such intracellular parasitism may be prolonged. There is, however, no evidence of a chronic carrier state or chronic infection. Debilitation, e.g. by immunosuppression or surgery, renders patients more prone to infections which are usually more severe than those encountered as sporadic cases infected in the community. The deterioration in body defences associated with ageing is another important factor, the disease being more common in the elderly.

Pontiac fever

Pontiac fever is a non-pneumonic, non-lethal form of legionella infection. Its pathogenesis is not understood but living legionella have been isolated from sources of infection associated with outbreaks of Pontiac fever and legionella antigen has been demonstrated in the urine of some cases with this illness, indicating that appreciable quantities of legionellae have been involved in the infection.

Almost all legionella infection is due to *L. pneumophila* SG1. Legionellae such as *L. micdadei* and *L. bozemanii*, as well as serogroups of *L. pneumophila* other than SG1, account for a small number of cases; other legionellae are recognized as very occasional causes of infection.

LABORATORY DIAGNOSIS

The tests used in the diagnosis of legionella infection are listed in Table 34.2. As in any case of pneumonia, respiratory secretions, i.e. sputum, bronchial aspirate or washings, as well as pleural fluid, lung biopsy or autopsy material, should be examined both by microscopy and culture. As legionellae stain poorly, Gram-stained films are of little value except to demonstrate the presence of other pathogens and organisms which may interfere with the isolation of legionellae.

The preferred diagnostic procedure is to look for legionellae with specific monoclonal or polyclonal antisera by an immunofluorescent staining technique. In the majority of infections, legionellae are infrequently present in the scanty sputum produced by most patients. Cultures for legionellae are specifically made on BCYE medium and also BCYE with antibiotics added to the medium to suppress other respiratory tract flora. Potentially contaminated material such as sputum or postmortem material may also be heated at 50°C for 30 min in order to diminish growth by other less heat-stable respiratory tract organisms which have an inhibitory effect on growth of legionellae in culture. In heavy infections, legionellae may appear on BCYE media, but not on standard media, after incubation for 48 h at 36°C in an atmosphere of air, preferably enriched with 2.5% carbon dioxide. Some of the less common legionellae may take longer to grow and cultures should not be discarded until after 10–14 d of incubation. Colonies having a 'cut-glass' appearance under plate microscopy or fluorescing blue-white under ultraviolet light are Gram-stained and single colonies are subcultured onto blood agar or cysteine-deficient medium to show that they will *not* grow on these media. Cultures are identified by use of specific antisera in an immunofluorescence test.

Table 34.2 Diagnostic tests for legionella infection

Nature of test	Test	Appropriate specimen
Detection of whole organism	Culture FAT Gene probes	Sputum or other pathological material
Detection of soluble antigen	ELISA	Urine
Detection of antibody	FAT RMAT ELISA	Serum

FAT, fluorescent antibody test; ELISA, enzyme-linked immunosorbent assay; RMAT, rapid micro-agglutination test.

A rapid diagnostic technique, available in some laboratories, is the examination of urine for legionella antigen by enzyme-linked immunosorbent assay (ELISA). This can be accomplished within a working day and is rapid and specific in identifying *L. pneumophila* SG1 as the likely cause of a pneumonia. Although antibodies take at least 8 d to develop after the onset of infection some cases may not reach hospital until this period has elapsed so that it is worthwhile to examine serum for antibodies to *L. pneumophila* on admission to hospital.

Further sera should be taken at intervals to show the development of antibodies or an increase in antibody titre. Although antibodies usually develop soon after 8–10 d of illness and then increase in titre, some patients may not produce any antibody for some weeks or, rarely, for several months. A four-fold or greater rise in antibody titre or an antibody level of 256 or higher in a typical clinical case indicates infection with legionella. However, in some cases proven by culture, lower levels of antibody may be found, especially when death occurs early in the illness. At the present time the only fully validated antibody test for legionella infection is that for infection by *L. pneumophila* SG1, although patients proven by bacterial culture to be infected by other legionellae produce antibodies to the infecting strain. Legionellae have occasionally been isolated from blood culture, but this is not a rewarding routine procedure.

TREATMENT

In the original outbreak of Legionnaires' disease due to *L. pneumophila* SG1 an association was observed between the use of erythromycin and the recovery of patients from infection; those treated with a range of other antibiotics fared less well. Animal experiments have since shown that erythromycin is effective in high dosage in the treatment of legionella infection and that rifampicin is even more effective. Ciprofloxacin is also very active in vitro, but does not appear to be as good as erythromycin or rifampicin in animal models.

In legionella pneumonia, high-dose intravenous erythromycin is the standard therapy. In severe cases, this may be supported by rifampicin and, possibly, by the addition of ciprofloxacin, although evidence for the value of this agent is not well documented.

EPIDEMIOLOGY

L. pneumophila was discovered in 1976 after a point source outbreak of 182 cases of pneumonia mainly affecting members of the American Legion at a convention in Philadelphia. Hence, this form of pneumonia became known as *Legionnaires' disease* and the bacterium associated with it as *L. pneumophila*. Since that time, legionella pneumonia has been recognized as the only acute *bacterial* pneumonia which may occur in outbreak form. This is due to the dissemination of the bacteria in aerosols. Outbreaks may occur on a fairly large scale in the community and the source of infection is invariably a cooling tower in which the bacteria are harboured in the water of the pond associated with this apparatus. Smaller outbreaks have been associated with domestic water supplies in hospitals, spas and hotels and also with whirlpool spas. So-called sporadic cases may on careful epidemiological examination, be shown to be associated with cooling towers in some instances. About a third of cases in the UK acquire their infection abroad, usually from domestic water supplies in hotels. Legionnaires' disease accounts for a small but significant number of pneumonias admitted to hospital. In any outbreak, or even one case occurring as a nosocomial infection, possible sources of an infectious aerosol must be examined by indirect immunofluorescence and cultured to try to identify the source so that it can be eradicated. The disease is most common in those over the age of 40 years with a peak in the 60–70 year age group. Predisposing factors are immunosuppression, smoking and hospitalization. The disease is more prevalent in the late summer and autumn. This may be due to an increase in bacterial numbers in warm water both in natural sources and cooling towers.

Pontiac fever may affect all age groups, including children, the route and source of infection being the same as in Legionnaires' disease. In Pontiac fever the attack rate is high with almost all of

joints. Such chronic brucellosis may follow an acute attack or develop insidiously over several years without previous acute manifestations.

LABORATORY DIAGNOSIS

Brucellosis is confirmed in man and animals by isolating the organisms from the blood and by serological and other tests.

Blood culture

When brucellosis is suspected, blood culture should be attempted repeatedly, not only during the febrile phase. Because the organisms may be scanty, at least 10 ml of blood should be withdrawn on each occasion, 5 ml being added to each of two blood culture tubes containing glucose–serum broth; one tube of each pair should be incubated in an atmosphere containing 10% carbon dioxide. Every few days subculture should be made onto serum–dextrose agar or onto selective media. Blood cultures should be retained for 6–8 weeks before being discarded as negative.

B. melitensis and *B. suis* are more readily isolated from blood than is *B. abortus*.

Serological tests

In the absence of positive blood cultures, the diagnosis of brucellosis depends on serological tests, the results of which tend to vary with the stage of the infection.

The tests used include: the standard agglutination test (SAT); the mercaptoethanol test; the complement fixation test and the anti-human globulin (Coombs') test.

Standard agglutination test (SAT)

This test usually becomes positive 7–10 d after infection. During the acute stage of the disease, levels of agglutination associated with both IgM and IgG immunoglobulins continue to rise. Since prozones may occur in the later stages with high titre sera, it is advisable to make a range of serum dilutions sufficiently great (e.g. to over 1 in 1000) to avoid false-negative results.

Mercaptoethanol test

Low-titre agglutination due to residual IgM may continue to be obtained for many months or even years after the infection has cleared. The mercaptoethanol test is carried out simultaneously and in the same manner as the SAT except that the saline diluent contains 0.05 M 2-mercaptoethanol. The agglutinating ability of IgM is destroyed by 2-mercaptoethanol and therefore agglutination in this test is indicative of the continuing presence of IgG and the likelihood of continuing infection.

Complement fixation test

As the disease progresses from the acute to the chronic form and the organisms become localized intracellularly in various parts of the body, the IgM antibodies decrease; the agglutination titre falls and may become undetectable even while the patient is still ill. The absence of agglutination therefore does not rule out the possibility of infection. IgG antibodies that remain present in the serum and are no longer capable of agglutinating may be detected by complement fixation tests.

In latent or chronic infection, the complement fixation test is likely to be positive whereas in cases of past infection it is negative.

Coombs' test

Non-agglutinating (IgG) antibodies may be detected with anti-human globulin serum as in the Coombs' test. This results in the agglutination of a brucella suspension that has been sensitized by the non-agglutinating antibodies in the patient's serum.

Table 35.2 summarizes the interpretation of serological tests.

It should be noted that in some rural communities the sera from a proportion of the normal population agglutinate brucellae in low dilutions because of previous inapparent or latent infections.

The sera of persons who have been immunized against cholera and of those who have antibodies to *Francisella tularensis* may give false-positive reactions in the agglutination test against brucella organisms.

Table 35.2   Results of serological tests used in the diagnosis of brucellosis

Type of brucellosis	Agglutination test	Complement fixation test	Anti-human globulin test
Acute	+	+	
Chronic	(−)	+	+
Past infection	(−)	−	(-)

(−), weak or negative.

Brucellin skin test

A delayed hypersensitivity reaction similar to the tuberculin test is sometimes used in the diagnosis of brucellosis, but its interpretation is difficult because, in communities frequently exposed to infection, there may be a high incidence of positive skin reactions as a result of latent infection.

Milk ring test

This is a screening test to detect the presence of brucella agglutinins in the milk of infected dairy cattle. It is sufficiently sensitive to be used for testing the bulked milk supply of a herd. A drop of a concentrated suspension of *B. abortus* stained with haematoxylin is added to a 1 ml column of well-mixed milk in a narrow test-tube. If agglutinins are present in the milk the bacteria are agglutinated and rise with the cream to form a blue line above the white skim-milk. In the absence of agglutinins the cream line is white above a blue milk column.

EPIDEMIOLOGY

Brucella melitensis

This organism was first isolated in 1886 from the spleens of fatal cases by David Bruce, an army doctor serving with the British army on the island of Malta. At that time the disease, known as Malta or Mediterranean fever, had a high incidence among army and navy personnel and among the island's civilian population. The name *Brucella* was subsequently given in honour of Bruce who established it as the cause of the disease by transmitting the infection to monkeys.

Twenty years later, Zammit, a Maltese bacteriologist, showed that the organism was transmitted to man in goats' milk. Goats' milk and goats' milk products were subsequently prohibited for services personnel and there followed a spectacular fall in the number of cases, whereas, among the civilian population, who continued to drink goats' milk, the incidence of the disease remained high with a correspondingly high fatality rate.

Brucella abortus

B. abortus infects cattle in many parts of the world. In humans the infection occurs mainly in farming communities and the disease it causes chiefly affects dairy farmers and veterinary surgeons, although persons who consume unpasteurized milk are also at risk.

In the UK five of the nine biotypes of *B. abortus* (biotypes 1, 2, 3, 4 and 9) have in the past been isolated from dairy herds in various parts of the country. However, since the introduction in 1967 of a compulsory scheme of testing and slaughter of infected animals, the disease has been eradicated. Human cases are now rare and are usually contracted abroad. In countries where the infection still exists, a history of close contact with cattle in a patient with a chronic febrile illness should give rise to a suspicion of brucellosis. However, persons who are no longer infected, but who are repeatedly exposed to brucella organisms, as a result of their work, may maintain high levels of IgG in their sera.

Brucella suis

Human brucellosis due to *B. suis* is almost entirely an occupational disease arising from contact with infected pigs or pig meat. It has been reported mainly from the USA, chiefly among those who handled raw meat shortly after slaughter. In some

European countries hares may act as reservoir hosts of *B. suis*.

TREATMENT AND CONTROL

Chemotherapy

Brucella infections respond to a combination of streptomycin and tetracycline or to rifampicin and doxycycline. Intensive treatment in the acute stage of the illness is advisable in order to prevent the infection from progressing to the chronic form which is less likely to respond to treatment. The effectiveness of therapy should be checked by measuring serum antibody titres during and after the course of treatment.

Vaccination

Vaccination of young cattle between 6 and 8 months of age with a single dose of *B. abortus* strain S19 protects them from abortion during the first and subsequent four or five pregnancies. Although vaccination cannot completely protect the animals against infection, it is beneficial in limiting its spread and thereby aids eradication.

Vaccination of man is not recommended because of undesirable side-effects and the possibility that hypersensitivity to brucella protein may develop.

Pasteurization

Pasteurization eliminates the risk of brucella infection arising from the consumption of infected milk or milk products. However, there remains the possibility of infection due to contact with infected cattle or their tissues. Veterinary surgeons and cattle farmers are particularly at risk.

Eradication

This depends on the elimination of the infection from domestic animals by a policy of compulsory testing of the animals and slaughtering positive reactors.

BARTONELLA BACILLIFORMIS

In the mountainous regions of Peru, Colombia and Ecuador in South America, *Bartonella bacilliformis* is responsible for outbreaks of a severe and often fatal disease of man, known as *Oroya fever*. The name was given after an epidemic of the disease in 1870 during the building of a railway between Lima and Oroya, when 7000 workmen died within a few weeks.

After recovery from Oroya fever the patient may suffer from a skin eruption known as *verruga peruana*. Individuals may act as reservoirs of infection long after recovery from the illness and also after asymptomatic infection.

Bart. bacilliformis is pathogenic only to humans. It belongs to the family Bartonellaceae, which includes animal pathogens of the genus *Grahamella*. These are found in the blood cells of moles, mice and other small mammals.

DESCRIPTION

Bart. bacilliformis is a small Gram-negative coccobacillus, $0.3–1.5 \times 0.2–0.5 \, \mu m$. The organisms occur singly, in pairs, chains or clumps. In older cultures they tend to be extremely pleomorphic. They are motile due to about 10 flagella situated at one end of the cell.

The organism is readily cultured in semisolid nutrient agar containing animal protein in the form of rabbit serum and haemoglobin, similar to that used for the culture of leptospires. *Bart. bacilliformis* is strictly aerobic; the optimum temperature for growth is 25–28°C. Growth is slow, taking up to 10 d to be visible.

PATHOGENICITY

After an incubation period of about 20 d, Oroya fever presents as a high fever followed by progressively severe anaemia due to blood cell destruction. There may be enlargement of the spleen and liver and haemorrhages into the lymph nodes.

The case fatality rate may be as high as 40%. Verruga peruana may occur without the initial attack of Oroya fever, or it may develop several weeks after recovery. It consists of a miliary-type skin eruption of round, elevated, hard nodules that may become secondarily infected, producing ulcers and haemorrhagic lesions. The rash may appear mainly on the legs, arms and face, although all parts of the body may be affected. The condition may persist for as long as a year but it is rarely fatal.

LABORATORY DIAGNOSIS

In both Oroya fever and verruga peruana, bartonellosis is confirmed by demonstrating the organisms in blood smears stained by Giemsa. They are seen packing the cytoplasm of the cells and adhering to the cell surfaces.

Blood culture should be carried out at all stages of infection, on semisolid medium containing rabbit serum. Growth is usually apparent within 10 d. It may be difficult to isolate the organisms from the blood when the verruga stage has developed and culture from the skin lesions is rarely satisfactory.

TREATMENT

Penicillin, streptomycin and chloramphenicol may be effective in the treatment of the infection and in reducing the mortality rate. Blood transfusion may be necessary in severe cases of anaemia.

CONTROL

Insecticides such as DDT are used to eliminate the sandfly vector, *Phlebotomus verrucarum*, in likely breeding sites inside and outside of houses and the surrounding areas. Since the insects bite only at night, individuals may protect themselves by withdrawing from affected areas at nightfall.

STREPTOBACILLUS MONILIFORMIS

Streptobacillus moniliformis is one of the causes of *rat-bite fever* in man, the other being *Spirillum minus* (Chapter 31). It is a normal inhabitant of the nasopharynx of rats and sometimes causes an epizootic disease of mice resulting in multiple arthritis and swelling of the feet and legs.

DESCRIPTION

S. moniliformis is Gram-negative, non-motile, non-capsulate and highly pleomorphic. The organisms appear as short bacilli, 1–3 μm in length, forming chains that are interspersed with long filaments that may show oval or spherical lateral swellings.

S. moniliformis is a facultative anaerobe that benefits from added carbon dioxide and a moist atmosphere. The optimum temperature for growth is 37°C and growth ceases at 22°C. The optimum pH is 7.6. Culture media must contain blood, serum or ascitic fluid. Loeffler's serum medium is satisfactory.

After incubation for 2 d, discrete, granular, greyish yellow colonies, 1–5 mm in diameter are visible on the surface, while minute colonies of 0.1–0.2 mm appear in the depth of the medium. The latter are L phase variants that have little or no virulence for laboratory animals. They develop spontaneously and are thought to have a defective mechanism for cell wall formation.

In liquid medium, e.g. serum broth, *S. moniliformis* produces no turbidity, but an abundant granular sediment develops, appearing like cotton wool balls that do not disintegrate on shaking.

S. moniliformis is catalase-, oxidase- and urease-negative. It produces acid from glucose. It does not produce indole.

Sensitivity

S. moniliformis is destroyed by a temperature of 55°C in 30 min. In culture it survives for only a few days although in serum broth at 37°C it may remain viable for as long as 1 week. With the exception of the L forms, *S. moniliformis* is susceptible to penicillin and both forms are sensitive to streptomycin.

PATHOGENICITY

In man the organism enters the body through the wound caused by a rat bite. It multiplies and invades the lymphatics and the bloodstream, causing a feverish illness with severe toxic symptoms and sometimes complications such as arthritis, endocarditis and pneumonia. Infection may also occur in epidemic form as a result of the ingestion of milk or other food contaminated by rats. This causes *Haverhill fever* a condition first described in the USA, which is characterized by fever, polyarthritis and erythema. The duration of the illness varies from a few days to several weeks. If untreated the mortality rate is about 10%.

LABORATORY DIAGNOSIS

S. moniliformis can be isolated in culture from the patient's blood during the acute phase of the illness and from the joint fluid of patients who develop arthritis. When growth occurs in a liquid medium the characteristic cotton wool balls are seen on the surface.

Mice are highly susceptible to intraperitoneal inoculation of patient's blood or joint fluid, as a result of which they develop a rapidly fatal generalized condition, or a more progressive disease with swelling of the feet and legs.

Specific agglutinins may be detected in the patient's serum as early as 10 d or as late as several weeks after the rat bite.

TREATMENT

Penicillin is effective in most cases.

RECOMMENDED READING

Ash J E, Spitz S 1947 Bartonellosis. *Pathology of Tropical Diseases*. W B Saunders, London, ch 3, pp 25–29
Kreier J P, Ristic M 1981 The biology of hemotrophic bacteria. *Annual Review of Microbiology* 35: 325–338
Madkour M M 1989 *Brucellosis*. Butterworths, London
Report 1986 Joint FAO/WHO Expert Committee on Brucellosis, 6th report *WHO Technical Report Series 740*. World Health Organization, Geneva
Washburn R G 1990 *Streptobacillus moniliformis*. In:

Mandell G L, Douglas R G, Bennett J E (eds) *Principles and Practice of Infectious Diseases*, 3rd edn. Churchill Livingstone, Edinburgh, pp 1762–1764
Weinman D 1965 The bartonella group. In: Dubos R J, Hirsch J G (eds) *Bacterial and Mycotic Infections of Man*, 4th edn. Pitman Medical, London, ch 34, pp 775–785
Williams E 1988 Brucellosis in humans: its diagnosis and treatment. *Acta Pathologica Microbiologica et Immunologica Scandinavica* suppl 3: 21–25

Yersinia, pasteurella and francisella

Plague; mesenteric adenitis; tularaemia

J. D. Coghlan

The organisms within these three genera are animal parasites that, under certain conditions, are transmissible to man, either directly or through insect vectors. They are Gram-negative coccobacilli which may show extreme variations in size and shape (*involution forms*), particularly in older cultures.

At one time these organisms were all contained within one genus, *Pasteurella*, but differences among the various strains are sufficient to warrant a division into separate genera, each with its own disease manifestations in man and animals.

The main distinguishing features of the most important species are shown in Table 36.1.

YERSINIA PESTIS
INTRODUCTION

Yersinia pestis (formerly *Pasteurella pestis*), the *plague bacillus*, is essentially a parasite of rodents. In certain parts of the world, burrowing animals such as gerbils and voles act as reservoirs of infection that may be transmitted by fleas to susceptible animals such as bandicoots, marmots and squirrels. The animals suffer from outbreaks of plague and their fleas may transmit the infection to man giving rise to sporadic disease referred to as *wild* or *sylvatic plague*. Farmers or trappers who come into contact with infected animals are at risk.

More serious for man, however, is the spread of infection among rats, especially the black rat, *Rattus rattus*, that at one time flourished around human habitation. Outbreaks of human plague, following epidemics in rats, have, in the past, sometimes developed into pandemics.

DESCRIPTION
Morphology

Y. pestis is a short coccobacillus, $1.5 \times 0.7\,\mu m$, occurring singly, in pairs or, when in fluid culture,

Table 36.1 Differentiating characters of *Yersinia*, *Pasteurella* and *Francisella* species

	Growth on nutrient medium	Growth on bile-salt medium	Motility at 22°C	Motility at 37°C	Acid (no gas) from: Maltose	Acid (no gas) from: Sucrose	Indole production	Urease activity
Y. pestis	+	+	−	−	+	−	−	−
Y. pseudotuberculosis	+	+	+	−	+	−	−	+
Y. enterocolitica	+	+	+	−	+[a]	+	−	+
P. multocida	+	−	−	−	−	+	+	−
P. haemolytica	+	+/−	−	−	−	+	−	−
P. pneumotropica	+	−	−	−	+	+	+	+
P. ureae	+	−	−	−	−	+	−	+
F. tularensis	−	−	−	−	+	−	−	−

[a] Late.

in chains. Pleomorphism is marked, especially in old cultures in which pear-shaped or globular cells, suggestive of yeast cells, may be seen. The organisms are Gram-negative, non-sporing and non-motile. In smears from exudates and in cultures grown at 37°C, instead of at the optimum temperature of 27°C, they are frequently capsulate. In smears from tissues stained by methylene blue they show characteristic bipolar staining.

Cultural characteristics

Y. pestis grows both aerobically and anaerobically but it is somewhat sensitive to oxygen and small inocula may not grow readily in ordinary culture media when grown aerobically. Growth occurs within a temperature range of 14–37°C.

Antigens

There are two main antigenic complexes that include many antigens associated with the virulence and immunogenicity of the organism. One is somatic and heat-stable, the other capsular and heat-labile. Two of the somatic antigens, V and W, appear to enable the organism to resist phagocytosis. The capsular antigen that contains the immunogenic fraction (F1) is necessary for efficient vaccine production.

Sensitivity

Y. pestis is killed at 55°C in 5 min and by 0.5% phenol in 15 min. It is sensitive to drying but may remain viable in moist culture for many months.

Y. pestis is sensitive to tetracycline, streptomycin and sulphonamides, but resistant to penicillin.

PATHOGENESIS

There are three severe forms of human plague: *bubonic, pneumonic* and *septicaemic* plague.

Bubonic plague

The transfer of *Y. pestis* from rats to man through the bites of infected fleas may occasionally result in a localized infection, known as *pestis minor*, with mild constitutional symptoms. More often the lymph nodes draining the area of the flea bite become affected and the adenitis caused results in painful swellings or *buboes* in the inguinal, axillary or cervical regions, depending on the position of the flea bite. From these primary buboes the plague bacilli may spread to all parts of the body. In the absence of adequate antibiotic therapy administered early in the course of the disease, the case fatality rate may be as high as 50%.

Pneumonic plague

This develops as a result of droplets infected with *Y. pestis* being passed from person to person. A severe bronchopneumonia develops. The sputum becomes thin and blood-stained. It contains numerous plague bacilli that are demonstrable by stained films or culture of the sputum. This type of plague is highly contagious and is usually fatal, unless treated early.

Septicaemic plague

This may occur as a primary infection or as a complication of bubonic or pneumonic plague. The plague bacilli spread throughout the body and the outcome is invariably fatal.

LABORATORY DIAGNOSIS

Plague is confirmed by demonstrating the plague bacillus in fluid from buboes in the case of bubonic plague, in the sputum in pneumonic plague and in blood films and by blood culture when septicaemic plague is suspected.

A smear of exudate or sputum is stained with methylene blue. Characteristic bipolar-stained coccobacilli are confirmed as *Y. pestis* by culturing some of the exudate on blood agar and incubating at 27°C. If some of the exudate is inoculated subcutaneously into guinea-pigs or white rats, or onto their nasal mucosa, infection follows and the animals die within 2–5 d.

In septicaemic plague the bacilli may be isolated in blood culture, or from smears of spleen tissue post-mortem.

Characteristic colonies growing on blood agar plates are identified as those of *Y. pestis* by various cultural and biological tests (Table 36.1) and by demonstrating the ability of the bacilli to form chains in broth culture and 'stalactite' growth from drops of oil layered on the surface of fluid medium.

Serology

The patient's serum may be tested by the complement fixation test or by haemagglutination of tanned sheep red cells to which the capsular antigen F1 has been absorbed.

TREATMENT

When plague is suspected, whatever the form, antibiotic therapy should be started without waiting for confirmation of the diagnosis. Tetracycline is the drug of choice. It should be given in large doses (4–6 g daily) for the treatment of bubonic and pneumonic plague, within 48 h of onset.

EPIDEMIOLOGY

History

Plague was introduced into Europe from Asia in the 13th century and led to the great pandemic known as the Black Death, when about a quarter of the population of Europe succumbed to the disease. The infection remained enzootic in European rats and continued to give rise to outbreaks of human plague. After the last major epidemic in England in 1665, plague disappeared spectacularly from Europe, perhaps because the black rat was displaced by the spread of the brown (sewer) rat, *Rattus norvegicus*. *R. norvegicus* is susceptible to plague, but does not commonly frequent human dwellings. Improvements in housing may also have played an important part in the elimination of plague from Europe.

A major outbreak of plague in Hong Kong in 1894 led to a new pandemic, with spread to most major seaports. It was during this outbreak that Yersin first described the plague bacillus.

Strict antirodent measures and the widespread use of DDT to destroy the fleas that transmit the infection have greatly reduced the incidence of urban plague. However, endemic foci of wild rodent plague continue to exist in many rural parts of the world, including North and South America, Africa, South-East Asia, China and the USSR (Fig. 36.1). Constant surveillance must be maintained to prevent its spread to urban populations, especially in areas where living conditions are below standard.

Bubonic plague

Bubonic plague is a zoonosis. The bacilli are transmitted from animal to animal and from animal to man by fleas, notably *Xenopsylla cheopis*, an ectoparasite of rats. In cool humid weather, fleas multiply and plague spreads readily among susceptible rats. Hot, dry weather, on the other hand, tends to limit the spread of infection because the fleas die out under those conditions.

When a flea feeds on the blood of a sick animal, plague bacilli are sucked into the insect's midgut where they multiply to such an extent that they block the proventriculus. On the death of the animal the flea seeks an alternative host which may be another rodent or man. Because the 'blocked' flea is unable to suck readily, some of the infected blood of the previous host is regurgitated and injected into the bite wound of the new victim.

When the epizootic among rats has reached a stage at which the number of susceptible animals has greatly decreased through death or immunity, it tends to die out, as does any human epidemic associated with it. The renewal of an epizootic and an epidemic in the following or later years depends on the growth of a fresh population of young susceptible rats and their heavy infestation of fleas. The infection may be introduced into this fresh population by an old surviving carrier rat with intermittent bacteraemia, or by other infected wild rodents.

Pneumonic plague

The sputum of persons suffering from pneumonic plague contains large numbers of plague bacilli and under favourable conditions the disease spreads rapidly through the community by droplet infection, independently of rodents or fleas. Epidemics are more likely to occur when overcrowding in

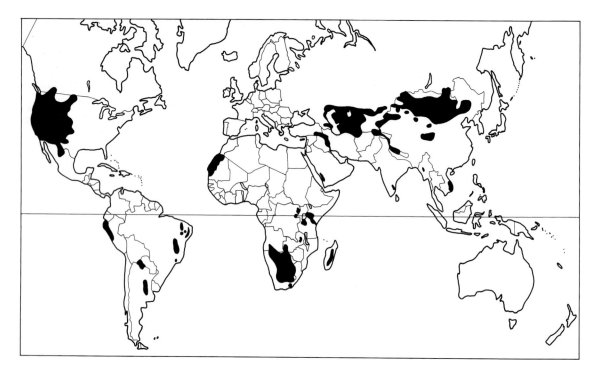

Fig. 36.1 Areas where endemic plague is known to have persisted during the 1980s.

unsanitary dwellings allows the infected droplets to spread readily from person to person.

CONTROL

Bubonic plague

In areas where the infection is endemic, periodic surveys are advocated to determine the prevalence of rodents and fleas so that control measures can be taken. Rats may be destroyed by rat poison and fleas by the liberal application of insecticide to rat runs.

Other control measures include the construction of rat-proof dwelling houses and buildings such as warehouses in dockland areas. The fumigation of ships and measures to prevent rats gaining access to ships help to prevent the spread of plague from one country to another.

Pneumonic plague

To control the spread of pneumonic plague, patients should be isolated if possible and over-

crowding of dwelling houses avoided. Sulphonamides administered to immediate contacts may afford some degree of protection.

Vaccination

Vaccination is sometimes used to protect persons who have been exposed to infection. Live vaccine prepared from avirulent strains of *Y. pestis*, and vaccine prepared from inactivated virulent organisms, are available. Neither can be relied upon to confer immunity of more than short duration, and revaccination is necessary after some months.

YERSINIA PSEUDOTUBERCULOSIS

Y. pseudotuberculosis causes acute mesenteric lymphadenitis in man and attacks many species of wild and domestic animals and birds, causing a fatal septicaemia.

DESCRIPTION

Morphology

Y. pseudotuberculosis is a small, ovoid Gram-negative bacillus which is slightly acid-fast. Like *Y. pestis* it grows on MacConkey's medium, although poorly. The organisms may be differentiated from *Y. pestis* by their motility when grown at 22°C and by their ability to produce urease.

Sensitivity

Y. pseudotuberculosis is sensitive in vitro to tetracyclines, streptomycin, sulphonamides and, unlike *Y. pestis*, penicillin.

Antigens

There are at least six serological types (and a number of subserotypes) that possess highly specific thermostable somatic antigens, one of which is common to all types, and thermolabile flagellar antigens present in cultures grown at 18–26°C. A somatic antigen common to all strains is shared with *Y. pestis* and the two species have many other antigens in common.

About 90% of all human cases appear to have been due to strains of serotype 1. An antigenic relationship exists between serotypes 2 and 4 and salmonellae of groups B and D.

PATHOGENESIS

Y. pseudotuberculosis may give rise to a subclinical infection or it may cause fatal septicaemia. Human infections occasionally result in a severe typhoid-like illness with fever, purpura and enlargement of the liver and spleen which is usually fatal. More frequently it causes mesenteric lymphadenitis, simulating acute or subacute appendicitis, with or without erythema nodosum. This mainly affects young males aged 5–15 years. They usually make an uneventful recovery.

LABORATORY DIAGNOSIS

Y. pseudotuberculosis infection in man is confirmed by isolation of the organism in culture from blood, local lesions or mesenteric glands, particularly the ileocaecal glands.

Specific antibodies in the patient's serum are detected and measured by tube agglutination tests carried out during the acute phase of the illness against smooth suspensions of strains of serotypes 1–6 grown at 22°C. The agglutinins decline rapidly and reach low levels within 3–5 months.

An intradermal test, similar to the tuberculin or brucellin tests, becomes positive during the acute infection and remains positive for many years afterwards.

TREATMENT

Mesenteric adenitis is usually self-limiting. Septicaemia demands parenteral treatment with ampicillin or tetracycline.

EPIDEMIOLOGY

The epidemiology of yersiniosis due to *Y. pseudotuberculosis* is still not clear. Many animal species suffer from the infection, but there is little proof of direct transmission to man. Human infections may result from skin contact with water polluted by infected animals, or the ingestion of contaminated vegetables or other food.

YERSINIA ENTEROCOLITICA

This species resembles *Y. pseudotuberculosis*; it causes gastro-enteritis in man, occasionally with more severe complications.

DESCRIPTION

Morphologically and culturally, *Y. enterocolitica* resembles *Y. pestis* and *Y. pseudotuberculosis* (see Table 36.1), but it differs from them antigenically and biochemically.

Antigenically the species is very complex; 34 different O-antigenic factors and 19 H factors have been identified, so that a large number of serotypes are recognized. Serotypes 3 and 9 account for most human infections in Europe, while serotype 8 is most common in the USA. Other serotypes have been isolated from healthy individuals and are probably non-pathogenic.

On the basis of bacteriophage typing some authorities have divided *Y. enterocolitica* into four different species: *Y. enterocolitica*, *Y. kristenseni*, *Y. intermedia* and *Y. frederikseni*.

PATHOGENESIS

Y. enterocolitica causes mild and severe gastroenteritis, mesenteric lymphadenitis, and septicaemia especially in the elderly. Secondary complications include erythema nodosum, polyarthritis, Reiter's syndrome and meningitis. It differs from *Y. pseudotuberculosis* in that it affects children and adults of both sexes. In young children the infection may produce fever, diarrhoea, abdominal pain and vomiting. The symptoms may last for several weeks.

In animals, *Y. enterocolitica* has been isolated from pseudotuberculosis-like lesions as well as from apparently healthy animals.

TREATMENT

Y. enterocolitica is sensitive to many antibiotics, including tetracyclines, aminoglycosides and chloramphenicol, but it is resistant to penicillins. Treatment is indicated only in severe infection. Tetracycline is probably the drug of choice; β-lactam agents are unreliable.

PASTEURELLA MULTOCIDA

Pasteurella multocida, previously known as *P. septica*, is a parasite of many species of domestic and wild animals and birds. Man occasionally becomes infected, especially following animal bites.

DESCRIPTION

Morphology

P. multocida organisms are aerobic and facultatively anaerobic coccobacilli, 0.7×0.3–$0.6\,\mu m$, i.e. smaller than those of *Yersinia* species. They are arranged singly, in pairs and small bundles, but are pleomorphic in culture. They are Gram-negative, non-motile, non-sporing and capsulate in culture at the optimum temperature of $37°C$. In smears of blood or tissue stained with methylene blue they show bipolar staining. *P. multocida* does not grow on MacConkey's medium.

Antigens

On the basis of 4 capsular antigens and 11 somatic antigens, 15 serotypes of *P. multocida* have been identified.

Sensitivity

P. multocida is killed rapidly at $55°C$ and by phenol (0.5%) in 15 min. The organisms may survive and remain virulent in dried blood for about 3 weeks and in culture or infected tissues for many months if kept frozen.

PATHOGENESIS

P. multocida can be extremely virulent to many species of animals and birds, causing haemorrhagic septicaemia which is usually fatal. It also causes respiratory infections.

The rare human infections take the form of:

1. A local abscess at the site of a cat or dog bite, with cellulitis, adenitis and, sometimes, osteomyelitis.

2. Meningitis following head injury.

3. Infections of the respiratory system such as pleurisy, pneumonia, empyema, bronchitis, bronchiectasis and nasal sinusitis, in which *P. multocida*, although not always the direct cause, may contribute to the severity and duration of the disease.

Cases of appendicitis, in which *P. multocida* has been isolated from pus in pure culture, have also been reported.

LABORATORY DIAGNOSIS

Swabs from bite wounds, from cerebrospinal fluid (CSF) in cases of meningitis and from the secretions in suppurative respiratory tract infections are cultured on blood agar. Identification of the organisms that produce colonies is made by various cultural and biochemical tests (see Table 36.1).

TREATMENT

P. multocida infections usually respond to treatment with penicillin. Tetracycline, erythromycin or co-trimoxazole offer suitable alternatives.

In cases of osteomyelitis following dog or cat bites, antibiotic therapy must be continued for at least 8 weeks.

EPIDEMIOLOGY

P. multocida is carried in the nasopharyngeal region of many species of wild and domestic animals, some of which remain healthy while others suffer septicaemic or respiratory diseases.

In human infections following animal bites, the organism passes directly to man in the animal's saliva. Man may also become infected through breathing an atmosphere contaminated by the coughing of animals suffering from respiratory infection.

P. multocida may be carried commensally in the human respiratory tract and may cause infection after surgical operation or cranial fracture.

OTHER PASTEURELLA SPECIES

P. haemolytica, *P. pneumotropica* and *P. ureae* differ from *P. multocida* in certain details of culture, biochemical characteristics and pathogenicity (Table 36.1). Their pathogenicity for man is not clear.

P. haemolytica causes pneumonia in sheep and cattle, septicaemia in lambs, and various diseases in domestic animals and poultry. It is apparently non-pathogenic for humans. It differs from *P. multocida* in forming haemolytic colonies on blood agar and by its ability to grow on MacConkey's medium.

P. pneumotropica is frequently isolated from the respiratory tract of laboratory animals. In man it has occasionally been isolated from cases of septicaemia, upper respiratory tract infections and from animal bite wounds.

P. ureae has been isolated from the sputum of humans suffering from chronic respiratory tract infection and from the CSF of cases of meningo-encephalitis. It is apparently non-pathogenic for laboratory animals.

FRANCISELLA TULARENSIS

Francisella tularensis produces a disease known as *tularaemia* in man and certain small mammals, notably rabbits and hares.

DESCRIPTION
Morphology

When first isolated from infected tissue, *F. tularensis* is seen as a very small, Gram-negative, non-motile, non-sporing, capsulate coccobacillus, $0.7 \times 0.2\ \mu m$. In culture it tends to be pleomorphic and larger, bacillary, even filamentous forms are present. It stains poorly with methylene blue but carbol–fuchsin (10%) produces characteristic bipolar staining.

Cultural characteristics

F. tularensis is strictly aerobic. It cannot be cultured on ordinary media but requires the addition of either egg yolk or pieces of sterile rabbit spleen. It also grows well on human blood agar containing 2.5% glucose and 0.1% cystine chloride.

Sensitivity

F. tularensis is killed by moist heat at 55°C in 10 min. It may remain viable for many years in culture maintained at 10°C, and for many days in moist soil and in water polluted by infected animals.

PATHOGENESIS

In animals suffering from tularaemia the organisms are present in large numbers within the cells of the liver and spleen, suggesting that they multiply intracellularly.

In man, cases are mostly sporadic, although occasional outbreaks have been reported. After an acute onset with fever, rigors and headache, the disease develops manifestations that vary according to the mode of infection; thus, glandular lesions and ulcers of the skin, sometimes with involvement of the eyes, may result from direct contact with infected animals, whereas indirect contact through tick bites, inhalation of infected dust or ingestion of contaminated meat or water is more likely to lead to typhoid-like or pulmonary illness.

LABORATORY DIAGNOSIS

Human infections are usually diagnosed by inoculating the discharge from local lesions onto a special enriched medium and identifying any small mucoid colonies characteristic of *F. tularensis*. Alternatively, the exudate may be inoculated into guinea-pigs or mice and the liver and spleen of the infected animals cultured post mortem. The patient's serum is tested for specific antibodies to *F. tularensis* by slide or tube agglutination tests. (Diagnostic antigens and antisera for use in the tests are available from Difco Laboratories.) Serum from cases of brucellosis may cross-react with *F. tularensis*.

TREATMENT

Streptomycin or gentamicin are the antibiotics of choice in tularaemia. Tetracycline or chloramphenicol are also effective, but relapse may occur with these bacteriostatic agents.

EPIDEMIOLOGY

Tularaemia has a world-wide distribution. Cases have been reported from North America, from several European countries including Scandinavia, and from Asia. It has not so far been identified in the UK. The infection, which is a typical zoonosis, is mainly tick-borne among the natural hosts, lagomorphs and rodents. It is transmitted to man either directly through the handling of infected animals, e.g. rabbits or hares, or indirectly through tick bites or inhalation of contaminated dust. The organism is highly infectious and laboratory workers are especially at risk through handling infected laboratory animals or cultures of the organism.

Tularaemia is sometimes water-borne as a result of pollution of water with the carcasses or excrement of infected rodents such as water rats or lemmings. Polluted water was probably the cause of the so-called *lemming fever* reported from Norway.

Man-to-man transmission of infection apparently does not occur.

RECOMMENDED READING

Adlam C, Rutter J M 1989 *Pasteurella and pasteurellosis.* Academic Press, London

American Public Health Association 1990 Plague. In: Benenson A S (ed) *Control of Communicable Diseases in Man*, 15th edn. American Public Health Association, Washington, pp 324–329

Cover T L, Aber R C 1989 *Yersinia enterocolitica. New England Journal of Medicine* 321: 16–24

Evans M E, Gregory D W, Schaffner W, McGee Z A 1965 Tularemia: a 30-year experience with 88 cases. *Medicine* 64: 251–269

Mair N S, Fox E 1986 *Yersiniosis; Laboratory Diagnosis, Clinical Features, Epidemiology*. Public Health Laboratory Service, London

Mansor-Bahr P E C, Bell D R (eds) 1987 Plague. *Manson's Tropical Diseases*, 19th edn. Baillière Tindall, London

Report 1983 Yersiniosis, report on a World Health Organization meeting, Paris, 1981. *EURO Reports and Studies 60,* Copenhagen

Tärnvik A 1989 Nature of protective immunity to *Francisella tularensis. Reviews of Infectious Diseases* 11: 440–451

Ziegler P 1969 *The Black Death*. Collins, London

38

Treponema and borrelia

A. Cockayne

Members of the genera *Treponema* and *Borrelia* are spirochaetes and belong to the family Spirochaetaceae.

DESCRIPTION

Spirochaetes are slender unicellular helical or spiral rods (Fig. 38.1) with a number of distinctive ultrastructural features used in the differentiation of the genera (Fig. 38.2). The cytoplasm is surrounded by a cytoplasmic membrane and a peptidoglycan layer contributes to cell rigidity and shape. In *Treponema* species, fine cytoplasmic filaments are visible in the bacterial cytoplasm (Fig. 38.3); but these are absent in *Borrelia* species. Members of both genera are actively motile and several flagella are attached at each pole of the cell and wrap around the bacterial cell body. In contrast to other motile bacteria, these flagella do not protrude into the surrounding medium but are enclosed within the bacterial outer membrane. Treponemal flagella are complex, comprising a sheath and core (Fig. 38.4), whereas those of *Borrelia* species are simpler and similar to those of other bacteria. The spirochaetal outer membrane is unusually lipid-rich and at least in some treponemes appears to be protein-deficient and to lack lipopolysaccharide. This may account for the susceptibility of these organisms to killing by detergents and desiccation.

Although the treponemes are distantly related to Gram-negative bacteria they do not stain by Gram's method and modified staining procedures are used in their examination. Moreover, the

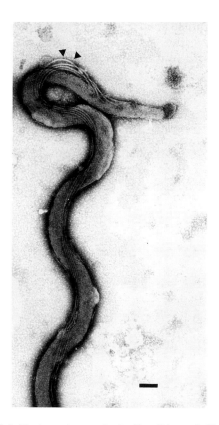

Fig. 38.1 Electron micrograph of a *T. pallidum* cell. The flagella (▼) are inserted at the tip and follow the helical contour of the bacterial cell enclosed within the outer membrane. Bar, 0.1 μm. (Photograph kindly provided by Dr C. W. Penn.)

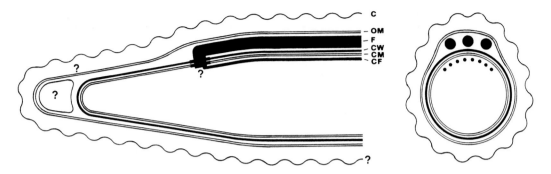

Fig. 38.2 Schematic representation of the structure of the spirochaete *T. pallidum* in longitudinal and cross-section: C, postulated capsular layer; OM, outer membrane; F, flagellum; CW, cell wall peptidoglycan layer; CM, cytoplasmic membrane; CF, cytoplasmic filaments (absent in borreliae). Areas of uncertainty concerning structure are indicated by question marks, and concern the existence and form of the capsular layer, the continuity or otherwise of the outer membrane over the tip of the organism, the nature and form of the tip structure, and the exact juxtaposition of the ends of the cytoplasmic filaments with the bacterial flagellar basal bodies. (Modified from Strugnell et al 1990 *Critical Reviews in Microbiology*, 17: 231–250.)

pathogenic treponemes cannot be cultivated in laboratory media and are maintained by subculture in susceptible animals. In contrast borreliae stain Gram-negative and many pathogenic species can be cultured in vitro in enriched, serum-containing media.

Importance of *Treponema* and *Borrelia* species as human pathogens

The principal human diseases caused by *Treponema* and *Borrelia* species are listed in Table 38.1. These include diseases such as syphilis that have

been known for thousands of years, and more recently recognized infections such as Lyme disease whose prevalence and geographical distribution is still being evaluated.

Treponemal infections may be spread from person to person by intimate physical contact, contact with infectious body fluids or, in some instances, by fomites. The treponemes infecting man are obligate human parasites and no other natural hosts are known. In contrast, borrelial infections are transmitted to man by biting insects

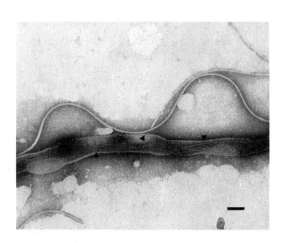

Fig. 38.3 Electron micrograph of a detergent-and protease-treated *T. pallidum* cell showing cytoplasmic filaments (▼) in the bacterial cytoplasm. Bar 0.1 μm.

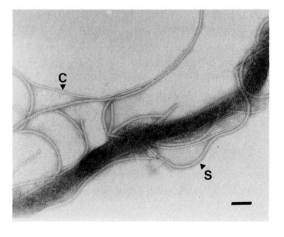

Fig. 38.4 Electron micrograph of a detergent-treated *T. pallidum* cell showing the complex structure of the treponemal flagellum. Both sheathed (S▼) flagella and the thinner flagellar cores (C▼) are visible. Bar, 0.1 μm.

Table 38.1 Principal human diseases caused by spirochaetes

Organism	Disease	Distribution	Primary mode of transmission	Animal reservoirs
T. pallidum	Syphilis	World-wide	Sexual–congenital	None
T. pertenue	Yaws	Humid tropics	Skin-to-skin contact	None
T. endemicum	Bejel	Arid, subtropical or temperate areas	Mouth-to-mouth via utensils	None
T. carateum	Pinta	Arid, tropical Americas	Skin-to-skin contact	None
B. recurrentis	Epidemic relapsing fever	Central, East Africa; South American Andes	Biting insects (lice)	None
Borrelia spp.	Endemic relapsing fever	World-wide[a]	Biting insects (ticks)	Yes
B. burgdorferi	Lyme disease	World-wide[a]	Biting insects (ticks)	Yes

[a] Distribution governed by presence of tick vectors.

(e.g. ticks or lice) infected with the spirochaete. The borreliae that cause Lyme disease and endemic relapsing fever also infect many other animal species which act as reservoirs of infection and man is an unfortunate incidental host in the natural history of these pathogens.

Characteristically, treponemal and borrelial infections occur in several distinct clinical stages. These may be separated by periods of remission and each stage may have a particular associated pathology. Commonly the causative organism is detectable in early lesions but is much more difficult to identify in later disease. The pathogen spreads from the initial site of infection to many organs via the bloodstream, and in some untreated cases these infections may be progressive, destructive and, in some instances (e.g. tertiary syphilis), may be fatal. In other cases, however, only the early symptoms are apparent and the later pathology is not seen.

With the exception of the relapsing fevers, in which antigenic variation contributes to bacterial virulence, the pathogenic mechanisms employed by spirochaetes are poorly understood. No extracellular toxins have yet been identified and the mechanisms that enable these organisms to persist in tissues despite vigorous immune responses remain unclear. It seems likely, however, that the later manifestations of these infections may involve auto-immune phenomena.

In addition to the pathogenic species, many other spirochaetes form part of the normal bacterial flora of the mouth, gut and genital tract. Morphological and antigenic similarities between pathogenic and commensal spirochaetes may cause problems in the clinical and serological diagnosis of spirochaetal infections.

TREPONEMA

Treponema species pathogenic for man include the causative agents of venereal *syphilis*, and the non-venereal treponematoses *yaws*, *bejel* and *pinta*. The spirochaetes causing these different infections are morphologically identical—tightly coiled helical rods, 5–15 µm long and 0.1–0.5 µm in diameter—and show only subtle antigenic differences. Differentiation of these organisms is based primarily on the clinical syndromes they cause and minor differences in the pathology induced in experimental animals.

Treponema pallidum ssp. *pallidum* (*T. pallidum*)

T. pallidum is the causative agent of syphilis and was first isolated from syphilitic lesions in 1905. Infection is usually acquired by sexual contact with infected individuals and is commonest in the most sexually active age group of 15–30 year olds. *Congenital syphilis* usually occurs following vertical transmission of *T. pallidum* from the infected mother to the fetus in utero but neonates may also be infected during passage through the infected birth canal at delivery. Infection in utero may have serious consequences for the fetus. Rarely, syphilis has been acquired by transfusion of infected fresh human blood.

Pathogenesis

Untreated syphilis may be a progressive disease with *primary*, *secondary*, *latent* and *tertiary* stages. *T. pallidum* enters tissues by penetration of intact mucosae or through abraded skin. The bacterium rapidly enters the lymphatics, is widely disseminated via the bloodstream and may lodge in any organ. The exact infectious dose for man is not known but in experimental animals less than 10 organisms are sufficient to initiate infection. The bacteria multiply at the initial entry site and a lesion characteristic of primary syphilis—a *chancre* —forms following an average incubation period of 3 weeks. The chancre is painless and most frequently on the external genitalia, but it may occur on the cervix, perianal area, in the mouth or anal canal. Chancres usually occur singly but in immunocompromised individuals, such as those infected with the human immunodeficiency virus (HIV), multiple chancres may develop.

The chancre heals spontaneously within 3–6 weeks, and 2–12 weeks later the symptoms of secondary syphilis develop. These are highly variable and widespread but most commonly involve the skin where macular or pustular lesions develop, particularly on the trunk and extremities. The lesions of secondary syphilis are highly infectious.

These lesions gradually resolve and a period of latent infection in which no clinical manifestations are evident but serological evidence of infection persists is entered. Relapse of the lesions of secondary syphilis is common and latent syphilis is classified as early (high likelihood of relapse) or late (recurrence unlikely). Individuals with late latent syphilis are not generally considered infectious but may still transmit infection to the fetus during pregnancy and their blood may remain infectious.

Late or tertiary syphilis, which may develop decades after the primary infection, is a slowly progressive, destructive inflammatory disease that may affect any organ. The three most common forms of late syphilis are *neurosyphilis, cardiovascular syphilis* and *gummatous syphilis*—a rare granulomatous lesion of the skeleton, skin or mucocutaneous tissues.

Treponema pallidum ssp. *pertenue* (*T. pertenue*)

T. pertenue is the causative agent of *yaws*, a disease that is endemic among rural populations in tropical and subtropical countries such as Africa, South America, South-East Asia and Oceania. The number of cases of yaws world-wide was estimated at over 50 million in the 1950s but eradication programmes sponsored by the World Health Organization reduced the number of cases to less than 2 million in the 1970s. Termination of these programmes has led to a resurgence of pockets of disease, particularly in West Africa.

Infection with *T. pertenue* is non-venereal, and occurs following contact of traumatized skin with exudate from early yaws lesions. Infection is usually acquired before puberty. Primary yaws has an incubation period of between 3 and 5 weeks and the initial lesions usually occur on the legs. The papular lesions enlarge, erode and usually heal spontaneously within 6 months. Eruption of similar lesions occurs weeks to months later and relapse is common. Secondary lesions of yaws may involve bones— particularly the fingers, long bones and the jaw. Late yaws is characterized by cutaneous plaques and ulcers and thickening of the skin on the palms and soles of the feet. Gummatous lesions may also develop. In contrast to syphilis, neurological and cardiovascular damage does not occur in late yaws. As affected individuals acquire infection early in life, they are essentially non-infectious at child-bearing age and congenital yaws is unknown.

Treponema pallidum ssp. *endemicum* (*T. endemicum*)

This organism causes a non-venereal, syphilis-like disease called *endemic syphilis* or *bejel*. Bejel is endemic in Africa, western Asia and Australia and is an infection which mainly affects children in rural populations where living conditions and personal hygiene are poor. Transmission is by direct person-to-person contact and by sharing of contaminated eating or drinking utensils.

The initial lesion is usually oral and may not be detected. Secondary lesions include oropharyngeal mucous patches, condyloma lata and periostitis. Late lesions involve gummata in the skin, nasopharynx and bones. As in yaws, the cardiovascular and central nervous systems are not involved and congenital infection is rare because of the early age of infection.

Treponema carateum

Unlike the other treponematoses, the manifestations of *pinta*, caused by *T. carateum*, are confined to the skin. Although these lesions are non-destructive, they do cause disfigurement with associated social problems for infected individuals. Pinta is probably the oldest human treponemal infection, whose distribution today is restricted to arid rural inland regions of Mexico, Central America and Colombia.

Spread of infection is by direct contact with infectious lesions and, following a 7–21 d incubation period, small, erythematous pruritic primary lesions develop most commonly on the extremities, face, neck, chest or abdomen. The primary lesions enlarge and coalesce and once healed may leave areas of hypopigmentation. Disseminated secondary lesions appear 3–12 months later and may become dyschromic. Recurrence of lesions is common up to 10 years after initial infection. The depigmented lesions are characteristic of the later stages of pinta but do not cause any serious harm.

Other infections associated with treponemes

There are several other human infections in which treponemes are implicated. Commonly, the microbial flora associated with these conditions is complex and the exact role of the spirochaetes in the aetiology of infection remains to be determined. Moreover, the true taxonomic status of some of these organisms is uncertain.

Oral infections

T.denticola and *T. socranskii* form part of the normal flora and numbers of these organisms increase in periodontal disease. *T. vincentii* (or Vincent's spirillum) is similarly associated with ulceromembranous gingivitis or pharyngitis, *Vincent's angina*. Several spirochaetes appear to be involved in the aetiology of a similar condition called *trench mouth*.

Gastro-intestinal infections

T. hyodysenteriae is the causative agent of *swine dysentery*, and a similar organism has been implicated as a rare cause of gastro-intestinal infection in humans.

Skin lesions

Tropical ulcer is a chronic skin condition in which spirochaetes of unknown identity have been implicated, usually in association with fusiform bacteria and other organisms.

LABORATORY DIAGNOSIS OF TREPONEMAL INFECTIONS

The inability to grow most pathogenic treponemes in vitro, coupled with the transitory nature of many of the lesions, makes diagnosis of treponemal infection impossible by routine bacteriological methods. Although spirochaetes are detectable by microscopy in primary and secondary lesions, diagnosis is based primarily on clinical observations and is confirmed by serological tests. For practical purposes, the serological responses to all these pathogens are identical and only their use in the serodiagnosis of syphilis will be considered here.

Direct microscopy

Treponemes can be visualized directly in freshly collected exudate from primary or secondary lesions by dark-ground or phase-contrast microscopy. Although this method allows a rapid definitive diagnosis to be made it may be rather insensitive because primary lesions may contain relatively few bacteria. In addition, care must be taken to differentiate between pathogenic and commensal spirochaetes that may occasionally contaminate such material. More sensitive and specific results may be obtained using fixed material in an immunofluorescence assay with an anti-treponemal antibody.

Serological tests

Infection with *T. pallidum* results in the rapid production of two types of antibodies:

1. Specific antibodies directed primarily at polypeptide antigens of the bacterium.
2. Non-specific antibodies that react with a non-treponemal antigen called *cardiolipin.*

The mechanism of induction of non–specific antibodies remains unclear. Cardiolipin is a phospholipid extracted from beef heart and it is possible that a similar substance, present in the treponemal cell or released from host cells damaged by the bacterium, may stimulate antibody production.

Assays for non-specific antibody, because of their low cost and technical simplicity, are routinely used as screening tests for evidence of syphilis infection. Since these tests have relatively low specificity, positive results are confirmed by detection of specific anti-*T. pallidum* antibody.

Non-specific serological tests for syphilis

The *Venereal Disease Reference Laboratory (VDRL)* test is a non-specific serological test for syphilis which uses a mixture of cardiolipin, cholesterol and lecithin as antigen. IgM or IgG antibody present in positive sera cause a suspension of this lipoidal antigen to flocculate, and the result can be rapidly read by eye. This is used as a screening test and is positive in approximately 70% of primary and 99% of secondary syphilitics, but is negative in individuals with late syphilis. This test can be used quantitatively, and increases in VDRL titre with time may be used to confirm a diagnosis of congenital syphilis.

Since a positive result in the VDRL test usually indicates active infection, it can also be used to monitor the efficacy of antibacterial therapy.

Tests for specific anti-treponemal antibody

Fluorescent treponemal antibody (FTA-Abs) test. The FTA-Abs test is an indirect immunofluorescence assay in which *T. pallidum* is used as antigen. Acetone-fixed treponemes are incubated with heat-treated sera and bound antibody is detected with a fluorescein-labelled conjugate and ultraviolet microscopy. The serum is first absorbed with a suspension of a non-pathogenic treponeme which removes non-specific cross-reactive antibodies that may be directed against commensal spirochaetes. The FTA-Abs is positive in approximately 80, 100 and 95% of primary, secondary and late syphilitics respectively, and, unlike the VDRL test, remains positive following successful therapy.

T. pallidum haemagglutination assay (TPHA). In this test, *T. pallidum* antigen is coated onto the surface of red blood cells and specific antibody in test sera causes haemagglutination. As in the FTA-Abs assay, sera are pre-absorbed with a non-pathogenic treponeme to remove antibody against commensal spirochaetes. The TPHA is less sensitive than the FTA-Abs in primary syphilis (positive in 65%) but both give similar results for secondary and late syphilis; the TPHA also remains positive for life following infection. This assay can also be used to detect localized production of anti-treponemal antibodies in cerebrospinal fluid, a marker of neurosyphilis.

Other antibody tests. Production of monoclonal anti-*T.pallidum* antibodies has permitted development of assay systems based on the detection of antibody responses to particular treponemal antigens. Such assays use enzyme-linked immunosorbent assay (ELISA) technology, allowing rapid screening of large numbers of samples with potentially enhanced specificity.

Problems in the serological diagnosis of syphilis

Occasionally, both the non-specific and specific tests produce false-positive results. The VDRL assay may give a transient positive result following any strong immunological stimulus such as acute

bacterial or viral infection or following immunization. More persistent false-positive results occur
in individuals with auto-immune or connective
tissue disease, in drug abusers and in individuals
with hypergammaglobulinaemia. False-positive results usually become apparent when negative
results are found in specific serological tests but
in some cases FTA-Abs results may also be
positive or borderline.

Rarely, the FTA-Abs test may be positive and
the non-specific VDRL test negative. Other
spirochaetal diseases such as relapsing fever,
yaws, pinta and leptospirosis may give positive
results in both specific and non-specific tests. Of
particular difficulty is the differential diagnosis of
syphilis and yaws in immigrants from areas in
which yaws is endemic.

Lyme disease (see below) induces antibodies
that react in the FTA-Abs but not in the VDRL
assay.

Direct detection of spirochaetal DNA in clinical
material by molecular methods, such as the polymerase chain reaction, may have a future role in
confirming a diagnosis of syphilis in difficult or
atypical cases.

TREATMENT

All the pathogenic treponemes are sensitive to
benzylpenicillin, and prolonged high-dose therapy
with procaine penicillin has been the traditional
method of treatment for primary and secondary
syphilis. So far there have been no reports of penicillin resistance. If penicillin allergy is a problem,
erythromycin, tetracycline or chloramphenicol
may be used. There are reports of treatment failure
with erythromycin and an erythromycin-resistant
variant of *T. pallidum* has been isolated. In late
syphilis, aqueous benzylpenicillin is used, as this
penetrates better into the central nervous system.

Antibiotic therapy of syphilitics, particularly
with penicillin, characteristically induces a
systemic response called the *Jarisch–Herxheimer
reaction*. This is characterized by the rapid onset
(within 2 h) of fever, chills, myalgia, tachycardia,
hyperventilation, vasodilation and hypotension.
This response is thought to be due to release of
an endogenous pyrogen from the spirochaetes.

EPIDEMIOLOGY AND CONTROL
Syphilis

The incidence of all venereal diseases, including
syphilis, increased dramatically during the Second
World War. The widespread introduction of antibiotic therapy shortly afterwards produced an
equally dramatic decrease in the incidence of
these diseases, but syphilis remained endemic
within the general population. Until the mid-
1980s most cases of syphilis in developed countries
occurred in male homosexuals. The advent of
HIV and acquired immune deficiency syndrome
(AIDS) in the 1980s reduced the incidence among
this group due to changes in sexual practices.
More recently, there has been a resurgence of
syphilis among the heterosexual population in the
USA, resulting in an increase in the incidence
among women and in the number of cases of
congenital syphilis. Several possibilities may have
accounted for this increase, including:

1. Changes in health care policies and abolition
   of screening of pregnant women in some states
2. Increased promiscuity associated with drug
   abuse
3. Changes in antibiotic prescribing for other
   sexually transmitted diseases which previously
   resolved many inapparent infections with
   T.pallidum.

Although the incidence of all forms of syphilis
in the UK is currently very low (fewer than 500
cases reported in 1988), this disease still has major
implications in relation to public health. In particular, the possibility of congenital infection and
the acquisition of syphilis by blood transfusion,
necessitates large and costly screening programmes
of all pregnant women and blood donations.

Control of syphilis is achieved by treating index
cases and any known contacts. Treatment of
contacts is important as some may be incubating
the infection even if they have no overt signs of
disease.

Other treponematoses

The incidence of the other treponematoses is
primarily influenced by socio-economic factors.

Prevention and control of these diseases therefore involves treatment of cases, individuals with latent disease and contacts, and improvement of living conditions and personal hygiene

BORRELIA

The two principal human diseases associated with borreliae are *relapsing fever*, caused by *Borrelia recurrentis* and several other *Borrelia* species; and *Lyme disease*, a multisystem infection caused by *B. burgdorferi*. The bacteria causing these infections are morphologically similar helical rods, 8–30 μm long and 0.2–0.5 μm in diameter, with 3–10 loose spirals. Antigenic differences are used in differentiation of the species.

RELAPSING FEVERS

Relapsing fevers occur virtually world-wide in endemic or epidemic forms. Both are transmitted to man by arthropod vectors. They are characterized clinically by recurrent periods of fever and spirochaetaemia.

Endemic or *tick-borne relapsing fever* is caused by several *Borrelia* species, including *B. duttoni*, *B. hermsii*, *B. parkeri* and *B.turicatae*, and is transmitted to man by soft-bodied *Ornithodorus* ticks. The natural hosts for these organisms include rodents and other small mammals on which the ticks normally feed. Endemic relapsing fever occurs world-wide, reflecting the distribution of the tick vector. In contrast, *B. recurrentis* is an obligate human pathogen, the sole cause of *epidemic* or *louse-borne relapsing fever* and is transmitted from person to person by the human body louse, *Pediculus humanus*. The incidence of epidemic relapsing fever is influenced by socio-economic factors such as lack of personal hygiene and, historically, increases during periods of social upheaval such as wars and famines. This disease still occurs in central and eastern Africa and in the South American Andes.

The spirochaetes causing the two forms of relapsing fever differ in their mode of growth in the insect vector and this influences the way infection is initiated in man. *B. recurrentis* grows in the haemolymph of the louse but does not invade tissues. As a result the excrement of the louse is non-infectious and the bacterium is not transferred transovarially to the progeny. Infection occurs in man when such lice are crushed, releasing the bacteria which then gain entry to tissues through damaged or intact skin or mucous membranes. Spirochaetes causing tick-borne relapsing fever invade all the tissues of the tick, including the salivary glands, genitalia and excretory system. Infection therefore occurs when saliva or excrement are released during feeding. Transovarial transmission to the tick progeny maintains the spirochaete in the tick population.

Pathogenesis of relapsing fever

In both forms of relapsing fever, acute symptoms, including high fever, rigors, headache, myalgia, arthralgia, photophobia and cough, develop about 1 week after infection. A skin rash may occur and there is central nervous system involvement in up to 30% of cases. During the acute phase there may be up to 10^5 spirochaetes per cubic millimetre of blood. The primary illness resolves within 3–6 d and terminates abruptly with hypotension and shock, which may be fatal. Relapse of fever occurs 7–10 d later and several relapses may occur. Each episode of spirochaetaemia is terminated as the result of development of specific anti-spirochaete antibody. Subsequent febrile episodes are caused by borreliae that differ antigenically, particularly in outer-membrane protein composition, from those causing earlier attacks. As the cycle of fever and relapse continues, the borreliae tend to revert back to the antigenic types that caused the original spirochaetaemia, and ultimate clearance of the infection appears to be due to antibody-mediated killing.

In general, louse-borne relapsing fever has longer febrile and afebrile periods than tick-borne infection, but fewer relapses. The case fatality rate varies from 4 to 40% for louse-borne infection and from 2 to 5% for tick-borne relapsing fever, with myocarditis, cerebral haemorrhage and liver failure the most common causes of death.

Laboratory diagnosis

Definitive diagnosis of relapsing fevers is made by detection of borreliae in peripheral blood samples.

Thick or thin blood smears may be stained with Giemsa, or other stains such as acridine orange.

Although antibodies to the borreliae are produced during infections, antigenic variation and the tendency to relapse complicates serological tests for these infections, and such tests are not widely available. Serological tests for syphilis are positive in 5–10% of cases.

Treatment

Tetracycline, chloramphenicol, penicillin and erythromycin have been used successfully. As in the treatment of syphilis, a Jarisch–Herxheimer reaction is produced following administration of antibiotics.

Prevention of these infections involves avoidance or eradication of the insect vector. Insecticides can be used to eradicate ticks from human dwellings but elimination from the environment is not feasible. Prevention of louse-borne infection involves maintenance of good personal hygiene and delousing if necessary.

LYME DISEASE

Lyme disease is a multisystem syndrome caused by *B. burgdorferi*. This disease was originally called *Lyme arthritis* and was recognized as an infectious condition in 1975, following an epidemiological investigation of a cluster of cases of suspected juvenile rheumatoid arthritis which occurred in Lyme, Connecticut, USA. A common factor in these cases was a previous history of insect bite, and the infectious agent, *B. burgdorferi*, was subsequently isolated from an *Ixodes* tick. Retrospective serological data suggests that Lyme disease was endemic in the USA as early as 1962, and the clinical manifestations of this infection have been known in Europe, including the UK, since the early 1900s. Lyme disease has now been reported in the USA, Europe and Scandinavia and, more recently, in the USSR, China, Japan and Australia.

The natural hosts for *B. burgdorferi* are wild and domesticated animals, including mice and other rodents, deer, sheep, cattle, horses and dogs. Infection in these animals may be inapparent, though clinical infection has been observed in cattle, horses and dogs.

B. burgdorferi is transmitted to man by ixodid ticks that become infected whilst feeding on infected animals. The principal vectors are, in the USA, *Ixodes dammini* and *I. pacificus* and, in Europe, *I. ricinus*. The life cycle of these ticks involves larval, nymph and adult stages, all of which are capable of transmitting infection, though the nymphal stage is most commonly implicated. In areas endemic for Lyme disease, 2–50% of ticks may carry *B. burgdorferi*. The bacterium grows primarily in the midgut of the tick and transmission to man occurs during regurgitation of the gut contents during the blood meal.

Lyme disease may be a progressive illness and is divided into three stages. Although there is general similarity, clinical manifestations may differ in the USA and Europe, possibly reflecting differences in strains of *B. burgdorferi* and genetic factors in the two populations.

Stage 1 Lyme disease is characterized by a spreading annular rash, *erythema chronicum migrans* (ECM), which occurs at the site of the tick bite 3–22 d after infection. The bacterium also disseminates to a variety of other organs. In the USA, secondary lesions similar to those of ECM are common. Malaise, fatigue, headache, rigors and neck stiffness may also be apparent. ECM and secondary lesions fade within 3–4 weeks and, weeks to months later, some patients develop cardiac or neurological abnormalities, musculoskeletal symptoms or intermittent arthritis, which are characteristic of *stage 2* Lyme disease. In general this arthritis is more often observed in the USA than in Europe, where neurological complications are more common. Patients with *stage 3* disease, which may occur months to years later, present with chronic skin, nervous system or joint abnormalities.

Congenital infection with *B. burgdorferi* may occur with serious, potentially fatal consequences for the fetus.

Laboratory diagnosis

Once a clinical diagnosis has been made, culture of the spirochaete from suitable biopsy material provides a definitive diagnosis but this is a specialized technique that is not widely available. In addition, the difficulty encountered in detecting the organism in histological sections means that serological tests are routinely used for the confirmation of Lyme disease.

Specific IgM antibodies develop within 3–6 weeks of infection. The earliest response appears to be against the bacterial flagellum and later against outer-surface proteins. Subsequently, IgG antibodies are produced and the highest titre is detectable months or years after infection.

An indirect immunofluorescence test is available, but ELISA is now widely used. Immunoblotting has been proposed as a method of confirming serological diagnosis. Serological diagnosis of early Lyme disease may still pose problems, as in some individuals antibodies to the bacterium are slow to develop and formation of immune complexes may affect the test results. Antibodies produced may cross-react with other spirochaetes and sera from Lyme disease patients may give a positive FTA-Abs test, though the VDRL test is negative.

Serological evidence of infection may also be detectable in the absence of overt disease in apparently normal individuals. The significance of these findings is not yet clear but the possibility that such individuals may develop late complications of Lyme disease merits consideration.

Treatment

Penicillins, erythromycin, and tetracyclines have all been used successfully in Lyme disease. Reports suggest that treatment with tetracyclines produces fewer later complications than penicillin therapy.

Approximately 15% of patients experience a Jarisch–Herxheimer reaction following antibiotic therapy. Despite antibiotic treatment, a number of patients still suffer from minor late complications of the disease, which may be immunologically mediated or may indicate low-level persistence of the organisms. An additional complication of antibiotic therapy is the reduction or abolition of the antibody response to the bacterium, which may interfere with the serological confirmation of infection.

Epidemiology and control

The geographical distribution of Lyme disease is governed by that of the tick vector and its associated animals hosts. Consequently, infection with *B. burgdorferi* occurs primarily in individuals who frequent these areas. Forestry workers and farmers are particularly at risk, but infection is also associated with recreational activities. In the UK, Lyme disease occurs in areas such as the New Forest, Thetford Chase, North Yorkshire and rural parts of Scotland, Wales and Ireland that support large populations of wild or domesticated animals on which ixodid ticks feed. In 1987 there were approximately 70 cases of clinically and serologically proven Lyme disease in the UK, and estimates suggest that now up to 1000 cases per year may occur in the UK. To date, about 25 000 cases have been diagnosed in the USA.

Prevention of infection involves avoidance of Lyme disease-endemic areas and education of the public regarding the possible risks of infection in these localities. Eradication of the tick vectors or mammalian hosts from such areas is not feasible.

RECOMMENDED READING

Barbour A G 1990 Antigenic variation of a relapsing fever *Borrelia* species. *Annual Review of Microbiology* 44: 155–171

Barbour A G, Hayes S F 1986 Biology of *Borrelia* species. *Microbiological Reviews* 50: 381–400

Holt S C 1978 Anatomy and chemistry of spirochetes. *Microbiological Reviews* 42: 114–160

Hudson M J 1991 The spirochaetes. In: Duerden B I, Drasar B S (eds) *Anaerobes in Human Disease*. Edward Arnold, London, pp 108–132

Schell R F, Musher D M (eds) 1983 *Pathogenesis and Immunology of Treponemal infections*. Marcel-Decker, New York

Steere A G 1989 Lyme disease. *New England Journal of Medicine* 321: 586–596

Szczepanski A, Benach J L 1991 Lyme borreliosis: host responses *to Borrelia burgdorferi*. *Microbiological Reviews* 55: 21–34

39

Leptospira
Leptospirosis; Weil's disease

J. D. Coghlan

Spirochaetes of the genus *Leptospira* are characterized by their slender appearance, numerous coils, hooked ends and active motility. Many different types exist; some are harmless to man and animals, while others are potential pathogens. The parasitic leptospires are normally carried in the kidneys of rodents and other small mammals and are excreted in the urine. In some parts of the world, wading birds, snakes, frogs and tortoises are infected, although they probably play only a minor role as carrier hosts. The organisms appear to cause no harm to their normal hosts but if they are transmitted accidentally to other animal species or to humans, they may give rise to clinical infections. The disease may be relatively mild or extremely severe. In man the most virulent types may cause spirochaetal jaundice, known as *Weil's disease* after the German physician who described the syndrome in 1886. In cattle, pigs, sheep, goats and horses, infection may give rise to abortions, or stillbirth in pregnant animals and mastitis in lactating cattle. Dogs suffer two forms of leptospirosis, one characterized by an acute and often fatal jaundice, the other a subacute or chronic nephritis, depending on the type of leptospire responsible.

DESCRIPTION

Classification

The genus *Leptospira* consists of two species, *Leptospira interrogans* and *L. biflexa*. The former includes the parasitic strains while the latter comprises the free-living saprophytic strains found in fresh water and occasionally in salt or brackish water.

The two species are indistinguishable morphologically but *L. biflexa* strains can grow in simple media without the addition of animal protein, which is normally essential for the growth of parasitic leptospires. Saprophytic strains can also grow at a temperature of 13°C and in the presence of 8-azaguanine, both of which are inhibitory to strains of *L. interrogans*. The two species may also be differentiated by their DNA composition.

Within the two species serological tests have revealed many antigenic variations, some of which are genus-specific, whereas others are restricted to certain strains. On the basis of these more specific antigens, many different serovars (serotypes) may be distinguished. Because of common antigens, certain serovars are collected into serogroups. Within *L. interrogans* 23 serogroups are now recognized, comprising over 170 serovars that have been isolated from man and animals.

Morphology

Leptospires are spiral bacteria, 6–20 μm long and 0.1 μm broad. They usually appear straight and rigid with one or both ends hooked, although unhooked forms are sometimes seen. The primary coils are so numerous and so closely set together that they are difficult to see in the living state except by dark-ground microscopy (Fig. 39.1). They are so thin that they are capable of passing

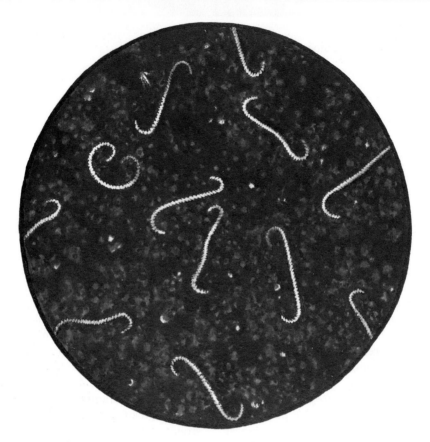

Fig. 39.1 The appearance of living leptospires as seen by dark-ground microscopy. Note the very fine coils and characteristic hooked ends. (From an original painting by Dr Cranston Low, in Low and Dodds 1947 *Atlas of Bacteriology* Livingstone, Edinburgh.)

through a membrane filter with a pore size of 0.22 μm.

Electron microscopy reveals a helicoidal protoplasmic cylinder surrounded by a cytoplasmic membrane and a peptidoglycan complex, the whole being enclosed in an outer envelope of at least three layers (Fig. 39.2). Between the cytoplasmic membrane and the outer envelope two flagella-like axial filaments are entwined around the organism, each attached subterminally, one at either end of the cell, to a basal body. The free ends of the axial filaments are directed towards the centre of the leptospire (Fig. 39.3).

Movement

In liquid medium leptospires rotate rapidly along their long axes and also glide across the field with either end foremost, occasionally forming secondary coils and then straightening again into the rigid form that is so characteristic of the group.

Staining

Leptospires stain poorly with the usual bacterial stains but they can be demonstrated by the silver impregnation techniques of Levaditi and Fontana and by fluorescent antibody techniques.

Cultural characteristics

Leptospires are obligate aerobes. The optimum growth temperature is 28–32°C, but for primary isolation from infected tissues incubation at 37°C may be advantageous. They grow best in a fluid

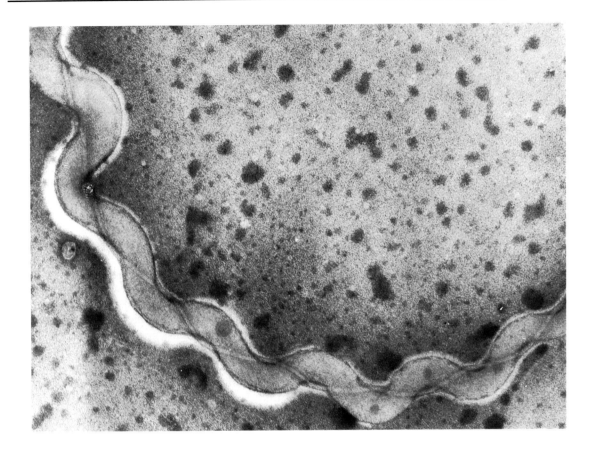

Fig. 39.2   Part of an intact leptospire, showing the protoplasmic cylinder, cell wall, outer envelope and axial filaments. (Transmission electron micrograph.)

medium of pH 7.2. Growth is slow, especially in primary culture, and may not be obvious until 2 or 3 weeks after inoculation.

L. interrogans strains require the addition of animal protein in the form of serum, or a fraction of bovine serum albumin (fraction V) with polysorbate (Tween 80), to supply the fatty acids that are their main source of energy. This medium, first devised by Ellinghausen and McCullough, is used in a modified form known as EMJH medium for culturing the strains that are used in serological diagnostic tests and for typing newly isolated strains.

A semisolid medium prepared by adding 0.2–0.5% agar to liquid medium is used for isolating leptospires from animal tissues.

Sensitivity

Leptospires are killed at a temperature of 50°C in 10 min and at 60°C in 10 s. They are susceptible to desiccation, to hypochlorite disinfectants and to pH values outside the range 6.2–8.0. They are especially sensitive to acid urine, non-aerated sewage and polluted water. Unlike saprophytic strains, they do not survive for long in salt or brackish water.

Pathogenic leptospires may survive for several days outside the animal body in moist conditions at a pH of not less than 6.8. They survive for a time in animal tissues kept at low temperature; thus, serovar *canicola* has been isolated from pigs' kidneys on sale in a butcher's shop.

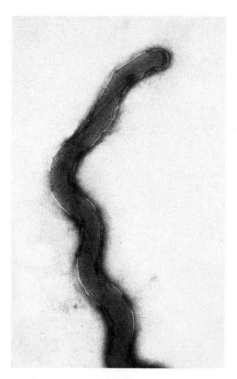

Fig. 39.3 One end of a leptospiral cell showing the axial filament attached to the basal body. × 70 000. (Transmission electron micrograph by courtesy of Dr Kari Hovind-Hougen.)

PATHOGENESIS

The pathogenic leptospires enter the body through cuts or abrasions of the skin or through the mucous membranes of the nose, mouth or eyes. They multiply in the blood and circulate to all parts of the body, affecting any organ, so that the signs and symptoms that characterize the disease vary considerably in their form and intensity. A mild influenza-like illness may develop, sometimes with meningitis and usually with some degree of renal involvement, indicated by albuminuria. *Canicola fever* is an example of this type of 'benign' leptospirosis. At the other extreme the disease may be severe and even fatal, characterized by jaundice and haemorrhages in the eyes, skin and mucous membranes. Any of the pathogenic serovars may cause benign leptospirosis, but the severe form, Weil's disease, is usually due to serovar *icterohaemorrhagiae*. In some parts of the world, other serovars, e.g. *andamana*, *australis*, *bataviae* and *pyrogenes*, may also cause spirochaetal jaundice.

LABORATORY DIAGNOSIS

Leptospirosis should always be considered as a possible cause of feverish illness, with or without jaundice, in patients whose work, recreation or living conditions are likely to expose them to infection from animal sources.

Examination of blood

After an incubation period of 5–12 d there is a phase of leptospiraemia that lasts for about a week, during which time live leptospires may be seen by dark-ground microscopy of the patient's blood. Care must be taken not to identify as leptospires the protoplasmic extrusions from red cells that are normally present in blood films and which may undulate, due to Brownian movement, in such a way that they resemble spirochaetes.

To confirm the diagnosis leptospires are cultured from the blood by inoculation of liquid medium, or by peritoneal inoculation of the blood into laboratory animals, followed some days later by culture of the animal blood obtained by cardiac puncture.

Examination of urine

Leptospires may be present in the urine during the 2nd week of illness and continue to be excreted intermittently for 4–6 weeks.

They may be seen by dark-ground microscopy in the deposit of centrifuged urine and may be cultured directly from the sediment in a semi-solid medium containing neomycin sulphate to control contaminants, or after animal inoculation. Because leptospires are very sensitive to acid urine, the urine should be examined immediately after being voided.

Identification of infecting strains

To identify the serovar of strains isolated from blood or urine, use is made of agglutination and agglutinin-absorption techniques that have been developed for the purpose. The results are compared with those obtained in parallel tests against reference strains of various serovars and their antisera prepared in rabbits. This is a specialized technique that is best carried out in one of the Leptospira Reference Laboratories recognized by the World Health Organization, to which all new isolates should be sent for identification.

Serological examinations

Specific antibodies are detectable in the patient's serum towards the end of the 1st week of illness; they continue to rise for several weeks, and then begin to decline. Residual agglutinating antibody may persist for many years. Serum should be examined during the early days of the illness and at 4–5 d intervals thereafter in order to detect the rise in antibody titre that is diagnostic of current infection.

Serological tests fall into two categories, viz. those that are genus-specific and those that are serogroup- (or serovar-) specific.

Genus-specific tests

These have the advantage of being able, in a single test, to detect, in human serum, antibodies resulting from leptospiral infection, whatever the serovar responsible. A complement fixation test with a genus-specific antigen prepared from a strain known as Patoc 1 of the saprophytic species *L. biflexa* has been widely used. Since complement-fixing antibodies of immunoglobulin class IgM decrease more rapidly than agglutinating IgG antibodies, the test is only suitable for diagnosing current infection, not for survey work.

Other genus-specific tests include the sensitized erythrocyte lysis test (SEL) and the slide agglutination test of Mazzonelli and Mailloux. In this simple test, a drop of the patient's serum is mixed with a drop of a dense suspension of a heat-killed culture of strain Patoc 1. Agglutination is clearly visible to the naked eye.

An enzyme-linked immunosorbent assay (ELISA) which is capable of detecting specific IgM and IgG leptospiral antibodies is useful for indicating the stage of the infection.

Serogroup-specific test

The microscopic agglutination test (MAT) has been widely used for many years to diagnose leptospirosis and to indicate the likely serogroup (and sometimes the serovar) of the infecting strain. A series of dilutions of the patient's serum is tested against a battery of reference strains of different serovars representing all serogroups to which the infecting strain might belong. The reactions are read by low-power dark-ground microscopy. In the early stages of infection the antibodies may cross-react with strains of different serogroups, but subsequent tests usually result in the highest titres being obtained against the specific serogroup and against the serovar that is most likely to be that of the infecting strain.

TREATMENT

Chemotherapy

Leptospirosis usually responds to treatment with antibiotics, provided the drugs are administered in large enough doses early in the infection. Penicillin is thought to be the most effective; patients allergic to penicillin may be treated with streptomycin, tetracycline or erythromycin. Benzylpenicillin should be administered intravenously for up to 7 d in a daily dose of 6–8 megaunits (3.6–4.8 g). Penicillin may cause a temporary exacerbation of the symptoms (Jarisch–Herxheimer reaction) but this should not prevent continuation of treatment.

Renal dialysis

When there is impairment of kidney function, as sometimes happens in Weil's disease, it may be necessary to resort to renal dialysis to counteract the uraemia which is the main cause of death in fatal cases of leptospirosis. Tetracyclines should not be used if there is evidence of renal failure.

EPIDEMIOLOGY

Leptospirosis is a zoonosis and man is an unnatural or 'end' host and does not transmit the infection further. Each leptospiral serovar appears to have its own particular animal host of election, usually a rodent, although some domestic animals, e.g. dogs, cattle and pigs, may also act as natural reservoirs of infection. Most reservoir hosts remain healthy carriers. Serovar *icterohaemorrhagiae* is normally carried by the brown rat, *Rattus norvegicus*, and serovar *hebdomadis*, first reported as the cause of seven-day fever of field workers in Japan, is carried by the field mouse, *Microtus montebelloi*. However, serovar *canicola*, which causes canicola fever in man, is carried by dogs and serovar *hardjo* by cattle; no rodent hosts having been found for these two serovars.

Leptospires are exceptional among pathogenic micro-organisms in being dependent on transmission in the host's urine. They localize in the kidneys, colonizing the convoluted tubules and are periodically washed out in the urine, thereby contaminating the environment. Cattle, pigs and horses become infected through grazing in fields or on fodder contaminated by infected urine. The infection may spread within the herd, again by means of the urine, resulting in herd epizootics. Man becomes infected mainly through contact with water, soil or vegetation contaminated by animal urine. Workers in certain occupations are particularly at risk: farmers, miners working in damp, rat-infested coal mines, sewer workers and fish handlers are all particularly liable to infection by serovar *icterohaemorrhagiae* because the conditions under which they work encourage rat infestation and the moist conditions allow the leptospires excreted in the rat urine to survive for a considerable time outside the animal body. Agricultural workers are especially at risk in countries where it is customary for them to go bare footed in the fields, as in the rice fields or sugar plantations of tropical countries. The leptospires readily penetrate the skin through cuts and abrasions of the feet and legs.

In the UK, as in other countries where serovar *hardjo* infects cattle, dairy farmers are liable to become infected through inhaling droplets of infected urine during milking.

CONTROL

Agricultural workers should protect their skin by wearing suitable gloves and boots when digging ditches, harvesting, cleaning out pig pens, cow sheds, kennels, etc. Buildings that house animals or act as work places should be rat-proofed and the floors and work benches kept in a good state of repair and cleanliness. They should be regularly washed down with sodium hypochlorite solution so that any leptospires will be killed.

Persons who seek recreation through water sports, such as bathing, paddling, wind surfing, canoeing or fishing in ponds, canals or rivers that may be fouled by rats or other animals, should be warned of the risk of infection. They should be encouraged to wear protective clothing and to cover any cuts or abrasions of the skin.

In parts of the world where the risk of infection is high among certain groups, e.g. rice field and sugar cane workers, vaccination against local leptospiral strains is being carried out successfully.

In the UK and some other countries, the incidence of human infection by serovars *icterohaemorrhagiae* and *canicola* derived from infected dogs has, in recent years, been reduced by the widespread vaccination of dogs against these two serovars.

RECOMMENDED READING

Alston J M, Broom J C 1958 *Leptospirosis in Man and Animals.* Livingstone, Edinburgh
Ellis W A, Little T W A (eds) 1986 *The Present State of Leptospirosis Diagnosis and Control.* Martinus Nijhoff Dordrecht
Faine S (ed) 1982 Guidelines for the control of leptospirosis. *WHO Offset Publication 67*, World Health Organization, Geneva

Gsell O 1990 The changing epidemiology of leptospirosis in Europe. *International Journal of Medical Microbiology* 273: 412–427
Palmer M F 1988 Laboratory diagnosis of leptospirosis. *Medical Laboratory Sciences* 45: 174–178

40

Chlamydiae
Genital infections; trachoma; psittacosis; pneumonia

I. W. Smith

Chlamydiae are small Gram-negative bacteria which are obligate intracellular parasites like viruses, but differ from them in that they have both RNA and DNA, ribosomes, a cell wall, and divide by binary fission. However, they differ from most true bacteria in that they have no peptidoglycan in their cell wall and lack the ability to produce their own ATP. They require to use the host ATP — hence the term *energy parasites*. The genus *Chlamydia* is the only one in the family Chlamydiaceae and the order Chlamydiales.

There are three species agreed by an international committee: *Chlamydia trachomatis. C. psittaci* and *C. pneumoniae* (previously known as the *TWAR agent*). *C. trachomatis* can be divided into three biovars:

1. Those causing trachoma and inclusion conjunctivitis (TRIC)
2. Those causing lymphogranuloma venereum (LGV)
3. The one causing mouse pneumonitis (MoPn).

Both the trachoma and LGV biovars which infect humans can be subdivided into serovars: trachoma has 14 (A–K) and LGV at least three (L1, L2, L3). Classic trachoma is caused by serovars A, Ba, B and C while inclusion conjunctivitis and genital infections are due to serovars D–K. *C. psittaci* will infect both mammalian and avian species and although there are both serological and nucleic acid differences this species has not as yet been subdivided. *C. pneumoniae*, the newest species, appears only to infect humans and so far seems serologically uniform.

DESCRIPTION
Morphology

Chlamydiae are small non-motile bacteria, 300–350 nm in size, which stain poorly with Gram's stain. They can, however, be demonstrated in preparations stained by Giemsa or other methods. These particles represent the extracellular, infectious, metabolically inert form of chlamydiae known as the *elementary body*. Once the organism infects its host cell it increases in size to 800–1000 nm. This non-infectious but metabolically active particle is known as the *reticulate body* (Fig. 40.1).

Chlamydiae may also be demonstrated by immunofluorescence when a specific antibody tagged with fluorescein isothiocyanate is applied to slides made from clinical material, e.g. from the cervix or urethra or from infected tissue culture material. The elementary bodies appear as discrete bright apple-green particles and intracellular inclusions may also be visualized in the ultraviolet microscope. By this technique it is possible to confirm chlamydial infection within 30 min of receiving a specimen.

The three species can be differentiated on the basis of:

1. Growth
2. Nucleic acid profile

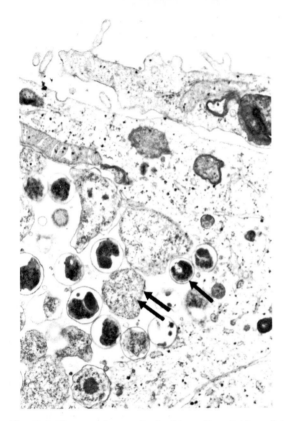

Fig. 40.1 Electron micrograph of a thin section of chlamydial inclusion: **a** ↑, small elementary body (EB); **b** ↑↑, 'reticulate' body (RB). × 15 000. (By courtesy of Dr Douglas R. Anderson, Miami.)

3. Presence of plasmids
4. The antigens they express
5. Inclusions in host cells which are morphologically different.

C. trachomatis produces a glycogen matrix in its inclusion which stains brown with iodine and has proved useful in diagnostic work.

Elementary bodies

The elementary bodies of *C. trachomatis* and *C. psittaci* are 300–350 nm in diameter with very little periplasmic space. *C. pneumoniae* is different in that it has a large periplasmic space, giving the elementary bodies a pear-shaped appearance (310 × 400 nm).

Freeze-replica techniques show that the surface of elementary bodies have flower-like structures through which a surface projection passes. This projection is internally anchored in the cytoplamic membrane and the strands of DNA appear to connect to this adhesion point (Fig. 40.2).

Reticulate bodies

The reticulate body of all three species is larger and circular in shape (800–1000 nm) with surface projections identical to those of the elementary body. As the reticulate bodies are metabolically active their internal structure will reflect the stage of replication. Early in the cycle many ribosomes are seen. Later the DNA is reorganized into cores for the progeny elementary body. Glycogen production in the reticulate bodies of *C. trachomatis* is detected in the electron microscope about 18 h post-inoculation and the inclusions are apparent at about 22 h. No glycogen production has been observed with *C. psittaci* or *C. pneumoniae*.

No peptidoglycan is demonstrable between the cytoplasmic membrane and cell wall, as is seen in Gram-negative bacteria.

Nucleic acid

The molecular weight of the nucleic acid content of chlamydiae has been estimated to be 660×10^6. The three species can be separated on the basis of homology as the intraspecies homology does not exceed 10%. Plasmid DNA is also found in most strains of *C. trachomatis* and *C. psittaci* but the ovine strains of *C. psittaci* and *C. pneumoniae* do not appear to have plasmids.

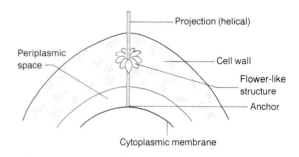

Fig. 40.2 Schematic diagram of a projection from the surface of an elementary body showing the flower-like structure and connection with the cytoplasmic membrane.

Protein

A small number of proteins are thought to be important to the understanding of antigenicity, pathogenesis and for possible vaccine production.

There are four outer-membrane proteins of which the major one has species-specific epitopes. These outer-membrane proteins are rich in cysteine and it is thought that the rigidity of chlamydial elementary bodies is due to disulphide bonding between cysteine residues of these proteins.

Chlamydiae have a heat shock protein, antibody to which cross-reacts with similar-sized proteins from unrelated micro-organisms, making the interpretation of serological responses to chlamydial infections difficult.

Lipopolysaccharide (LPS)

Genus-specific chlamydial antigen may be obtained by the methods used for extraction of LPS from Gram-negative bacteria. This material has three epitopic sites, only one of which is specific for chlamydiae. The LPS contains 2-keto-3-deoxyoctonic acid (KDO) and lipid A. These epitopes cross-react with mutants of *Escherichia coli, Proteus mirabilis* and *Salmonella typhimurium* and with LPS derived from *Acinetobacter* species. As the LPS is the antigen used in both the complement fixation test and in certain of the enzyme-linked immunosorbent assay (ELISA) detection tests, care must be taken in the interpretation of results.

LABORATORY PROPAGATION

In the 1930s Bedson, while studying the replication of the psittacosis strain in mice, was able to elucidate the growth cycle and establish that the organism divided by binary fission. In 1957 *C. trachomatis* was isolated in the yolk sac of embryonated hens' eggs. The presence of the organism in the moribund eggs was confirmed by staining. Although this method is not now widely used for isolation it is used to produce antigen, especially for the micro-immunofluorescence test. Tissue culture isolation was first successful in 1965. For growth of chlamydiae, tissue cultures have to be modified to allow productive inter-

action of the organism and its host cell. This is done by centrifuging the organism onto the cells and inhibiting the host cell by irradiation or by addition of 5-iodo-2'-deoxyuridine or cycloheximide to the medium. Giemsa stain will detect all types of chlamydiae, and iodine can be used to detect the glycogen containing inclusions of *C. trachomatis*. Immunofluorescence with appropriate antisera can detect either genus-specific or species-specific antigens. The different species of chlamydiae have slightly different requirements for growth but *C. pneumoniae* is the most difficult to cultivate in both eggs and tissue culture.

GROWTH CYCLE

Initially the organism must attach to the host cell. Specific binding proteins have been sought and it is tempting to speculate on the possible role of the protein appendages on the surface of the elementary bodies. Not all species of chlamydiae interact easily with their host cells. *C. psittaci* and LGV attach and saturate the host cell surface but *C. trachomatis* and *C. pneumoniae* are unlikely to do so. This appears to be due in part to the net negative charge of the organism and host cells, causing repulsion at a distance. To overcome this, the addition of a polycation, such as DEAE dextran, increases the adsorption of *C. trachomatis*, while centrifuging *C. trachomatis* or *C. pneumoniae* with their host cells allows hydrophilic bonds to be formed and increases the attachment of both species. These interactions, though successful in vitro, probably do not reflect the situation in vivo.

Once the chlamydiae and host cell have come into contact the organism enters the cell within a vesicle (Fig. 40.3). Viable chlamydiae entering the host cell cytoplasm inhibit fusion with lysosomal vesicles and so escape degradation.

In the vesicles the elementary body loses its dense DNA core. The cell wall becomes less rigid due to breaking of the disulphide bonds; the particle increases in size and becomes a reticulate body. The reticulate bodies have no cytochrome and lack the ability to produce ATP, which must be supplied by the host. In the vesicle the reticulate body divides by binary fission to yield

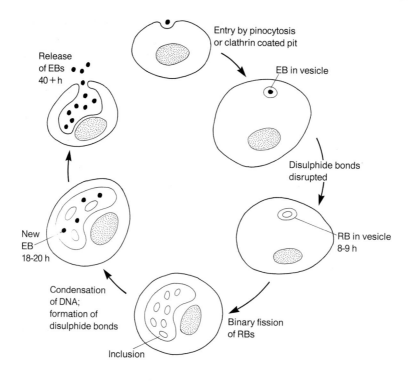

EB = elementary body; RB = reticulate body

Fig. 40.3 The chlamydial growth cycle.

pleomorphic organisms. At 18–20 h the DNA condenses, disulphide bonds are formed in the outer-membrane proteins and new elementary bodies are generated within the endosomal vesicle. The release of elementary bodies follows autolysis of the host cell, but whether release is the cause or the effect of autolysis is uncertain.

The need of chlamydiae for specific amino acids may lead to an inhibition of growth which can be reversed on the addition of the essential amino acid. This obviously gives the opportunity for latency since an amino acid-starved infection may lie dormant for a period but reappear on the addition of the essential building block.

IMMUNOLOGICAL RESPONSE AND PATHOGENESIS

Infections with chlamydiae give rise to both humoral and cell-mediated immune responses,

which play varying roles in the recovery from infection, resistance to reinfection and immunopathological sequelae. Human infections cannot be studied easily experimentally and although animal models have been developed for human infections the reactions may not be typical of those in humans. However, two natural infections, guinea-pig inclusion conjunctivitis (GPIC) and mouse pneumonitis have been exploited. Recovery is delayed if the guinea-pigs are immunosuppressed with either cyclophosphamide or anti-lymphocytic serum, indicating that both humoral and the cell-mediated immune responses are required in recovery from GPIC.

Initial host response

In human infections chlamydiae have a predilection for either squamous epithelial cells or for the macrophages of the lung or gastro-intestinal tract. Such infections invoke an inflammatory response with infiltration of neutrophils during the acute stage. The intracellular destruction of chlamydiae by the neutrophils occurs in cells with oxygen-dependent or oxygen-independent enzyme systems. Subsequently, monocytes and lymphocytes appear in the infiltrate. Chlamydiae do not replicate in monocytes but when these cells become macrophages both *C. psittaci* and LGV can escape the phagolysosomal fusion and produce high titres of organisms. *C. trachomatis* can also replicate in macrophages but to a lesser extent. It has been suggested that the infected macrophages may be a vehicle for the spread of the chlamydiae within the host.

Antibody response

Antibody production follows the normal sequence of IgM then IgG, the level of antibody production being dose-dependent. Serum IgA is produced and secretory IgA (S-IgA) is found in the mucosal fluids. The higher the level of S-IgA, the less successful is the isolation of chlamydiae from a genital site. The development of IgM and IgG antibody to *C. pneumoniae* is delayed 6–8 weeks compared with 2–3 weeks following genital infection — a factor which must be considered when using serology for diagnosis.

The importance of mucosal antibody (or rather the lack of it) is seen in neonates who have maternal IgG. Of those infected with *C. trachomatis* in the birth canal a proportion develop conjunctivitis, despite maternal IgG. If the infection is not appropriately treated, a proportion of these babies develop pneumonitis at 4–12 weeks of age. This is when the maternal antibody is waning and neonates are beginning to produce their own IgM and IgG. The presence of IgM antibody or a rising IgG titre is taken as evidence of chlamydial infection of the respiratory tract of neonates.

Although specific antibody can neutralize chlamydiae in vitro there is little protection against reinfection of the ocular and genital mucous membranes in patients with circulating IgG antibody. In second or subsequent infections there is a very swift infiltration of neutrophils and lymphocytes. The plasma cells produce antibody, making it difficult to recover the organism. This lack of protection has implications for attempts to produce a successful vaccine.

Cellular response

Antibody is not the only factor to be considered in reinfection. The cell-mediated response also plays a part which may or may not be of advantage to the host. Whole live chlamydiae, heat-killed organism or even LPS can stimulate the production of lymphokines such as γ-interferon and interleukin-1.

In trachoma, the acute infection results in an inflammatory response with infiltration of neutrophils and lymphocytes. These lymphocytes may clump together and produce a follicle. The centre of the follicle is composed of B cells and macrophages surrounded by T cells and all are enclosed in a thin layer of epithelial cells. These epithelial cells are sloughed off as the follicle becomes necrotic and regeneration of fibrotic tissue stimulated by interleukin-1 leads to scarring. With reinfection or restimulation with chlamydial antigen the inflammatory response is quicker, leading to more follicle formation and scarring.

A similar situation pertains in the genital tract where ascending infection can lead to salpingitis. This results in an inflammatory response with infiltration of neutrophils and lymphocytes, deciliation of the epithelium and destruction of the epithelial cells near to the lymphocytes. Repeated infection causes severe tubal damage with follicle formation, more damage to the epithelium and scarring, leading to the obstruction of the fimbriated end of the fallopian tube. Such damage can result in infertility due to interruption of ovum transport and to chronic pelvic inflammatory disease.

INFECTION OF HUMANS

Table 40.1 summarizes the chlamydial infections of the eye, genital and respiratory tracts.

Ocular infection

Trachoma has been known for thousands of years and during the 19th century was still found in

Table 40.1 Human chlamydial infections

Site of infection	Disease	Organism (serovars)
Eye	Trachoma	*C. trachomatis* (A, B, Ba, C)
	Inclusion conjunctivitis	*C. trachomatis* (D–K)
	Ophthalmia neonatorum	*C. trachomatis* (D–K)
Genital tract		
Male	Urethritis, epididymitis, proctitis	*C. trachomatis* (D–K)
Female	Urethritis, cervicitis, proctitis, salpingitis perihepatitis, peri-appendicitis, infertility	*C. trachomatis* (D–K)
	Abortion, stillbirth	*C. psittaci* (ovine strains)
Male and female	Lymphogranuloma venereum	*C. trachomatis* (L1–L3)
Respiratory tract	Pneumonitis of infants	*C. trachomatis* (D–K)
	Pharyngitis, pneumonia	*C. pneumoniae*
	Psittacosis	*C. psittaci* (avian strains)
	Pneumonia	*C. psittaci* (ovine strains)

Europe. The improvement in hygiene led to a decrease in the incidence of the disease in industrially developed countries, but it is still found in countries where standards of sanitation and hygiene are poor and flies abound. *C. trachomatis* A, B, Ba and C are the usual causal agents and in endemic areas children are often infected before their second birthday. Blindness due to this cause is still a problem in the 'trachoma belt', which stretches from North Africa to South-East Asia. Re-infection and secondary infections play a part in the progression to blindness, which may take 25–30 years. To compare the progress of the disease in different areas a grading scheme was produced for the World Health Organization. Five selected key signs were recorded to illustrate the progression of the disease:

1. Medium trachomatis inflammation in the conjunctiva with follicular inflammation
2. Intense inflammation with diffuse thickening of the conjunctiva
3. Scarring of tarsal conjunctiva
4. Inturned eyelashes
5. Corneal opacity.

The disease is spread by eye-seeking flies, or fingers, from one patient to another (Table 40.2). The children also shed the organism from the respiratory and gastro-intestinal tract, thus constituting another mode of spread.

Adult inclusion conjunctivitis (paratrachoma) is caused by serotypes D–K. It is most prevalent in sexually active young people and is spread from genitalia to eye. In the acute stage it presents as follicular conjunctivitis, which, if not treated, persists, together with a mucopurulent discharge. Although some patients develop scarring, corneal lesions or pannus formation, the disease is visually self-limiting and is not thought to lead to blindness.

Chlamydial ophthalmia neonatorum (inclusion blennorrhoea) develops in infants 5–21 d after birth. Follicles are not usually seen but the disease presents as a swelling of the eyelids, hyperaemia and a purulent infiltration of the conjunctiva. If untreated the disease can linger up to 1 year and secondary bacterial infection may cause ocular damage and even blindness. A proportion of these untreated neonates develop pneumonia. The source of infection is the infected genital tract of the mother, and the child is infected during passage through the birth canal (Table 40.2).

Genital Infection

Males

C. trachomatis serovars D–K are the commonest cause of non-gonococcal urethritis in males, accounting for at least 30% of cases (Table 40.3).

Table 40.2 Modes of spread of chlamydial infections

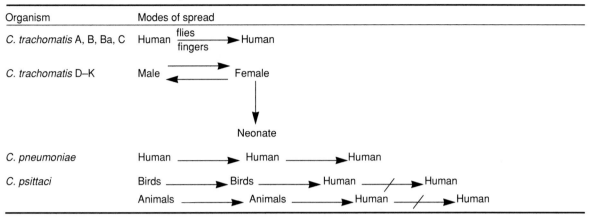

Varying amounts of mucopurulent discharge are produced in symptomatic patients and, although the condition is usually localized, some may progress to epididymitis, especially in those aged under 35 years. The effect on infertility is not known although acute epididymitis may result in a transient subfertility. *C. trachomatis* may also be isolated from males who do not have clinical signs or symptoms. Unless such patients are identified by laboratory screening they will form an untreated pool of infection.

Members of this group of chlamydia have also been isolated from the rectum of homosexual males and are associated with some cases of proctitis. Rectal pain, rectal bleeding, mucopurulent discharge and diarrhoea have all been described with chlamydial proctitis.

Lymphogranuloma venereum

C. trachomatis serovars L1–L3 can cause LGV in both males and females, with the majority of reported cases in males. It is found in the tropics and subtropics, though isolated cases are imported elsewhere. The disease begins with a genital ulcer followed by lymphadenopathy of the regional lymph nodes. Buboes are seen in men and, should the infection persist, it can spread to the gastrointestinal and genito-urinary tract, causing strictures and, in some cases, penoscrotal elephantiasis.

Females

In females *C. trachomatis* D–K can cause mucopurulent cervicitis and urethritis. It has also been associated with a proportion of cases of vaginitis and vaginal discharge. Many apparently asymptomatic females harbour the organism in their cervix. If untreated, such patients are not only a risk to their sexual partners or offspring (Table 40.2) but also to themselves, as ascending infection can occur. This results in endometritis and salpingitis, which singly or together may be referred to as *pelvic inflammatory disease*. Tubal damage

Table 40.3 Frequency of isolation of *C. trachomatis* from the genital tract

Heterosexual males		Females	
Primary diagnosis	Range (%)	Primary diagnosis	Range (%)
Non-specific urethritis	30–58	Contacts of chlamydia-positive males	45–67
Gonorrhoea	26–32	Contacts of chlamydia-negative males	4–18
Asymptomatic	3–7	Gonorrhoea	27–63
		Attending genito-urinary clinic	12–30
		Attending other clinics	1–19
		Requesting termination of pregnancy	10–23

from such infections can result in ectopic pregnancy and infertility. Peri-appendicitis and perihepatitis *(Fitz-Hugh-Curtis syndrome)* may follow salpingitis.

Infection in pregnancy

There have been a few reported cases in the UK of *C. psittaci* infection in pregnancy leading to miscarriage or intra-uterine death. The patients developed a febrile prodrome a few days to 2 weeks after contact with sheep. One infant delivered vaginally yielded *C. psittaci* from the liver, lungs and heart. The organism seems to have a predilection for the placenta, causing placentitis. The confirmed infections were all in patients who had been in contact with sheep, so women should be counselled to avoid contact with sheep during pregnancy. Also, as two cases of abortion have occurred at 14 weeks, there is a potential hazard to nursing or medical staff when dealing with unsuspected cases due to the heavy load of organisms in the placenta.

C. trachomatis has also been isolated from abortion products but its role in abortion, stillbirth, premature birth and premature rupture of membranes is uncertain. A number of patients who yielded *C. trachomatis* from abortion products have subsequently developed salpingitis and possible infertility. Similarly, a proportion of patients seeking therapeutic abortion have been shown to harbour the organism pre-evacuation and these are also at risk of more serious infection. Thus, all such patients should be screened and, if necessary, treated before and during surgical manipulation.

Respiratory infections
Chlamydia pneumoniae

In 1983 a chlamydia strain was isolated from a throat swab of a student at the University of Washington, Seattle. This organism proved to be the same as one isolated in 1965 from the eye of a patient in Taiwan during a trachoma study. These two organisms, originally called TWAR, differed from *C. trachomatis* and *C. psittaci* and have now been classified as *C. pneumoniae*. During

the period 1983–87, 650 students with acute respiratory infection were examined in Seattle. Twenty students showed serological evidence of an acute infection with *C. pneumoniae*, which was isolated from 12 cases who presented with sore throat that progressed after 2–3 weeks to pneumonia. Recovery was slow, with a residual cough for 1–2 months, but was accelerated with appropriate antibiotic therapy. Since then various serological surveys have shown that, in hospitalized patients in North America, *C. pneumoniae* was the third most common cause of pneumonia following *Streptococcus pneumoniae* and *Haemophilus influenzae*. Patients who had been treated initially with penicillin or ampicillin had a recurrence of their pneumonia 3 weeks to 3 months later. Radiological evidence showed that a different part of the lung was affected at the second episode. These patients developed a high IgG response but no IgM response, so the pneumonia was thought to be due to either reactivation or reinfection. Thus, *C. pneumoniae* not only causes acute respiratory infections, it also gives rise to recurrences. Serological surveys have shown that there is a 40–50% prevalence in a number of countries. The antibody to *C. pneumoniae* does not decline with age, in contrast to the findings with *C. trachomatis* infections of the genital tract. *C. pneumoniae* has not yet been shown to have any other animal host and so, unlike *C. psittaci*, it presumably spreads by the respiratory route between humans (Table 40.2).

Chlamydia psittaci

Psittacosis (ornithosis) in man is caused by infection with avian strains of *C. psittaci*. The incubation period is about 10 d and the illness ranges from an 'influenza-like' syndrome with general malaise, fever, anorexia, rigors, sore throat, headache and photophobia, to a severe illness, with typhoidal state, delirium and pneumonia with numerous well-demarcated areas of consolidation; these may resemble bronchopneumonia, but the bronchioles and larger bronchi are involved as a secondary event and sputum is scanty. Although the pneumonic form of the illness may focus clinical attention, the organism is blood-borne

Table 40.4 Examples of the range of diseases caused by *C. psittaci* in natural hosts

Host	Conjunctivitis	Intestinal infections	Respiratory infections	Placental infection & abortion	Seminal infection	Infertility	Polyarthritis	Meningo-encephalitis	Mastitis
Birds	+	+	+	−	−	−	−	+	−
Sheep	+	+	+	+	+	−	+	−	+
Cattle	+	+	+	+	+	+	+	+	+
Goats	−	+	+	+	−	−	−	−	+
Cats	+	+	+	−	−	−	−	−	−
Guinea-pigs	+	−	−	−	−	+	−	−	−
Koala bears	+	−	−	−	−	+	−	−	−

through the body and there may be meningo-encephalitis, arthritis, pericarditis or myocarditis, or a predominantly typhoidal state with enlarged liver and spleen and even a rash resembling that of enteric fever. Subacute endocarditis resembling that complicating Q fever has also been described. The ovine strain of *C. psittaci* has caused respiratory infection of shepherds and a proportion of neonates develop pneumonitis due to *C. trachomatis*.

INFECTION OF BIRDS AND MAMMALS

Table 40.4 shows some examples of natural hosts infected and the range of diseases reported to date. Non-human infections are important economically and as a source of infection to humans. Agricultural economy is affected as psittacosis is not confined to psittacine birds: outbreaks have been reported in turkeys, geese and ducks. Abortion in ewes can occur in one-third of a previously uninfected flock and a continuing 1–2% abortion rate is found in infected flocks. Genital and eye infections of koala bears have been reported in Australia, giving rise to speculation that the species could become endangered due to chlamydia-induced infertility.

Birds with respiratory and intestinal infections shed the organism in nasal secretions and droppings. The nasal secretions contaminate the feathers, where they dry and produce an infected dust in which the organism can survive for months. There are import controls in many countries to restrict the movement of birds which are rendered more infectious by stress.

Similarly, the organism has been found in sheep droppings, in the milk, and on the placenta and fleece of sheep. Aerosols can be produced and are a hazard to shepherds, who may develop a respiratory infection, and to pregnant women who have miscarried.

EPIDEMIOLOGY OF HUMAN CHLAMYDIAL INFECTIONS

Unlike *C. psittaci*, for which there is a non-human reservoir of infection, *C. trachomatis* and *C. pneumoniae* only appear to infect humans (Table 40.2). *C. psittaci* infections of humans are not usually spread from person to person.

In areas hyperendemic for trachoma, such as sub-Saharan Africa and the Middle East, nearly all children become infected with *C. trachomatis* but the severity of the infection appears to be dependent on the poverty level of the families.

Chlamydial *ophthalmia neonatorum* is caused by the D–K serovars responsible for the sexually transmitted disease which is prevalent in sexually active young people world-wide and can be found in association with gonorrhoea and other sexually transmitted diseases.

C. pneumoniae has only recently been recognized but there have been outbreaks in military establishments and in student populations, indicative of aerosol spread. Serological studies have shown that there is a difference in the age profile of the infection. In the Far East 10–15% of children under 5 years have evidence of infection, while there is little serological evidence in children in the western world until they start school. After that the attack rate rises steadily till the late teenage years and reaches 50% by middle age.

LABORATORY DIAGNOSIS

Cultivation

Chlamydiae may be isolated in either embryonated eggs or tissue culture. However, McCoy cells treated with cycloheximide are the most widely used, although *C. pneumoniae* grows better in HeLa or monkey kidney cells. The presence of the organism is detected by staining for inclusions or elementary bodies. The disadvantage of culture is that it only detects viable organisms. This requires specimens to be sent quickly to the laboratory in a suitable transport medium (containing no penicillin) at 4°C or after freezing the sample in liquid nitrogen.

Antigen detection

To overcome the problems of culture, several direct tests have been developed. Staining of smears by fluorescent antibodies will demonstrate elementary bodies and the ELISA test can detect chlamydial antigens. While these tests have the advantage of not requiring special transport conditions they do suffer from false-positive results due to cross-reactions with antigens of other bacteria. In the ELISA test it is especially important to confirm positive results by the blocking test or by fluorescent staining of a deposit from the specimen.

DNA probes

In certain chlamydial infections (or, more correctly, chlamydia-stimulated immunopathological reactions) it is not possible to isolate viable organisms, so either an antigen detection method (as above) or a DNA probe has to be used. This has been successfully used in the study of trachoma and it has been suggested that such probes might be used to seek evidence of chlamydial infection of the rectum. Specimens from the rectum are difficult to examine due to the presence of contaminating bacteria and extraneous particles;

these may fluoresce and confuse the interpretation of the direct immunofluorescence test or cross-react with ELISA antigen.

Serology

Serology has also been used, especially in respiratory infections. Atypical pneumonia due to *C. psittaci* produces high levels of complement-fixing antibody in serum from patients. This antibody is directed against group antigen and, until recently, adults with high or rising titres were thought to have psittacosis although contact with psittacine birds could not be established in all cases. Now that *C. pneumoniae* has been isolated, it is clear that a number of these cases of 'psittacosis' were in fact due to *C. pneumoniae*. To detect species-specific and serovar-specific antibody, the micro-immunofluorescence test is used with antigens from all chlamydial strains. Serology is also used to confirm the diagnosis of pneumonitis due to *C. trachomatis* in neonates. A high level (>64) of IgM and a rising or high titre of IgG are taken as diagnostic.

TREATMENT AND CONTROL

Immunization

To date, vaccines have not been very successful. The agent used against ovine abortion in sheep does not give complete protection and a suitable replacement is being sought. There are several problems: serum antibody is not completely protective in vivo; mucosal antibody is also required; and the question of cell-mediated immunity must be addressed. Another problem is the choice of antigen: should a genus-specific antigen which stimulates antibody to all three species of chlamydia be used, or should it be a strain-specific antigen with a much narrower spectrum? For a rapid response to challenge, the immune response should be to exposed epitopes.

Chemotherapy

Antibiotic can be used in the treatment of chlamydial infections. The antibiotics of choice are tetracycline in adults and erythromycin in babies. Penicillin should *not* be used as it is chlamydiastatic. The dangers of using penicillin in chlamydial infection have been shown in some respiratory cases in which the patient appeared to improve on penicillin, but later relapsed with pneumonia. Similarly, chloramphenicol eye drops, which have been used to treat sticky eyes in babies, are chlamydiastatic and there is a risk of the baby developing pneumonitis when the drug is discontinued. Because chlamydiae have a prolonged replication cycle and may be suppressed, not eradicated, by short courses of antibiotics, treatment must be given for a minimum of 7 d. Many authorities advocate treatment of 3 weeks duration, especially for ascending and complicated genital infections in women. Unfortunately, many patients receive inadequate antimicrobial therapy.

Contact tracing

Tracing partners of index cases of chlamydial infection is very important as it is useless to treat the index case only to leave the patient exposed to a risk of reinfection from an untreated partner. Genital infections can be insidious, not causing clinical signs and symptoms. It is therefore essential that the partner should be screened for chlamydiae and treated even if clinically normal. In cases of neonatal infection both parents should be examined and treated.

Animal contact

Control of infection may mean avoidance of contact with well-known sources of infection, e.g. sheep at lambing, milking and shearing. Pregnant women are particularly at risk from such infection and so should avoid contact with sheep during pregnancy. The control of importation of psittacine birds has reduced the risk of psittacosis in pet owners and bird fanciers in the UK, although the increasing popularity of exotic pets has lead to an increase in numbers of cases.

Hygiene

The effect of improved hygiene has been shown by the decrease in trachoma in the western world so that, in addition to extending medical care, improving standards of hygiene and sanitation should be a prime objective in developing countries.

RECOMMENDED READING

Barron A L 1988. *Microbiology of Chlamydia.* CRC Press, Boca Raton
Grayston J T, Wang S P, Kuo C C, Campbell L A 1989 Current knowledge of *Chlamydia pneumoniae*, strain TWAR, an important cause of pneumonia and other acute respiratory diseases. *European Journal of Clinical Microbiology and Infectious Disease* 8: 191–202
Mårdh P-A, Paavonen J, Puolakkainen M 1989. *Chlamydia.* Plenum, New York
Ridgway G L and Taylor-Robinson D 1991 Current problems in microbiology: I Chlamydial infections: which laboratory test? *Journal of Clinical Pathology* 44:1–5

Schachter J 1988 The intracellular life of *Chlamydia. Current Topics in Microbiology and Immunology* 138: 109–139.
Treharne J D and Ballard R C 1990. The expanding spectrum of the *Chlamydia*—a microbiological and clinical appraisal. *Reviews in Medical Microbiology* 1: 10–18
Treharne J D 1991 Recent developments in the biology of the chlamydiae. *Reviews in Medical Microbiology* 2: 45–49

41

Rickettsiae Typhus; spotted fevers; Q fever

K. L. Gage and D. H. Walker

Few diseases have had a greater impact on the course of human history than epidemic typhus. Hans Zinsser's classic book *Rats, Lice and History* provides a graphic account of how *Rickettsia prowazekii*, the aetiological agent of this louse-borne disease, has caused millions of deaths and much human suffering in conditions of famine, poverty and war. Epidemic typhus has become relatively rare as world conditions have improved, but various other rickettsial diseases are still widely distributed (Tables 41.1 and 41.2).

As currently classified, the Rickettsiaceae include a diverse group of organisms that share such common features as intracellular growth and use of arthropod vectors, but these traits are almost surely the result of evolutionary convergence rather than descent from a common ancestral line.

Rickettsiae are typically defined as obligate, intracellular Gram-negative bacteria that require an arthropod vector as part of their natural cycle. This definition excludes some organisms that are traditionally considered to be members of the family Rickettsiaceae. For example, *Rochalimaea quintana*, the louse-borne aetiological agent of trench fever, is a cell-associated bacterium that can be grown in cell-free culture. Another exception is *Coxiella burnetii*, an obligate, intracellular bacterium that can be isolated from arthropods, but does not require an arthropod vector to maintain itself in nature.

RICKETTSIA

DESCRIPTION

The genus *Rickettsia* includes organisms responsible for numerous diseases in many parts of the world (Table 41.1). The pioneering research of Ricketts and others in the early 20th century led to the demonstration of the rickettsial aetiology of Rocky Mountain spotted fever. A number of other diseases, including epidemic and murine typhus, were later shown to be rickettsial infections. The discovery of a hitherto unrecognized Japanese form of spotted fever as recently as 1984 and the subsequent isolation of the aetiological agent, *R. japonica*, indicates that much remains to be learned about these organisms. In addition to species known to be associated with human disease, there are a number of presumably non-pathogenic rickettsiae which have been isolated primarily from arthropods and are poorly understood.

Rickettsia species are small (0.3–0.5×0.8–$1.0\,\mu m$) Gram-negative bacilli. They are obligate intracellular parasites that reside in the cytosol of host cells (Fig. 41.1). All are associated with an arthropod vector. Species that are pathogenic for humans parasitize endothelial cells almost exclusively.

The genus *Rickettsia* is currently divided into three antigenically distinct groups: the typhus group,

Table 41.1   Human diseases caused by *Rickettsia* species

Species and disease	Geographical distribution	Means of transmission	Primary vectors	Important vertebrate hosts
Typhus group				
R. prowazekii (epidemic typhus)	Extant foci in Africa, North and South America	Louse faeces	*Pediculus humanus*	Humans, possibly other mammals (flying squirrels)
R. typhi (murine typhus)	Primarily tropics and subtropics	Flea faeces	*Xenopsylla cheopis* and other fleas	Rodents and other small mammals
Spotted fever group				
R. akari (rickettsialpox)	USA, USSR, Korea	Bite of mouse mite	*Liponyssoides sanguineus*	House mice (*Mus musculus*), possibly other rodents
R. australis (Queensland tick typhus)	Australia	Bite of tick	*Ixodes holocyclus*	Small marsupials
R. conorii (boutonneuse fever)	Europe, Africa, Middle East, India	Bite of tick	*Rhipicephalus*, etc.	Rodents; possibly dogs and other small mammals
R. japonica (Oriental spotted fever)	Japan	Probably tick	Unknown	Unknown
R. rickettsii (Rocky Mountain spotted fever)	North and South America	Bite of tick	*Dermacentor*, etc.	Rodents and other small mammals
R. sibirica (north Asian tick typhus)	Northern Asia	Bite of tick	*Dermacentor*, etc.	Rodents and other small mammals
Scrub typhus group				
R. tsutsugamushi (scrub typhus)	Asia, Australia, islands of SW Pacific and Indian Oceans	Bite of larval mite	Chiggers (*Leptotrombidium*)	Rodents (particularly rats)

the spotted fever group, and the scrub typhus group. Typhus and spotted fever group rickettsiae appear to be closely related, as indicated by DNA–DNA hybridization studies; both have a typical Gram-negative bacterial cell wall, including a bilayered outer membrane that contains the lipopolysaccharide antigens that distinguish the two groups. External to the outer membrane there appears to be a slime layer, probably composed of polysaccharides. Electrophoresis has demonstrated a number of distinct proteins in typhus group rickettsiae. The immunodominant antigen has a molecular weight of approximately 120 000 in both *R. prowazekii* and *R. typhi* and contains both cross-reactive and species-specific epitopes. The spotted fever group rickettsiae differ slightly in that two surface proteins with molecular weights in the range 100 000–190 000 are immuno-dominant.

The scrub typhus rickettsiae appear to be fundamentally different. There is no indication of close genetic relationships or antigenic similarities between *R. tsutsugamushi* and other members of the genus. The cell wall lacks lipopolysaccharide, peptidoglycan or a slime layer and appears to derive its structural integrity from proteins linked by disulphide bonds. *R. tsutsugamushi* exhibits three or four major antigenic proteins with both strain-specific and cross-reactive epitopes. The three standard laboratory strains of *R. tsutsugamushi*

Table 41.2 Human diseases caused by members of the Rickettsiaceae other than *Rickettsia* species

Species and disease	Geographical distribution	Means of transmission	Primary vectors	Important vertebrate hosts
Genus *Coxiella*				
Coxiella burnetii (Q fever)	World-wide	Aerosol of animal products or tick faeces	Usually airborne but possibly tick-borne (*Dermacentor* spp.)	Wild and domestic ungulates and other mammals, possibly birds
Genus *Ehrlichia*				
E. sennetsu (Sennetsu ehrlichiosis)	Japan, Malaysia	Unknown	Unknown	Unknown
E. canis or closely related species	USA	Probably tick bite	Probably ticks	Uncertain, probably dogs
Genus *Rochalimaea*				
R. quintana (trench fever)	World-wide	Louse faeces	*Pediculus humanus*	Humans

(Karp, Kato and Gilliam) appear to be distinct enough from one another to be designated as separate species.

Studies of rickettsial metabolism have revealed that these organisms are highly specialized parasites that are capable of synthesizing adenosine triphosphate (ATP) and proteins. Transport of ATP, amino acids and metabolic intermediates from the cytoplasm of the host cell also occurs.

PATHOGENESIS
Invasion and destruction of target cells

Rickettsiae normally enter the body through the bite or faeces of an infected arthropod vector. They enter endothelial cells by induced phagocytosis, multiply intracellularly and eventually destroy their host cells. Observations of rickettsiae

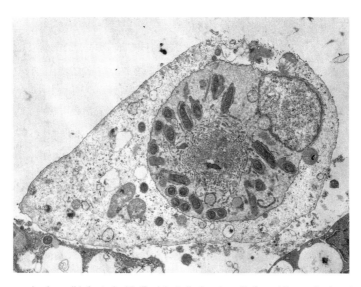

Fig. 41.1 Electron micrograph of a cell infected with *R. rickettsii*, showing dilation of the endoplasmic reticulum of host cells that occurs as a result of injury associated with infection by spotted fever group rickettsiae.

in cell culture systems suggest that the mechanisms of destruction of the host cell differ among the three serogroups. Following infection of *R. prowazekii* or *R. typhi*, the rickettsiae continue to multiply until the cell is packed with organisms (Fig. 41.2) and then bursts, possibly as a result of phospholipase A activity; before lysis, host cells have a normal ultrastructural appearance.

Spotted fever group rickettsiae behave differently: they seldom accumulate in large numbers and do not cause lysis of the host cells, but appear to induce the formation of filopodia, which the rickettsiae enter and from which they escape (Fig. 41.3). Infected cells exhibit signs of membrane damage caused by an influx of water, which is sequestered within cisternae of dilated, damaged rough endoplasmic reticulum (Fig. 41.1). The means by which rickettsiae damage host cells is uncertain but there is experimental evidence to suggest a role for protease or phospholipase.

Scrub typhus rickettsiae also escape from host cells soon after infecting them, but little is known about the mechanism(s) by which these organisms damage cells.

Pathological lesions

All members of the genus *Rickettsia* cause widespread microvascular injury leading to the destruc-

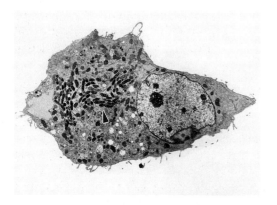

Fig. 41.2 Electron micrograph of a cell infected with *R. prowazekii*. The rickettsiae will continue to multiply within the cell until it is completely packed with organisms and bursts. In contrast to cells infected with spotted fever group rickettsiae, the ultrastructural appearance of cells infected with typhus group rickettsiae will remain normal until the cell lyses. The region of the cell containing rickettsiae is indicated by the arrow.

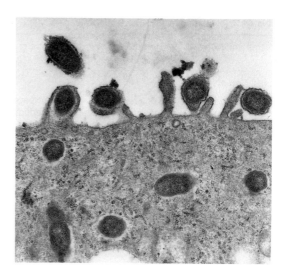

Fig. 41.3 Electron micrograph of *R. conorii* escaping from a host cell. Note the location of the rickettsiae within host cell filopodia.

tion of infected endothelial cells. The resulting pathological manifestations are probably due to direct rickettsial injury rather than immunopathology, inflammation-mediated injury, disseminated intravascular coagulation, or endotoxin. Interference with normal circulation following damage of blood vessels can cause life-threatening encephalitis and non-cardiogenic pulmonary oedema.

Clinical aspects of rickettsial diseases
Epidemic typhus

Initial symptoms of the disease are headache and fever 6–15 d after being exposed to *R. prowazekii*. A macular rash, often noted 4–7 d after patients become ill, first appears on the trunk and axillary folds and then spreads to the extremities. In mild cases the rash may begin to fade after 1–2 d, but in more severe cases it may last much longer and become haemorrhagic. Severe cases may also develop pronounced hypotension and renal dysfunction. The mental state of the patient may progress from dullness to stupor and, in very severe cases, even coma. Although the prognosis is grave for comatose patients, prompt treatment may be life-saving.

Individuals who survive a primary infection of louse-borne typhus may develop a mild reactivation of latent infection many years later. This is referred to as recrudescent typhus or *Brill–Zinsser disease*. Such individuals are nevertheless immune to a second louse-borne infection.

Murine typhus

Patients infected with *R. typhi*, the aetiological agent of murine typhus, develop symptoms similar to those of epidemic typhus. Fatal cases are rare but occasionally do occur, particularly in the elderly. Although the disease is much milder than epidemic typhus, it is still severe enough to require several months of convalescence.

Tick-borne spotted fever

There are many clinical similarities among the tick-borne rickettsioses of the spotted fever group. Although all can be life-threatening, the most severe is Rocky Mountain spotted fever. Patients become ill within 2 weeks of being bitten by an infected tick. Early symptoms include fever and severe headache, often accompanied by myalgia, anorexia, vomiting, abdominal pain, diarrhoea, photophobia, and cough. An eschar frequently occurs at the site of the tick bite in all spotted fever group infections except Rocky Mountain spotted fever. A maculopapular rash usually develops within 3–5 d. The rash of spotted fever usually develops first on the extremities rather than on the trunk. Absence of a rash does not exclude rickettsial infection since a disproportionate number of fatal cases of Rocky Mountain spotted fever are of the 'spotless' variety. Spotted fever group rickettsiae are found almost exclusively within the endothelial cells of vertebrate hosts, but *R. rickettsii* is also capable of invading vascular smooth muscle.

Vascular damage in severe cases may result in haemorrhagic rash, hypovolaemia, hypotensive shock, non-cardiogenic pulmonary oedema and impairment of central nervous system function. A fulminant form of Rocky Mountain spotted fever sometimes kills the patient within 5 d of the onset of symptoms; this form of the disease is more common in black males who are deficient in glucose-6-phosphate dehydrogenase and may be a result of haemolysis in these patients. Infection with spotted fever group rickettsiae confers long-lasting immunity.

Rickettsialpox

Rickettsialpox is a relatively mild infection transmitted by mites. The clinical course is similar to other spotted fever group infections and includes development of fever, headache and an eschar at the site where the infected mite fed. The rash is initially maculopapular but becomes vesicular. Fever lasts about a week and patients usually recover uneventfully.

Scrub typhus

Human infection with scrub typhus rickettsiae may be inapparent or fatal, depending on host factors and the virulence of the infecting strain. Symptoms develop 6–18 d after being bitten by infected mite larvae (*chiggers*). An eschar is often apparent at the site of the bite with enlargement of local lymph nodes. Progression of the disease may be accompanied by interstitial pneumonitis, generalized lymphadenopathy, splenomegaly and rash. Death may result from encephalitis, respiratory failure and circulatory failure. Patients who survive generally become afebrile after 2–3 weeks, or sooner if treated. Scrub typhus confers only a transient immunity and reinfection may occur.

LABORATORY DIAGNOSIS

Timely and accurate diagnosis of rickettsial disease followed by administration of an appropriate antibiotic may mean the difference between death of the patient and uneventful recovery. The lack of widely available, reliable diagnostic tests that can detect the disease in its early stages remains a problem, particularly as symptoms are often non-specific. The rash may appear at a late stage in the infection and may resemble exanthemata of many other diseases. The presence or significance of an eschar, if present, is also commonly overlooked.

Methods of laboratory diagnosis

Laboratory methods can be divided into: serological tests; isolation of rickettsiae from blood and tissues; and detection of rickettsiae in tissue samples.

Serological methods

The oldest and most widely used laboratory method is the *Weil-Felix* test, which relies on agglutination of the somatic antigens of non-motile *Proteus* species. Although widely available, this test is not recommended because of unacceptably low levels of sensitivity and specificity.

More reliable diagnostic tests for detecting antibodies to rickettsiae include indirect haemagglutination, immunofluorescence, latex agglutination, micro-agglutination, complement fixation, and enzyme immuno-assay. Of these techniques, the micro-agglutination assay and the enzyme immuno-assay are currently unavailable for general use because of difficulties in obtaining sufficient quantities of purified rickettsial antigens. The complement fixation test is the least sensitive of all the serological tests and is highly dependent on the quality and quantity of antigen used. The indirect haemagglutination, immunofluorescence and latex agglutination assays appear to have the greatest clinical applicability. Each is capable of detecting both IgG and IgM antibodies, and commercial kits are available for the immunofluorescence and latex agglutination assays.

The detection of specific antibody early in the course of rickettsial infections remains a problem. Serological diagnosis is usually achieved only after the patient is on the way to recovery; in fatal cases death may occur before detectable levels of antibody are present.

Isolation of rickettsiae

Isolation of the organism in cell culture or susceptible laboratory animals, such as mice or guinea-pigs, provides conclusive proof of rickettsial infection. However, it is seldom attempted because of lack of facilities or expertise and because of the presumed danger to laboratory personnel of handling rickettsiae-infected tissues. Such dangers have been overemphasized in this era of antibiotics, but use of containment facilities is appropriate.

Detection of rickettsiae in tissue

Skin biopsies from the centre of petechial lesions can be examined for rickettsiae by immunofluorescence. This technique is virtually 100% specific but has a sensitivity of 70%. Rickettsiae can be visualized for up to 48 h after the administration of antirickettsial drugs. Formalin-fixed, paraffin-embedded specimens can also be examined for rickettsiae using immunohistological methods. This approach is particularly effective for diagnosing rickettsial infection post-mortem.

TREATMENT

Owing to the difficulties of accurate diagnosis and the risks involved in misdiagnosis, empirical antirickettsial therapy is appropriate for patients who have a fever for 3 d or more and a history consistent with the epidemiological and clinical features of rickettsial disease. Rickettsial infections may be treated with tetracyclines or chloramphenicol. Both are rickettsiostatic and allow the patient's immune system time to respond and control the infection. Sulphonamides should not be administered as they exacerbate rickettsial infections. Intensive nursing care, management of fluids and electrolytes, replacement of platelets to compensate for those consumed as part of the patient's haemostatic response, and administration of red blood cells to patients that develop anaemia may be needed. Surgery may also be necessary to remove digits and extremities that develop ischaemic necrosis.

EPIDEMIOLOGY

Typhus group infections

Epidemic typhus

R. prowazekii is transmitted from human to human by the body louse, *Pediculus humanus*; the

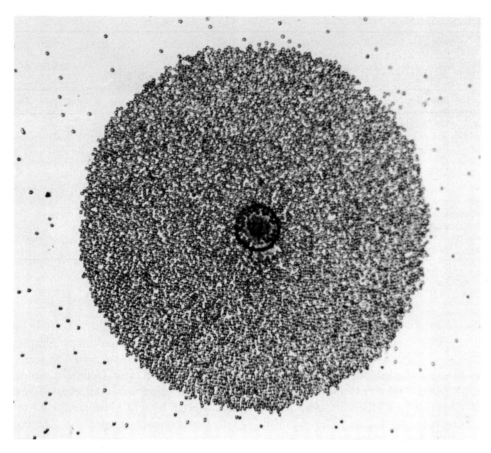

Fig. 42.6   Colony of *M. agalactiae* (caprine origin) covered completely by adherent guinea-pig erythrocytes (phenomenon of haemadsorption.)

linkages in the mucopeptide molecule, results in the formation of bacterial variants that have no cell wall or a modified one. If given osmotic protection, those variants are able to multiply and are termed *L-phase variants*. They are designated as unstable if they revert to the normal bacterial form on removal of the inducer, or stable if they do not revert. The colonies of L-phase variants in solid media may bear a close resemblance to those of mycoplasmas, probably a reflection of the lack of cell wall in both types of organism. This has led to the suggestion that mycoplasmas might be bacteria in their stable L-phase. However, the evidence is strongly against this because suspected relationships have not been confirmed by DNA base ratio or nucleic acid homology studies.

PATHOGENESIS

Eleven species in the genus *Mycoplasma*, two in the genus *Acholeplasma* and one in the genus *Ureaplasma* have been isolated from humans (Table 42.1), mostly from the oropharynx. Only three unequivocally cause disease, namely *M. pneumoniae*, *M. hominis* and *U. urealyticum*.

Respiratory infections

Pneumonias not attributable to any of the common bacterial causes were recognized over 50 years ago and labelled as *primary atypical pneumonias* (PAPs). In one variety of PAP associated with the development of cold agglutinins, a filtrable micro-organism (the *Eaton agent*) was isolated in

Table 42.1 Some properties of mycoplasmas of human origin

Mycoplasma	Frequency of isolation from		Metabolism of	Preferred pH of medium	Aerobic reduction of tetrazolium	Phosphatase activity	Haem-adsorption (chick RBCs)	Susceptibility to thallium
	Respiratory tract	Urogenital tract						
M. buccale	Rare	Not reported	Arginine	7.0	−	+	−	−
M. faucium	Rare	Not reported	Arginine	7.0	−	−	+	−
M. fermentans	Not reported	Rare	Glucose and arginine	7.5	−	+	−	−
M. genitalium	Rare	Rare	Glucose	7.5	W	−	+	+
M. hominis	Rare	Common	Arginine	7.0	−	−	−	+
A. laidlawii	Rare	Not reported	Glucose	7.5	W	−	−	−
M. lipophilum	Rare	Not reported	Arginine	7.0	−	?	−	−
M. orale	Common	Not reported	Arginine	7.0	−	−	+	−
M. pneumoniae	Rare[a]	Very rare	Glucose	7.5	+	−	+	−
M. primatum	Not reported	Rare	Arginine	7.0	−	+	−	−
M. salivarium	Common	Rare	Arginine	7.0	−	−	−	−
M. spermatophilum	Not reported	Rare	Arginine	7.0	−	W	−	−
U. urealyticum	Rare	Common	Urea	≤6.0	−	+	+[b]	+

W, weak; RBCs, red blood cells.
[a] Rare, except in disease outbreaks
[b] Serotype 3 only

embryonated eggs. Serious doubts about the possibility of the agent being a virus arose when its growth was found to be inhibited by chlortetracycline and gold salts, and cultivation on cell-free medium by Chanock and others in 1962 finally clinched its mycoplasmal nature. The organism was subsequently named M. pneumoniae and its importance as a cause of respiratory disease was confirmed by numerous studies based on isolation, serology, volunteer inoculation, and vaccine protection.

Apart from M. pneumoniae, no other mycoplasma has been shown to cause acute respiratory disease in children and adults, although M. hominis and the ureaplasmas have been implicated in the newborn. M. genitalium has been isolated, together with M. pneumoniae, from the respiratory secretions of a few adults, but its role in respiratory disease is still uncertain. Furthermore, although M. hominis produced sore throats when given orally to adult volunteers, it does not seem to be a cause of naturally occurring sore throats in children or adults.

Epidemiology

Infection with M. pneumoniae is world-wide. Although endemic in most areas, there is a preponderance of infection in late summer and early autumn in temperate climates; in some countries, such as the UK and Denmark, epidemic peaks have been observed about every 4 years. Spread is fostered by close contact, e.g. in a family. M. pneumoniae is responsible for only a small proportion of upper respiratory tract disease: overall, it may cause about one-sixth of all cases of pneumonia but in certain populations, e.g. military recruits, it has been responsible for almost half the cases of pneumonia. Children are infected more often than adults and the consequence of infection is also influenced by age. Thus, in persons 9–14 years old, about a quarter of infections culminate in pneumonia, whereas, in young adults, fewer than 10% do so. Thereafter, pneumonia is even less frequent, but severity tends to increase with the age of the patient.

Clinical features

M. pneumoniae infections often have an insidious onset with malaise, myalgia, sore throat or headache overshadowing and preceding chest symptoms by 1–5 d. Cough, which starts around the 3rd day, is characteristically dry, troublesome and sometimes paroxysmal. Physical signs, such as rales, become apparent, frequently after radiographic evidence of pneumonia. Most often this amounts to patchy opacities, usually of one of the lower or middle lobes. About one-fifth of patients suffer bilateral pneumonia, but pleurisy and pleural effusions are unusual. The course of the disease is variable, but cough, abnormal chest signs, and radiographic changes may extend over several weeks and relapse is a feature. A prolonged paroxysmal cough simulating the features of whooping cough may be a feature in children, and very severe infections have been reported in adults, usually in those with immunodeficiency or sickle cell anaemia, although death is rare.

Disease is limited usually to the respiratory tract, but various extrapulmonary conditions have been observed. These include the Stevens–Johnson syndrome and other rashes, arthralgia, meningitis/encephalitis (and other neurological sequelae), haemolytic anaemia, myocarditis and pericarditis. Haemolytic anaemia with crisis is an auto-immune phenomenon brought about by cold agglutinins (anti-I antibodies). Some of the other complications, such as the neurological ones, may arise in a similar way, although *M. pneumoniae* has been isolated.

Laboratory diagnosis

Because the clinical manifestations of *M. pneumoniae* infections are not sufficiently distinct to make a definitive diagnosis, laboratory help is required. A specific (often complement fixation) or non-specific (cold agglutinin) serological test is usually relied upon. Isolation of the organism is not often attempted because the procedures are specialized and lengthy. For culture, mycoplasmal broth is supplemented with penicillin and glucose, and with phenol red as a pH indicator. After inoculation with sputum, throat washing, pharyngeal swab, or other specimen, the fluid medium is incubated at $37°C$ and a colour change (red to yellow), which may take up to 3 weeks or longer, indicates fermentation of glucose due to multiplication of the organisms. The broth is then subcultured onto agar medium for specific identification. Detection of antigen in respiratory exudates by enzyme immuno-assays and detection of DNA by commercially available probes are, as

yet, insufficiently sensitive to be of value as diagnostic methods.

A four-fold or greater rise in antibody titre in a complement fixation test, with a peak at about 3–4 weeks, is indicative of a recent infection, and occurs in about 80% of cases. Furthermore, a single antibody titre of 64 or more, in a suggestive clinical setting, should be acted upon. If necessary, this can be supported preferably by an ELISA for IgM antibody, the presence of which, allied to a declining titre, indicates a current or recent infection.

Treatment

M. pneumoniae, like other mycoplasmas, is most sensitive to the tetracyclines in vitro, but is more sensitive to erythromycin than some of the other mycoplasmas of human origin. In practice these antibiotics have proved less effective for treating pneumonia than they have in planned trials, probably because disease is often well established before treatment begins. Nevertheless, administering a tetracycline to adults is worthwhile, as is erythromycin to children and pregnant women. Despite this, the organisms may persist in the respiratory tract long after clinical recovery and, in hypogammaglobulinaemic patients, they may do so for months or years. The antibiotics only inhibit multiplication of the organisms and do not kill them, which probably explains the slow eradication and relapse in some patients. Antibiotic treatment should start as soon as possible, based on clinical suspicion rather than waiting for laboratory confirmation, and a 3 week course is justified, particularly if supported by serological or other evidence of infection.

Infection in the newborn

M. hominis and ureaplasmas occasionally cause respiratory disease in the newborn, particularly in those of very low birth weight, the infections often being acquired in utero. Infants of less than 1000 g with a ureaplasmal respiratory tract infection within 24 h of birth are twice as likely to die or to develop chronic lung disease than uninfected infants of similar birth weight, or heavier infants.

Urogenital infections

Seven *Mycoplasma* species (*M. fermentans*, *M. genitalium*, *M. hominis*, *M. pneumoniae*, *M. primatum*, *M. salivarium*, *M. spermatophilum*) and *U. urealyticum* have been isolated from the urogenital tract; *M. hominis* and ureaplasmas occur most frequently.

Non-gonococcal urethritis (NGU)

Although *M. hominis* may be isolated from about one-fifth of patients with NGU, it has not been incriminated as a cause; nor has *M. genitalium* been established as important. On the other hand, there is evidence to implicate ureaplasmas as one of the causes of non-chlamydial NGU. This comes mainly from animal and human volunteer inoculation studies in which disease has been produced, and observations on immunocompromised patients, together with serological and controlled antibiotic studies. The proportion of cases for which ureaplasmas are responsible remains unclear, but their occurrence in the urethra of asymptomatic men suggests that only certain serotypes are pathogenic or that predisposing factors, such as impaired mucosal immunity, exist in those who develop disease. There is no evidence that mycoplasmas are a cause of acute or chronic prostatitis, but the isolation of ureaplasmas from an epididymal aspirate of a patient suffering from non-chlamydial, non-gonococcal epididymitis, together with an antibody response, suggests that they may occasionally cause the disease. It is not thought that ureaplasmas are a cause of male infertility.

Urinary infection and calculi

M. hominis has been isolated from the upper urinary tract of patients with symptoms of acute pyelonephritis, often accompanied by an antibody response. It probably causes about 5% of such cases. Ureaplasmas do not seem to be involved in pyelonephritis. However, the fact that they produce urease, induce crystallization of struvite and calcium phosphates in urine in vitro and produce calculi experimentally in animal models raises the question of whether they cause calculi in the human urinary tract. The occurrence of ureaplasmas more often in the urine and calculi of patients with infective stones than in those with metabolic stones suggests that they may have a causal role.

Reproductive tract disease and sequelae in women

M. hominis organisms and, to a lesser extent, ureaplasmas are found in much larger numbers in the vagina of women who have bacterial vaginosis than in healthy women and, with various bacteria, may contribute to the condition. However, evidence that ureaplasmas contribute to the development of the urethral syndrome is weak.

M. hominis is a likely cause of pelvic inflammatory disease (PID), although the proportion of cases attributable to it is probably small. Ureaplasmas have also been isolated directly from affected fallopian tubes, but the absence of antibody responses and failure to produce salpingitis in subhuman primates make them a much less likely cause of disease. The minor part that *M. hominis* plays in PID makes its role, if any, in infertility inevitably small and somewhat speculative.

Diseases associated with pregnancy and the newborn

M. hominis and ureaplasmas have been isolated from the amniotic fluid of women with severe chorio-amnionitis who had preterm labour. Similarly, ureaplasmas have been isolated from spontaneously aborted fetuses and stillborn or premature infants more frequently than from induced abortions or normal full-term infants. The ability to isolate ureaplasmas from the internal organs of aborted fetuses, together with some serological responses and an apparent diminished occurrence following antibiotic therapy, have supported a role for these organisms in abortion. Nevertheless, whether it occurs because ureaplasmas invade the fetus to cause its death, or whether the fetus dies for some other reason and is then invaded, is a question that remains unanswered. So too is the question of whether genital mycoplasmas, particularly ureaplasmas, cause low birth weight in otherwise normal infants. The association of ureaplasmas with low birth weight is supported by serological data and by a study in which women given erythromycin in the third trimester delivered larger babies than those given a placebo. However, it has not been excluded that women who are predisposed to smaller babies for some reason are selectively colonized. Although there is uncertainty surrounding this problem, premature infants are prone to invasion of the cerebrospinal fluid by both *M. hominis* and ureaplasmas within the first few days of life, causing meningitis.

After an abortion, *M. hominis* occasionally appears to be a cause of fever. Thus, it has been isolated from the blood of about 10% of such febrile women, half of them exhibiting an antibody response, but not from that of aborting afebrile women, nor from normal pregnant women. In addition, *M. hominis* has been recovered from the blood of about 5–10% of women with postpartum fever but seldom from the blood of afebrile women. Similar observations have been made for ureaplasmas and it seems that both microorganisms induce fever by causing endometritis.

Infections in immunocompromised patients

A small proportion of hypogammaglobulinaemic patients develop suppurative arthritis for which mycoplasmas, particularly those in the urogenital tract, are responsible. In some of the cases involving ureaplasmas, the arthritis has been associated with subcutaneous abscesses, persistent urethritis, and chronic cystitis. Although responding sometimes to tetracyclines, it is not unusual for the organisms and disease to persist for many months even though treatment with these and other antibiotics has been coupled with anti-inflammatory and γ-globulin replacement therapy. Septicaemia due to *M. hominis* has occurred after trauma and genito-urinary manipulations and the mycoplasma has been found in brain abscesses and osteomyelitis, but haematogenous spread leading to septic arthritis, surgical wound infections and peritonitis seems to occur more often after organ transplantation and in other patients on immunosuppressive therapy. Particularly common are sternal wound infections caused by *M. hominis* in heart and lung transplant patients.

Laboratory diagnosis of urogenital mycoplasmal infections

Testing swabs from the urethra or vagina for genital mycoplasmas is a little more sensitive than testing urine specimens. Clinical material is added to separate vials of liquid mycoplasmal medium containing phenol red and 0.1% glucose, arginine or urea. *M. genitalium* metabolizes glucose and changes the colour of the medium from red to yellow. *M. fermentans* does likewise but, in addition, converts arginine to ammonia, as do *M. hominis* and *M. primatum*. The ureaplasmal urease also breaks down urea to ammonia. In each case, the pH of the medium increases and there is a colour change from yellow to red. The colour change produced by ureaplasmas usually occurs within 1–2 d, while that for *M. genitalium* may take 50 d or longer. Subculture to agar medium results in the formation of characteristic colonies. On ordinary blood agar *M. hominis*, but not ureaplasmas, produces non-haemolytic pinpoint colonies. *M. hominis* also multiplies in most routine blood culture media; the mycoplasma-inhibitory effect of sodium polyanethol sulphonate, included as an anticoagulant, can be overcome by the addition of gelatin (1% w/v). Definitive identification of the genital mycoplasmas is based on the same serological procedures that are used to identify *M. pneumoniae* and other mycoplasmas.

There has been some progress in the development of DNA probes for the genital mycoplasmas, but those for both *M. hominis* and *U. urealyticum* have, so far, proved less sensitive than cultural procedures. However, *M. genitalium*, which is difficult to culture, has been detected in urethral specimens from men with NGU by means of a DNA probe.

Genital mycoplasma infections stimulate antibody responses which may be used for diagnostic purposes but utmost caution should be exercised in regarding a single elevated titre as diagnostic.

Treatment of urogenital mycoplasmal infections

Chlamydiae, even more than ureaplasmas, are a cause of NGU (see Chapter 40), so that patients should receive one of the tetracyclines which inhibit both groups of micro-organisms. However, at least 10% of ureaplasmas are resistant to tetracyclines and patients who fail to respond to such therapy should then be treated with erythromycin, to which most tetracycline-resistant ureaplasmas are sensitive. A tetracycline should also be included for the treatment of PID so that chlamydiae and *M. hominis* strains are covered. However, since about 20% of *M. hominis* strains are resistant to tetracyclines, other antibiotics, such as lincomycin and clindamycin, may need to be considered. Fever following abortion or childbirth often settles within a few days but if it does not do so, tetracycline therapy should be started while, at the same time, keeping tetracycline resistance in mind.

MYCOPLASMAS AND CELL CULTURES

Mycoplasmal contamination of cell cultures is a common occurrence. Whereas only about 1% of primary cell cultures become infected, continuous cell lines do so frequently. The observed effects of mycoplasmal contamination include those caused by mycoplasmal gene products, enzymes and toxins, and those resulting from the utilization of media components, or from changes in pH. Mycoplasmal infection of cell cultures, despite the existence sometimes of 10^8 organisms per millilitre of culture fluid, may have an insignificant effect on viral propagation. On the other hand, it may decrease the yield, or increase it, the latter being seen with, for example, vaccinia virus in *M. hominis*-infected cells.

The procedures described to eliminate mycoplasmas from cell cultures fall into several categories: antibiotic treatment, use of specific mycoplasmal antisera, and treatment with agents selectively toxic to mycoplasmas, e.g. 5-bromouracil. No procedure, however, is consistently successful and, whenever possible, it is easier to discard contaminated cell cultures, replace them with mycoplasma-free cells and adhere to simple guidelines to prevent contamination.

RECOMMENDED READING

Barile M F, Razin S (eds) 1979 *The Mycoplasmas. Cell Biology*. Academic Press, New York, vol I

Cassell G H (ed) 1986 Ureaplasmas of humans: with emphasis upon maternal and neonatal infections. *Pediatric Infectious Disease* 5(suppl) S221–S354

Cassell G H, Waites K B, Crouse DT et al 1988 Association of *Ureaplasma urealyticum* infection of the lower respiratory tract with chronic lung disease and death in very-low-birth-weight infants. *Lancet* ii: 240-245

Chanock R M, Hayflick L, Barile M F 1962 Growth on artificial medium of an agent associated with atypical pneumonia and its identification as a pleuropneumonia-like organism. *Proceedings of the National Academy of Sciences of the USA* 48: 41–49

Glatt A E, McCormack W M, Taylor-Robinson D 1990 The genital mycoplasmas. In: Holmes K K et al (eds) *Sexually Transmitted Diseases*, 2nd edn. McGraw Hill, New York, p. 279

McGarrity G J, Kotani H 1985 Cell culture mycoplasmas. In: Razin S, Barile M F (eds) *The Mycoplasmas. Mycoplasma Pathogenicity*. Academic Press, New York, vol 4, p 353

Mårdh P-A, Møller B R, McCormack W M (eds) 1983 *Mycoplasma hominis* – a human pathogen. *Sexually Transmitted Diseases* 10 (suppl)

Razin S, Barille M F (eds) 1985 *The Mycoplasmas. Mycoplasma Pathogenicity*. Academic Press, New York, vol 4

Razin S, Tully J G (eds) 1983 *Methods in Mycoplasmology. Mycoplasma Characterization* Academic Press, New York, vol I

Taylor-Robinson D 1985 Mycoplasmal and mixed infections of the human male urogenital tract and their possible complications. In: Razin S, Barile M F (eds): *The Mycoplasmas. Mycoplasma Pathogenicity*. Academic Press, New York, vol 4, p 27

Taylor-Robinson D, McCormack W M 1980 The genital mycoplasmas. *New England Journal of Medicine* 302: 1003–1010 and 1063–1067

Taylor-Robinson D, Furr P M, Webster A D B 1986 *Ureaplasma urealyticum* in the immunocompromised host. *Pediatric Infectious Disease* 5(suppl): S236–S238

Tully J G 1985 Newly discovered mollicutes. In: Razin S, Barile M F (eds) *The Mycoplasmas. Mycoplasma Pathogenicity*. Academic Press, New York, vol 4, p1

Tully J G, Razin S (eds) 1983 *Methods in Mycoplasmology. Diagnostic Mycoplasmology*. Academic Press, New York, vol 2

Tully J G, Whitcomb R F (eds) 1979 *The Mycoplasmas. Human and Animal Mycoplasmas*. Academic Press, New York, vol 2

Whitcomb R F, Tully J G (eds) 1979 *The Mycoplasmas. Plant and Insect Mycoplasmas*. Academic Press, New York, vol 3

PART 4

Viral pathogens and associated diseases

43

Adenoviruses   Respiratory disease; conjunctivitis; gut infections

C. R. Madeley and J. S. M. Peiris

Adenoviruses have been described as the weeds in the virological garden; always present, not valued for themselves, sometimes decorative and felt to be of only limited interest to serious clinical virologists. As all gardeners will know, a plant is only a weed if it is in the wrong place and much of the interest in a wild area is provided by 'weeds'. They can also be valued for themselves and, with increasing doubts that viruses are always pathogens, the epidemiology of adenoviruses is becoming of greater interest.

They were named from their original source, *adenoid tissue* removed at operation and cultured as explants in vitro. Cellular outgrowth occurred readily, but this often deteriorated rapidly a week or 10 d later. The cause of the deterioration was found to be *adenovirus(es)* present in the original tissue and which replicated enthusiastically in the new cells growing from the explant.

This discovery initiated much research which established that there were a considerable number of serotypes, or species, and that they were most-ly associated with mild *upper respiratory tract infections*. In addition, there were occasional serious (and even fatal) childhood *pneumonias* and infrequent *eye infections*. There were also infections, mostly in children and not always symptomatic, which could persist for weeks or months. The focus of adenovirus research then shifted away from clinical virology with the discovery that some species could cause malignancies in laboratory rodents. As a result, virologists have thoroughly investigated adenovirus structure, replicative mechanisms and oncogenicity during the last 20 years.

Clinical interest revived in the middle 1970s with the discovery of two new serotypes (subsequently numbered types 40 and 41) linked (with several other previously unknown viruses) to that previously elusive entity '*viral gastro-enteritis*'. This revival of clinical interest has now been extended by the discovery in rapid succession of six new species (numbered 42–47), most of them in patients with acquired immunodeficiency syndrome (AIDS). This was unexpected, the more so because it is only rarely that adenoviruses have been noted as opportunist invaders of immuno-suppressed patients. Why they do not exploit more the vulnerability of these patients is unknown at present. Although often present in the stools of congenitally immunodeficient children, adenoviruses rarely damage their human hosts seriously, but their activities and epidemiology should have important lessons for medicine, and investigations into their interactions with our immune mechanisms are overdue.

DESCRIPTION

Adenovirus virions provide a very good example of an *icosahedron*, a 20-sided regular solid with triangular faces. This provides the basic model for most cubic (spherical) viruses but the adenovirus exemplifies this best in both symmetry and form. Figure 43.1a shows a group of typical adenovirus particles while Fig. 43.1b and c

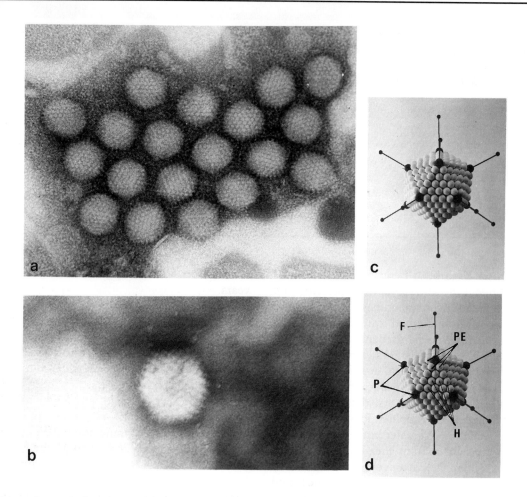

Fig. 43.1 a Group of adenovirus particles from a stool extract. These show the typical adenovirus morphology, although apical fibres are not visible. Individual capsomers are visible as surface 'knobs'. These particles should be compared with the model seen in **c**. Negative contrast, 3% potassium phosphotungstate, pH 7.0. × 160 000. **b** Single adenovirus particle showing some of the apical fibres. This is an uncommon finding. Negative contrast, 3% potassium phosphotungstate, pH 7.0. × 280 000. **c** Photograph of a model of an adenovirus for comparison with the electron micrograph. **d** The same model with pentons (P), peripentons (PE) and hexons (H) indicated. Note that the fibres (F) are attached to the penton.

compares a single virus particle, as seen in the electron microscope, with a model. The particles in Fig. 43.1a lack the fibres projecting from the apices (they are rarely seen in situ in the electron microscope but otherwise the particles in Fig. 43.1a and b resemble the model closely. Indeed, the adenovirus is one of the few viruses of which a convincing model can be made.

The virion is 70–75 nm in size, depending on whether it is measured across the 'flats' or the apices, and there are probably minor variations between preparations and, possibly, serotypes.

The surface has 252 visible surface knobs, the capsomers: 12 apical capsomers, each surrounded by five others are known as *pentons*; 60 peripentons surround the pentons and 180 other capsomers make up the major part of the faces (Fig. 43.1d). Except for the pentons, all the other capsomers are surrounded by six others, and are therefore called *hexons* while the apical capsomers are called pentons by the same logic.

From each penton projects an apical *fibre*. The fibres vary greatly in length between 9 and 31 nm but are rarely seen in position on intact particles by electron microscopy. However, collapse of particles on storage or on exposure to some negative stains can release visible fibres in large amounts. The explanation of this paradox is not known but may be due to the three-dimensional structure of intact particles, which may keep the fibres clear of the puddle of stain. Alternatively, they may be retractable but this is speculative at present. Some avian types have double fibres but human strains all have single ones.

Breakdown of adenovirus particles releases amorphous material, which can be shown to contain thread-like structures, presumably DNA.

Adenoviruses contain double-stranded DNA with a relative molecular weight of approximately 20×10^6, equivalent to 33–45 kilobase pairs. This codes for a considerable number of proteins with molecular weights between 7500 and 400 000. They include both structural and non-structural proteins. The 10 structural ones include three polypeptides which make up each hexon, one which forms the penton base and a glycoprotein for the fibre. These lie on the surface of the particle while the others are internal.

The pentons and fibres bear antigenic determinants that are 'type' specific, and antibody binding to them results in neutralization of virus infectivity. The hexons also have some type-specific antigenic determinants, but carry group-specific antigens as well. The same group antigens are found on all the mastadenoviruses (see below), the genus to which the medically important human adenoviruses belong. These group-specific antigens provide a basis for tests to detect adenoviruses and antibodies to them (by immunofluorescence, enzyme immuno-assays, complement fixation, etc. — see below).

Classification

The adenoviruses belong to two genera:

1. Mastadenoviruses, which infect mammalian species, including man
2. Aviadenoviruses, which infect avian species.

The two genera are completely distinct antigenically. Human adenoviruses are further subdivided into six subgenera (A–F) (Table 43.1), based on DNA homology. By definition, those with >50% homology are members of the same subgenus, while those of different subgenera have <20% homology.

Within each subgenus, adenovirus serotypes are defined by cross-reactivity in neutralization

Table 43.1 Properties and classification of adenoviruses of subgenera A–F

Subgenus[a]	Serotypes	No of Small fragments[b]	Haemagglutination pattern[c]	Oncogenicity in newborn hamsters	Tissues most commonly infected
A	12, 18, 31	4–5	IV	High	Gut (no symptoms)
B	3, 7, 11, 14, 16, 21, 34, 35	8–10	I	Low	Respiratory tract Kidney
C	1, 2, 5, 6	10–12	III	None	Respiratory tract Lymphoid tissue (tonsils and adenoids)
D	8, 9, 10, 13, 15, 17, 19, 20, 22–30, 32, 33, 36–39, 42–47	14–18	II	None	Conjunctiva Gut Respiratory tract (?)
E	4	16–19	III	None	Conjunctiva Respiratory tract
F	40, 41	9–12	IV	None	Gut

[a] > 50% DNA homology between members.
[b] Restriction endonuclease digestion. Some small fragments probably not included.
[c] I, complete agglutination of monkey erythrocytes; II, complete agglutination of rat erythrocytes; III, partial agglutination of rat erythrocytes; IV, agglutination of rat erythrocytes only after addition of heterotypic serum.

tests. There are 47 recognized serotypes of human adenoviruses at present, of which types 40–47 have only been recognized within the last 10 years. There may yet be more types to be discovered. Some virologists refer to *species* rather than *serotypes*, but most clinical virologists refer to serotypes, and this term will be used here.

REPLICATION

The virus attaches to susceptible cells by the apical fibres and is then taken into the cell, losing both fibres and pentons in the process. It then passes to the nucleus, losing the peripentons at the nuclear membrane. Inside the nucleus the DNA is released and the process of replication initiated.

The first messenger RNAs (mRNAs) code for non-structural proteins which shut off most host cell activities while switching on the host cell DNA-dependent DNA polymerase, which is required to replicate viral DNA. About 20 of these 'early' proteins are produced, most of which are not incorporated in new particles (i.e. they are non-structural).

Following production of new viral DNA, the remaining genes are transcribed from it to form 'late' proteins. These are produced in quantity in the cytoplasm, are mostly structural and are later transported back to the nucleus where new virus particles are assembled, normally as crystalline arrays. They are assembled on a scaffold protein, initially as empty shells into which the nucleic acid is inserted afterwards. The effects of the shutting down of the host cell metabolism and the accumulation of thousands of new virions results in rupture (lysis) and death of the infected cell with release of the particles.

In cell cultures this process causes the cells to round up, swell and aggregate into clumps resembling bunches of grapes. The cells then disintegrate as they lyse.

CLINICAL FEATURES

Table 43.2 lists the more common associations of serotypes with disease. However, this does not tell the whole story. On the one hand, the great majority of infections with adenoviruses are probably undiagnosed and the full extent of pathogenesis is not known. On the other hand, virus infection and replication is not invariably associated with disease. For example, a wide variety of serotypes are isolated from faeces without evidence of gut pathology, and prolonged tonsillar carriage in children is common. However, some well-recognized disease syndromes are caused by adenovirus infections.

Respiratory disease

In childhood

These are usually mild upper respiratory tract infections with fever, a runny nose and cough.

Table 43.2 Disease associated with adenovirus serotypes

Disease	Those at risk	Associated serotypes
Acute febrile pharyngitis		
Endemic	Infants, young children	1, 2, 5, 6
Epidemic	Infants, young children	3, 4, 7
Pharyngoconjunctival fever	Older school-age children	3, 7
Acute respiratory disease	Military recruits	4, 7, 14, 21
Pneumonia	Infants	1, 2, 3, 7
Follicular conjunctivitis	Any age	3, 4, 11
Epidemic keratoconjunctivitis	Adults	8, 19, 37
Haemorrhagic cystitis	Infants, young children	11, 21
Diarrhoea and vomiting	Infants, young children	40, 41
Intussusception	Infants	1, 2, 5
Disseminated infection	Immunocompromised, e.g. AIDS, renal, bone marrow and heart–lung transplant recipients	5, 34, 35, 43–47

The majority are due to types 1–7, although higher serotypes may be involved sporadically. Types 1, 2, 5 and 6 are more commonly associated with endemic infections while types 3, 4 and 7 are more epidemic. In Newcastle upon Tyne, in the period March 1989 to March 1990, types 1, 2, 5 and 6 accounted for 71 of 103 adenovirus infections (69%), types 3, 4 and 7 for 12 (12%) and other types for 20(20%). The associated clinical diagnoses included 'upper respiratory tract infection (URTI)', 'increased secretions', 'wheezy', 'cold and cough' and 'failure to thrive'.

These infections are rarely serious but, occasionally, and unpredictably, may progress to a pneumonia which is both extensive and frequently fatal. The majority of these pneumonias occur in young children.

In older children and young adults

A proportion of these will be labelled as 'colds' but epidemics of adenoviral infection with respiratory symptoms and fever are common in, for example, US military recruit camps, where violent exercise and close proximity combine to make the victims more vulnerable and facilitate spread. These outbreaks can be severe in both numbers and extent of disease; severe enough, in fact, to warrant preparation of a trial vaccine. Eye involvement is a common feature (see below), leading to such outbreaks being called pharyngoconjunctival fever. Types 3 and 7 are associated with these outbreaks but other serotypes are found from time to time.

Adenovirus infections are said to mimic whooping cough in some patients and dual infections with *Bordetella pertussis* have been found. There is little doubt that genuine whooping cough is due to the bacterium.

Eye infections

Adenoviruses have been associated with several outbreaks of conjunctivitis in the UK, frequently referred to as 'shipyard eye' because it was originally thought to be caused by steel swarf thrown up from welding and grinding. It was later shown that adenovirus was being transmitted through fluids, eyebaths and other instruments used to treat eye injuries in the shipyard first aid clinic and which had become contaminated by virus from the index case. Use of properly sterilized instruments and single-dose preparations of eye ointment have now made this uncommon. Most such outbreaks were due to adenovirus type 8 (although types 19 and 37 may also be involved). This is not one of the easiest types to isolate and sporadic cases may not be identified as readily as outbreaks, which inevitably attract a more concentrated effort at diagnosis. Eye infections with type 8 do not usually cause systemic symptoms.

As indicated above, conjunctivitis caused by other serotypes may form part of outbreaks of pharyngoconjunctival fever. It is a follicular conjunctivitis which resembles that due to chlamydiae, from which it should be differentiated, but the usual marked adenovirus respiratory symptoms provide a clue.

Gut infections

The common respiratory serotypes (1–7) are frequently isolated from faeces and, in young children, the same serotype may be recovered from both ends of the child. Despite some anecdotal reports there is little evidence to link such isolates with disease of the gut. However, when faecal extracts from children with diarrhoea were examined by electron microscopy, typical adenoviruses were seen in a proportion of cases, often in very large numbers. Surprisingly, these morphologically typical viruses could not be isolated in cell culture. It is now clear that these belonged to two hitherto unknown serotypes, 40 and 41. These are associated with a significant proportion of endemic cases of childhood diarrhoea and, in numbers of cases, are second only to rotaviruses. Estimates of the proportion vary between different laboratories but they may contribute up to a third of such cases in which a virus is found. As with other viruses found in diarrhoeal faeces, such adenoviruses may also be present less frequently in the faeces of apparently normal babies, but there is no doubt of their pathogenic potential for the gut. How they differ from the other types non-pathogenic in the gut is unknown, nor is it known whether they cause respiratory infections.

The role of adenovirus(es) in mesenteric adenitis and intussusception is uncertain. Even when the former is identified at laparotomy it is not usual to excise a node for diagnosis and direct evidence is lacking. Finding a coincidental adenovirus in faeces is not proof of involvement, nor is it clear how often adenitis precedes (and possibly initiates) intussusception. Where any such temporal association has been recorded it has involved the common serotypes 1, 2, 5 and 6. Probably the appropriate verdict is the old Scots one of 'not proven'!

Recently, six new serotypes (42–47) have been found, five of them (43–47) in the faeces of patients with AIDS. The sixth was isolated from the faeces of a normal child. Chronic diarrhoea is, in any case, a feature of AIDS and the role of these adenoviruses, if any, in causing it awaits further investigation. Interestingly, these new serotypes were isolated and identified in cell culture, suggesting they are indeed 'new'. If so, their origin and significance are both unknown.

Other diseases

Infrequently there have been reports of adenovirus (types 11 and 21 mostly) recovered from the urine of children with haemorrhagic cystitis. Finding virus provides a (possible) retrospective cause.

There are reports in the literature of recovery of adenoviruses from both the male and the female genital tracts. They may be sexually transmitted but are not the cause of a major sexually transmitted disease.

There is no good evidence of adenoviruses being involved in central nervous system disease nor in human tumour production. Experimentally, adenoviruses may induce transformation of hamster cells in culture and such transformed cells will produce tumours in laboratory animals. There is no evidence that this can occur in man although it has been diligently sought. Under laboratory conditions adenoviruses can also form hybrids with SV40, a simian papovavirus which contaminated early stocks of polio vaccine grown in monkey kidney cells. The hybrids, carrying part of the SV40 genome, are neither pathogenic nor oncogenic in man.

PATHOGENESIS

Adenoviruses are mostly infectors of mucosal surfaces (respiratory tract, gut, eye) but it is clear that by no means all such infection leads to overt disease. Different serotypes appear to prefer different regions. It is not known what this means at a molecular or cellular level but it may reflect the presence or absence of particular receptors. Infection of an individual cell will cause its death but several studies have documented prolonged respiratory and gut excretion in healthy children lasting weeks or months. Such respiratory 'carriage' is probably in lymphoid tissue (tonsils and adenoids) and gut carriage may be in the equivalent Peyer's patches, although this has not been documented.

Most infections with adenoviruses, whatever the primary site, probably spread to include the gut. 'Respiratory' strains are frequently recovered from faeces and it seems very improbable that this results solely from overflow from the upper respiratory tract. It is much more likely that faecal excretion follows a secondary gut infection, albeit asymptomatic in most cases.

The role of the five newly discovered serotypes (43–47) in patients with AIDS is not known at present. All were recovered from faeces by culture and had not been identified before. They extend the unanswered questions about adenoviruses to include where new types could come from and whether they can arise by mutation and/or recombination.

LABORATORY DIAGNOSIS

Direct demonstration of 'virus'

Electron microscopy

Virus particles may be seen directly in stool extracts by *electron microscopy*, although this will not identify serotypes. Nonetheless, where virus is seen this will usually be types 40 or 41, particularly where large numbers are present (the level may reach $>10^{10}$ particles per gram of faeces). Finding virus in faeces by electron microscopy does not mean that virus must also be present in the nasopharynx or eye.

Virus antigen

The presence of viral antigen in the nasopharynx may be identified by *immunofluorescence* using group-specific antibodies (polyclonal or monoclonal) directly on aspirates (*not* swabs), provided they contain respiratory cells. The presence of such infected cells usually indicates a significant infection, in contrast to asymptomatic carriage. Alternatively, viral antigen may be detected by *enzyme immuno-assays*. However, these detect virus antigen alone without indicating where it was located. Hence they cannot distinguish between a significant presence in respiratory cells (indicating invasion of the mucosal surface) and mostly silent (and clinically insignificant) carriage, probably in the tonsils and adenoids.

Viral DNA

It is also possible to detect viral DNA directly from faeces by *polyacrylamide gel electrophoresis*. The intact DNA forms a single band found near the top of the gel but its identity as definitely adenovirus in origin can be confirmed only after digestion with restriction endonucleases and repeat electrophoresis. A characteristic 'ladder' of DNA fragments separated by size confirms the diagnosis, distinguishes between types 40 and 41 (and identifies others) and can also indicate subtypes. This approach is particularly useful to identify types 40 and 41, which are difficult or impossible to isolate in cell culture, and for laboratories without access to electron microscopy.

Culture

Virus can be grown in *cell culture* from respiratory specimens (nasopharyngeal aspirates, nose and throat swabs) eye swabs, faeces and, occasionally, urine. The speed of isolation can provide a pointer to the significance of the finding. If it takes longer

than 12 d it is less likely to be clinically significant, particularly with types 1, 2, 5 and 6.

Isolation of an adenovirus in cell culture from the faeces of patients with diarrhoea is by itself of little significance. As mentioned earlier, diarrhoea-causing adenoviruses are not readily isolated in culture and cultivable adenoviruses in the stool are not usually those associated with diarrhoea.

Serology

A rise in antibody levels indicates recent infection (though not its site or nature) but absence does not exclude it, especially in babies. Complement fixation is the test most frequently used, and it provides only a group-specific diagnosis. Group- and type-specific enzyme immuno-assays have also been developed but are not used widely. Neutralization tests are both type-specific and more sensitive, but are not available as routine tests; neither is haemagglutination inhibition widely available. However, both tests may be used by reference laboratories or in research.

TREATMENT

There are no antiviral drugs available for the treatment of adenoviral infections. Since adenovirus infections are usually self-limiting and there is no evidence that they provide major problems in the immunocompromised, demand is likely to be insufficient to warrant development of a drug for treatment.

EPIDEMIOLOGY

Adenoviruses are endemic and types 1–7 spread readily between individuals, presumably by droplets. Faecal–oral transmission can also occur and probably does in underdeveloped areas, particularly where there is also overcrowding. However, it is probable that types 40 and 41, which are widespread causes of diarrhoea even in highly developed countries, also spread via droplets. Perhaps spread of most serotypes, including those so far only isolated from the gut, is by droplets.

Subtyping, which has shown, for example, eight subtypes of adenovirus type 7 (the prototype 7p, and seven variants 7a–7g) has also shown geographical variations in their distribution. Such detailed analysis is not done routinely, however, and no information on subtype distribution of type 41 is available.

It is probable that only a minority of adenovirus infections are diagnosed virologically. What is known about their epidemiology is therefore only the tip of a considerable iceberg. Using the earlier analogy to weeds, like them they will always be with us, providing a more luxuriant overgrowth from time to time as circumstances allow. It is probable that some individuals are more vulnerable than others to their activity, e.g. some young children who develop pneumonia, and, possibly, patients with AIDS. There is a need for more information about these viruses whose range of activities is wide.

CONTROL

For the same reasons discussed earlier under treatment, there is little demand for a vaccine. How well it would work can be questioned because circulating antibody may not prevent reinfection, although volunteer studies indicate that reinfection rarely results in disease. Nevertheless, the problems the US armed forces encountered with adenoviruses in recruit camps led them to experiment with a live virus vaccine administered orally in enteric capsules. It provided adequate protection from disease and was licensed for use but only for military personnel. The plethora of serotypes, their widespread presence and their generally benign outcome makes extension to the general public unlikely to be worthwhile.

A careful and rigorous attention to aseptic technique and single-dose vials of materials for use in the eye is the best approach to preventing outbreaks of adenovirus eye infections. As a component of pharyngoconjunctival fever, conjunctivitis is not preventable.

ADENOVIRUS-ASSOCIATED VIRUSES (AAV)

These are members of the parvoviridae. They are about 22 nm in diameter, appear to be more hexagonal than circular in outline and contain insufficient single-stranded DNA to replicate on their own. They form a genus, dependoviruses, indicating their *dependence* on adenoviruses (or herpes simplex virus) to provide the missing functions.

True AAV (also known as adenovirus satellite virus) has not been implicated in clinical disease. However, as with any other virus found in faeces, large numbers of parvovirus-like particles have been seen in extracts of diarrhoeal faeces, sometimes (but not invariably) combined with smaller numbers of adenoviruses. Neither virus grows in cell culture, leaving the significance of these observations obscure (see Chapter 48 on parvoviruses).

RECOMMENDED READING

Madeley C R 1986 The emerging role of adenoviruses as inducers of gastroenteritis. *Pediatric Infectious Disease* 5(suppl 1): 563–574

Wadell G 1990 Adenoviruses. In: Zuckerman A J, Banatvala J E, Pattison J R (eds) *Principles and Practice of Clinical Virology*, 2nd Edn. Wiley, Chichester

44

Herpesviruses

Herpes simplex; varicella–zoster; cytomegalovirus infections; infectious mononucleosis; Burkitt's lymphoma; nasopharyngeal carcinoma; exanthem subitum; herpes B

M. M. Ogilvie

The herpesviruses, a large family infecting many animal species, share a number of features, including their structure and mode of replication and the capacity to establish lifelong latent infections from which virus may be reactivated.

Latent infection. This has been defined as 'a type of persistent infection in which the viral genome is present but infectious virus is not produced except during intermittent episodes of reactivation'.

Reactivation. Reactivation from the latent state may be restricted to asymptomatic virus shedding.

Recurrence or recrudescence. These terms are used when reactivated virus produces clinically obvious disease.

At present six human herpesviruses are recognized and infection with each has been shown to be common in all populations:

1. Herpes simplex virus 1   HSV-1
2. Herpes simplex virus 2   HSV-2
3. Varicella–zoster virus   VZV
4. Epstein–Barr virus   EBV
5. Cytomegalovirus   CMV
6. Human herpesvirus 6   HHV6

The herpes B virus of monkeys can be transmitted to man accidentally. These viruses, the infections caused by them, and associated diseases will be described here.

DESCRIPTION

Herpesviruses have a characteristic morphology visible in electron microscopical studies (Fig. 44.1).

Negative staining reveals the *icosahedral protein capsid* of average diameter 100 nm, consisting of 162 hollow hexagonal and pentagonal capsomeres, with an electron-dense core containing the DNA genome. Beyond the capsid in mature particles is an amorphous proteinaceous layer, the *tegument*, surrounded by a lipid *envelope* derived from cell membranes. Projecting from the trilaminar lipid envelope are *spikes* of viral glycoproteins. Recent cryo-electron micrographs indicate that the capsid is organized into at least three layers, with viral DNA inserted in the innermost layer. The average enveloped particle diameter is approximately 200 nm.

The genome of herpes virions is linear double-stranded DNA, varying in length from 125–240 kilobase pairs (kbp), with base content ranging from 42 to 69 G + C mol % for the human herpesviruses. The presence of long and short unique regions bounded by repeated and inverted short segments allows recombination and isomeric forms in some cases (Fig. 44.2). The DNA sequences for EBV, HSV-1 and VZV have been published and much of HSV-2 and human CMV is known. Genes coding for the glycoproteins, major capsid proteins, enzymes involved in DNA replication and some associated with latency have been identified. Conserved sequences appear in certain regions, and some genes show homology with regions of human chromosomes. Restriction endonuclease analysis permits epidemiological comparison of strains ('fingerprinting') within herpes species.

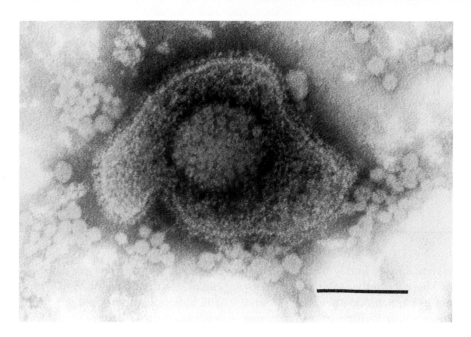

Fig. 44.1 Electron micrograph of HSV. Negative staining (2% phosphotungstate). Bar, 100 nm. (Prepared by Dr B. W. McBride.)

Some human herpesviruses are predominantly neurotropic (HSV, VZV) or lymphotropic (EBV).

Biological classification

The herpesviruses can be classified into three broad groups:
1. Alphaherpesviruses, e.g. HSV, VZV, B virus; rapid growth, neuronal latency
2. Betaherpesviruses — CMVs; slow growth, restricted host range
3. Gammaherpesviruses, e.g. EBV; growth in lymphoblastoid cells.

The viruses are relatively thermolabile and readily inactivated by lipid solvents such as alcohols and detergents.

Replication

After attachment to receptors, the envelope of herpes virions fuses with the cell membrane. The nucleocapsids cross the cytoplasm to the nuclear membrane; replication of viral DNA and assembly of capsids takes place within the nucleus. With HSV, it is known that tegument protein trans-activates early genes. Between 65 and 80 viral proteins are synthesized, in an orderly sequence or cascade.

These proteins are of three types:
1. Immediate early (α) — mainly regulatory functions
2. Early (β) — includes many enzymes involved in DNA replication

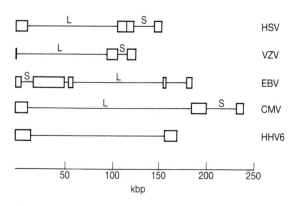

Fig. 44.2 Diagrammatic comparison of herpesvirus DNAs. Lines indicate long (L) or short (S) unique sequences, and repeated regions are boxed.

3. Late (γ) — structural proteins of capsid, glycoproteins.

The viral capsid proteins migrate from the cytoplasm to the nucleus where capsid assembly occurs and new viral DNA is inserted and located in the inner shell. Viral glycoproteins are processed in the Golgi complex and are incorporated into cell membranes from which the viral envelope is acquired, usually from the inner layer of the nuclear membrane as the virus buds out from the nucleus (Fig. 44.3). It then passes through nuclear pores to reach the cell surface. Productively infected cells generally do not survive.

HERPES SIMPLEX VIRUS (HSV)

HSV is ubiquitous, infecting the majority of the world's population early in life and persisting in a latent form from which reactivation with shedding of infectious virus occurs, thus maintaining the transmission chain.

Description

The virus has the general structure and chemical composition already described. In contrast to other members of the group, HSV can be grown in cells from a wide variety of animals relatively easily, so that far more extensive studies have been undertaken with this virus.

There are two distinct types of HSV, named type 1 (HSV-1) and type 2 (HSV-2). These two types are generally (but not exclusively) associated with different sites of infection in patients (see below); type 1 strains are associated primarily with the mouth, the eye and the central nervous

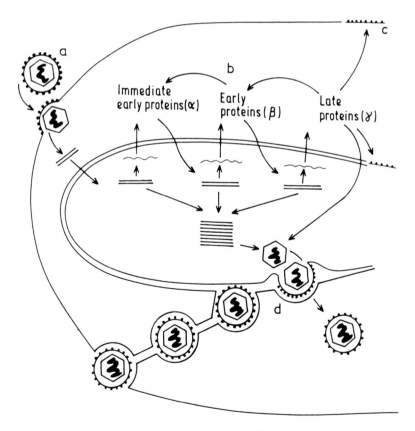

Fig. 44.3 A summary of events in herpesvirus replication: **a** entry; **b** viral DNA transcription and replication, showing cascade of proteins synthesized; **c** glycoprotein expression on cell membranes; **d** assembly and egress of new virions. (Courtesy of J. P. Vestey, Dermatology, Royal Infirmary, Edinburgh.)

system, whilst type 2 strains are found most often in the genital tract and nearby sites of infection.

HSV glycoproteins

The envelope of HSV contains several glycoproteins which have been studied in detail both at the structural and functional level. Gold labelling and high-resolution electron microscopy have revealed three distinct structures labelled with monoclonal antibodies to three of the major glycoproteins, gB, gC and gD. At least four further glycoproteins, gE, gH, gG and gI, are known. Three of the glycoproteins are essential for production of infectious virions — gB and gD, which are involved in adsorption to and penetration into cells, and gH, involved in the release of virus. Some of the glycoproteins have common antigenic determinants shared by HSV-1 and HSV-2 (gB, gD) whilst others have specific determinants for one type only.

Pathogenesis

Primary infection

The typical lesion produced by HSV is the *vesicle*, a ballooning degeneration of intra-epithelial cells. The underlying layer of basal epithelium is usually intact, vesicles only occasionally penetrate the subepithelial layer. The base of the vesicle contains *multinucleate cells* (sometimes called Tzanck cells, seen in Giemsa-stained preparations) and infected nuclei contain eosinophilic *inclusion bodies*. The roof of the vesicle breaks down and an ulcer forms: this happens rapidly on mucous membranes and non-keratinizing epithelia; on the skin the ulcer crusts over, forming a scab, and then heals. A mononuclear reaction is normal, with the vesicle fluid becoming cloudy, and cellular infiltration in the subepithelial tissue. After resorption or loss of the vesicle fluid the damaged epithelium is regenerated. Natural killer cells play a significant role in early defence. Synthesis of herpesvirus glycoproteins during the virus growth cycle is followed by the insertion of the glycoproteins into the cell membranes, and some are secreted into extracellular fluid. gE and gI form a cell membrane receptor for

the Fc part of human immunoglobulin G and gC can bind complement C3b. The infected host responds to all these foreign antigens, producing cytotoxic T cells (CD8+), and helper T lymphocytes (CD4+), which activate primed B cells to produce specific antibodies and are also involved in the induction of delayed hypersensitivity. The different glycoproteins have significant roles in generating these various cell responses; probably all of them induce neutralizing antibody.

During the replication phase at the site of entry in the epithelium, virus particles enter through the sensory nerve endings which penetrate to the parabasal layer of the epithelium and are transported, probably as nucleocapsids, along the axon to the *nerve body* (neurone) in the sensory (dorsal root) ganglion by retrograde axonal flow. Virus replication in a neurone ends in neuronal cell death; however, some of the herpesvirus reaching the ganglion cells is able to establish a *latent infection* in which the neurones survive but continue to harbour the viral genome. Neurones other than those in sensory ganglia can be the site of herpes latency. Whether true latency occurs at epithelial sites is not yet clear; there is some evidence of persistence of virus at peripheral sites, but this may be due to a reactivation with a low level of virus replication.

Antibody does reduce the severity of infections, although it does not prevent recurrences. Neonates receiving maternal antibody transplacentally are protected against the worst effects of neonatal herpes. HSV-2 infection seems to protect against HSV-1, but prior HSV-1 infection only partly modifies HSV-2 disease.

Latent infection

Latent infection of sensory neurones is a feature of the neurotropic herpesviruses HSV and VZV. Most of the information available about the latent state has been obtained from studies of HSV-1 latency. Of the latently infected neurones, only a small proportion (about 1%) of cells in the affected ganglion carry the viral genome which is in a different state to that found in virions. In latency, viral DNA exists as free circular *episomes* — perhaps about 20 copies per infected cell. Very

and much less informative. Indeed, in recurrent episodes the antibody titre may not vary. Sensitive assays for IgG antibody, including type-specific antibody, have an important place in prospective testing.

Herpes virus detection

Direct diagnosis of HSV infection is available, and should be sought in cases where there is any doubt as to the clinical diagnosis, or where rapid confirmation is required to support the choice of therapy or other management. Virus isolation is suitable for most common herpes infections, direct diagnosis being reserved for the atypical or serious situations.

Isolation of HSV from an infected patient is now most usually attempted in cultures of human diploid fibroblast cells, although other fibroblast lines and epithelial cells can all support its growth. Growth is rapid and within 24 h a cytopathic effect (CPE) may be visible, presenting as rounded, ballooned cells in foci (later detaching to leave plaques) which expand and eventually involve the whole cell sheet. Some virus strains may give rise to fusion of infected cells — syncytium formation. This is most commonly seen with the HSV-2 strains. Virus is released from infected cells into the culture fluid, hence the rapid spread of infection from the initial foci.

Herpes virions may be demonstrated by *electron microscopy* in vesicle fluid or tissue preparations; the negative-staining technique can provide an answer within an hour. Detection of viral antigens in cells also provides a same-day diagnosis by testing cells scraped from the base of lesions, or tissue preparations. Unfortunately, in the most serious infections it is often not possible to have easy access to the site of infection. Examination of brain biopsy tissue is still the most reliable method for diagnosis of acute herpes encephalitis as virus does not usually appear in the CSF except in neonatal cases. Detection of excreted viral antigens and DNA in CSF may be useful but further evaluation is needed. In the case of suspected neonatal herpes without skin lesions, nasopharyngeal secretions, CSF and blood lymphocytes should be cultured.

Antibody tests for HSV

Complement fixation tests are still useful in the diagnosis of primary infections when a significant change in antibody titre can be expected. The titre of antibody may not be greater than 32, especially in genital infection, and the test measures total antibody, not differentiating type-specific antibodies. In the case of herpes encephalitis when no brain biopsy has been done, a diagnosis depends on demonstration of *intrathecal antibody* to HSV. Complement fixation tests can be used, testing serum and CSF in parallel against HSV antigens and another unrelated antigen. In health there is no antibody detectable by such tests in the CSF. If the serum antibody:CSF antibody ratio is diminished from the normal 200:1 to 40:1 (or less), and the blood–CSF barrier integrity is confirmed by other antibody (or albumin) being excluded from the CSF, intrathecal antibody synthesis is demonstrated. It is also helpful to check for the possible transfer of antibody from blood to CSF by means of an IgG index performed on the same serum and CSF samples by the biochemists or immunologists. Tests on serum alone cannot confirm HSVE.

Enzyme immuno-assays are much more sensitive and specific than complement fixation tests, although not so useful for demonstrating seroconversion. When type-specific antigen preparations based on glycoprotein G are used, type-specific antibody can be detected. Immunoblotting can similarly demonstrate type-specific antibody, and can be used to study changes in the profile of antibodies seen in sequential samples at intervals after infection. Therapy often results in delay in these type-specific antibodies appearing, and late convalescent samples, at 6 weeks, should be included. One of these sensitive assays for IgG antibody should be used for determination of previous herpes experience, i.e. to show that the patient is latently infected.

Treatment

Specific antiviral therapy has revolutionized the management of HSV infections in the last decade. Prior to the development of agents for systemic use, topical application of the relatively non-selective *idoxuridine* was used successfully in the treatment of eye and skin infections. The newer agents *vidarabine* and *acyclovir* have better therapeutic ratios and have been proven effective, when used early enough, in appropriate dosage, for the whole range of acute HSV infections. Latency is not eradicated by these agents, which inhibit viral DNA synthesis. Prophylactic use of acyclovir is now an established part of the management to prevent reactivation in the immunocompromised, e.g. transplant recipients. Long-term suppressive therapy with acyclovir has been successful in the management of frequently recurring genital herpes and HSV-related erythema multiforme. Patient-initiated early treatment can also abort or modify recurrences.

Acyclovir is the most widely used antiherpes treatment, having an excellent safety record and being available in preparations for topical, oral and intravenous use. Use in pregnancy continues to be monitored for any adverse outcome in the infant. Topical cream or ointment is suitable only for mild epithelial lesions, such as recurrent cold sores or genital herpes or corneal ulcers. Oral or intravenous therapy with acyclovir should be given for:

1. Any deeper lesions
2. Disease in immunocompromised hosts
3. Any of the serious manifestations.

Intravenous therapy is required for central nervous system and other systemic infection.

Dosage varies considerably, depending on the site of infection and whether the aim is suppression or therapy of established disease. Because the level of acyclovir achieved in the CSF is only half that in plasma, the dosage for the treatment of encephalitis has to be twice that for other systemic disease. It is important to maintain therapy until clinical signs indicate a favourable response. In serious systemic disease, or in the severely immunocompromised, therapy will need to continue for 2 weeks or longer.

Resistance to acyclovir does develop in some instances; so far this has not been a significant clinical problem in relation to strains with *altered thymidine kinase* (TK), which are unable to phosphorylate acyclovir, but it is increasing. The first resistant virus isolated with altered DNA polymerase was associated with clinical disease. With increasing use of acyclovir, more resistant strains may be expected to arise and monitoring of antiviral sensitivity of herpes isolates will be necessary. Strains resistant to acyclovir may need to be controlled with a TK-independent agent, such as vidarabine, or by different dosage schedules of acyclovir. Several new agents are under development.

Epidemiology

HSV is probably transferred by *direct contact*. Many children, especially in overcrowded conditions, acquire oral HSV-1 infections in the first years of life. Spread may not occur so readily in better social conditions with the result that primary infection is delayed to young adulthood. This is the usual time of exposure to genital herpes and, as a result, primary infections may be HSV-2 or HSV-1.

Sensitive immuno-assays have shown that 60–90% of adults have had HSV-1 infections. Type-specific serology has also revealed that many more women have had HSV-2 infection than give a history of genital herpes. However, neonatal herpes is still a rare complication in the UK; the British Paediatric Surveillance Unit reported 37 confirmed neonatal herpes infections over a period of 42 months. Eleven of the infants died within the 1st month and several of the survivors suffered adverse sequelae. The rate of cases has increased in some populations as genital herpes has become more common. Herpes encephalitis outside of the neonatal period occurs sporadically at a rate of about 1 per 500 000 per annum.

The role of HSV in human carcinomas, particularly carcinoma of the cervix, is not clear; the ability of the virus to transform cells in vitro is well known, although permissive cells are usually destroyed before any effect can be shown.

Control

Transmission of herpes simplex can be reduced by alleviating overcrowding, practising simple hygiene, and education regarding the infectious stages. Sexual transmission may be significantly reduced by the use of condoms. Exposure of the infant at birth can be avoided if delivery by caesarean section is performed in the early stage of labour, but this is only to be recommended when lesions are present in the mother or virus has been demonstrated at that time. Reference has already been made to the use of prophylactic antiviral regimens to control predictable recurrence. Progress in understanding latency and reactivation will provide approaches to preventing reactivation. Protection from ultraviolet light and the use of inhibitors of prostaglandin synthesis may be useful in this context.

Experimental vaccines are under investigation, but none is licensed for use in the UK at present. Research into subunit vaccines based on the viral glycoproteins or other significant viral proteins may lead to an appropriate preparation to elicit the immune responses important in control of herpes simplex.

VARICELLA–ZOSTER VIRUS (VZV)

Infection with VZV presents in two forms. The primary infection *varicella* (or chickenpox), is a generalized eruption, whereas the reactivated infection *zoster* (or shingles), is localized to one or a few dermatomes.

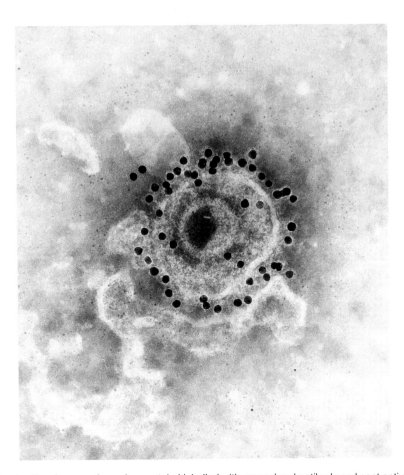

Fig. 44.4 VZV showing the virus envelope glycoprotein I labelled with monoclonal antibody and goat anti-mouse IgG conjugated with 15 nm colloidal gold. × 150 000. (Taken by C. Graham, supplied by Dr E. Dermott, Department of Microbiology and Immunobiology, Queen's University, Belfast.)

Description

The viruses isolated from varicella or zoster are identical and this has now been confirmed by molecular epidemiological studies on viruses isolated from individual patients. The virus has the morphology of all herpesviruses. The sequence of the 125 kbp VZV DNA is fully established. Seventy genes code for 67 different proteins, including five families of glycoprotein genes. The glycoproteins gpI, gpII and gpIII are particularly abundant in infected cells and are present in the viral envelope (Fig. 44.4).

Virus replication takes place in the nucleus, and histological examination of infected epidermis reveals typical nuclear inclusions and multinucleate giant cells identical to those of herpes simplex. Human fibroblast cell cultures are most often used for isolation, but VZV can grow in a variety of human and simian cell cultures. The enveloped virions released from the nucleus remain closely attached to microvilli along the cell surface, and this 'cell-associated' characteristic, with infection being passed from cell to cell, has limited studies with this virus compared to the lytic HSV. The typical cytopathic effect appears in cell cultures in 3 d to 2 or 3 weeks.

There is only one antigenic type of VZV known, but 'fingerprinting' of the DNA can be used in some cases to identify isolates from epidemiologically linked sources. Antibodies to the three main glycoproteins all neutralize virus infectivity. One of these glycoproteins (gpII) has a common sequence shared with glycoprotein B of HSV, and this accounts for the cross-reactive *anamnestic* antibody response that may be detected during infections with either virus.

Pathogenesis

Varicella

This is a disease predominantly of children, characterized by a vesicular skin eruption. Virus is thought to enter through the upper respiratory tract, or conjunctivae, and multiply in local lymph tissue for a few days before entering the blood and being distributed throughout the body. Following replication in reticulo-endothelial sites, a second viraemic stage precedes the appearance of the skin and mucosal lesions. Mucosal lesions are less noticeable and ulcerate early, and the skin rash is readily recognized.

These vesicles lie in the middle of the epidermis and the fluid contains numerous free virus particles. Within 3 d the fluid becomes cloudy with the influx of leucocytes; fibrin and interferon are also present. These pustules then dry up, scabs form, and they desquamate. It is a noticeable feature that lesions in all stages are present at any time while new ones are appearing. The clearance of virus-infected cells is dependent on functional *cell-mediated* immune mechanisms, cytotoxic T cells and antibody-dependent cell cytotoxicity in particular. Persons deficient in these responses and in interferon production have prolonged clear-vesicle phases and great difficulty in controlling the infection.

Zoster

The pathogenesis of Zoster is not so well established as that of HSV recurrence. Nucleic acid probes have revealed VZV sequences in sensory ganglia, and explant cultures of ganglia produce some VZV proteins, although not fully infectious virus. The latent virus is found in neurones and in satellite cells in sensory ganglia, and more than one region of the genome is transcribed, but the state of the latent VZV is not known. It seems likely that virus reaches the ganglion from the periphery by travelling up nerve axons, as HSV does, but there is also the possibility that during viraemia some virus enters ganglion cells. Another difference from HSV latency lies in the persistent VZV expression which has been detected in some mononuclear cells, which may have a role in VZV disease such as post-herpetic neuralgia (see below).

Reactivation of VZV manifested as zoster can occur at any age in a person who has experienced a primary infection which may or may not have been clinically apparent. The rate is much increased in persons aged 60 years or over and, as most primary infection takes place before the age of 20 years, there is usually a latent period of several decades. However, a much shorter latent period is seen in immunocompromised patients, and also in those who acquired primary infection in utero (see below). More than one episode of zoster is uncommon in any individual. The stimulus to reactivation is not known, nor the details, but virus does appear to travel from sensory ganglia to the peripheral site. The zoster is usually limited to one dermatome and, in adults, this is most commonly in the thoracic or upper lumbar regions or in the area supplied by the ophthalmic division of the trigeminal nerve. This distribution is thought to be related to the density of the original varicella rash. There are associations with preceding trauma to the dermatome — injury or injections for instance with an interval of 2–3 weeks before the zoster appears. (An inquiry usually elicits some such association in immunocompetent hosts.) There is an associated suppression of specific cell-mediated responses in acute zoster, but rapid secondary antibody responses are usually found. Reactivation occurs more commonly in T cell immunodeficiency states.

Viraemia may occur in the course of zoster but is not usual, pre-existing immunity normally being rapidly boosted. In the immunocompromised, however, viraemia leads to dissemination of zoster, either to internal organs or in a generalized manner similar to varicella.

Clinical features

Varicella

The incubation period averages 14–15 d but may range from 10 to 20 days. The patient is infectious for 2 d before and up to 5 d after onset, while new vesicles are appearing.

The rash of varicella is usually centripetal, being most dense on the trunk and head. Initially macular, the rash rapidly evolves through papules to the characteristic clear vesicles ('dew drops').

Presentations vary widely — from the clinically inapparent to only a few scattered lesions, or to a severe febrile illness with a widespread rash, especially in secondary cases in older members of a household. Whilst commonly a relatively mild infection in the young child, the complications of varicella are serious and account for significant morbidity, requiring hospitalization of normal children and adults, unlike the other herpesvirus infections.

Secondary bacterial infection of skin lesions is the commonest complication, mainly in the young child, and it increases the amount of residual scarring. *Thrombocytopenic purpura* occurs, especially in immunocompromised hosts. A variety of organs may be affected, producing myocarditis, arthritis, glomerulonephritis and appendicitis. The two most frequent problems are related to the lungs and the central nervous system.

Pneumonia. In varicella, viral *pneumonitis* is a most serious complication, even in normal people. It occurs as a subclinical feature evident only by radiography in a proportion of adults, but is increasingly being recognized for the danger it brings, especially to smokers. Cough, dyspnoea, tachypnoea and chest pains begin a few days after the rash. Nodular infiltrates are seen in the lungs on radiography. Specific antiviral therapy is only successful if used early in sufficient dosage, and should be instituted at the first sign of pneumonia in an adult with chickenpox. Early investigations (radiography and gas exchange) are indicated in all smokers with chickenpox. Immunocompromised patients are even more at risk of varicella pneumonia.

Central nervous system. Neurological complications include the common but benign cerebellar ataxia syndrome. Acute encephalitis is rare but more serious, and occurs more commonly in immunocompromised patients. This may be confused with post-infectious encephalopathy, which with other post-infectious manifestations, such as transverse myelitis or Guillain–Barré syndrome, is immunologically mediated and not related to viral cytopathogenicity. Varicella has also been noted for its association with the metabolic encephalopathy, Reye's syndrome. Now that salicylate use is contra-indicated in febrile children, that association should diminish, and the true incidence of varicella encephalitis will become apparent.

Varicella in pregnancy. Varicella virus can cross the placenta following viraemia in the pregnant woman, and infect the fetus. The infection may be more serious for the mother herself in pregnancy, with pneumonia the major problem. Two types of intra-uterine infection are noted.

1. *The congenital varicella syndrome* is a consequence of fetal infections with VZV in the first half of pregnancy. The birth of infants so infected has been rarely reported but the features include characteristic scarring of the skin, hypoplasia of limbs, and chorioretinitis. The maternal infection is usually varicella but in one case at least it was disseminated herpes zoster. Fetal infection is not inevitable. Silent intra-uterine infection can also occur: no damage is seen, but the baby is born with latent VZV infection, having recovered from infection.

2. *Neonatal varicella* occurs when varicella develops within the first 2 weeks of life, following maternal varicella in late pregnancy, depending on the interval between maternal viraemia and delivery of the baby. If the rash in the mother begins 7 d or more prior to delivery, her antibody response will have developed and been transferred across the placenta so that the baby does not develop disease. However, varicella occurring 6 d or less before delivery (or up to 2 d after) allows viraemic spread across the placenta, without any antibody being transferred, and places the infant at serious risk. Because the usual respiratory entry route has been bypassed, the incubation period is reduced to 10 d on average. If infection occurs, disseminated disease with *pneumonitis* and *encephalitis* may be found. The rate of transmission is 1 in 3 but there is no way of knowing which mother will transmit, and in this situation protection of the neonate with passive immunity (see VZIG, p. 496) and early antiviral therapy is indicated.

Zoster

This is the manifestation of reactivated VZV infection. It takes the form of a *localized eruption*, and is unilateral and typically confined to one dermatome. Prodromal paraesthesia and pain in the area supplied by the affected sensory nerve is common before the skin lesions develop; these are identical to those of varicella except in their

distribution. The evolution of the rash is similar, with some new vesicles appearing while the earliest ones are crusting; however, the whole episode in the majority of cases is confined to the affected dermatome and heals in 1–3 weeks. Acute pain is not always a feature, but its presence should alert to the possibility of zoster, and a search for early lesions, perhaps internal, is indicated. Occasionally there are no skin lesions — 'zoster sine herpete'.

Dissemination of zoster is indicated by lesions appearing in the skin at distant sites or, more seriously, by involvement of internal organs such as the lung and brain. In the immunocompromised this results in severe disease, with occasional fatalities.

Post-herpetic neuralgia (PHN). This is the most common complication of zoster, and results in significant morbidity in around 20% of patients aged over 60 years. PHN is defined as intractable pain persisting for 1 month or more after the skin rash. Constant pain at the site, or stabbing pains or paraesthesiae may continue over 1 year or much longer in a number of individuals. This is an exhausting and disabling condition for which no satisfactory cure has been found. The indications are that adequate early antiviral therapy may reduce the incidence.

Ophthalmic zoster. Involvement of the ophthalmic division of the trigeminal nerve occurs in up to one-quarter of zoster episodes, with ocular complications in more than half the patients. Corneal *ulceration*, stromal *keratitis* and anterior *uveitis* may result in permanent scarring, so this complication may threaten sight when the nasociliary branch is involved. Ocular complications are reduced in patients given oral acyclovir early in ophthalmic zoster. A contralateral hemiparesis due to granulomatous cerebral angiitis in the weeks following acute zoster is a recognized neurological complication. Other post-infection manifestations are seen, and more acute ones such as the *Ramsay–Hunt syndrome* (facial palsy with aural zoster vesicles) suggest that motor neurones can also be involved. Sympathetic ganglia may also be the site of latency, as indicated by cases where the initial recrudescence has been in gastric mucosa, with subsequent dissemination.

Recurrent and chronic VZV. Immunodeficient patients, most particularly those with CD4$^+$ lymphopenia due to HIV infection, may develop *recurrent* and *chronic* infection. New lesions continue to appear, or reappear after acyclovir therapy, which needs to be prolonged. Acyclovir-resistant VZV has been isolated in this situation.

Laboratory diagnosis

Typical presentations of varicella or zoster seldom need laboratory confirmation; however, atypical presentations merit investigation, especially in the immunocompromised. Vesicular rashes due to enterovirus are sometimes confused with varicella and, in compromised patients, various vesicular lesions may be mistaken for zoster. A common misdiagnosis is the assumption that localized vesicular lesions other than on the face or genitalia are due to zoster. In fact, many are due to herpes simplex recurrences, and this is readily shown by virus isolation.

Virus detection

Vesicle fluid is the sample of choice, and it can be collected in a capillary tube or aspirated with a fine needle and syringe. Direct examination by *electron microscopy* will reveal herpes particles; some of the fluid can be diluted in virus transport medium and inoculated into tissue culture for virus isolation, which takes from 5 d to 3 weeks. More rapid detection is possible with centrifuged cultures stained for virus antigens after 24 h. If cells from the base of lesions are available, or biopsy tissue, virus antigens may be sought directly in them. Monoclonal antibodies are now making this a reliable test, and also provide the means of identifying isolates as VZV.

Serological diagnosis

Antibody testing with varicella–zoster antigens is useful in confirming a diagnosis of varicella by demonstration of *seroconversion* or *rising titres* of antibody between acute and convalescent serum samples; complement fixation is still a useful test for this purpose. However the test is not sufficiently sensitive to determine past infection and, to assess immune status, assays need to be based on enzyme or radiolabelled methods, or immunofluorescent staining of varicella–zoster-infected cells. For demonstration of IgM antibody, IgM capture systems have been shown to be useful. IgM to VZV is detectable in both varicella and zoster, appearing early in zoster. (Infants with congenital varicella syndrome may have lost varicella–zoster IgM by birth, and do not have virus detectable by isolation.) Immunoblotting is used to determine the antibody reaction with separate viral proteins, which may have a bearing on protection.

Treatment

Both *acyclovir* and *vidarabine* given intravenously are effective in the treatment of varicella and zoster in immunocompromised patients. Oral acyclovir can be used to accelerate healing and reduce new lesion formation in zoster in healthy patients if given early enough and may lower the rate of post-herpetic neuralgia. Trials of the prophylactic use of oral acyclovir in patients at high risk from reactivation are under way. VZV is not as sensitive to acyclovir as HSV, with 50% inhibitory dose (ID$_{50}$) values ranging from 4 to 17 µM acyclovir compared with 0.1–1.6 µM acyclovir for HSV, so higher dosage is required. For the intravenous preparation this means 10 mg/kg given every 8 h (or 15 mg/kg if the central nervous system is involved). Oral therapy has to be with the high-dose 800 mg five times a day regimen. These doses require that adequate urine flow is maintained and that the dose is adjusted if any renal function impairment is present. Acyclovir-resistant VZV has been isolated very rarely as yet. Newer experimental antivirals may offer better therapeutic regimens. Treatment of VZV infection is given primarily to all 'high-risk of complication' groups:

1. Neonates (within the first 3 weeks of life)
2. Immunocompromised patients
3. Those with ophthalmic zoster

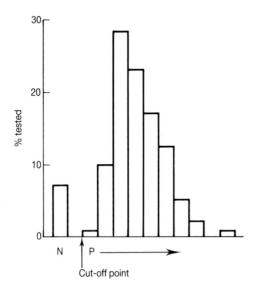

Fig. 44.5 Distribution of antibody (IgG) to VZV in young adult population (southern England). Percentage confirmed negative (N) was 7.8%; P →, increasing positive result

4. Healthy patients with varicella when there is an additional complicating factor such as smoking or pneumonia.

Epidemiology

Varicella is partly seasonal, being spread mainly by the *respiratory route* in winter and early spring. Some cases which result from contact with zoster occur sporadically at any season. The majority of children contract varicella between the ages of 4–10 years in western countries, with around 8% of young adults remaining susceptible (Fig. 44.5). However, a much higher proportion of young adults remain susceptible in developing countries. Mortality from varicella is surprisingly high in normal adults, particularly smokers, who develop pneumonia. The mortality rate in the immuno-compromised was between 7 and 15% prior to the use of acyclovir or vidarabine for varicella. Zoster is associated with decreased T cell function, and occurs with increasing incidence in *old age*, the pre-AIDS (acquired immune deficiency syndrome) phase of *HIV infection*, and after organ *transplantation* and *chemo-* or *radiotherapy* for lymphomas or leukaemia.

Control

Passive immunization

Passive immunity is partly protective for varicella, as seen in infants with maternal antibody or patients given *varicella–zoster immunoglobulin* (VZIG) within 72 h of exposure. VZIG (in the UK) or another similar high-titre antibody preparation is available for neonates, non-immune pregnant contacts or immunocompromised contacts at risk of varicella. As the majority of pregnant contacts will in fact be immune, testing for antibody after exposure may prevent unnecessary use of VZIG. Current preparations will seldom prevent infection, but will modify disease. More specific antibody preparations may be required to produce better protection.

Varicella vaccine

A live attenuated varicella vaccine has been in use for some years in Japan and more recently has been licensed in several European countries, but not yet in the UK or USA. This vaccine, given by intramuscular injection, has been found to be immunogenic in children with leukaemia in remission and in healthy children and adults; vaccinees have resisted infection on close exposure to varicella. Some symptoms are noted around 10 d post-vaccine, and vesicles can occasionally develop. Immunization does not necessarily prevent latency developing after exposure to another VZV strain. However, the incidence of zoster in vaccinees is not increased. Whether vaccination will ever boost immunity to prevent zoster is not yet known. Subunit vaccines would remove the risks of transmission, latency and potential oncogenicity inherent in the live vaccine.

EPSTEIN–BARR VIRUS (EBV)

Epstein, Barr and Achong in 1964 described herpesvirus particles in cells from a common lymphoma in African children studied by Burkitt, who suspected a viral aetiology of the tumour. The link between that new herpesvirus — the Epstein–Barr virus — and a variety of lymphoproliferative diseases is now clearer. EBV is, however, most often involved in asymptomatic infections early in childhood or in the classical infectious mononucleosis ('*glandular fever*') of adolescents in the developed world. Humans are the only natural host, but EBV infection can be transmitted to some subhuman primates.

Description

The characteristic morphology seen on electron microscopy placed EBV with the herpesviruses. This virus cannot be grown in human fibroblast or epithelial cell lines and there is no completely productive or permissive system for culture of EBV.

Replication

The full replication (productive, or lytic) cycle of EBV is now known to take place in differentiated epithelial cells. EBV receptors (the CD21 molecule, also the receptor for the C3d component of complement) are expressed on mature resting *B lymphocytes*, and on cells of the basal layer of stratified squamous epithelium — in the oropharynx, salivary glands and ectocervix for instance. Viral production, however, is restricted to the differentiated cells of the *granular layer* and above, and virus is shed from the *superficial* cells. Technical difficulties in growing differentiating epithelia in culture have limited these studies to date, and most work on the lytic cycle of EBV has been done in lymphoblastoid cell lines, in which a proportion of the EBV-infected cells can be induced to produce virions. One such line of marmoset cells, B95-8, produces the transforming, infectious virus strain used in much experimental work. A range of Burkitt lymphoma-derived cell lines is used for a variety of tests; one line (P$_3$HR$_1$) produces viral capsid antigens and infectious virions but a genetic deletion renders the virus non-transforming.

The genome of EBV is about 186 kbp. The organization of the genome differs from HSV and some genes are present in one and not the other. Approximately 80 proteins are encoded; some glycoproteins are known, including the major glycoprotein gp 350/220, which mediates attachment to CD21, and gp 85, which is involved in membrane fusion. The latent (non-productive) state of EBV infection is maintained in B lymphocytes, which have been extensively studied, and perhaps in certain basal epithelial cells (as described above). In the B lymphocytes the EBV genome is maintained as multiple full-length copies in the form of circular episomes. A variable number of EBV genes are expressed in the latent state; these are principally genes coding for nuclear antigens (EBNAs) and a gene encoding a latent membrane protein which hardly extends beyond the plasma membrane but may be involved in recognition by immune T cells. It may also have a role in cell transformation.

The Epstein–Barr nuclear antigen (EBNA 1) is responsible for maintaining the replication of the EBV episome. EBNA 2 is necessary for transformation of B lymphocytes; there are two alleles of this gene, giving EBNA 2A and EBNA 2B. EBV strains with EBNA 2B have been found mostly in Africa, with EBNA 2A found worldwide. The genes of the latent EBV are replicated by host cell DNA polymerase.

The full lytic cycle of EBV replication is accompanied by production of virus structural antigens and assembly of virions. EBV does have a viral thymidine kinase and it can be shown that acyclovir is phosphorylated in cells producing EBV. The viral polymerase is sensitive to acyclovir triphosphate and treatment with acyclovir will reduce EBV production, but has no effect on latency or the proliferation induced by the virus.

Pathogenesis

Infection of oropharyngeal epithelial cells occurs initially, then infection of B lymphocytes, which disseminate through the circulation, with the potential to enter a productive phase and release virus elsewhere in the body. Most shedding of virus, however, takes place in the oral cavity and this can be detected regularly in the saliva of asymptomatic hosts, increasing in immunosuppressed states. How B cells become infected is not proven, but there are opportunities for close contact between lymphocytes and epithelial cells in the nasopharynx.

A proportion of infected B lymphocytes undergo transformation and continue to proliferate in vitro as a lymphoblastoid cell line (*'immortalization'*). Activated B lymphocytes secrete immunoglobulin, and EBV is a potent polyclonal activator of antibody production by B cells, independent of any accessory cells. IgM-producing lymphocytes predominate, and IgM antibody is found in high levels, but detectable IgG (especially the IgG3 subclass), IgA and IgD have also been found.

Recovery from primary EBV infection is associated with humoral and cellular responses; any delay in cellular control, or over-vigorous responses contribute to the 'disease' associated with the infection. Thus, large initial infective doses result in high numbers of circulating infected B lymphocytes, followed by a marked T cell response. The polyclonal activation of B cells results in transient antibodies (predominantly IgM) appearing, directed against a wide range of self and heterophile antigens. The cellular response is detected as large numbers of 'atypical lymphocytes' in the blood and infiltrating many tissues. These cells have been shown to be mainly cytotoxic/suppressor T cells. The suppression is

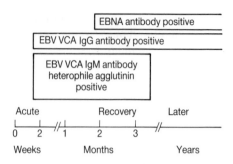

Fig. 44.7 Appearance and duration of diagnostic antibodies following primary EBV infection.

manifested as a general depression of immune responses. The cytotoxic elements carry the ability to kill EBV-infected cells, and this is not entirely human leucocyte antigen (HLA) restricted (Fig. 44.6).

Antibody responses following EBV infection make a characteristic pattern, with the initial IgM response to virus capsid antigens persisting for some months. The EBNA complex elicits antibodies in late convalescence only, perhaps after release from B cells lysed by the cytotoxic T cells (Fig. 44.7). Failure to produce antibody to EBNA is a feature of immunodeficiency states. This may be associated with increased levels of antibodies to EBV lytic cycle antigens (EA, early antigen and VCA, viral capsid antigen), reflecting a high virus replication rate. High IgA levels to EBV VCA are found in those at risk of developing nasopharyngeal carcinoma (see later).

Clinical features

Primary infection with EBV is usually mild and unrecognized in the vast majority who acquire it in the first years of life.

Infectious mononucleosis

The disease known as *infectious mononucleosis*, or *glandular fever*, is a primary EBV infection seen predominantly in the 15–25 year age group. The incubation period is 30–50 d and the onset is abrupt with a *sore throat, cervical lymphadenopathy* and *fever*, accompanied by *malaise, headache,*

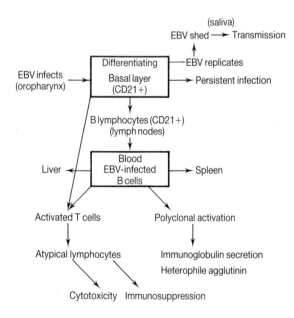

Fig. 44.6 Simplified outline of EBV infection of cells in oropharynx and interaction with lymphocytes.

sweating and gastro-intestinal discomfort. Pharyngitis may be severe, accompanied by a greyish white membrane and gross tonsillar enlargement. Lymphadenopathy becomes generalized, often with splenic enlargement and tenderness, mild hepatomegaly in some cases and clinical jaundice in 5–10%. Intermittent fevers with drenching sweats occur daily over 2 weeks. A faint transient morbilliform rash may be seen; a maculopapular rash may follow ampicillin administration due to immune complexes with antibody to ampicillin. The illness can last several weeks and fatigue and lack of concentration are common in the aftermath.

Complications of glandular fever

Complications are rare but some are serious. Acute airway obstruction may occur as a result of the lymphoid enlargement and oedema; this merits emergency tracheostomy in some cases, but usually responds well to corticosteroids. Splenic rupture is also rare. Neurological complications include meningitis, encephalitis and Guillain–Barré syndrome.

EBV infections, immunodeficiency and tumours

X-linked lymphoproliferative syndrome

This rare genetic immune response defect is found in male members of certain families (and occasional sporadic cases) and is specific to EBV. Primary infection is not controlled, resulting either in early death from fulminant B cell infection or a more prolonged B cell lymphoproliferation with associated hypogammaglobulinaemia and later lymphoma.

Burkitt's lymphoma

This lymphoma is seen in regions of *equatorial Africa* and *New Guinea* and is associated with an early age of EBV infection, hyperendemic malaria, contributing to immunosuppression, and a translocation of chromosomal material from chromosome 8 to chromosomes 14, 2 or 22. The activation of the oncogene c-myc is thought to be the origin of this malignant B cell lymphoma, with EBV infection and immunosuppression as cofactors. The African tumour is seen commonly in children, affecting the jaw and abdominal organs.

B cell lymphomas

Patients who are immunodeficient as the result of transplantation or HIV infection may develop B cell lymphomas associated with EBV. In the early stages proliferation is polyclonal and intervention with acyclovir may be of some benefit, but later lymphoma therapy will be required.

Oral hairy leukoplakia

This condition is seen in HIV-infected patients, and affects the tongue and buccal epithelium. This is a productive infection, and capsids of EBV are found in the affected tissue.

Lymphocytic interstitial pneumonitis

EBV is associated with this presentation in HIV-infected children.

Nasopharyngeal carcinoma

This has an even stronger association with EBV than Burkitt's lymphoma. This undifferentiated carcinoma of nasopharyngeal epithelium contains EBV DNA and EBNA, and patients have high levels of antibody to the lytic cycle antigens, especially IgA antibody. The disease is common in people from southern China, Eskimos and Greenlanders, and there are possibly chemical co-factors.

Laboratory diagnosis

Infectious mononucleosis is accompanied by production of *heterophile agglutinins* which may be readily detected by a rapid slide agglutination test or the *Paul-Bunnell* test. Agglutination of horse or sheep red cells by serum absorbed to exclude natural antibody is the basis of this test. *Atypical lymphocytes*, accounting for 20% of the lymphocytosis common in this condition, are seen in blood films. Definitive diagnosis requires the demonstration of IgM antibody to the EBV viral capsid antigen (VCA), or seroconversion if an earlier serum lacks IgG antibody. These tests, using indirect immunofluorescence, are generally available. Other serological tests are applicable in special situations.

EBV isolation is generally confined to research laboratories. Saliva or throat washings are suitable specimens. Tissues can be stained for EBNA, or probed for EBV DNA but these approaches are not yet routinely available.

Treatment

Acyclovir therapy does reduce EBV shedding in acute infections, and there may be a place for it in patients suffering from, or at risk of, complications associated with an ongoing viral lytic cycle.

Epidemiology

Infection with EBV is known to be transmitted by saliva, and requires intimate oral contact. Transmission has rarely been reported following transfusion of fresh blood to seronegative recipients. Transplacental transmission, whilst theoretically possible, is unlikely and has not been identified. The recent evidence showing EBV infection of the ectocervix presents another source of infection, at least to the neonate. Infection is widespread, with most of the population infected from early in life, even in developed countries.

Control

A subunit vaccine, based on the major membrane glycoprotein gp 350/220 is undergoing trials. It has been shown to protect marmosets against tumour-inducing doses of EBV. Screening for IgA to EBV VCA is used in populations at risk of nasopharyngeal cancer to detect preclinical cases.

CYTOMEGALOVIRUS (CMV)

There are CMVs specific to other animals, and the full name for the virus infecting man is human cytomegalovirus (HCMV). This will be used only in the description where features of HCMV

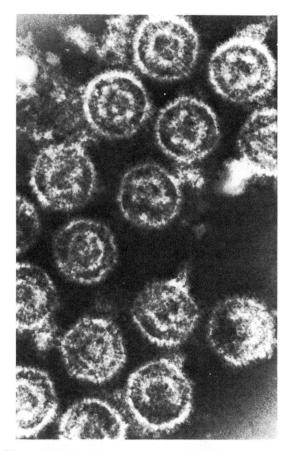

Fig. 44.8 CMV. Virions from cultured cells; none have envelopes, most show a 50 nm core. (From Madeley C R 1972 *Virus Morphology*, Churchill Livingstone, Edinburgh.)

specifically are given, otherwise the more usual CMV will be used. The name cytomegalovirus was chosen on account of the swollen state of infected cells as seen in culture and in tissues. Nuclei of productively infected cells contain a large inclusion body, giving a typical 'owl's eye' appearance.

Description

The CMVs have the same general structure as other members of the herpes group (Fig. 44.8).

Human fibroblast cells are required for isolation of HCMV in vitro, but in vivo the virus replicates in *epithelial cells* — in *salivary glands, renal* and *respiratory epithelium* particularly. CMV remains highly cell associated, and is sensitive to freezing

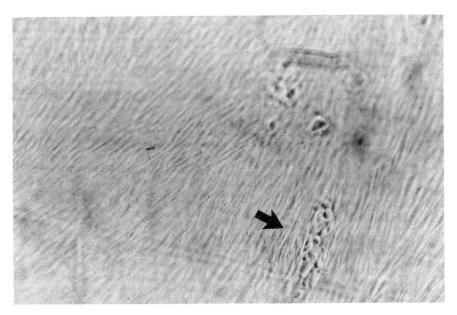

Fig. 44.9 A focus of CMV infection (arrowed) in a tissue culture monolayer of human embryo fibroblasts.

and thawing. Virus shed in urine is stable at 4°C for many days.

Replication

The temporal regulation of viral protein synthesis in the growth cycle is more obvious in laboratory culture of the slower-growing CMV than with HSV. Early (non-structural) proteins appear in nuclei within 16 h of inoculation, whilst late (virion-structural) proteins are produced after DNA synthesis and the typical cytopathic effect is often not recognizable for 5–21 d. Foci of swollen cells slowly expand as infection passes from cell to cell (Fig. 44.9). Passage and storage of virus is best achieved by trypsinization and passage as infected cells.

HCMV does not produce a detectable virus-specified thymidine kinase. As a consequence there is no selective phosphorylation of acyclovir in CMV-infected cells, however, some inhibition of CMV replication is seen when high levels (>30 μM) of acyclovir are used. During CMV replication, host cell synthesis is initially stimulated and a cellular enzyme deoxyguanosine kinase is produced. This enzyme phosphorylates the anti-

viral agent ganciclovir, which, as a triphosphate, inhibits CMV DNA polymerase.

There are several families of glycoproteins in CMV, and these are important antigenic targets. One potential glycoprotein gene has homology with the cellular class I HLA α chain gene. HCMV binds to the host cell protein β_2-microglobulin (which associates with HLA class I) and can use the class I HLA molecule as an additional receptor for cell attachment and infection. Virions of CMV excreted in urine are coated with β_2-microglobulin, which appears to be attached to the tegument protein. Like HSV, CMV induces a receptor for the Fc portion of human IgG on cells (Fig. 44.10). This enables complexes, e.g. HIV–antibody, to gain entry to cells lacking (HIV) receptors.

Pathogenesis

Primary infection with CMV may be acquired at any time, possibly from conception onwards.

CMV persists in the host for life. *Reactivation* is common and virus is shed in body secretions such as urine, saliva, semen, breast milk and cervical fluid. Mononuclear cells are thought to carry the

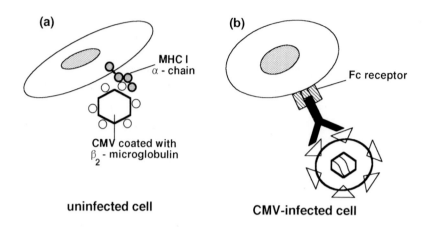

Fig. 44.10 **a** CMV coated with β_2-microglobulin associated with class I HLA expressed on cell surface. **b** CMV-induced Fc receptor on human fibroblast cells mediating entry of HIV–antibody complex.

latent virus genome since viral RNA transcripts of early genes have been detected in them, but the nature and site of latency is not yet clear. Whether any virus persists in epithelial cells is not known.

Recurrent infections may follow reactivation of latent (endogenous) virus, or reinfection with another (exogenous) strain. Isolates can be distinguished by restriction endonuclease analysis.

Intra-uterine infection

Maternal viraemia may result in fetal infection in approximately one out of three cases of primary CMV during pregnancy, and this may lead to disease in the fetus. Infection may also be acquired in utero when the mother has a reactivation, but this rarely results in disease. Transplacental infection is probably carried by infected cells.

Perinatal infection

This is predominantly acquired from infected maternal genital tract secretions or from breast feeding (3–5% of pregnant women in Europe reactivate CMV). Rarely, perinatal blood transfusion is the source.

Postnatal infection

This can be acquired in many ways. Saliva containing CMV is profusely distributed amongst young children, and shared by intimate kissing. Semen can have high titres of virus, and may be a source of sexual transmission or artifical insemination-associated infection. Blood transfusion and donated organs are important sources of CMV. As it is not known which donors are most likely to transmit infection, all antibody-positive ('seropositive') donors are considered potential transmitters as the presence of antibody implies the presence of persistent virus.

Host responses

The host response to primary CMV includes IgM, IgG and T cell responses. Some of the T cell responses may contribute to immunopathology by reacting with HLA molecules induced by CMV. CMV early genes transactivate other viral and cellular genes and this may be an important interaction with HIV, leading to the production of HIV from latently infected cells. Because CMV infects mononuclear cells, there is a degree of immunosuppression associated with the acute infection. Cell-mediated responses are crucial to control of CMV, as shown by the serious consequences of disseminated infections in those deficient in effector cell functions. The incubation period for primary infection is 4–6 weeks; reactivation, post-transplantation for instance, appears a little later.

Clinical features

Congenital CMV infection

This is *asymptomatic* in 95% of infected babies, but around 15% of these will go on to show sensorineural *deafness* or *intellectual impairment* later. Progression of the persistent CMV infection may be involved. All congenitally infected infants excrete abundant virus in urine during the first year. The 5% symptomatic infants have 'cytomegalic inclusion body disease'. Growth retardation, hepatosplenomegaly, jaundice and thrombocytopenia are common to various congenital infections. Central nervous system involvement is the significant problem with CMV; *microcephaly, encephalitis* and *retinitis* may be noted at birth. Some changes may even be detectable on ultrasound scanning in utero.

Mononucleosis

Postnatal infection with CMV is seldom recognized clinically, unless virus is isolated. Respiratory tract infection is common in infancy. A *mononucleosis syndrome* is seen occasionally, especially in young adults or when CMV is acquired from blood transfusion. Hepatitis, fever and atypical lymphocytosis are noted, but pharyngitis and lymphadenopathy are unusual and heterophile agglutinins are not found (see EBV — infectious mononucleosis). This syndrome is also seen in some HIV-infected patients before the development of AIDS and should prompt HIV-related investigations.

Infection in the compromised patient

Immunocompromised patients may develop symptoms as the result of primary or recurrent CMV infection. Dissemination of the virus in the blood as indicated by a hectic fever is a bad prognostic sign. The complications of disseminated CMV infection include:

1. Pneumonitis — has a high mortality in bone marrow allograft recipients
2. Encephalitis — like pneumonitis this may be fatal
3. Retinitis — which may occur on its own (10% of AIDS patients)
4. Colitis — 5–10% of AIDS patients
5. Hepatitis
6. Pancreatitis or adrenalitis.

Primary CMV infection in transplant recipients is a significant cause of morbidity and loss of graft. Mortality is high (Fig. 44.11), particularly in allogeneic marrow recipients who develop pneumonitis associated with graft versus host disease.

Laboratory diagnosis

Detection of CMV is the objective, and, if possible, to show its presence at the site of disease. Samples should include urine, saliva, broncho-alveolar lavage fluid or biopsy tissue if available, and peripheral blood collected into preservative-free heparin. In the neonate, urine samples taken in the first 2 weeks of life are sufficient for diagnosis of congenital infection.

Virus detection

Rapid diagnostic methods will detect virus DNA in the samples or CMV early antigen in cell cultures 24 h post-inoculation (Fig. 44.12), while conventional culture will be used to isolate virus. High titres of CMV will produce a cytopathic effect very quickly, but most cultures require 2–3 weeks. CMV isolation from urine does not of course prove that the virus is the cause of the disease being investigated. To demonstrate congenital infection, virus must be shown in a sample taken within the first 2 weeks of life; later samples may reflect postnatally acquired virus. Additional confirmation that CMV is related to a disease process comes from showing that the virus is replicating in the affected tissues (perhaps by cytology), and in some cases that a primary infection has occurred.

Serology for CMV

This is increasingly important and sensitive screening tests are more widely available. Complement

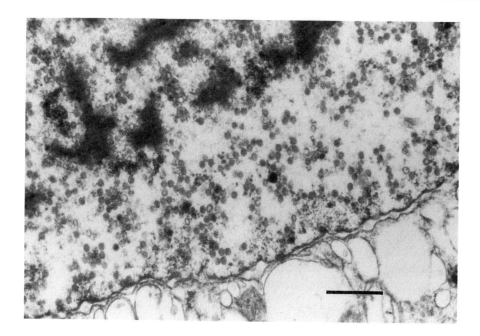

Fig. 44.11 Electron micrograph of ultrathin section of post-mortem lung from a child with leukaemia infected with CMV acquired from blood transfusion. Numerous herpes virions can be seen within the nucleus. Bar, 1000 nm.

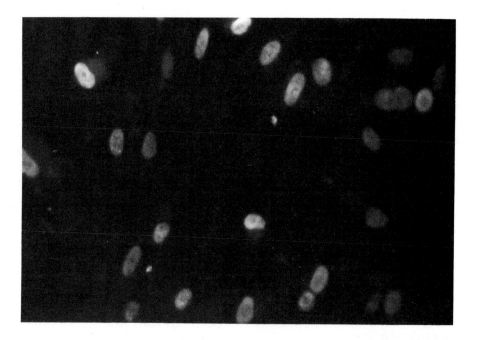

Fig. 44.12 CMV early antigen demonstrated in nuclei of human embryo fibroblasts by immunofluorescence after incubation for 24 h following centrifuge-assisted inoculation.

fixation tests are adequate for showing *seroconversion* after primary infection in competent hosts. To screen for '*seropositive*' status a more sensitive assay, such as enzyme immuno-assay for CMV IgG antibody or latex agglutination assay, is appropriate. These tests can be done urgently for donor–recipient assessment. CMV IgM testing is not always helpful in the situations where it is most important to detect recent infection and IgM-capture methods are not wholly satisfactory. It is not always possible to detect IgM in the neonate or immunocompromised patient.

Treatment

Some antiviral agents for CMV infections are available but serious side-effects limit their use to life- or sight-threatening complications. *Ganciclovir* is the agent most often used for serious CMV disease, given intravenously twice a day. Marrow toxicity results in *neutropenia*, and there is a potential for long-term loss of spermatogenesis. Clinically, treatment has been successful in *CMV colitis, encephalitis* and *pneumonitis*, and progression of CMV *retinitis* in AIDS has been controlled with prolonged maintenance therapy. Ganciclovir-resistant virus has been found. *Foscarnet* (phosphonoformate) is an experimental alternative agent (licensed in some countries) that inhibits viral DNA replication. Acylovir is not effective therapy for CMV, but some benefit from high-dose prophylaxis of CMV in bone marrow recipients is noted.

Epidemiology

Primary CMV infection is acquired by 40–60% of persons with limited exposure by mid-adult life, and by over 90% of those with multiple intimate exposures. Less than 5% of units of blood from seropositive donors result in transmission to seronegative recipients, whilst 80% of kidneys transmit infection from seropositive donors. The full extent of congenital CMV disease is not known, but this infection occurs in approximately 3 out of 1000 live births in the UK.

Control

Some preventive action is undertaken by way of screening organ donors and recipients to avoid, where possible, a seronegative recipient receiving an organ from a seropositive donor. This has been shown to reduce morbidity and mortality significantly in all forms of allogeneic transplant. Blood donor screening to select CMV seronegative units for support of patients in the transplant programmes is important but not always available. The heavy demands for blood do not allow for such a provision generally, but a special case can be made for any seriously compromised host or any very premature baby to receive screened blood (from CMV seronegative donors) or leucocyte-depleted blood.

No CMV vaccine is licensed for use. Experimental live attenuated vaccines have been tried, but hopes rest on subunit vaccines.

HUMAN HERPESVIRUS 6 (HHV6)
Description

This, the most recently recognized herpesvirus infecting humans, was first isolated in 1986 from the blood of patients with lymphoproliferative disorders. Electron microscopy revealed a virus with characteristic herpes group features. Hybridization studies with cloned DNA fragments have shown HHV6 to be distinct from the other human herpesviruses, but closer to HCMV, with which it has some homology. HHV6 is now known to be associated with a common disease of infancy called *exanthem subitum* (roseola infantum).

Pathogenesis and clinical features
Exanthem subitum

This was long considered to be an infection caused by a virus, and transmission by blood was confirmed experimentally years before HHV6 was isolated. The infection is extremely common in the first years of life, presenting between 6 months and 3 years of age with a sudden onset of fever (40°C). The child is not usually ill, remaining alert and playful, with some throat congestion and cervical lymphadenopathy. Sometimes more pronounced respiratory symptoms occur and febrile convulsions have been reported. Fever persists for 3 d, when the temperature suddenly falls, and a widespread *macular rash* appears in around a third of cases. HHV6 has been isolated from peripheral blood in the acute febrile phase, in patients who subsequently produced a rash and some who did not. Seroconversion from an antibody-negative to antibody-positive state is noted in convalescence, confirming a primary infection with HHV6.

Laboratory diagnosis

Isolation involves co-cultivation of peripheral blood lymphocytes with cord blood lymphocytes. The infected B cells do survive for some time but are not immortalized. Very large refractile cells are produced in culture, and many intact enveloped virions are released into the culture medium. CD4+ T cells can also be infected with HHV6 and where there is a dual infection with HIV-1 this results in increased expression of HIV and cell death. There is no confirmation that this occurs in vivo.

Laboratory diagnosis of HHV6 is currently available only from specialist laboratories. Antibody tests will become more widely applied in the near future.

Treatment

HHV6 is sensitive to ganciclovir, but requires high doses of acyclovir to inhibit its replication in vitro.

Epidemiology

Antibody analysis to date has been based on immunofluorescence studies using HHV6-infected cells as antigen. High antibody titres are found in young children in the first 4 years of life, reflecting recent primary infections in this group. Primary infection, with viraemia and seroconversion, has also been detected in seronegative

transplant recipients of liver or kidney from seropositive donors. Possible transmission by blood transfusion has not been excluded. Older persons have lower levels of antibody, and more sensitive tests will be required to establish just how common seropositivity is in different age groups and populations. The spectrum of disease associated with this virus and the extent of asymptomatic shedding also remain to be established. Virus has been isolated from saliva of asymptomatic adults. Latency may be in epithelial sites, as it does not appear to be in lymphocytes.

CERCOPITHECINE HERPESVIRUS 1 (B VIRUS)

Description

This virus, antigenically related to HSV, commonly infects Old World (Asiatic) macaque monkeys, causing a mild vesicular eruption on the tongue and buccal mucosa analogous to primary herpetic stomatitis in man. The infection rate in monkeys increases markedly if they are kept in crowded conditions and, whilst relatively benign in the monkey, this virus is highly pathogenic for humans.

Human infection with B virus is rare. It has usually been acquired from a bite or from handling infected animals without appropriate protective wear. In one instance the wife of an infected monkey handler became infected through contact with her husband's vesicles, and B virus has also been transmitted in the laboratory from infected monkey cell cultures. Within 5–20 d of exposure local inflammation may appear at the site of entry, usually on the skin, accompanied by some itching, numbness and vesicular lesions. Ascending myelitis or acute encephalomyelitis may follow. Delay in specific therapy leads to a high mortality rate and serious neurological sequelae in survivors.

Diagnosis and treatment

Diagnosis is by isolation of the virus, which is readily grown in a range of cell cultures (e.g. monkey kidney, rabbit kidney). Virus can be grown from blood, vesicle fluid, conjunctival swabs and CSF. Herpes group particles may be detectable on electron microscopy of vesicle fluid. Definitive identification of the virus is available in special reference laboratories. Demonstration of specific antibodies is complicated by cross-reacting HSV antibody. B virus is not as sensitive to acyclovir as HSV, requiring concentrations equivalent to those used for VZV. Treatment needs to be given promptly to be effective, and high-dose intravenous acyclovir (15 mg/kg over 1 h every 8 h) for 14 d or longer is recommended. Ganciclovir may also be useful. Because of the small number of cases the best therapeutic regimen is not well established.

Prevention of B virus infection

Guidelines have been issued for the protection of those handling monkeys or monkey tissues. These include: recommendations for training to prevent exposure; safe handling and protective wear procedures; care of wounds; and information as to the risks and nature of the infection. Prophylaxis in the event of possible exposure involves wound washing, cleansing with 10% iodine in alcohol, and a course of oral acyclovir (high dose, 800 mg five times a day for 3 weeks) with a prolonged observation period, as the onset of infection may be delayed.

RECOMMENDED READING

Epstein M A, Achong B G 1986 (eds) *The Epstein–Barr virus: Recent Advances.* Heinemann, London
McGeoch D J 1989 The genomes of the human herpesviruses; contents, relationships and evolution. *Annual Review of Microbiology* 43: 235–265

Nahmias A J, Keyserling H, Lee F K 1989 Herpes simplex viruses 1 and 2. In: Evans A S (ed) *Viral Infections of Humans,* 3rd edn. Plenum Press, New York
Stevens J G 1989 Human herpesviruses: a consideration of the latent state. *Microbiological Reviews* 53: 318–332

45

Poxviruses

Smallpox; molluscum contagiosum; parapoxvirus infections

T. H. Pennington

The world's last naturally occurring case of small-pox was recorded in Merca, Southern Somalia, in October 1977. This momentous event marked the end of a long campaign against smallpox, which in its 'modern' phase started with the introduction of vaccination by Edward Jenner at the end of the 18th century. With the eradication of smallpox — which has joined the dodo and the great auk by becoming extinct in the wild at the hand of man — the importance of poxviruses in medical practice may appear to be much diminished, as the other naturally occurring viruses in this family that infect man nearly always restrict themselves to causing self-limiting and trivial skin lesions. Smallpox, on the other hand, caused a generalized infection with high mortality, and fell into that small group of viruses (including viral haemorrhagic fevers and, now, human immuno-deficiency virus) which differ from the majority — which usually cause mild or subclinical infections — because their infections are commonly severe and frequently lethal. Notwithstanding their minor role today as human pathogens, poxviruses retain their importance, and their place in this book, for three reasons.

Firstly, the successful smallpox eradication campaign is important in its own right as a major achievement. It is also important because it highlights the principles and problems associated with projects that aim to control infections by eradicating the pathogen. Smallpox was the first disease to fall to this approach and remains the only successful example to date.

Secondly, work on the molecular biology of poxviruses has led to the identification of distinctive properties and the development of techniques and approaches which have made it possible to move significantly towards constructing single-dose vaccines which protect simultaneously against a wide range of diseases. Genes coding for foreign non-poxvirus antigens have been inserted into the poxvirus genome so that the antigens are expressed during virus infection and induce immunity.

Thirdly, no account of virus diseases in general and poxvirus infections in particular is complete without consideration being given to the events which followed the introduction of myxomatosis into Australia, by far the best studied example to date of the evolution of a new virus disease in real time.

DESCRIPTION

Classification

A large number of different poxviruses have been described. They infect a wide range of vertebrate and invertebrate hosts. The subfamily chordo-poxvirus contains all the viruses that infect vertebrates; it is divided into six genera, each containing related viruses which generally infect related hosts. Thus, members of the genus *leporipoxvirus* infect rabbits and squirrels, *avipoxvirus* members infect birds, *capripoxvirus* members infect goats and sheep, *suipoxvirus* members infect swine, and *parapoxvirus* members infect cattle and sheep.

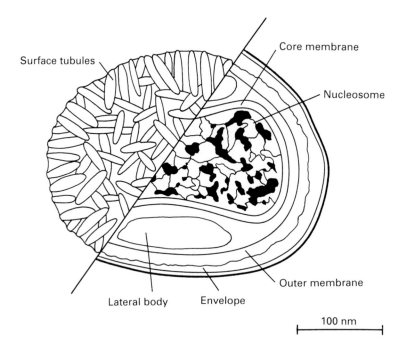

Fig. 45.1 The structure of the vaccinia virion. Right-hand side, section of enveloped virion; left-hand side, surface structure of non-enveloped particle. (Reproduced with permission from Fenner F et al 1988 *Smallpox and its Eradication*. World Health Organization, Geneva.)

Some viruses, including that of molluscum contagiosum, which infects man, remain unclassified. By far the most intensively studied poxvirus is vaccinia virus, the Jennerian smallpox vaccine virus. This virus has been placed in the genus *orthopoxvirus* together with smallpox virus and some viruses which infect cattle and mice.

The virion

Poxviruses are the largest animal viruses. Their virions are big enough to be seen as dots by light microscopy after special staining procedures. They are much more complex than those of any other viruses (Figs. 45.1 and 45.2). They are also distinctive in that they do not show any discernible symmetry. The core contains the DNA genome and 15 or more enzymes which make up a transcriptional system whose role is to synthesize biologically active polyadenylated, capped and methylated virus messenger RNA (mRNA) molecules early in infection. The core has a 9 nm thick membrane, with a regular subunit structure. Within the virion, the core assumes a dumb-bell shape because of the large lateral bodies. The core and lateral bodies are enclosed in a protein shell about 12 nm thick — the outer membrane — the surface of which consists of irregularly arranged tubules, which in turn consist of a small globular subunits. Virions released naturally from the cell are enclosed within an envelope which contains host cell lipids and several virus-specified polypeptides, including the haemagglutinin; they are infectious. Most virions remain cell-associated and are released by cellular disruption. These particles lack an envelope so that the outer membrane constitutes their surface; they are also infectious. More than 100 different polypeptides have been identified in purified virions.

The genome

Their DNA genomes range in mass from 85 MDa (parapoxviruses) to 185 MDa (avipoxviruses). The

a

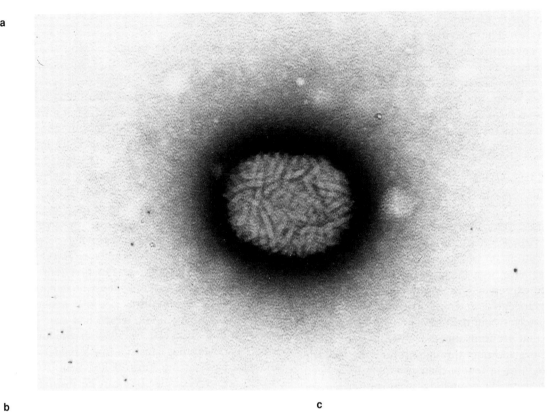

b

c

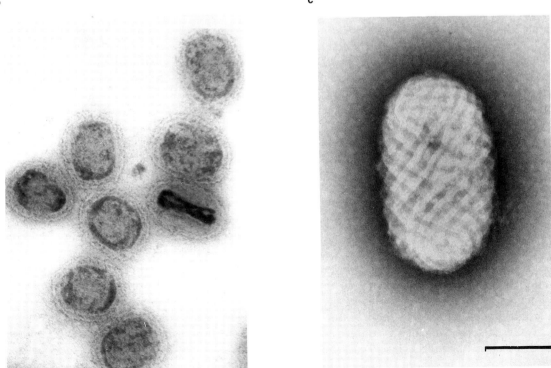

Fig. 45.2 Electron micrographs of poxviruses. **a** Molluscum contagiosum virus (MCV). × 15 000. **b** MCV showing internal structure. × 75 000. (Prepared by N. Atack) **c** Parapoxvirus: orf. Bar, 100 nm. (Courtesy of Dr D. W. Gregory.)

vaccinia virus genome has 186 000 base pairs (123 MDa). The poxvirus genome is distinctive in that covalent links join the two DNA strands at both ends of the molecule, the genome thus being a single uninterrupted molecule that is folded to form a linear duplex structure. The occurrence of inverted terminal sequence repetitions is also a characteristic feature, identical sequences being present at each end of the genome.

REPLICATION

Poxviruses are unique among human DNA viruses in that virus RNA and DNA synthesis takes place in the cytoplasm of the infected cell. Because of this they have been intensively studied by workers on gene expression. After entry into the cell the core is uncoated. It starts to synthesize mRNA immediately. About half the genome is transcribed. Genes that are transcribed at this time are called early genes and map throughout the length of the genome. Only a few of their products have been characterized. They include enzymes needed for replication and transcription of viral DNA, such as DNA polymerase. Virus DNA replication starts at about 90 min after infection and goes on for several hours. It takes place in well-defined areas in the cytoplasm called factories. As soon as DNA replication starts, a dramatic change in viral gene expression occurs. Nearly all the genome now becomes available for transcription, and regulatory mechanisms come into play which lead to the synthesis of a new class of gene product, the late polypeptides. Soon after the onset of synthesis of these polypeptides the expression of most of the early genes is turned off. Most virion structural polypeptides are made late. Virion assembly takes place in the cytoplasm and proceeds in a series of steps which include the formation of spherical immature particles. The onset of virus macromolecular synthesis is accompanied by irreversible inhibition of host protein synthesis due to the functional inactivation and degradation of host cytoplasmic RNA molecules. It is probable that this effect on the host, which leads to the death of infected cells, is a major factor in the causation of tissue damage during infection.

CLINICAL FEATURES

Smallpox virus had no animal reservoir and spread from person to person by the *respiratory route*. After infecting mucosal cells in the upper respiratory tract without producing symptoms it spread to the regional lymph nodes and, after a transient viraemia, infected cells throughout the body. Multiplication of virus in these cells led to a second and more intense *viraemia* which heralded the onset of clinical illness. During the first few days of fever the virus multiplied in skin *epithelial cells* leading to the development of focal lesions and the characteristic *rash*. Macules progressed to *papules, vesicles* and *pustules*, leaving permanent pockmarks, particularly on the face. Two kinds of smallpox were common in the first half of the 20th century. These were called *variola major* and *variola minor*, or alastrim. Variola major virus caused classical smallpox, which had case fatality rates varying from 10 to 50% in the unvaccinated. Variola minor caused a much milder disease and had case fatality rates of less than 1%. The viruses are very similar but can be distinguished in the laboratory by restriction enzyme fragment length polymorphisms of their genomes.

CONTROL OF SMALLPOX
Before vaccination

Before the introduction of vaccination, the control of smallpox relied on two approaches, variolation and isolation. Variolators aimed to induce immunity equivalent to that after natural infection. Susceptible individuals were deliberately infected with smallpox pus or scabs by scratching the skin or by nasal insufflation. Although the virus was not attenuated, infections had lower case fatality rates (estimated to be 0.5–2%) and were less likely to cause permanent pockmarks than those acquired naturally. Variolation was first recorded in China nearly 1000 years ago, and was practised in many parts of the world. Variolators were active until very recent times. In Afghanistan, Pakistan and Ethiopia their activities caused problems towards the end of the smallpox eradication programme in the 1970s because they spread virus in a way which evaded the measures erected to control natural virus transmission.

Vaccination

Edward Jenner vaccinated James Phipps with cowpox virus on the 14 May 1796 and challenged him by variolation some months later. He repeated this 'trial', as he called it, in other children, and the description of these events in his 'Inquiry' in 1798 led to the rapid world-wide acceptance of vaccination. Introduction of the vaccine virus into the epidermis led to the development of a local lesion and the induction of a strong immunity to infection with smallpox virus which lasted for several years. Although the essentials of *Jennerian* vaccination remained unchanged for the rest of its history, early vaccinators developed their own vaccine viruses, which became known as vaccinia. The origin of these viruses is obscure and modern vaccinia viruses form a distinct species of orthopoxvirus, related to but very clearly distinct from the viruses of both cowpox and smallpox.

The eradication campaign

Routine vaccination of children — compulsory in some countries — combined with outbreak control by isolation and selective vaccination gradually brought smallpox under control in Europe, the USSR, North and Central America, and Japan, and the virus had been eradicted from all these areas by the mid-1950s. In 1959 this achievement prompted the World Health Organization (WHO) to adopt the global eradication of smallpox as a major goal. At this time 60% of the world's population lived in areas where smallpox was endemic. A slow reduction in disease was maintained for the next few years, but epidemics continued to be frequent. Consequently the WHO initiated its Intensified Smallpox Eradication Programme. This started on 1 January 1967 when the disease was reported in 31 countries. It had the goal of eradication within 10 years. The goal was achieved in 10 years, 9 months and 26 days. From a starting point of 10–15 million cases annually (Fig. 45.3) and against a background of civil strife, famine and floods, success came

because of a major international collaborative effort — aided by some virus-specific factors (Table 45.1). At the beginning of 1976 smallpox occurred only in Ethiopia (Fig. 45.4). Transmission was interrupted there in August of that year, although an importation of virus into Somalia and adjacent countries had occurred by then. This was the last outbreak. The last case occurred on 26 October 1977. In the final years of the programme its emphasis moved from mass vaccination to a strategy of surveillance and containment. This strategy rapidly interrupted transmission. It was possible because cases were easy to detect due to the characteristic rash, because patients usually transmitted disease to only a few people — and only to those in close face-to-face contact —, because only persons with a rash transmitted infection, and because outbreaks could be successfully contained in most areas by isolation of cases and vaccination of contacts and people in the immediate vicinity. The WHO Global Commission for the Eradication of Smallpox formally certified that smallpox had been eradicated from the world on 9 December 1979.

OTHER POXVIRUS INFECTIONS OF MAN

Molluscum contagiosum

The lesions of this mild disease are small copper-coloured warty papules which occur on the trunk, buttocks, arms and face. It is spread by direct contact or by fomites. The lesion consists of a mass of hypertrophied epidermis which extends into the dermis and protrudes above the skin. In the epithelial cells very large hyaline acidophilic granular masses can be observed. They crowd the host cell nucleus to one side, eventually filling the whole cell. When material from the lesions is crushed, some of the inclusions burst open and from them large numbers of virions escape. These have the size, internal structure and morphology of vaccinia virus. The infection has been transmitted experimentally to human subjects, but the virus has not been grown in cultured cells. The

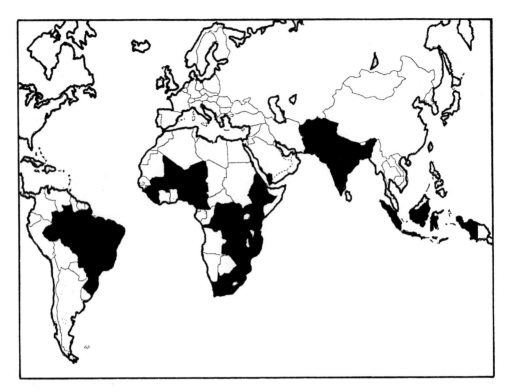

Fig. 45.3 Smallpox in the world, 1967. The map shows the 31 countries with endemic smallpox. (From Fenner et al 1988 with permission.)

Table 45.1 Features of smallpox that facilitated its eradication

Feature	Importance
Disease severe	Ensured strong public and governmental support for eradication programme
characteristic rash and subsequent development of facial pockmarks	
Slow spread and poor transmissibility	Facilitated containment of outbreaks by vaccination/isolation
Transmission by subclinical cases not important	Meant that control of spread by isolation of cases was an effective procedure
No carrier state in man	Meant that control of spread by isolation of cases was an effective procedure
No animal reservoir	Meant that control of spread by isolation of cases was an effective procedure
Vaccine technically simple to produce in large amounts, in high quality and at low cost (in skin of ungulates)	Meant that vaccine availability was not an important constraint in the eradication programme
Vaccine delivery simple and optimized by use of reusable, cheap, specially designed needles to deliver a standard amount of vaccine to scratches in skin	Meant that failure at the point of vaccination was not an important constraint in the eradication programme
Freeze dried vaccine stocks were heat-stable with very long shelf life in tropics	Meant that vaccine viability under adverse environmental conditions was not an important constraint in the eradication programme

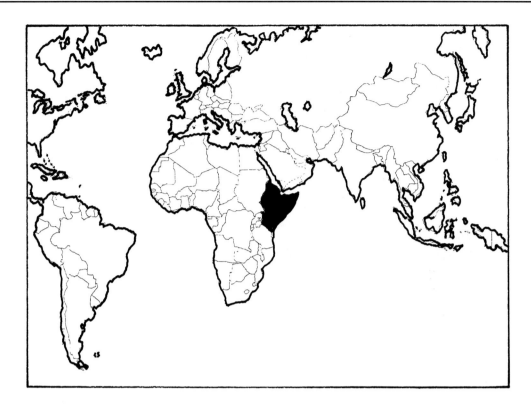

Fig. 45.4   Smallpox in the world, 1976–77. (From Fenner et al 1988, with permission)

development of immunity is slow and uncertain. Lesions can persist for as long as 2 years and re-infection is common.

Monkeypox

This has been occasionally implicated in a smallpox-like condition in equatorial Africa. It may be fatal in unvaccinated individuals, but is less transmissible from person to person than smallpox.

Parapoxvirus infections

The virions of parapoxviruses are characterized by a criss-cross pattern of tubes in the outer membrane (Fig. 45.2 c), and genomes that are considerably smaller — 85 MDa — than those of other poxviruses. They infect ungulates and cause the occupational diseases in man of *orf* and *milker's nodes*. The lesions of orf (which causes a

disease in sheep known as contagious pustular dermatitis) are often large and granulomatous. Erythema multiforme is a relatively frequent complication. The lesions of milker's nodes are highly vascular hemispherical papules and nodules. Both diseases are self-limiting, are commonest on the hands and are contracted by contact with infected sheep (orf) or cows (milker's nodes). They are occupational diseases, and are mainly seen in farm workers such as shepherds, slaughter house workers or butchers.

VACCINIA VIRUS AS A VACCINE VECTOR

The vaccinia virus genome can accommodate sizeable losses of DNA in certain regions, to the extent that as many as 25 000 base pairs can be lost without lethal effect. By replacing this non-essential DNA with foreign genes it has been possible to construct novel *recombinant virus strains* which express the foreign genes when they infect cells. These genes have been inserted into the vaccinia genome by standard gene manipulation techniques, recombination and transfection.

When a cell is infected with more than one poxvirus strain, recombination can take place between them if they are closely related genetically. Recombination takes place even if one of the poxvirus genomes enters the cell in the form of naked DNA: techniques exist that optimize this process, which is known as transfection. Recombination has been used to insert foreign genes into the region of the vaccinia genome that codes for the non-essential enzyme thymidine kinase (TK). A fragment of vaccinia virus DNA containing this gene is taken and by use of gene manipulation techniques the foreign gene is inserted into the TK region, with a vaccinia virus promoter next to it to ensure gene expression. This DNA is then introduced by transfection into cells infected with wild type (TK +) vaccinia virus. Recombination takes place at the TK gene, producing viruses whose genomes now contain the foreign gene. Because this is inserted into the TK gene the latter is non-functional (TK -). Selection procedures for the absence of TK activity are now applied, aiding the identification of recombinant viruses. Recombinant vaccinia strains containing as many as four foreign genes, coding for combinations of bacterial, viral and protozoal antigens, have been constructed.

The advantages of this ingenious way of developing new vaccines are its applicability to many different antigens, the possibility of constructing multivalent vaccines that could give protection against several diseases after a single 'shot', and the ease of administration and cheapness of vaccinia as a vaccine. Serious disadvantages remain, however. These are primarily those associated with vaccinia virus itself, whose use carried with it a number of serious complications. The most important of these were *progressive vaccinia*, a fatal infection which occurred in immunodeficient individuals, *eczema vaccinatum*, a serious spreading infection which occurred in eczematous individuals, and *post-vaccinal encephalitis*, which, although rare, was severe and occurred in normal healthy individuals. These

disadvantages preclude the use of vaccinia as a vector for foreign antigens in man, and work is being done on the modification of its virulence, the optimization of foreign gene expression and the enhancement of its immunizing power to get round these problems. Recombinant vaccinia virus is, however, being used in animals. A strain which expresses the rabies glycoprotein antigen is being used in Europe to protect foxes. Bait is dosed with the virus and left in the wild.

MYXOMATOSIS: AN EVOLVING DISEASE

As a rule, virus infections are mild and self-limiting. Viruses are obligate parasites and it is easy to understand that it is not in their interests to cause the extinction or massive reductions in size of host populations. It is reasonable to suppose that the type of disease caused by a virus reflects the outcome of a process in which host and virus have co-evolved to levels of resistance and virulence optimal for the maintenance of their respective population numbers. The high mortality of classical smallpox is considered by some to have been a major factor in the restriction of human population size, and this has been used to support the hypothesis that the association between smallpox and man has been established — in evolutionary terms — only in recent times, co-evolution of the relationship being a long way from equilibrium. It is impossible to test this hypothesis directly, but a dramatic example with many parallels has been provided by the relationship between another poxvirus — myxoma virus — and the rabbit in Australia. This is the only example of co-evolution where changes in an animal host and virus and the evolution of a disease have been studied in real time.

Myxoma virus is South American. It causes a benign local fibroma in its natural host, the rabbit *Sylvilagus brasiliensis*, but causes *myxomatosis* in the European rabbit, *Oryctolagus cuniculus*. This is a generalized infection with a very high mortality rate. Field trials to test its efficacy as a measure for controlling the European rabbit were done in Australia in 1950. The virus escaped and caused enormous epidemics in the years that followed. The original virus caused infections with a case mortality rate greater than 99%, and rabbits survived less than 13 d. Within 3 years virus isolates from epidemics had become much less virulent, causing infections with mortality rates of 70–95% and survival times of 17–28 d. Changes in the resistance of the rabbit also occurred, with mortality rates of infection falling (from 90% to 25% following challenge with strains of virus with modified virulence, for example) and symptomatology becoming less severe. In myxomatosis natural selection favoured virus strains with intermediate virulence because such strains are transmitted more effectively than highly virulent strains, which kill their hosts too quickly, and non-virulent strains, which are poorly transmitted.

RECOMMENDED READING

Baxby D 1981 *Jenner's Smallpox Vaccine*. Heinemann, London

Fenner F 1990 Poxviruses. In: Fields B N, Knipe D M, (eds) *Virology* 2nd edn. Raven, New York, pp 2113–2133

Fenner F, Henderson D A, Arita I, Jezek Z, Ladnyi I D 1988 *Smallpox and its Eradication*. World Health Organization, Geneva

Fenner F, Ratcliffe F N 1965 *Myxomatosis*. Cambridge University Press, Cambridge

Jenner E 1798 *An Inquiry into the Causes and Effects of the Variolae Vaccinae*. Sampson Low, London

Moss B 1990 Poxviruses and their replication. In: Fields B N, Knipe D M, (eds) *Virology* 2nd edn. Raven, New York, pp 2079–2111

46

Papovaviruses

Warts: warts and skin cancers; progressive multifocal leuco-encephalopathy

P. Ward and D. V. Coleman

The *papillomavirus*, *polyomavirus* and simian virus 40 (SV40), the *vacuolating* virus of rhesus monkeys, are a group of small DNA viruses which are currently classified as 2 genera of the papovaviruses, whose name is derived from the first two letters of the names of each of the family members. They were placed in the same family because they are all small DNA tumour viruses with icosahedral capsid structure but it is now recognized that their molecular biology differs considerably.

Papillomavirus. These are species-specific DNA viruses that infect the squamous epithelia and mucous membranes of higher vertebrates, including man. They are responsible for the many varieties of *warts* and fibropapillomas. Although the lesions are usually benign, their association with *tumours* of man and other animals is now well documented. Most of the evidence for the oncogenic properties of the viruses comes from study of the virus types infecting animal species. In the 1930s Shope found that the cottontail rabbit papillomavirus caused benign warts and that 25% of the lesions underwent malignant change within a year. Application of tar to the lesions led to more rapid malignant change; moreover, viral DNA was detectable in the malignant tumours. Bovine papillomavirus (BPV) has been implicated in the production of tumours of the oesophagus, stomach and bladder in cattle fed on a diet containing bracken. The tumours are preceded by papillomatosis in the affected organs and the benign lesions contain BPV type 4 DNA,

although the virus is not detected after malignant transformation.

Polyomavirus. The name is derived from 'poly' (many) and 'oma' (tumour); the viruses are also species-specific, although experimental animals may be infected with human viruses by direct inoculation. Tumour induction is well described in experimental animals, but there is to date no documented association of any of the viruses with any naturally occurring tumour of man. Recognized members of this group include the mouse polyomavirus, SV40 of monkeys and two viruses of man — JC virus and BK virus. JC virus was first isolated from the brain of a male patient (his initials were JC) with Hodgkin's disease who developed progressive multifocal leuco-encephalopathy. BK virus was isolated from the urine of a renal transplant recipient and was named after his initials.

PAPILLOMAVIRUSES

Description

The papillomaviruses are 52–55 nm in diameter and have an icosahedral capsid composed of 72 capsomeres (Fig. 46.1). The genome is a supercoiled double-stranded circle of DNA with a molecular weight of approximately 5×10^6 and consists of about 8000 base pairs (bp).

There are over 50 types of the human papillomavirus (HPV), which are distinguished on the basis of the homology between their genomes

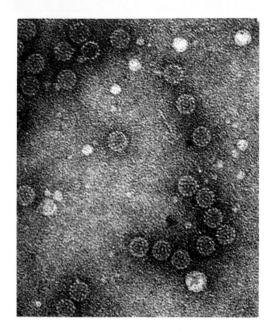

Fig. 46.1 Electron micrograph of wart virus from a plantar wart. PTA stain. × 100 000. (Courtesy of Dr M. M. Ogilvie.)

ation. The L (late) region contains two ORFs which code for the two proteins of the virus capsid. The third region is the long control region (LCR), which does not code for proteins but is concerned with the control of transcription. This is achieved by interaction between the protein products of the E2 ORF and an enhancer site in the LCR. Binding of the whole E2 gene product at this site increases transcription from the downstream ORFs, particularly those of the E6/7 ORFs thought to be responsible for transformation of the infected host cell.

Viral DNA can be found in the *basal cells* of the epithelium but whole virions are found only in the uppermost cell layer in the terminally differentiated *keratinocyte*. This close alignment of viral replication with tissue differentiation has prevented the development of tissue culture systems. Viral DNA can be found in *episomal* form or may be *integrated* at random sites into the host chromosomes. Transformation of cells has been demonstrated with cloned HPV 16 DNA.

measured by cross-hybridization between the separated DNA strands. A new type will show less than 50% cross-hybridization with any other known type. The appearance of the lesions produced or the tissues commonly infected can be associated with virus type. Thus, HPV types 6, 11, 16, 18, 33, 34 and 57 are found in lesions of the genital tract and are commonly referred to as the *genital wart viruses*. Types 1, 2, 3 and 4 commonly infect the keratinized epithelium of the hands and feet, producing the *common warts* frequently seen in young children and adolescents. Type 7 is found in skin warts affecting *meat workers* (butchers' warts). Table 46.1 shows the lesions associated with different viral types.

Replication

The human papillomaviruses cannot be grown in cell culture and, thus, understanding of the events in the replication cycle is deduced from knowledge of comparable viruses. The E (early) region of the viral DNA contains open-reading frames (ORFs), most of which code for proteins concerned with genome replication and transform-

Clinical features and pathogenesis

Cutaneous warts

These are the commonest wart virus lesions and are found most frequently in childhood. Viruses associated with cutaneous lesions are HPV types 3, 10, 26 and 28 (flat warts), 1 and 4 (plantar warts), and 2, 27 and 29 (verrucae) (Table 46.1). Histologically, the lesions are benign with *hypertrophy* of all the layers of the dermis and *hyperkeratosis* of the horny layer (Fig. 46.2). The lesions will usually disappear spontaneously within 2 years of onset but may be resistant to treatment. Regrowth of the lesions after treatment is thought

Table 46.1 Lesions associated with HPV types

Lesion	HPV type
Plantar warts	1, 4
Verruca vulgaris	2, 27, 29
Flat warts	3, 10, 26, 28
Macular lesions (epidermodysplasia verruciformis)	5, 8, 9, 12, 13, 15, 17, 19, 20, 21, 22, 23, 24, 25
Genital warts and tumours	6, 11, 16, 18, 30, 31, 33, 39, 57

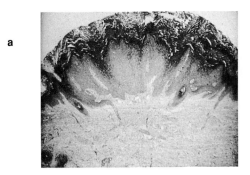

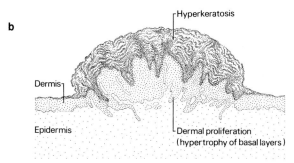

Fig. 46.2 Histology of a wart.

to be due to *persistence* of the virus in the skin surrounding the original wart.

The importance of the immune response, especially cell-mediated immune reactions is illustrated by two groups of patients. Persons suffering from the rare skin disorder epidermodysplasia verruciformis have large persistent planar warts which are associated with virus types not found in the normal population. In addition to their skin condition these people have a defect of the immune system which leads to an inability to eradicate the virus. Renal allograft recipients are immunosuppressed and up to 40% develop cutaneous warts within a year of the graft. This is a much higher incidence than found in an age-matched population, suggesting that there is either a *recrudescence* of latent disease or that *reinfection* is common.

Genital warts

These lesions (also known as condyloma acuminata) are commonest in sexually active adults. In women they are found on the *vulva*, within the *vagina* and on the *cervix*. Vulvar and vaginal warts are usually plainly visible, but on the cervix they may be indistinguishable from the normal mucosa without the aid of a colposcope, to magnify the cervical epithelium. The application of 5% acetic acid causes whitening of epithelium in which there is a high concentration of nuclear material and under these conditions the wart lesions are revealed as areas of densely white whorled epithelium known as flat or non-condylomatous warts while normal mucosa remains pink.

Latent infection of the genital tract is documented and may become clinically apparent if the immune response is disturbed. During pregnancy warts may appear on vulvar epithelium and disappear post-partum. It is not known whether this is a hormonal effect or due to the alteration of the immune response that occurs during pregnancy.

In men the favoured sites for lesions are the shaft of the penis, peri-anal skin and the anal canal. Subclinical infection of the genital tract may also occur in men and will be visible only if the penis is painted with 5% acetic acid and examined with a magnifying glass or a colposcope.

HPV types 6 and 11 are commonly isolated from benign vulval or penile warts. Cervical and anogenital warts may be due to HPV types 16 or 18, both of which are associated with malignant and premalignant lesions of the cervix and anogenital tract.

Recurrent respiratory papillomatosis

This condition is characterized by the presence of benign squamous papillomas on the mucosa of the respiratory tract, most commonly on the *larynx*. The condition has a bimodal age distribution with peaks of incidence in children under 5 years of age and adults after the age of 15 years. It is caused by infection of the respiratory mucosa with HPV types 6 and 11. Children acquire the disease by passage through an infected birth canal, while adults acquire the disease from orogenital contact with an infected sexual partner. The transmission rate is low. Recurrence following treatment is common. Recurrent respiratory papillomatosis presents with hoarseness of voice or, in children, with an abnormal cry. As the lesions grow they may cause *stridor* and upper airway obstruction which will require treatment. Extension of the disease to the bronchial tree may occur, particularly after tracheostomy. Involvement of the alveolar membrane, causing the formation of multiple cysts, is uncommon but is usually fatal. *Malignant conversion* of laryngeal papillomas has been described, usually after radiotherapy to treat the initial lesion.

Oral papillomatosis.

This condition occurs in adults: subclinical lesions can be detected on the oral mucosa of normal people after the application of acetic acid. The virus types are those more commonly found in the genital tract and infection is acquired during orogenital contact with an infected sexual partner. Multiple lesions may develop on the buccal mucosa, a condition known as oral florid papillomatosis. Malignant coversion of oral papillomas has been observed. HPV DNA is also found in association with *hairy leukoplakia* of the tongue in patients infected with human immunodeficiency virus (HIV) but the Epstein–Barr virus is also implicated in the development of the condition.

Human wart viruses and cancer

Premalignant lesions of the genital tract. Malignant disease of the cervix is preceded by neoplastic change in the surface epithelium, a condition known as *cervical intra-epithelial neoplasia* (CIN). A similar pattern of events takes place in other sites in the genital tract of both men and women, known respectively as penile (PIN), vulval (VIN) or vaginal (VaIN) intra-epithelial neoplasia. The initial transforming event takes place in the deepest layer of the epithelium, the germinal layer, and abnormal cells spread through the surface layers. This condition increases in severity from grade 1 to grade 3 (Fig. 46.3), which is characterized by the presence of abnormal cells in all layers of the epithelium with loss of stratification and differentiation. Mitotic figures are present in the uppermost layers of the epithelium. CIN3 has been shown in two prospective studies to progress to *invasive cancer* in 35–50% of affected individuals over a period of 10 years. Lesser degrees of CIN have a lower malignant potential than this and *regression* may occur spontaneously at all stages. HPV DNA can be detected in all grades of the premalignant lesions of the

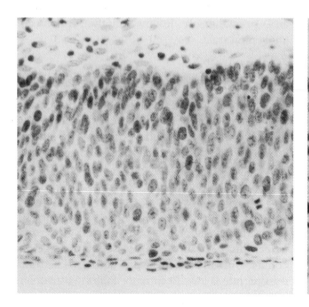 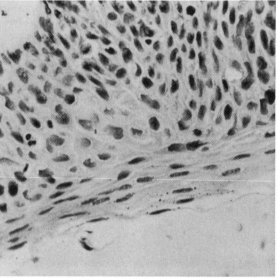

Fig. 46.3 Histological appearances of CIN1 (left) and CIN3 (right).

female and male genital tract. HPV types 6 and 11 are most commonly found in the minor grades (CIN, VIN, VaIN and PIN 1 and 2) whereas HPV types 16 and 18 are more commonly associated with lesions of greater severity and invasive cancer. In pre-invasive lesions the HPV DNA commonly exists in an *extrachromosomal* form (episome), whereas in invasive cancers it is frequently *integrated* into the host chromosomal material.

Squamous cell carcinomas. There is a well-documented association of the wart viruses with invasive cancers of the skin, larynx and genital tract. Malignant conversion of skin warts in patients suffering from epidermodysplasia verruciformis occurs usually on skin exposed to *sunlight* and in lesions containing HPV types 5 or 8. Malignant conversion of vulval condylomata has been documented in immunosuppressed women.

Individuals with recurrent respiratory papillomatosis may develop laryngeal carcinoma after *radiation* therapy. HPV type 30 has been isolated from a laryngeal carcinoma.

The commonest association with invasive cancer, however, is with tumours of the *anogenital tract*; HPV types 16, 18 and 31 have been detected in 60–100% of cervical cancers (Table 46.1). However, the proportion of cancers containing the different HPV types varies around the world. In the UK, HPV type 16 is the most common but types 18 and 31 are more often found in the USA. HPV 57 has been isolated from a cervical cancer biopsy in Japan. In-situ DNA hybridization of tumour biopsies has shown that the HPV DNA is unevenly distributed throughout the tumour, suggesting that these cancers are polyclonal in origin. However, it is not yet certain that infection of the cervix with HPV types is necessary for malignant conversion. Thus, the incidence of HPV type 16 infection in the normal female population has been reported to be high — up to 80% — but cervical carcinoma remains a relatively rare disease.

In most animal cancers associated with papillomavirus there is an identifiable *cofactor*. In humans, the genetic background of the individual, smoking, seminal fluid factors and immune status, have all been implicated as cofactors in HPV-associated genital tract malignancies. Thus, CIN is commoner in relatives of affected women than in the population at large and women who smoke are at increased risk of CIN and cancer of the cervix. The prevalence of CIN is increased in renal allograft recipients and women who are immunosuppressed; many of these lesions are associated with HPV types not usually found in the genital tract.

Summary. In humans, the suggested cofactors in the development of squamous carcinomas are:

1. Genetic background
2. Radiotherapy
3. Ultraviolet irradiation
4. Smoking
5. Immunosuppression.

Laboratory diagnosis

HPV infection may be recognized by the appearance of the typical clinical lesions. Subclinical infection is not uncommon, however, especially in the genital tract. The diagnosis may be made by histological and cytological methods and by electron microscopy, immunocytochemistry or DNA hybridization methods.

Histological examination of a biopsy taken from an identifiable lesion will show the characteristic features of HPV infection (Fig. 46.2). These include *papillomatosis, hyperkeratinization* of the surface layer, *hypertrophy* of the basal layers and a degree of disorganization of the epidermal structure (*acanthosis*). Cellular changes seen in the epithelium include the presence of vacuolated cells with atypical enlarged hyperchromatic nuclei described as *koilocytes*; multinucleate cells are also seen. Electron microscopical examination shows that virions are readily seen in most warts but are less plentiful in genital warts. Viral antigens have been demonstrated in cervical smears and tissues. Although a humoral response can be demonstrated, serological tests do not have a role in diagnosis.

DNA hybridization

At present the only means of accurately determining the specific HPV type present in a lesion is to undertake hybridization, in which DNA extracted from a biopsy or from a cytological preparation is screened with type-specific radio-labelled HPV probes. This approach to diagnosis is not widely available. The polymerase chain reaction (PCR) allows the detection of small amounts of DNA by amplification, using primers specific for regions of the genome; this is a rapid method of considerable potential.

Treatment

In most cases warts are a cosmetic nuisance which will disappear spontaneously. In pregnant women, vaginal warts may occasionally grow to such a size that the birth canal is obstructed and surgical removal is required. CIN is, however, a potentially premalignant condition, and intervention is advisable.

There are many possible methods of treating warts. Chemicals such as trichloroacetic acid, salicylic acid and podophyllin can be applied directly to the wart. Alternatively, warts may be destroyed by cryotherapy with dry ice or liquid nitrogen or by electrodiathermy or laser evaporation. At any site, warts can be removed surgically. All of these treatments will remove the lesions but do not eradicate the virus from surrounding normal epithelium. Specific antiviral drugs directed against the wart viruses do not yet exist but some agents such as interferon or inosine pranobex may assist the immune system to eradicate the virus and decrease the likelihood of recurrence. In particular, interferons have been used to treat recurrent CIN or laryngeal warts after reduction of tumour load by laser vaporization or surgery. Interferon can be applied in creams, or given by intralesional or intravenous injections. Unfortunately patients have to be maintained on interferon to prevent the development of new lesions.

Transmission and epidemiology

There is a lack of information on the epidemiology of the various HPV types in man. Clinical studies of the incidence of skin warts show that infection is common in early childhood and is acquired by *direct contact* with an infected person. Studies of genital warts in patients attending genito-urinary medicine clinics show that transmission occurs during *sexual activity*. It has been estimated that up to two-thirds of the partners of an infected person will develop genital warts.

Direct transfer has been recorded in wrestlers and rugby players. Fomites may also be important, as shown by outbreaks of hand warts from the use of *gymnastic apparatus* and plantar warts acquired in *swimming baths*. Mild shearing trauma may be necessary to allow the virus to reach the basal layers of the skin. The laryngeal mucosa of children suffering from recurrent respiratory papillomatosis has been found to contain HPV types 6 and 11, which are most commonly found in genital mucosa. It is thought that these individuals acquire their infection during passage through their mothers' infected birth canal.

Latency

Studies of apparently normal people have shown that the papillomaviruses can be latent in that they may be present in normal epithelia in the absence of lesions. Viral DNA may be detected in up to 80% of cytologically normal cervices using the most sensitive methods of detection and even in cervices that are colposcopically and cytologically normal.

Control

Prevention of spread of wart viruses can be achieved by avoiding contact with affected individuals; thus, the use of condoms will diminish the risk of spread of genital warts. Although HP virus DNA has been found on vaginal specula, no woman has been shown to have been infected by this route. Autoclaving of vaginal specula will also protect against warts.

Although there are a number of vaccines available for animal use, no vaccine against HP virus is yet on trial.

POLYOMAVIRUSES
Description

The virions are 42–45 nm in size with a 72 capsomere icosahedral capsid. The genome has a molecular weight of 3.4×10^6 and is of the order of 5000 bp in length. Like the papillomaviruses, it is a double-stranded supercoiled loop of DNA but both strands code for virus proteins.

Replication

The replicative cycles of both BK virus and JC virus have been extensively studied. JC is not only species- but tissue-specific, replicating only in human embryo glial cell cultures. After infection, the first antigens (small t and large T) are detectable in the nucleus and arise from genes in the early region of the DNA. There is an accumulation of these antigens and then a switch to transcription of the late region and production of the structural proteins VP1, 2, 3. The growth cycle in culture is 36–44 h long and the release of mature virus particles follows lysis of the cell.

Clinical features

Minor childhood illnesses

Primary polyomavirus infection is a rare diagnosis, but has been made in children with acute respiratory infection and haemorrhagic cystitis.

Malignant tumours

Although experimental animals infected with polyomaviruses develop a variety of malignant tumours, there is as yet no association of any of the viruses with naturally occurring tumours in man.

Progressive multifocal leuco-encephalopathy (PML)

This condition was first described in 1958 and usually affects people with an abnormal immune response due to therapy or disease. The patients in whom the illness was originally described suffered from *Hodgkin's disease* and *chronic lymphocytic leukaemia*, but PML is recognized in *renal allograft* recipients and other *immunosuppressed* patients. PML patients have multiple foci of demyelination, usually in the cerebral hemispheres, but occasionally in the cerebellum and brain stem. The oligodendrocytes surrounding these areas are enlarged and have swollen, hyperchromatic nuclei which occasionally contain large basophilic inclusions. Oligodendrocytes are absent or rare in the centre of the lesion but the astrocytes have an almost neoplastic appearance. Malignant gliomas and lymphomas have been described in these patients and are usually found near the areas of demyelination. Replication of the virus occurs in the nucleus of the oligodendrocyte, causing cell destruction and breakdown of the myelin sheath. Virus has not been seen in the abnormal astrocytes.

The clinical features depend on the areas affected and the disease evolves gradually, with deteriorating vision, mental function and speech. Thereafter, progression is rapid with the onset of coma. Death usually occurs within 6 months of the disease first becoming manifest.

JC virus is consistently associated with PML and is the cause of the demyelination. It is not confined to the central nervous system, however, and renal infections occur in patients with and without PML. It has been isolated from the urine of immunosuppressed individuals but, although the genome is detectable in skin sites, virus has not been cultured from sites other than the brain. Polyomavirus infection is quite common in pregnancy. Viruria has been detected in 3–7% of women, usually beginning in the second and third trimesters.

Polyomavirus infection and transplant recipients

In renal transplant recipients, polyomavirus infection of the transplanted ureter results in cell proliferation leading to *ureteric stenosis* or occasionally to obstruction. Both BK and JC viruses have been implicated in this condition. The obstruction occurs within 300 d postoperatively and in 50% of the patients the cause is not recognized until nephrectomy is performed or at post-mortem examination. Polyomavirus infection appears to be as common as cytomegalovirus infections in transplant recipients. Most infections are due to reactivation of BK virus, but primary infection with JC virus has been recognized. Half of the cases occur between 4 and 8 weeks after transplantation but reactivations of virus occurring up to 12 months after transplantation are not uncommon. Polyomavirus infection is associated with a transient decrease in graft function. If this is wrongly interpreted as being a rejection episode and managed by further immunosuppression, complications such as ureteric stenosis may occur. In bone marrow transplant recipients, 38% of a study group in the USA were found to be excreting polyomavirus in their urine. Although not associated with graft versus host disease, some patients had a transient post-transplant hepatitis.

Pathogenesis

Infection with BK virus was first associated with ureteric stenosis in the transplanted ureter. BK virus has since been isolated from the urine of immunosuppressed patients and from pregnant women. The virus has only rarely been isolated from people with normal immune systems, but not live virus, and most of these are children probably experiencing their first infection. BK virus DNA has been detected in tonsils, spleen, lymph node and lung.

Laboratory diagnosis

The diagnosis of infection with the polyomaviruses is possible by assays of specific antibody. Haemagglutination inhibition is the normal method used; rising titres and the presence of IgM are diagnostic of recent infection. Electron microscopy of urine deposits or tissues may be used, as may virus isolation. Cytological examination of cells in the urine may show transitional cells with the typical inclusions. Histological examination may show similar changes. In the brain the oligodendrocytes are swollen with foamy cytoplasm and enlarged nuclei. Viral DNA can be detected by hybridization using specific probes.

Treatment

There is no established treatment for PML, although many antiviral agents have been tried. Reducing the level of immunosuppression is likely to be beneficial, but this may not be possible because of the underlying disease.

Epidemiology

Serological studies in the UK show that BK virus infection is a relatively common event in early childhood. By 3 years of age 30% of children have antibody to the virus and this rises to 90% by the age of 5 years. The pattern of infection is similar in other countries.

Serological evidence suggests that JC virus circulates independently of BK virus in the community. In the UK, 5% of the pre-school population have antibody, this proportion rising to 30% by the age of 17 years and to 60% in adults. In the USA and Japan, infection is more widespread, rising to 75% and 90%, respectively, in adults.

Transplacental transmission

This has been reported in Japan where IgM antibodies to BK virus were found in 7.5% of pregnant women and in cord samples from their babies. However, other studies from the UK and USA have failed to confirm this finding. The methods of transmission and maintenance of BK and JC viruses within the community are unknown.

RECOMMENDED READING

Coleman D V, Evans D M D 1988 *Biopsy Pathology and Cytology of the Cervix.* Chapman and Hall, London
Grudzinskeas J G, Breedham T 1989 *Treatment and Prognosis: Obstetrics and Gynaecology.* Heinemann, London
Howley P, Schlegar R 1988 The human papillomaviruses: an overview. *American Journal of Medicine* 85(2A): 155–158

McCance D J, Gardner S D 1987 Papovaviruses: papillomaviruses and polyomaviruses. In: Zuckerman A J, Banatvala J E, Pattison J R (eds) *Principles and Practice of Clinical Virology.* Wiley, Chichester
Shah K 1986 Papovaviruses. In: Spector S, Laucz G, (eds) *Clinical Virology Manual.* Elsevier, Cambridge

47

Hepadnaviruses

Hepatitis B infection; delta virus infection; hepatitis C infection

J. F. Peutherer

The hepadnavirus family includes the human hepatitis B virus (HBV) and the woodchuck, ground squirrel and Pekin duck viruses: others have been identified, but these are the best known and studied. The viruses share a number of important features in relation to the structure of their virions and associated particles, the size, nature, organization and replication of the DNA genome, their ability to cause both acute and chronic infections in their natural hosts and their association with hepatocellular carcinoma. Only HBV can infect man, although study of the other members of the family has yielded important insights relevant to our understanding of HBV. One of the major problems in working with HBV is the lack of a suitable laboratory system of virus culture.

PROPERTIES

Structure

Three different particles can be seen in the blood in HBV infection (Figs. 47.1 and 47.2). The predominant form is a small, spherical particle with a diameter of 22 nm. Filaments also occur, which vary in length, but have a diameter of about 22 nm. Both types of particle are composed of lipid, protein and carbohydrate; they are not infectious and consist solely of surplus virion envelope. The particles carry the hepatitis B surface antigen (HB$_s$Ag). The third type of particle, the virion or *Dane particle*, has a diameter of 42 nm: enclosed within the envelope is the core

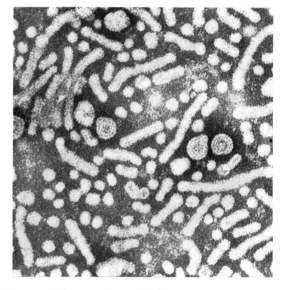

Fig. 47.1 Electron micrograph of the particles in the blood of a patient infected with HBV. ×130000. (Courtesy of Dr A. Keen, University of Cape Town.)

(27 nm), which contains the viral DNA and polymerase within a shell composed of hepatitis B core antigen (HB$_c$Ag). There may be as many as 10^{13} of the small particles and filaments per millilitre. The virions are present in much smaller numbers, usually by a factor of 10 000 or more and the proportion varies considerably in different stages of the disease. The viral DNA is about 3200 nucleotides long in the form of a circle (Fig. 47.3). The long strand is complete, but there is a gap of variable length of about 1000 nucleotides

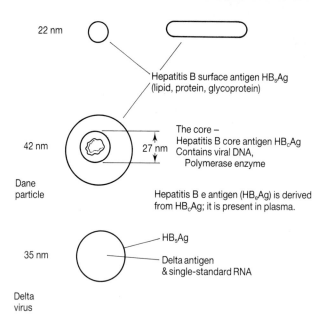

Fig. 47.2   The particles and antigens of hepatitis B and delta viruses.

in the complementary strand: this can be closed via the action of the virion polymerase.

There are four overlapping genes coding for the core, surface and polymerase proteins and an X protein which may act as an activator of transcription. The hepatitis B e antigen (HB$_e$Ag) which is associated with the virion is also found free in the plasma, especially at times when there is active viral replication reflected by the presence of Dane particles in the plasma. HB$_e$Ag is derived from the core protein and is thus virus coded although there is no separate e gene. The surface antigen gene is transcribed to produce 3 mRNAs, L, M and S. These are translated to give 3 proteins: each contains the S protein. The product of the M mRNA consists of the S and pre-S$_2$ proteins. The protein from the L mRNA comprises pre-S$_1$, pre-S$_2$ and S. The L product is present only in the virion, while the M and S proteins are found in each type of particle.

Antigenic and sequence overlap can be shown among the members of the hepadnavirus family, particularly in the core and polymerase proteins. The surface particles are more type-specific al-

though, within HBVs, antigenic diversity is recognized in the surface antigens. Thus HB$_s$Ag particles contain a common 'a' antigen, linked to two sets of mutually exclusive determinants, 'd' or 'y' and 'w' or 'r', giving the four main types — adw, adr, ayw and ayr. These phenotypic variations reflect genomic differences and can be used in epidemiological studies. There are differences in the geographical distribution of the types and also to some extent with the means of transmission in that, in the UK, adw is the most frequent type found in homosexual men while ayw is associated with parenteral drug misusers. No differences in infectivity or pathogenicity can be associated with each type. However, the 'a' determinant is dominant and immunity induced by one phenotype will protect against other types. This means that only one antigenic type is needed in vaccines.

Stability

It is difficult to assess the stability of HBV due to the lack of a suitable laboratory culture system.

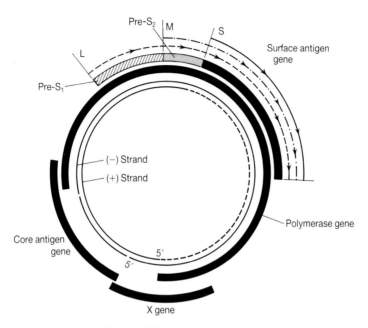

Fig. 47.3 The gene organization of hepatitis B virus DNA.

Inoculation of the chimpanzee can be used to test for virus but obviously only a few studies have been reported.

Indirect evidence has been obtained from the study of recipients of blood products treated in various ways. Thus, it was established that heating to 60°C for 10 h inactivates virus by a factor of 100 to 1000 fold. Chimpanzee inoculation experiments show that treatment with hypochlorite (10 000 p.p.m. available chlorine) and 2% glutaraldehyde for 10 min will inactivate virus 100 000 fold. Studies based on the survival of HB$_s$Ag show that this is much more resistant to destruction.

Replication

Replication of viral nucleic acid starts within the hepatocyte nucleus where viral DNA can be either free, extra-chromosomal or integrated at various sites within the host chromosomes. However, integration is not essential for viral replication. There are some parallels between the hepadnaviruses and the retroviruses, in that:

1. Both synthesize DNA from an RNA template
2. There is base sequence homology between the enzymes involved.

To replicate hepadnavirus DNA, a full-length RNA copy is enclosed in core protein in the hepatocyte nucleus. This is copied to DNA by the polymerase, the RNA is destroyed and the DNA copied, to form double-stranded DNA, as the virion matures.

CLINICAL FEATURES

The broad range of clinical features associated with HBV infection is summarized in Fig. 47.4. The incubation period varies widely from 40 d to 6 months, but is often about 2–3 months. A prodromal illness occurs in some patients, who complain of malaise and anorexia accompanied by weakness and myalgia. Arthralgia also occurs and may be accompanied by an urticarial or maculopapular rash. These features may be related to circulating immune complexes containing HB$_s$Ag, which have been implicated in the rarer complications of polyarteritis nodosa and glome-

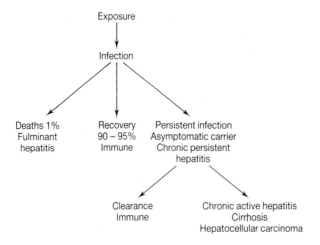

Fig. 47.4 The outcome of hepatitis B infection.

rulonephritis. Complexes are usually present also in the plasma in cases of fulminant hepatitis B. In an acute case, hepatocellular damage is detectable biochemically before the onset of jaundice and persists after it has resolved. The patient usually begins to feel better when the jaundice appears, accompanied by pale stools and dark urine. Carriers of HBV are initially symptom-free, and many will remain so. If virus replication continues, some carriers develop the clinical features of chronic hepatitis and cirrhosis, and eventually hepatocellular carcinoma.

PATHOLOGY

All types of viral hepatitis produce similar changes at the histological level. In the acute stage there are signs of inflammation in the portal triads: the infiltrate is mainly lymphocytic. In the liver parenchyma, single cells show ballooning and form acidophilic (*Councilman*) bodies as they die. In healthy carriers, the inflammatory response is mild and the affected hepatocytes are pale-staining and glassy.

In chronic hepatitis, damage extends out from the portal tracts, giving the piecemeal necrosis appearance. Some lobular inflammation is also seen. As the disease progresses fibrosis develops and, eventually, cirrhosis.

Pathogenesis

Acute disease

HBV replicates in the hepatocyte, reflected in the detection of viral DNA and HB$_c$Ag in the nucleus and HB$_s$Ag in the cytoplasm and at the hepatocyte membrane. However, HB$_c$Ag is also present at the cytoplasmic membrane as a result of the function of a short pre-core sequence which allows the HB$_c$Ag to link with the endoplasmic reticulum and the cell membrane. Both B and T cell responses are induced by the core and surface antigens; damage to the hepatocyte could result from both antibody-dependent and cytotoxic T cell action. However, the major factor causing cell damage is the action of cytotoxic T cells specific for HB$_c$Ag in the cell membrane, although natural killer cells may assist. Expression of MHC class I antigens is poor in hepatocytes but can be enhanced as interferons are produced in response to the infection. This in turn leads to increased antigen recognition and lysis of the infected hepatocytes. The released HB$_s$Ag may induce tolerance, a feature of the acute and chronic stages of hepatitis B. This may be due to a specific suppression of lymphocytes or to the impairment of function of peripheral blood mononuclear cells due to the presence of HBV in these cells. It can be concluded that HBV is non-cytocidal without the assistance of the host's immune system and in fact the disease is usually milder in the immunocompromised. In the asymptomatic carrier there may be no evidence of cell damage, despite the presence of integrated HBV DNA and HB$_s$Ag in the liver and HB$_s$Ag in the plasma. The lack of production of HB$_c$Ag in the hepatocytes of such patients is probably significant. In contrast, cell-mediated responses to HB$_c$Ag are often detectable in patients with chronic active hepatitis, who usually show evidence of continued viral replication, indicated by the presence of HB$_c$Ag in the hepatocyte and virus in the plasma. Auto-immune reactions may also contribute to the damage as various liver-specific antigens are induced as the result of HBV infection. Superinfection with the delta virus (see later) may predispose to progression to cirrhosis.

It is not yet clear what determines that an individual will progress to the carrier state. The absence, or relative inefficiency, of the immune system is important, as shown by the increased likelihood of the carrier state in the very young. In the Far East, 90% of children born to infectious mothers will become carriers although acute hepatitis is uncommon in this age group. In the neonate, infection occurs in the presence of maternal IgG anti-HB$_c$. This will have the effect of masking HB$_c$Ag on hepatocyte membranes and thus will prevent its recognition by cytotoxic T cells. This mechanism will prevent liver cell destruction and hepatitis but will favour virus persistence.

Persistence of hepatitis B

1. Is indicated by HB$_s$Ag present for more than 6 months
2. Occurs in 5–10% of adult, 30% of childhood and 90% of newborn infections
3. Is more frequent in males
4. Is more likely in the immunocompromised.

The presence of HBV in peripheral blood mononuclear cells and in precursor cells in the marrow may also be important. This is associated with diminished function which can be improved in the presence of interferon. It has been suggested that genetic factors may be important and that an inadequate interferon response may be one such factor. In support of this, an increase in hepatocellular damage can be measured when chronically infected cases are treated with interferon.

Hepatocellular carcinoma (HCC)

HCC is one of the 10 most frequent tumours in the world and there is considerable evidence that chronic infection with HBV is an important aetiological factor. Thus, the highest rates of HCC are found in areas where HBV is highly endemic and where infection occurs at a very early age. This is necessary as there may be an interval of 30–40 years between infection and tumour development. Integrated viral DNA can be found in the tumour cells but the site differs in different tumours, although the tumour is clonal in origin in each individual. The integrated DNA is extensively rearranged and regions may be deleted: the patient is usually negative for HB$_c$Ag and other indications of ongoing viral replication. The mechanism of carcinogenesis is not yet clear, although it is usually associated with cirrhosis. As with other tumours, infection with the virus, HBV, may be only one factor and others, such as genetic or chemical, may be necessary.

LABORATORY DIAGNOSIS

The virology laboratory can test for a wide range of HBV antigens and antibodies, using radioimmunoassays and enzyme-linked immunosorbent assays (ELISAs). The standard test is for HB$_s$Ag, which if present in the serum indicates that the patient is infected with HBV, either as a recent acute infection or as a carrier.

Acute infection

In an acute case (Fig. 47.5), HB$_s$Ag is present for some weeks before the onset of symptoms and is at maximum titre at the height of liver damage. In most cases HB$_s$Ag cannot be detected beyond 3–4 months. In a few (5–10%) patients, antigenaemia is of short duration and may not be detectable at the onset of clinical symptoms. In such cases the presence of anti-HB$_c$, especially

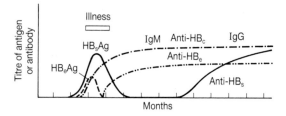

Fig. 47.5 Hepatitis B virus antigens and antibodies in a patient recovering from acute infection.

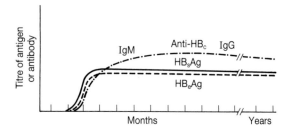

Fig. 47.6 The sequence of events in a patient who becomes a carrier of hepatitis B virus.

IgM anti-HB$_c$, and anti-HB$_e$ may be the only indications of HBV infection. If successive serum samples are examined, the development of anti-HB$_s$ will confirm the timing of the infection, although there is considerable variation in the appearance of this antibody.

Typical responses shown by at least three-quarters of cases are outlined in Fig. 47.5. HB$_e$Ag is produced when virus is replicating and thus it is usually found soon after HB$_s$Ag. IgM anti-HB$_c$ is the next response to be detected. The association of HB$_e$Ag with viral replication is not absolute, but it is correlated strongly with the detection of viral DNA, virions and viral DNA polymerase in the serum. IgM anti-HB$_c$ is a transient response and if present in high titre is a clear indication of a recent acute infection. The response declines with time and is usually absent by 6 months. Tests for HB$_e$Ag and anti-HB$_e$ during an acute infection can be helpful in that the disappearance of HB$_e$Ag and replacement with anti-HB$_e$ indicates that the patient is responding to the infection and will clear HB$_s$Ag. Ninety per cent of patients develop anti-HB$_s$; in a few cases it is present at the same time as HB$_s$Ag, but usually there is a gap of up to 6 months before the anti-HB$_s$ appears. Once present, the patient is immune to further infection with HBV.

There have been reports that some patients may be infected with a variant of HBV. Infection may be detected by assays for HB$_s$Ag, but some do not react in current assays for anti HB$_c$. These variants arise in recipients of vaccine and presumably arise by the selection pressure of the antibody response.

Chronic infection

A patient becomes a carrier if HB$_s$Ag is detectable beyond 6 months. As illustrated (Fig. 47.6), a carrier is almost always HB$_e$Ag-positive beyond 6 months. During this time IgM anti-HB$_c$ will disappear, to be replaced by IgG anti-HB$_c$. This is typical of the early replicative phase of chronic infection. It may be succeeded by the loss of HB$_e$Ag and the appearance of anti-HB$_e$ (Fig. 47.7): the change happens at a variable time, but each year from 5 to 20% of HB$_e$Ag-positive carriers will convert, when there is often biochemical evidence of a short-lived increase in liver damage. Eventually, 1–2% of carriers clear HB$_s$Ag each year.

TREATMENT

Much effort has been focused on the treatment of the chronic carrier with the twin aims of preventing progression of liver disease and of reducing the possibility of transmission to others.

Only long-term follow-up will establish the full benefit of treatments but there is evidence that

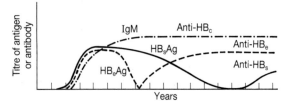

Fig. 47.7 The sequence of events in a hepatitis B carrier who clears the virus.

liver pathology can be improved. Immunosuppression and anti-inflammatory treatment are not indicated in the long-term management of chronic hepatitis B, but various regimens involving interferon and antiviral compounds are under study. As such treatment can only inhibit viral replication it is usual to select patients with evidence of chronic active hepatitis and continuing viral replication with HB_eAg, viral DNA and DNA polymerase in the serum. The response to therapy varies: in some there is transient loss of serum HBV DNA and DNA polymerase during therapy; in others there is a permanent cessation of HBV replication, but antigenaemia continues and, least often, there is a complete response and DNA replication ceases, HB_sAg disappears and anti-HB_s develops. Adenine arabinoside monophosphate has induced transient responses, but therapy is complicated by the toxicity of the drug. Interferons have shown promise, particularly synthetic α–interferons. If a response occurs this is usually signalled by exacerbation of liver cell damage after 6–10 weeks of therapy. However, response rates vary, although 30–40% of patients may show reduced or absent viral replication after at least 3 months of treatment. The factors associated with a favourable response to therapy are:

1. Recent infection (less than 2 years)
2. Adult patient
3. Caucasian
4. Heterosexual
5. Chronic viral replication
6. Healthy immune system
7. Therapy maintained for more than 4 months.

If patients are selected according to these criteria, a response to interferon can be expected in 50% of patients.

If this success rate is confirmed, it will be important to monitor patients with acute infection to identify those who became carriers and who show the features of continued virus replication. An alternative approach is liver transplantation: this has been undertaken for patients with acute fulminant disease who are not suitable for antiviral therapy due to the extent of liver damage.

EPIDEMIOLOGY

HBV is present in the blood and also in body fluids such as semen, vaginal secretions and saliva, although the level is only about one-thousandth of that in blood. Even so, this may still represent a large number of virions. It was recognized from a very early stage that there was a type of hepatitis related to blood transfusion or the use of blood products — hence the name *serum hepatitis*. In fact, it was also apparent that very small quantities of blood could transmit infection as occurs in needlestick injuries. Sexual transmission is also recognized, as is that which occurs between family members, siblings, peers and residents in institutions for the mentally handicapped. In these circumstances there will be frequent contact with blood and saliva: the virus will gain entry through cuts and abrasions or across mucous membranes. Biting and scratching are also important.

Vertical transmission from mother to child is one of the most important routes. Transmission probably occurs when maternal blood contaminates the newborn mucous membranes during birth. Transplacental infection is thought to be quite rare.

The prevalence of HBV infection varies widely in different parts of the world:

Highest rates: HB_sAg 10–15% anti-HB_s 70–90% in South-East Asia, China, equatorial Africa, Oceania and South America. Vertical and horizontal transmission are common.

Intermediate rates: HB_sAg 5%: anti-HB_s 30–40% in eastern Europe, around the Mediterranean, South America and the Middle East.

Lowest rates: HB_sAg 0.1–0.5%: anti-HB_s, not more than 5% in Western Europe, North America and Australia.

Overall, it is estimated that there are 200–300 million carriers in the world, with a preponderance of male carriers in all populations. In areas of low endemicity it is easy to demonstrate that the risk of infection varies widely in different groups according to behaviour (Table 47.1). Most cases occur in parenteral drug injectors who share scarce needles and syringes: sexual transmission by both homosexual and hetero-

Table 47.1 Factors predisposing to increased risk of hepatitis B infection

1. Parenteral drug injection
2. Many sexual partners — both homosexual and heterosexual
3. Geography: highly endemic in various parts of the world
4. Patients in residential homes for the mentally handicapped
5. Patients in haemodialysis, haemophilia and other units
6. Sexual partner has one of the above risk factors
7. Babies born to mothers who are at risk
8. Health care personnel, especially those in surgery, obstetrics, dental surgery and those caring for patients in categories 4 and 5

Relative importance of each category varies in different parts of the world and also within countries.

sexual routes is also important. Screening of all blood donations has virtually eliminated transmission by transfusion and blood products. Some groups of patients are at increased risk of infection and of becoming carriers. These include patients on maintenance haemodialysis and in homes for the mentally handicapped. Finally, health care personnel and laboratory workers are at risk, although the degree of risk varies with the nature of their work and the care with which it is performed (Table 47.2).

The reduction in the rate of reported acute hepatitis B infections in the period 1985–88 probably reflects an increased awareness of the need to adopt good working practices and the introduction of active immunization (see below).

Table 47.2 Acute hepatitis B in health care workers in England[a]

Staff	1975–79	1980–84	1985–88[b]
Surgeons	12	25	0
Physicians	12	11	2
Laboratory staff (medical)	27	16	0
Laboratory staff (scientific)	18	37	10
Nurses	7	4	2
Mental handicap staff	31	27	10
Dentists	17	17	16

[a] Rate per 100 000 per annum.
[b] Public Health Laboratory Service Communicable Diseases Report (unpublished).

Surgery, including dental surgery, obstetrics and procedures involving sharp instruments, etc., and the spilling of patient's blood all increase the risk of transmission. The proportion of staff with evidence of infection rises with age. Changes can also occur with time: in the UK, cases of hepatitis B linked to drug abuse increased to a peak from 1980 to 1984. This may be reflected in the increased experience of hepatitis B in surgeons and laboratory workers from 1975 to 1984. Patients are also at risk from staff, and several episodes have been identified where a surgeon, gynaecologist, dentist or other staff member has transmitted the virus to their patients during invasive procedures, especially in difficult operations where needles and instruments are guided by touch. Apart from small outbreaks linked to a common source, such as surgery or haemodialysis, epidemics of hepatitis B are rare. In the past, before specific tests were available, a few outbreaks were described following the use of blood products prepared in bulk from large numbers of donations. There was a large outbreak in the US armed forces during the Second World War due to the use of yellow fever vaccine stabilized with infectious human plasma.

CONTROL

Broadly, there are two approaches to the prevention of infection with HBV. Firstly, the possibility of transmission can be reduced or removed by modifying risky behaviour of the type described above in the section on epidemiology. The measures are the same as those widely advocated to prevent the spread of the human immunodeficiency virus (HIV) and include the reduction of the number of sexual partners, the use of condoms and avoidance of sharing needles by injecting drug misusers. Occupationally, health care personnel are at risk through exposure to the blood and other body fluids of patients. Implementation of sensible control of infection policies can reduce the risks considerably. Patients are also at some risk, particularly if they require frequent transfusion or blood products, or their treatment requires frequent vascular access or they are immunologically deficient, usually as the result of disease or therapy. It is essential, of course, that blood for transfusion is screened. However, there are limits to these approaches, and immunization, both passive and active, offers many advantages, not least in situations where the prevention of infection is otherwise difficult or impossible. Such conditions exist among the patients and staff in homes or institutions for the mentally handicapped. In areas of high endemicity the prevention of transmission of HBV from mother to child and between young children can only be attempted by large-scale immunization programmes, which present considerable problems, not least in the cost of vaccine.

Passive immunization

Hyperimmune hepatitis B immunoglobulin (HBIG) is prepared from donors with high titres of anti-HB_s. Doses of 300–500 IU in 3 ml are given intramuscularly after accidental exposure, as may occur by needlestick or when broken skin and mucous membranes are splashed with blood from a patient who is positive for HB_sAg.

HBIG must be given as soon as possible after the incident and preferably within 48 h: some protection may be possible after an interval of up to 1 week but such delay should be avoided if at all possible. A second dose is usually given 4 weeks after the first. Such a regimen does not provide absolute protection but an efficacy of 76% has been reported. Serological studies of patients protected by passive immunization show that a transient antigenaemia can occur but the patient remains well. Protection against the development of the carrier state is also provided. The most obvious protective effect has been shown after exposure by needlestick whereas protection after sexual exposure has been harder to demonstrate. Passive immunization is also effective in reducing the risk of the carrier state in babies born to infected mothers, in particular those who are also positive for HB_eAg. Again, HBIG must be given as soon as possible, preferably at birth but no later than 12 h after birth. When this is repeated at monthly intervals for up to 6 months, the proportion of babies who become carriers can be reduced by about 70%. However even greater

protection is provided by combined passive and active immunization in post–exposure prophylaxis. It is advisable, however, to give the injections into different sites. Babies have been shown to respond to the vaccine and the first dose of the course of active immunization can be given at the same time as the HBIG; the protective efficacy of this combined treatment is 90%. Passive immunization is still necessary for those exposed to HBV if they have not been actively immunized; have not yet completed the course; have failed to respond to the full course of vaccine; or several years have elapsed since the completion of the course of vaccine.

Active immunization

Much effort has been devoted to the development of vaccines for long-term protection against hepatitis B. Two preparations have been used. The first contained the small 22 nm particles of HB_sAg purified from the plasma of carriers. The particles were separated by ultracentrifugation and treated with proteinase, 8 M urea and formaldehyde.

The product is immunogenic and safe, as the various steps in its preparation inactived hepatitis B virions and viruses of all other groups. There were fears, however, that HIV might be present in the donors of the plasma and that it might contaminate the vaccine. There is no foundation for this fear as, even if present in the pooled plasma, HIV could not survive the manufacturing process. Current hepatitis B vaccines are produced by cloning the surface antigen gene in yeast cells. The product is particulate and resembles the small particles seen in patients, and although not glycosylated it is claimed to be as immunogenic as the plasma-derived vaccine. Both vaccines are administered with alum as adjuvant and are injected intramuscularly; care should be taken to avoid injection into fat as this can produce poorer seroconversion rates. For this reason, injection into the deltoid muscle of the upper arm is recommended. Both vaccines are free from major side-effects; local swelling and reddening may occur in up to 1 in 5 recipients with a slight fever in only a few cases.

Three doses of vaccine are given at 0, 1 and 6 months. The seroconversion rate is dependent on a number of factors, the most important of which are the age and sex of the vaccinee. Rates in excess of 95% are seen in young women, whereas the rate may drop to 80% in older men. Immunosuppressed patients show even lower rates, e.g. only 50–60% in patients on maintenance dialysis. Because virus challenge doses and the infectivity of sources can vary considerably it is impossible to define a minimum protective level of anti-HB$_s$ but levels should be greater than 50 IU/l. In areas of low endemicity, vaccine is used selectively to protect particular groups in the population. In these circumstances it seems reasonable to check that vaccinees have responded by testing within a few months of the third dose of vaccine. The duration of the response to vaccine is variable and dependent on the level of anti-HB$_s$ after the completion of the course. Vaccinees whose anti-HB$_s$ titres are in excess of 1000 IU/l are likely to maintain adequate levels for at least 4–5 years. If the initial response is greater than 10 but less than 1000 IU/l, this cannot be guaranteed to persist. Booster doses may help in some, but the improvement may be short-lasting. Low or non-responders need to be identified and told that they are not protected and that they must seek prophylaxis by passive immunization if they suffer accidental exposure. Those who are known to have responded can be given a booster if they are exposed to the virus, although the need for this will depend on the level of anti-HB$_s$ and the interval since completion of the course. It would seem reasonable to give all vaccinees a booster dose after 5 years.

Who should be immunized?

The aim of immunization is to prevent transmission of HBV by the routes described in the epidemiology section. In the UK, vaccine is offered to: health care personnel, especially those in direct contact with blood and sharp instruments, etc.; patients and staff in homes and hospitals for the mentally handicapped; sexual partners of those known to be infected with HBV; individuals with many sexual partners; parenteral drug misusers; some members of the police, fire and ambulance services; patients at particular risk, e.g. those requiring frequent blood transfusion and blood products and on maintenance dialysis. The introduction of active immunization may already have contributed to the observed reduction in reported cases of hepatitis B in most groups of health care workers (Table 47.2). In the UK and other areas where the prevalence of anti-HB$_s$ is low, it is not cost effective to test for anti-HB$_s$ before immunization. However, it may be useful to test potential vaccinees who are at increased risk for a particular reason such as drug misuse, as many will already be immune. Babies born to infected mothers are an important group to identify as transmission is likely to lead to the carrier state and all its complications. Mothers may be at risk because of their geographical or ethnic origin, by the misuse of drugs or by sexual exposure; they can be defined by selective testing or by routine screening of all antenatal patients. The greatest risk of transmission occurs with carrier mothers who are HB$_e$Ag-positive or develop acute hepatitis B late in pregnancy. Combined passive and active immunization should be started at birth or within 24 h. Active immunization alone has an efficiency of 70–85%. There is less risk of transmission if the mother is negative for HB$_e$Ag, but it may be advisable to immunize all babies born to mothers who are HB$_s$Ag-positive as there may be another source, either father or sibling in the immediate family. In areas of moderate and high endemicity, the main approach must be widespread use of the vaccine. In the East, where neonatal transmission is common, vaccine should preferably be given to all babies at birth. Studies in Africa indicate that many children are infected at a later age and, in this situation, immunization of infants can be expected to reduce the carrier rate in the population. Eradication of hepatitis B is a desirable objective, but there are considerable financial and organizational problems to be overcome before it can be achieved. Alternative vaccines are also under development. Incorporation of the pre-S$_1$ and pre-S$_2$ proteins and HB$_c$Ag has been proposed, as this might enhance the range and scope of the response. Alternative approaches such as the use of synthetic peptides and hybrid virus vaccines are also under investigation.

THE DELTA AGENT (HEPATITIS DELTA VIRUS, HDV)

When first discovered, the delta (δ) antigen was thought to be another antigen of HBV. It is now known that it is part of another virus which cannot replicate without assistance from HBV (or other hepadnavirus). The virus is a small (35–37 nm) enveloped particle containing a single small circular molecule of RNA of 1.7 kilobase pairs. The internal protein — the δ antigen — has a molecular weight of 68 000. The envelope of the virus is the same as that of HBV (Fig. 47.2). The origin of the virus is unknown and it is has no homology with HBV DNA. The closest relatives are the satellite viruses of plants.

Clinical features and pathogenesis

HDV can only infect simultaneously with HBV or as a superinfection of a chronic HBV carrier. The symptoms are similar to those of acute and chronic hepatitis B. There is agreement that the presence of HDV may increase the severity of the clinical features compared with those seen with HBV alone. This is reflected in a 10% risk of fulminant hepatitis with simultaneous HBV and HDV infection and a 20% risk in superinfections.

Overall, HDV can be found in up to half of all cases of HB$_s$Ag-associated fulminant hepatitis B. In about 1 in 10 cases co-infection with HDV and HBV results in a biphasic illness. HDV superinfection of an HBV carrier can cause clinical acute hepatitis and may lead to persistence of both HBV and HDV. The risk of chronic liver disease is increased if this occurs — even to the extent of 50–90% of cases in areas where HDV is common. The rate of progression of the liver disease is also increased so that cirrhosis may be apparent within 5 years.

Diagnosis

Tests are available for delta antigen and antibody. The sequence of appearance of the various

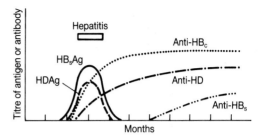

Fig. 47.8 Test results in a patient simultaneously infected with hepatitis B and D viruses.

markers in a patient co-infected with HBV and HDV is illustrated (Fig. 47.8). The initial antibody to HDV is of the IgM class. In cases of superinfection, the test results are as illustrated (Fig. 47.9). During the episode of acute hepatitis there may be a drop in the HB$_s$Ag titre and, although it is usually still detectable, it may disappear temporarily in a few cases. This can cause some confusion if the episode is the first presentation of the patient. As illustrated, when the clinical features improve, HB$_s$Ag recovers.

Epidemiology

HDV is not a new virus as there is evidence of infection in the 1930s at least. Overall the prevalence of HDV reflects that of HBV, except that it is low in the East. The highest prevalence (1 in 5 carriers of HBV) has been seen in South America in the Amazon basin but there is considerable variation and HDV is not found uniformly throughout the population. Infection is important also in Italy and the Middle East and some parts of Africa. In areas of low HBV endemicity, HDV

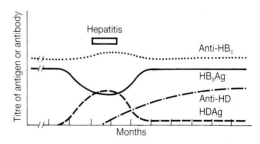

Fig. 47.9 Test results in a hepatitis B carrier superinfected with hepatitis D virus.

is associated with drug misusers in whom the prevalence in HBV carriers may be 50% or more. Sexual transmission is recognized but does not appear to be as frequent as via blood, e.g. in drug misusers and haemophiliacs. In a number of episodes HDV has spread rapidly among a population of HBV carriers, causing hepatitis, death from fulminant hepatitis and chronic illness.

Treatment and control

There is no established treatment for HDV infection although there is evidence that interferons may induce a temporary improvement in δ antigen levels. The same general control measures for HBV are also relevant to HDV. HBV vaccines will prevent HDV co-infection but there is no means of protecting existing HBV carriers against the potentially serious consequences of super-infection with HDV. Only the avoidance of exposure can help.

NON-A, NON-B (NANB) HEPATITIS; HEPATITIS C VIRUS (HCV)

Once reliable diagnostic tests for hepatitis A and B infection had been developed it was evident that there were other, presumed viral, causes of hepatitis. The cumbersome name non-A, non-B hepatitis was coined for these conditions. Epidemiological studies have established that there are two routes of transmission of NANB hepatitis; thus, it is possible to identify enteric and parenteral forms of NANB hepatitis. Hepatitis C virus is now recognized as the major cause of the parenteral type. Viruses with very different properties are linked to NANB hepatitis and they will be classified in different families. However, for the present NANB infections will be presented together in this section.

Enteric NANB hepatitis. This form of NANB hepatitis was first recognized in India as the cause of large outbreaks of hepatitis apparently transmitted by the faecal–oral route. Sporadic cases are also known. Apart from India, infection has been identified in Asia, the Middle East, North Africa, and Mexico. Within these areas enteric NANB hepatitis may account for 30–50% of cases of acute hepatitis. In contrast to hepatitis A, which mainly infects children, there is a preponderance of cases in young adults. Severe infections are seen in pregnant women in the third trimester, when mortality rates can reach 30%. The wide age range of the patients infected in epidemics suggests that while the virus may be endemic in many areas considerable numbers of children and adults must avoid infection early in life. As with other viral infections the clinical attack rates are lower in children than in adults by a factor of at least 10.

The incubation period is 10–40 d and the pattern of virus excretion is similar to hepatitis A. The comparison with hepatitis A extends to the absence of a carrier state. A small round virus with a diameter of about 27 nm can be seen in the faeces: it appears to have the features of a calicivirus. The name hepatitis E has been suggested.

Parenteral NANB hepatitis; hepatitis C virus (HCV). Parenteral NANB hepatitis viruses share a number of features with HBV, in particular an association with blood as a source of infection and the ability to produce the carrier state and associated chronic hepatitis. Epidemiological, clinical and experimental studies indicate that there must be more than one type of virus. Infection can be transmitted to the chimpanzee and the most consistent experimental finding is the presence of tubular structures in the hepatocyte cytoplasm. Studies of the tubule-forming agent showed that it has a diameter of no more than 80 nm and that it can be inactivated with organic solvents. These features are similar to those of the togavirus or flavivirus families.

Plasma from infected chimpanzees was the starting point for the definition of hepatitis C virus. The plasma was extracted, and the enzyme reverse transcriptase used to produce a DNA copy of any RNA present; this was then cloned and expressed in *Escherichia coli*. Numerous clones had to be tested before one was found whose protein product reacted with antibody present in well-documented NANB hepatitis sera. It is this antigen which is used in assays for antibody. The original sequence cloned is part of a non-structural gene and further genes have now been identified. The cloning evidence is that the genome is positive stranded and approximately 10 000 nucleotides long. These features, together with the gene arrangement, the size and presence of an envelope, confirm that hepatitis C virus is probably a flavivirus and, indeed, there is some base sequence homology with members of the family. Further characterization is awaited.

There is some evidence that a virus, perhaps a picornavirus, is another, rarer, cause of parenteral NANB.

Clinical features

The disease has an incubation period of 6–10 weeks and is usually mild and may often be detected only by biochemical studies. Up to one-third of patients develop jaundice and fulminant hepatitis occurs in about 1–2% of cases. Chronic infection varies in severity and typically runs a variable course with fluctuations in the extent of liver damage, as measured by the levels of aminotransferases in the plasma. Chronic liver damage may occur in 20–50% of patients and can progress to cirrhosis over a period of only a few years. A role in the development of hepato-cellular carcinoma has also been suggested. How the virus persists is unknown. Plasma may contain 10^5–10^6 or more infectious units per millilitre, considerably lower than the titres found in patients with hepatitis B. The mechanism of liver damage is also unknown.

Diagnosis

Two approaches to diagnosis have been described, based on the detection of antibody (anti-HCV) or viral RNA. ELISAs for the detection of antibody to the virus are available and have been shown to be useful in the investigation of NANB hepatitis. Sequential studies of samples indicate that, in the acute stage, no more than 20% of patients have seroconverted: this rises to about 60% by 6 months and almost 100% by 1 year. Thus, the test in its present form can be used for epidemiological studies and for the diagnosis of chronic infections but may have limited use in the early stages of acute infection. New versions of the test are able to detect antibody earlier in the infection. Viral RNA can be detected by reverse transcription followed by amplification of the DNA by the polymerase chain reaction using synthetic primers derived from the known base sequence. This test has established that most patients who have antibody to the virus have viral RNA in their plasma. This suggests some patients eliminate the virus or that not all who are infected are viraemic. Another possibility is that some antibody results are not specific.

Confirmatory immunoblot assays with several different viral proteins are now available.

Treatment

Interferon therapy has shown promise in that many patients show improved liver function when treated with quite small doses of α-interferon: in about half of the cases the remission is maintained after treatment is stopped.

Epidemiology and transmission

Hepatitis C is world-wide in distribution and has been claimed to be the cause of 10–50% of all cases of acute hepatitis. It is associated especially with transfusion and the use of blood products. There are obviously considerable variations in the prevalence of infection in different groups in different parts of Europe and the USA (Table 47.3). In blood donors the highest prevalences recorded so far are in Italian cities. Haemophiliacs are uniformly infected, although there is evidence that the heat treatment step introduced to inactivate HIV also kills HCV as patients who have only received heat-treated factor VIII are sero-negative. Intravenous drug misusers are infected in both Europe and the USA. The evidence of sexual transmission is less clear. In the UK,

Table 47.3 Prevalence of anti-HCV in Europe and the USA

Group	Prevalence (%)
Blood donors	less than 1
Haemophiliacs	66–90
Intravenous drug misusers	32–80
Acute NANB hepatitis	20–30
Post-transfusion NANB chronic hepatitis	45–90

infection of homosexual men appears to vary according to HIV status; thus, only 4% of those not infected with HIV have anti-HCV compared with 28% in the group positive for anti-HIV. The association with NANB and post-transfusion NANB hepatitis is very clear and establishes that HCV is the major cause of this form of hepatitis. HCV may also be the cause of about one-third of cases of sporadic hepatitis. The association with hepatocellular carcinoma is interesting: the mechanism is unknown but could be related to the established association of NANB hepatitis with chronic infection and cirrhosis.

Control

Some of the routes of transmission are known but further information is needed before rational control measures can be defined. As there are many similarities with hepatitis B, application of the same cross-infection measures is appropriate until the routes of transmission can be assessed.

RECOMMENDED READING

Bonino F, Smedile A, Verme G 1987, Hepatitis delta virus infection. *Advances in Internal Medicine* 32: 345–358
Davis L G, Webster D J, Lemon S M 1989 Horizontal transmission of hepatitis B virus. *Lancet* i: 889–893
Expert Advisory group on AIDS: Guidance for clinical health care workers: protection against infection with HIV and hepatitis viruses. HMSO: London
Hoofnagle J H 1981 Type B hepatitis: virology, serology and clinical course. *Seminars in Liver Disease* 1: 7–14
Neurath A R, Jameson B A, Huima T 1987 Hepatitis B virus proteins eliciting protective immunity. *Microbiological Sciences* 4: 48–51
Polakoff S, Vandervelde E M 1988 Immunisation of neonates at high risk of hepatitis B in England and Wales: national surveillance. *British Medical Journal* 297: 249–253

48

Parvoviruses
B19 infection; erythema infectiosum

J. R. Pattison

There are three genera in the parvovirus family. The *densoviruses* infect insects but do not infect man or other vertebrates. The *dependoviruses* infect a number of species and serology shows that adeno-associated viruses 1–4 are common human infections although they have not yet been associated with any human disease.

The *autonomous* parvoviruses are widespread in nature and frequently cause disease in their natural hosts (Table 48.1). Some of these viruses (FPV and CPV) are so important in veterinary medicine that immunization against them is a routine practice in developed countries. At present there is only one parvovirus (B19) that is important in human medicine, although in the future some of the small round viruses seen in human faeces may be shown to be parvoviruses and may prove to be pathogenic.

Table 48.1 The autonomous parvoviruses, their natural hosts and the diseases they cause

Virus	Host	Disease
H1	Rat	Subclinical
Minute virus of mice (MVM)	Mice	Subclinical
Feline parvovirus (FPV)	Cat	Enteritis Leucopenia Cerebellar ataxia
Mink enteritis virus (MEV)	Mink	Enteritis
Canine parvovirus (CPV)	Dog	Enteritis Myocarditis
Porcine parvovirus (PPV)	Pigs	Reproductive failure
Aleutian disease virus (ADV)	Mink	Pneumonitis Hypergammaglobulinaemia Renal failure
B19	Man	Respiratory tract illness Aplastic crisis Erythema infectiosum Hydrops fetalis

DESCRIPTION

Parvovirus virions (Fig. 48.1) are uniform isometric particles 20–25 nm in diameter lacking an envelope. They have a characteristic buoyant density in caesium chloride, ranging from 1.41 to 1.45, and the capsid consists of two or three proteins. The genome consists of a single strand of DNA which has a characteristic structure. There is a linear coding region bounded at each end by terminal palindromic sequences. Throughout the parvoviruses there is variation in the size of the genome and whether plus and minus strands are packaged into mature virions. In the case of B19 the genome is 5.5 kilobase pairs in length, making it one of the largest parvovirus genomes, and both plus and minus strands are packaged with equal efficiency so that the DNA spontaneously anneals into a double-stranded form when extracted from the virions.

Many animal parvoviruses can be grown in cell culture, but this is not yet true of the human virus. With those that can be replicated in vitro the appearance of intranuclear inclusions is

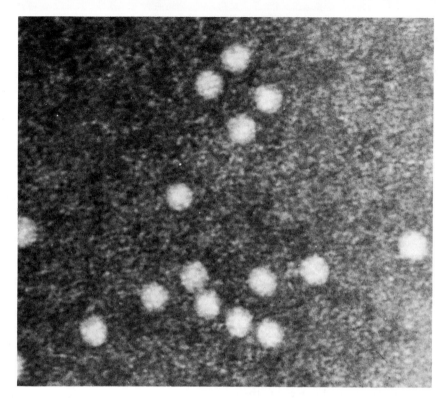

Fig. 48.1 Parvovirus B19 particles in the serum of a child with sickle cell anaemia suffering an aplastic crisis. × 300 000.

characteristic and such inclusions can be seen in B19-infected tissue specimens (see below).

The individual parvoviruses appear to be very host-specific, although MEV is very closely related to FPV, and CPV more distantly so. These viruses are probably a set of host range variants of the same virus. Otherwise, each species, including man, is affected by a genetically and antigenically stable virus. As a consequence, infection with B19 virus is followed by life-long immunity in normal individuals.

PATHOGENESIS

Autonomous parvoviruses are so called because they do not require the presence of a helper virus for replication. However, they do depend on certain cellular helper functions which are expressed transiently in the cell during the late S or early G_2 phase of mitosis. Therefore, virus replication will be relatively extensive in *rapidly dividing*

tissues and it is not surprising that diseases of the intestine, the haemopoietic system and the fetus feature frequently as consequences of parvovirus infections in animals. There is also evidence that susceptibility to parvovirus infection is related to a particular stage of differentiation of the cell. Thus, very distinct clinical syndromes such as cerebellar ataxia in kittens and aplastic crisis in humans are also a feature of parvovirus infection.

Animal diseases

With the closely related parvoviruses FPV, MEV and CPV an explanation is required for the occurrence of similar diseases (enteritis) in a variety of species in addition to a number of very distinct illnesses such as ataxia in kittens and myocarditis in puppies.

In the cat FPV causes ataxia in kittens if infection occurs in the perinatal period, since the cells of the external granular layer of the cerebellum are dividing rapidly at this stage and become a target for virus-induced damage. In newborn kittens there is a relatively low turnover of intestinal cells. This increases as the animals are weaned after which time the crypt epithelial cells have a cell cycle time of 8–12 h and are thus susceptible to FPV. As a consequence, infection is associated with enteritis.

In the dog the distinct clinical syndrome of perinatal infection by CPV is myocarditis, since in the very young pup there is rapid growth of the myocardium and the mitotic index is high. If infection occurs in older puppies, enteritis is a consistent feature. The white blood cells are also a target for infection by FPV and CPV, and so kittens and puppies of 2–4 months of age tend to suffer leucopenia and enteritis.

In mink infected with MEV, severe enteritis is the most consistent feature and there is not a distinct clinical syndrome associated with perinatal infection. However, mink are the natural host of another parvovirus, Aleutian disease virus (ADV). With this virus there is a distinct disease in newborn kits, an acute respiratory disease due to infection of type II alveolar cells, which are only susceptible to productive infection in the early stages of life. In later life ADV establishes a persistent infection in the germinal centres of lymph nodes. This results is a plasmacytosis in many organs, hypergammaglobulinaemia and death due to chronic renal failure as a consequence of immune complex glomerulonephritis. The reason it is called Aleutian disease is because it occurs earlier and more regularly in Aleutian mink than in any other variety. This is due to the linkage of the Aleutian coat colour gene to a gene associated with a lysosomal abnormality of the Chédiak–Higashi type, leading to a failure to destroy immune complexes following phagocytosis.

In rodents, parvoviruses appear to be asymptomatic in their natural hosts and the same was thought to be true of PPV, a very common infection of pigs. However, the virus was found in tissue, vaginal and seminal samples from pig herds affected by reproductive failure and it was subsequently shown that infection in early pregnancy leads to transplacental infection, stillbirth, mummification or resorption of the piglets.

Human disease

Volunteer studies

Experimental infection of healthy volunteers has revealed the steps in the pathogenesis of B19 infection (Fig. 48.2). The virus is infectious when given in the form of nasal drops. One week later there is an intense viraemia and virus is excreted in the nasal secretions. The viraemia lasts for only a few days before there is a brisk antibody response, initially of the IgM class but followed rapidly by the appearance of IgG antibody.

Haematological changes take place in the 2nd week following inoculation. Erythroid precursors are absent from the bone marrow of normal individuals 10 d after inoculation and there is consequent disappearance of reticulocytes from the peripheral blood and a small fall in haemoglobin (Fig. 48.2). Lymphocytes, neutrophils and platelets sometimes fall transiently but this is not due to lack of precursors in the bone marrow. Studies with cultured bone marrow cells confirm the in-

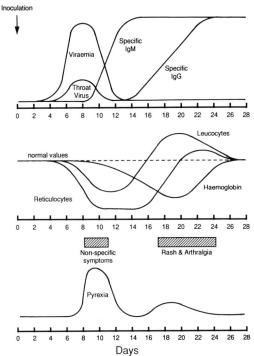

Fig. 48.2 The virological (upper trace), haematological (middle trace) and clinical events (lower trace) following inoculation of B19 virus. (Reproduced with permission of Wiley, Chichester.)

vivo observations. B19 selectively inhibits erythroid colony formation but has no effect on the cells of the myeloid series.

The *rash* and *arthralgia* associated with B19 infection occur in infected volunteers during the 3rd week after inoculation. As yet there are no studies of the pathology of either of these features, but since they follow the disappearance of the viraemia and occur at a time when there is an easily detectable immune response it is assumed that the rash and arthralgia are immune mediated.

The viraemia that is characteristic of B19 infection gives ample opportunity for infection of the placenta and fetus if it occurs during pregnancy. In infected fetuses there appears to be a persistent infection with damage to haematopoietic cells, leading to anaemia, which is one of the factors responsible for *hydrops fetalis*. The other situation in which persistent infection occurs is in the immunosuppressed. The reason is that such individuals produce only small amounts of antibody in response to infection and none of it is capable of neutralizing the virus.

Clinical diseases due to B19

There is a spectrum of clinical consequences of B19 infection (Table 48.2). These depend in part on the natural variation in symptomatology that occurs with common childhood infections and in part on recognizable host factors.

Minor illness. In children, in whom B19 infection is most common, asymptomatic infection accounts for about half of all infections. Non-specific respiratory tract illness is the next most common illness, at least in boys. This can

Table 48.2 Spectrum of disease due to B19 related to host factors

Disease	Host
Asymptomatic Respiratory tract illness Rash illness Arthralgia	Normal
Severe anaemia	Chronic haemolytic anaemia Immunosuppressed Intra-uterine infection

mimic influenza and coincides with the viraemic phase of the infection.

Rash illness. B19 virus causes an erythematous maculopapular rash, which in its most clinically distinct form is called *erythema infectiosum* (EI). EI is common in children aged 4–11 years and is sometimes called fifth-disease since it was the fifth of six erythematous rash illnesses of childhood in an old classification. Classically, it starts with an intense erythema of the cheeks, hence another of its names — '*slapped-cheek disease*'. The rash then proceeds to involve the trunk and limbs. It lasts only a day or two, although transient recrudescences may occur when the individual is hot. The rash on the limbs tends to have a lacy or reticular appearance. There may be associated lymphadenopathy and joint symptoms.

It is now clear that B19 is a cause of rash illness world-wide, but such illnesses are not always diagnosed clinically as EI. The erythematous rash illness is often very similar to rubella. Erythema of the cheeks is not always prominent and the rash often does not have a lacy appearance. It sometimes occurs on the palms and soles. In the absence of laboratory tests the most frequent clinical diagnoses made are rubella, allergy or 'viral illness', unless there is an outbreak in young children associated with red cheeks in which case the diagnosis of EI is often made. In a few cases of B19 infection the rash is purpuric in nature. In most of these the platelet count is normal but a transient thrombocytopenia occasionally occurs.

Joint disease. Symptoms and signs of joint involvement occur frequently in B19 infection. Approximately 80% of adult females will report joint symptoms, although the figure is only approximately 10% in childhood cases. Like the rash, the arthropathy of B19 infection is very similar to that seen with rubella, being a *symmetrical arthralgia* or *arthritis* involving the small joints of the hands with wrists, knees and ankles affected in some cases. There is a tendency for the arthropathy to be more severe in children. The symptoms and signs usually resolve within 2 weeks but in a few cases they will persist for months and very occasionally for years. Some of these patients may be classified clinically as early benign rheumatoid arthritis but they will be found to be rheumatoid factor-negative and B19 virus is not related to rheumatoid arthritis in any way.

Aplastic crisis. An aplastic crisis is a transient, acute event which complicates chronic haemolytic anaemia. There is a fall in haemoglobin from steady-state values, a disappearance of reticulocytes from the peripheral blood and a virtual absence of red blood cell precursors in the bone marrow at the beginning of the crisis. The cessation of erythropoiesis lasts 5–7 d and patients present with symptoms of worsening anaemia. Blood transfusion is required in the acute phase, but after a week or so the bone marrow recovers rapidly, there is a reticulocytosis and the haemoglobin concentration returns to steady-state values.

Throughout the world B19 infection is responsible for 90% of cases of aplastic crisis. It most commonly occurs in children with sickle cell anaemia but also in patients with hereditary spherocytosis, pyruvate kinase deficiency, β thalassaemia intermedia and a dyserythropoietic anaemia (hereditary erythroblastic multinuclearity with a positive acidified serum; HEMPAS).

B19 infection in the immunosuppressed. Cases of persistent B19 infection have been described in patients with underlying immunodeficiency states (Nezelof's syndrome, acute lymphatic leukaemia and human immunodeficiency virus (HIV)-positive individuals). The illness is characterized by either persistent anaemia or a remitting and relapsing anaemia. Viraemia occurs and recurs in periods of anaemia and only a weak humoral immune response can be detected. The bone marrow picture is typical of that seen in aplastic crisis complicating haemolytic anaemia.

B19 in pregnancy. No evidence of B19 infection can be found in sera taken during the 1st month of life from infants with birth defects and as yet there is no evidence of late developmental abnormalities in children exposed to B19 in utero. However, early studies of B19 infection in women known to be pregnant suggested that the spontaneous abortion rate was high. Recent studies indicate that there is not an excess number of abortions in the first trimester of pregnancies complicated by B19 infection compared to controls. However, approximately 1 in 10 of pregnancies complicated by B19 infection end in *spontaneous abortion* during the second trimester and this is approximately 10 times the incidence in controls. The pregnancy is lost, on average, 4–6 weeks after the onset of symptoms of EI in the mother.

The majority of pregnancies complicated by B19 continue to full-term delivery of normal infants. However, damage sometimes occurs as a consequence of second or third trimester infection and in these cases *fetal hydrops* appears to be a consistent feature. Maternal B19 infection appears to occur 2–12 weeks prior to the diagnosis of hydrops fetalis. There is a chronic infection in the fetus which leads to anaemia, which is one of the factors responsible for the hydrops. Overall, B19 infection probably accounts for 10% of cases of non-immunological hydrops fetalis.

LABORATORY DIAGNOSIS OF B19 INFECTION

In acquired infection the diagnosis of B19-associated disease follows the classical principles for acute systemic virus infections. The viraemia and throat virus excretion coincide with haematological changes and detection of virus is a useful diagnostic test in cases of aplastic crisis. Rash and arthralgia occur some days after the end of the short period of circulation and excretion of virus, so in these cases diagnosis by the detection of virus-specific IgM antibody is the best method.

Detection of virus

Serum is the specimen of choice for the detection of virus since the highest concentrations (up to 10^{11} particles per millilitre) of virus are found in this fluid and, if virus is not detected in the sample, it can serve as an acute-phase serum for antibody assays. Counterimmuno-electrophoresis (CIE) using a human convalescent serum as the detector antibody is a simple and rapid technique and detects virus in 30% of sera taken within 3 d of the clinical presentation of aplastic crisis. The more sensitive techniques of immuno-assay or nucleic acid hybridization will increase this percentage to 60% in such samples.

Antibody detection

In the vast majority of cases of rash and arthralgia virus is not detectable in the serum at the time of the illness. Most cases have detectable B19-specific IgM within a day or two of the onset of the rash, although in some cases it is necessary to wait for 7 d after the onset in order to be able to demonstrate such antibody in convincing amounts. Once B19-specific IgG has appeared in the serum it rapidly reaches peak concentrations and persists in decreasing amounts for 2–3 months. High concentrations of IgM antibody are usually found a month or two after infection and in most instances detectable IgG antibody persists for life. Diagnosis of recent infection can also be made by demonstrating seroconversion or increasing amounts of IgG antibody.

Infection in the fetus

The diagnosis of B19 in a fetus depends upon the detection of virus in fetal specimens. Maternal infection is likely to have been some weeks previously and there may be no specific IgM in maternal serum. In most instances the infected fetuses have not been specific IgM-positive, but there is frequently a persistent viraemia. Thus, the diagnosis can be made by detection of virus in fetal blood samples or in fetal tissues taken at autopsy from which DNA has been extracted or detected by in-situ hybridization on formalin-fixed, paraffin-embedded tissue sections.

TREATMENT

Most cases of B19 infection are mild and self-limiting and specific treatment is not required. However, there are three situations (Table 48.2) in which severe anaemia occurs as a consequence of B19 infection and in each of these blood transfusion is indicated. In cases of aplastic crisis the transfusion tides patients over the relatively short period of erythroid aplasia before the immune response rapidly clears the virus infection. In the immunosuppressed there is a failure to produce neutralizing antibody so treatment consists of transfusion plus the administration of human normal immunoglobulin for 10 d. This leads to disappearance of the viraemia, sometimes permanently, sometimes only temporarily. The failure of the fetus to eliminate the virus is presumably associated with its inability to mount an immune response. Intra-uterine transfusion has been used to correct the anaemia and the full-term delivery of normal infants has followed in these cases.

EPIDEMIOLOGY

B19 infection has been found in all countries (Europe, North America, Scandinavia, Australia and Japan) in which appropriate diagnostic tests have been applied and it is almost certainly world-wide in distribution. Diseases due to B19 infection cluster in childhood, although some complications such as arthralgia occur more commonly in adult cases. Serological studies indicate that infection is most commonly acquired between 4 and 10 years of age and at least 60% of adults are seropositive. B19 virus infections are endemic throughout the year in temperate climates but there is a seasonal increase in frequency in late winter, spring and early summer months. There are also longer-term cycles of B19 infection with a periodicity of about 4–5 years. The majority of B19 infections are transmitted by the *respiratory route*, but the occurrence of high-titre viraemia creates the possibility of transmitting this infection by *blood* or blood products and this has been shown to occur in haemophiliacs.

CONTROL

Prevention of disease by isolating susceptible individuals is impractical since infections may be subclinical and symptomatic individuals are infectious before any sign of illness. Theoretically, susceptible individuals with chronic haemolytic anaemia or immunocompromised children could be temporarily protected by the administration of human immunoglobulin but this has not been tried. There is as yet no vaccine against B19 disease but, by analogy with the animal viruses, such a strategy would be very effective once sufficient quantities of viral antigen capable of stimulating neutralizing antibody are produced.

tain polioviruses, particularly when there is infection in a community. Enteroviruses can survive for several months in river water, but are unlikely to survive in chlorine-treated water or swimming pools where the recommended level of chlorination (without protein contamination) is achieved. The association with the summer and autumn is not always found as outbreaks have occurred in winter among Eskimos, but this probably results from the isolation of the people and their lack of immunity to many viruses. Flies and cockroaches have been found to harbour viruses but their role in transmission is minimal. Close contact and hygienic standards remain the most important factors.

Prevention and control

After natural infection immunity is permanent. Virus-neutralizing antibodies are formed early during the disease (often before the 7th day) and persist for several decades. Virus types 1 and 2 give each other some cross-protection. In response to the intestinal infection, there is a considerable amount of secretory IgA produced as well as IgG in the blood. There is some doubt about the duration of immunity to some of the coxsackieviruses, although there is long-lasting immunity to many.

Immunization

Active immunization against poliovirus infection can be produced by the use of:

1. Inactivated polio vaccine (Salk) or
2. Live attenuated polio vaccine (Sabin).

Inactivated polio vaccine (IPV). IPV (Salk) was introduced in 1956 for routine immunization. The vaccine contains strains of the three types of virus grown in monkey kidney cell culture and inactivated by exposure to formaldehyde. The batches of vaccine are tested for the presence of residual live poliovirus and must be free of bacteria, fungi, mycoplasmas and SV40 (simian virus 40) virus, which is oncogenic in hamsters. Inactivated vaccines are used almost exclusively in Sweden, Finland, Iceland and Holland. With acceptance rates in excess of 90%, these countries have virtually eliminated poliovirus. The circulation of poliovirus in the community has been dramatically reduced despite the fact that inactivated vaccine does not induce much secretory IgA in the alimentary tract. A high rate of immunization is necessary and antibody levels need to be maintained because it has been shown in children that the outcome of exposure to virus is directly related to the level of antibody at the time of exposure. In the recent outbreak of poliomyelitis in Finland, the strains of poliovirus type 3 were antigenically slightly different from the type 3 poliovirus vaccine strains. Finland has recently introduced a higher-potency vaccine which has been shown to produce a good immunological response to all three poliovirus types and it seems likely that this vaccine will give good, long-lasting protection. It was concluded that the outbreak was not due to failure of inactivated vaccine in general but to the poorly immunogenic preparation previously used. The vaccine should be administered by deep subcutaneous or intramuscular injection and is not associated with local or general reactions. A course of three injections given with intervals of 6–8 weeks between the first and second doses and 4–6 months between the second and third doses produces long-lasting immunity to all three poliovirus types. Inactivated vaccine is recommended for *immunocompromised individuals* and their contacts and others for whom a live vaccine is contra-indicated.

IPV may be used simultaneously with the triple vaccine for diphtheria, pertussis and tetanus. Booster doses of polio vaccine can be given at the same time as diphtheria/tetanus and also with the combined mumps, measles, rubella (MMR) vaccine.

Live attenuated polio vaccines (OPV). Attenuated live oral (Sabin) vaccine replaced the Salk vaccine for routine use in the UK in 1962 and is used extensively in many other countries. It contains live but *attenuated* strains of poliovirus types 1, 2 and 3, grown either in cultures of monkey kidney cells or human diploid cells. The strains were obtained by growing less virulent polio viruses which had been isolated in the wild and, after passage, selecting strains which had lost their neurovirulence. The strains most commonly used were developed by Sabin in 1959.

The vaccine is administered orally and parallels natural infection with stimulation of both local *secretory IgA* in the pharynx and alimentary tract and *circulating IgG*, thereby producing local resistance to subsequent infection with wild poliomyelitis viruses. Herd immunity is important in preventing the circulation of the wild-type virus and high levels of immunization uptake are necessary. This is aided by the wide circulation of vaccine virus, which helps to maintain immunity in the community. However, vaccine strains are not completely stable and studies of sequential isolates of virus from vaccine recipients show that changes can be detected very rapidly. There is therefore the theoretical possibility that vaccine virus, attenuated by serial passage in culture, could revert to neurovirulence with multiple rounds of replication in the vaccinee and after transmission to contacts. Cases of vaccine-associated poliomyelitis have been reported in recipients of OPV at a rate of 1 in 2 million doses: it has also been seen in contacts of recipients. It is not possible to predict who will become affected, although the extended replication which occurs in the immunocompromised should be avoided as the rate of vaccine-associated poliomyelitis in such patients is 10 000 times greater than in normal people. Non-immunized parents and household contacts of children receiving primary immunization should be immunized against poliomyelitis at the same time as the children.

OPV is recommended for infants from 2 months of age. The primary course consists of three separate doses given at the same time as diphtheria/tetanus/pertussis vaccine (see Chapter 68). Each dose contains all three strains. In infants three drops are dropped from a spoon directly into the mouth, which may be open in response to the simultaneous administration intramuscularly or subcutaneously of diphtheria/tetanus/pertussis vaccine. Breast feeding does not interfere with the antibody response to OPV and should continue. A reinforcing dose is given to the children at school entry, but it is not necessary for adults unless they are at special risk, e.g. through travel or occupational exposure. The effectiveness of live vaccine is shown by the experience in the USA where the number of paralytic cases has dropped from 21 000 to 5–10 per annum. In the UK, an average of three cases per annum have been notified in recent years.

When a case of paralytic poliomyelitis is diagnosed a dose of OPV should be given to all persons in the immediate neighbourhood of the case who are immunocompetent, whether or not they have a history of previous vaccination against poliomyelitis. This should be followed by completion of the primary course in those not immunized. If the source of the outbreak is uncertain it should be assumed to be a 'wild-type' virus until proven otherwise.

Poliovirus immunization in the tropics. Serological studies in Africa have shown that children will have been infected with two or three types of poliovirus by the age of 5 years. The rate of paralytic disease is low in young children, but significant numbers occur as the infection is widespread. The disease is known as *infantile paralysis*. Through the expanded programme on immunization the World Health Organization has increased the rate of polio immunization chiefly with the use of OPV. Although this is cheaper than IPV, it must be stored at 0–4°C and thus requires the existence of an effective cold chain to ensure successful immunization. Apart from inactivation of the vaccine, other explanations for low rates of seroconversion include interference from other enteroviruses, malnutrition and the presence of inhibiting factors in the gastro-intestinal contents. It is likely, however, that failure to control poliomyelitis in under-privileged countries is also due partly to failure to reach a sufficiently high proportion of the population, and thus is due to a failure of organization rather than vaccine. Recent experience in Brazil, where a national programme of OPV vaccine distribution has resulted in a dramatic decrease in disease, supports this possibility.

Prospects for the future. When the incidence of poliomyelitis falls dramatically, as in the USA for example, the proportion of cases attributable to vaccine becomes increasingly significant. Recent work has identified the amino acid sequence of antigenic sites which are important for neutralization of the virus. Information concerning the viral factors necessary for virulence is also available. Therefore, it may be possible to develop modified vaccine viruses which cannot revert to neurovirulence. For use in under-privileged countries, it may also be possible to prepare vaccines which are stable and which will not need to be kept under refrigeration.

Enterovirus 72; hepatitis A virus (HAV)

Epidemic jaundice has been recognized for centuries; many large epidemics have occurred related to wars, including the Second World War. The virus was first detected by electron microscopical examination of faeces from cases. In the laboratory, infection can be transmitted to the marmoset.

HAV, the causative agent of *infectious hepatitis*, is now classified as enterovirus 72. It is an unenveloped virus, containing linear, single-stranded RNA. It has similar polypetides to the four major polypeptides of the enterovirus family and shares the same properties of resistance to physical and chemical agents. Recently, it has been adapted to cell culture; it will grow only in cells of primate origin.

Clinical features

The illness caused by HAV is usually mild, and occurs after an incubation period of 14–45 d (median, 28 d). There is a prodrome of malaise, muscle pain and headache and there may be a low-grade fever. The symptoms usually improve and disappear as jaundice develops. Serological tests show that many patients have a subclinical illness, but fulminating hepatitis and liver failure can also occur (overall, less than 0.5%). There are no carriers of the virus. Infection is mildest in young children, often accompanied only by nausea and malaise. Of children under 3 years of age, only 5% develop jaundice, but this rises progressively to more than 50% in adults. The fatality rate also rises with age to about 2%. Some patients develop diarrhoea and some appear to have a relapse a few weeks after the onset. Arthritis and aplastic anaemia are rare complications.

Pathogenesis

Like other enteroviruses, HAV probably infects cells in the gut and then spreads to the liver via the blood. The histopathology is similar to that of hepatitis B, with periportal necrosis and infiltration of mononuclear cells; viral antigens are seen in the cytoplasm of the hepatocytes. Virus is excreted via the bile into the gut from about 1–2 weeks before the onset of jaundice, excretion then declines rapidly over the next 5–7 d. Virus is also present in the urine of clinical and subclinical cases during the same period.

Laboratory diagnosis

Although the virus has been grown in cell culture, it is not possible to do this routinely from the faeces of cases. Diagnosis relies on the demonstration of specific *IgM antibody* to HAV, which develops very early in the course of infection and is generally present by the time the patient is investigated. It is detectable in the serum for 2–6 months after the onset of symptoms (Fig. 49.3). IgG antibody usually persists for many years and is a useful indicator of immunity.

Epidemiology

Only one major type of HAV has been recognized. Serological tests have made it possible to study the rate of infection in different populations throughout the world. Such studies confirm that, since the virus is spread by the faecal–oral

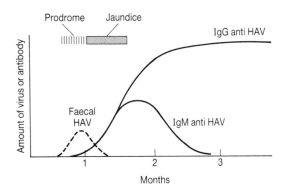

Fig. 49.3 Events in hepatitis A infection

route, it is prevalent in countries where sanitation is poor, and children are infected early in childhood. Serological studies also show that, even in developed countries, more than half the population have been infected with HAV. However, lower rates may also be seen, and are reflected in the appearance of increased numbers of acute cases. In young adults and older patients there may be a history of recent travel to an endemic area.

Outbreaks of HAV infection have been associated with certain foods. Shellfish such as mussels have been incriminated, particularly when they are harvested from coastlines adjacent to sewage outlets, as the mussel is a filter feeder and can concentrate the virus. Shellfish are eaten raw or partially cooked, thus protecting the virus. Contaminated raspberries were incriminated in another notorious outbreak in which uncooked frozen raspberries were eaten many months after picking. Infection is assumed to have come from an infected raspberry picker. Because there is only a transient viraemic phase, only a few infections have been recognized after blood transfusion.

Prevention and control

Vaccines are at present under evaluation and should be available shortly. Passive immunization with normal human immunoglobulin (NIG) gives protection to seronegative individuals for a limited period of up to 6 months. NIG has also been used in the control of outbreaks in institutions such as homes for the mentally handicapped. Prophylaxis with NIG is recommended for travellers to highly endemic areas unless they have been tested for IgG antibody to HAV and are known to be immune.

RHINOVIRUSES

The viruses of this genus are responsible for the most frequent of all human infections, the 'common cold'. Most people suffer from two to four colds every year and, although the primary infection is not a severe one, secondary bacterial infection often follows with symptoms that may be more severe than the original cold. Sinusitis and otitis media are quite common. These viruses cause the loss of many million man-hours of work.

Properties

As the name rhinovirus implies, the genus is associated with the nose. They can be distinguished from the enteroviruses by their acid lability and thus their inability to reach and infect the intestinal tract. There are over 100 serotypes of rhinoviruses; all are fastidious in cell culture. Electron microscopy cannot differentiate them from other family members (Fig. 49.4). Some primates may be susceptible to human viruses and there are related viruses in cattle, cats and horses. The genomes of some rhinoviruses have 45–60% homology with polioviruses in hybridization tests.

The capsid of rhinoviruses appears to be less rigid than that of the enteroviruses. This loose packing is consistent with its greater buoyant density and sensitivity to acid.

Cultivation

Rhinoviruses show a distinct preference for cells of human origin, especially fetal lung or kidney. Previously, they were divided into three groups according to the source of the cells in which the virus had been grown. Thus 'M' strains grew in both *m*onkey and human cells, the 'H' strains grew only in *h*uman cells and lastly the 'O' strains could only be grown in *o*rgan cultures of nasal or tracheal ciliated epithelium. Since many of the 'H' strains could be adapted to grow in monkey cells and many of the 'O' strains could be adapted to grow in human cells this classification was abandoned.

Stability

Inactivation of rhinoviruses occurs below pH 6.0 and is more rapid the lower the pH. Complete inactivation occurs at pH 3.0.

Some rhinoviruses may survive heating at 50°C for 1 h. They are relatively stable in the range from 20–37°C and can survive on enviromental surfaces such as door knobs for several days. They can be preserved at –70°C.

Rhinoviruses are resistant to 20% ether and 5% chloroform, but are sensitive to aldehydes and hypochlorites.

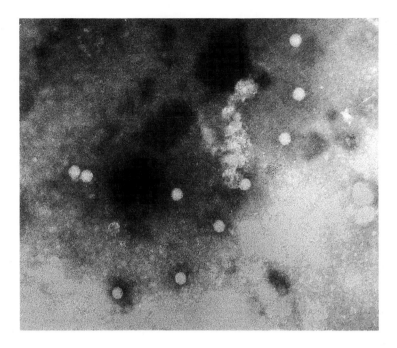

Fig. 49.4 Human rhinovirus. This virus is indistinguishable in appearance from other picornaviruses. Approximate size 25–30 nm. (Reproduced with permission from Madeley C R, Field A M 1988 *Virus Morphology*, 2nd edn. Churchill Livingstone, Edinburgh.)

Replication

Rhinoviruses attach to cell receptors that are sensitive to proteolytic enzymes. Most types appear to use the same receptor. The viruses replicate in the cytoplasm of infected cells to give a CPE which coincides with release of the virus in the same way as other picornaviruses. If the infected cultures are incubated at 37°C the yield is reduced to 30–50% of that at 33°C.

Clinical features and pathogenesis

The typical illness is generally referred to as a common cold. The onset, after contact with infection, is usually within 2–3 d, sometimes as long as 7 d. There is a clear watery nasal discharge which often becomes mucoid or purulent due to secondary bacterial infection and sneezing and coughing are common. Sore throat, headache and malaise may occur. The symptoms are most severe for 2–3 days when nasal virus titres are maximal and, although recovery is usually com-

plete within a week, symptoms can persist for 2 weeks or longer. The ratio of symptomatic to asymptomatic infection is about 3:1 and the illness is generally worse in cigarette smokers. Rhinoviruses have frequently been isolated from patients during acute exacerbations of chronic obstructive airway disease and they are the most common viruses to be associated with wheeze in pre-school children.

It should be remembered that all respiratory viruses may cause the symptoms of the common cold and that laboratory diagnosis is necessary to establish the aetiological agent.

Experimental rhinovirus infection in healthy human volunteers and studies on rhinovirus-infected organ cultures have helped to show their pathogenic potential. Man has proved to be the more sensitive assay as illness can occur when virus cannot be detected by culture in the inoculum. In organ cultures, it has been shown that the virus settles on the ciliated nasal epithelial cells, enters, infects and spreads from cell to cell in the epithelium. The cilia become immobilized and both cilia and cell degenerate as the virus replicates. In man it is likely that bacterial invasion of the damaged epithelium is responsible for the purulent nasal discharge which develops in many cases. Interferon is usually detectable shortly after the peak of virus shedding and probably plays a part in recovery. When specific antibody is first detected in nasal secretions virus shedding ceases, suggesting that this may be the main factor leading to recovery. Little is known of the importance of cell-mediated immunity. The symptoms probably relate to the local inflammatory response and interferon release. Rhinoviruses have been recovered in pure culture from sinus fluids collected from patients with acute sinusitis, but secondary bacterial infection is thought to be the usual cause.

It is not certain that rhinoviruses can infect the lower respiratory tract. They can be recovered from sputum but this may be due to contamination with secretions from the upper airways. It is suggested that lower respiratory tract infection may occur on some occasions since (1) patients with colds may also have lower respiratory tract symptoms with abnormal lung function, (2) children who develop colds may develop wheeze and (3) adults with colds may suffer exacerbations of chronic obstructive airway disease.

Immunity

After the acute illness, circulating antibodies, mainly IgG, can be detected by neutralization tests. There is a good correlation between the titre of neutralizing antibody in the blood and resistance to small doses of homologous virus. Neutralizing antibody, both in serum and nasal secretions, may continue to rise in titre for 4–5 weeks after infection and persist for up to 4 years, although some infections may provoke only a poor response, leaving the patient susceptible to the same serotype after a few weeks or months.

Laboratory diagnosis

Culture

Nose and throat swabs in virus transport medium are the specimens of choice for the recovery of

virus from all age groups. Nasopharyngeal aspirates are excellent specimens from children. Specimens of sputum may also be studied but may often be toxic for cell cultures or contaminated with antibiotic-resistant organisms. Specimens should be taken as early in the illness as possible, preferably within the first 3 d.

Cell cultures of human origin such as MRC5 or WI38 are preferred for the isolation of rhinoviruses. Organ cultures are also susceptible but difficult to obtain and are not used routinely. Cultures are incubated at 33°C and observed microscopically for a cytopathic effect (CPE).

The majority of isolates are apparent within 2 weeks of inoculation although some may take longer. Identification of an isolate as a rhinovirus may be made by considering the cells in which the CPE develops, the appearance of the CPE and the demonstration of acid lability. Isolates are not generally typed with specific neutralizing antisera.

Serology

Serological methods cannot be used in the routine diagnosis of rhinovirus infections because of the multiplicity of serotypes and the lack of a common antigen.

Epidemiology and transmission

Rhinoviruses can be isolated from patients with respiratory illnesses throughout the year but in temperate climates the incidence of colds due to rhinoviruses increases in the autumn and spring and is at its lowest in the summer months. In the tropics the peak incidence occurs in the rainy season. Deliberate exposure of volunteers to wet and chilling does not increase their susceptibility to colds. Rhinoviruses may be transmitted by inhalation of droplets expelled from the nose of a patient. However, during the acute phase of the illness high concentrations of virus are present in nasal secretions and may contaminate the fingers, whence infection may be transmitted by finger-to-finger contact or finger-to-door-knob-to-finger, and thereafter the contaminated finger may touch the eye or nasal mucosa. Colds in the home are often introduced by pre-school children in whom the incidence of rhinovirus infections is highest. People who are in contact with young children appear to suffer from more colds than others.

Colds are mostly trivial and are an inconvenience; however, they do cause considerable morbidity and absence from work.

Treatment and control

Although inactivated vaccines can be produced, there remains the considerable problem of deciding on the antigenic composition. Much effort has been devoted to the development of suitable antiviral therapy and although compounds such as those related to the benzimidazoles have antiviral activity, no useful drugs are available. Isolation of the infected person, although perhaps desirable, is not a practical method of preventing the spread of infection. Attention to personal hygiene in those with colds and their contacts might help.

RECOMMENDED READING

HMSO 1988 *Immunisation against Infectious Disease*. Her Majesty's Stationery Office, London
Grist N R, Bell E J 1984. Paralytic poliomyelitis and Non-polio Enteroviruses. Studies in Scotland.

Reviews of Infectious Diseases 6 (suppl 2.): S385–S386
Roebuck M O 1976 Rhinoviruses in Britain. *Journal of Hygiene*. 76: 137–146

50

Orthomyxoviruses Influenza

J. M. Inglis

The orthomyxoviruses comprise influenza A, B and C viruses, which infect man. Formerly the orthomyxoviruses and the paramyxoviruses were grouped together in the Myxovirus (Greek, *myxa* = mucus) family. While there are some general similarities in structure and the diseases they cause, the viruses differ in a number of fundamental features. For this reason they were separated into the two families — the Orthomyxoviridae and Paramyxoviridae.

Influenza A viruses can infect a variety of different host species, an ability that is of great importance in determining their ability to cause pandemic infection in man. Influenza B only infects man. Influenza C is little studied, and although assumed to be primarily a human infection, it has recently been isolated from pigs in China.

Influenza virus type A was the first to be isolated, this being achieved in 1933 by the unlikely process of intranasal instillation in the ferret. Thereafter, type B was isolated along with type A in cell culture in 1940. One of the most prominent features of the influenza viruses is their ability to change antigenically either gradually over years (*antigenic drift*) or suddenly (*antigenic shift*). Only influenza A virus has the potential to shift whereas all three types may drift antigenically, although only very minor changes have been demonstrated in influenza C.

DESCRIPTION

The virions are spherical, 80–120 nm in diameter, but may be filamentous, sometimes up to several micrometres in length (Fig. 50.1). They have a helical nucleocapsid with a core of eight segments of single-stranded RNA with a total molecular weight of 5×10^6, which is wound tightly to form a rounded mass and corresponds to the 'S' or 'soluble' antigen. Also present within the virion is the viral RNA-dependent RNA polymerase: this is essential for infectivity as the virion RNA is of negative sense and therefore has to be transcribed to produce viral messenger RNA (mRNA). An envelope which contains lipids derived from the plasma membrane of the cell surrounds the virion. From the envelope project *spikes* (Fig. 50.2) which attach the virion to cell receptors; as a result they are able to agglutinate erythrocytes from certain species and are thus termed *haemagglutinins* (H). They are about 10 nm in length, with a molecular weight of 225 000, and consist of trimers of identical glycoprotein subunits, each consisting of two polypeptide chains, HA1 and HA2. HA1 contains 328 amino acids and HA2, 221. The two polypeptides are linked in each subunit by a single disulphide bond between residues 14 of HA1 and 137 of HA2. In the virus particle the haemagglutinin molecule is associated with the lipid membrane by a hydrophobic region near the carboxyl terminus of HA2. Influenza viruses bond to cells by the haemagglutinin interacting with membrane receptors containing *N*-acetylneuraminic acid (NANA). Antigenic changes in the haemagglutinin have been studied by protein and nucleic acid sequencing techniques.

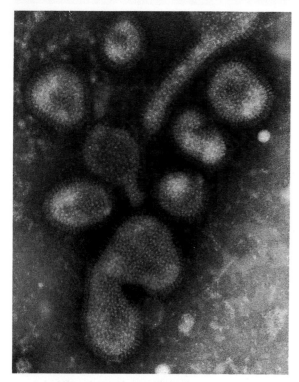

Fig. 50.1 Infuenza A/Dunedin/27/83 H_1N_1 virus. Spikes which make up the fringe are also seen in the end-on view, covering the surface of the virus particles and giving them a 'spotty' appearance. Approximate size 80–120 nm. (Reproduced with permission from Madeley C. R. and Field A.M. 1988 Virus Morphology, 2nd edn. Churchill Livingstone, Edinburgh.)

which it is embedded in the viral membrane. The enzyme catalyses the cleavage of NANA and an adjacent sugar residue in glycoproteins found in mucus. This action allows the virus to permeate mucin and escape from these so-called 'non-specific' inhibitors. The neuraminidase also destroys the haemagglutinin receptors on the host cell. Neuraminidase activity is also thought to be important in the final stages of release of new virus particles from infected cells. NANA is always present in newly synthesized virions and its removal by neuraminidase prevents the new virus particles agglutinating, thus increasing the number of free virus particles and hence spread of the virus from the original site of infection. The viral genes and their functions are shown in Table 50.1.

Nomenclature

In 1980 the World Health Organization (WHO) revised the system of nomenclature. This includes the host of origin, geographical origin, strain number and year of isolation; then follows in parentheses the antigenic description of the haemagglutinin and the neuraminidase, e.g. A/swine/Iowa/3/70 (H_1N_1). If isolated from a human host the origin is not given, e.g. A/Scotland/42/89 (H_3H_2). There are 13 different H antigens and nine N antigens. Only H_{1-3} and N_{1-2} have been found so far in viruses from man, the others being recovered from animals and birds.

This has shown that the antigenic changes are related to mutation of the RNA, causing amino acid substitutions. These changes can be located in the three-dimensional structure of the molecule and are found only at a few well-defined sites close to the attachment site. These changes will of course affect antibody binding and hence the ability of the virus to infect people who have been infected, and become immune to the previous antigenic variant.

Between the haemagglutinin spikes there are mushroom-shaped protrusions of *neuraminidase* (N). The head is box-shaped and is assembled from four roughly spherical subunits attached to the stalk containing the hydrophobic region by

Cultivation

For primary isolation the most suitable cells are primary monkey kidney or human embryo kidney cells, but since these tissues are scarce most laboratories now use secondary baboon kidney cells. Embryonic chick cells and those from various species of mammals are susceptible but the rate of growth and the cytopathic effects vary with different strains. If continuous cell lines are used the cycle of viral multiplication is often abortive. Although isolation may be made in the amniotic or allantoic cavity of embryonated hens'

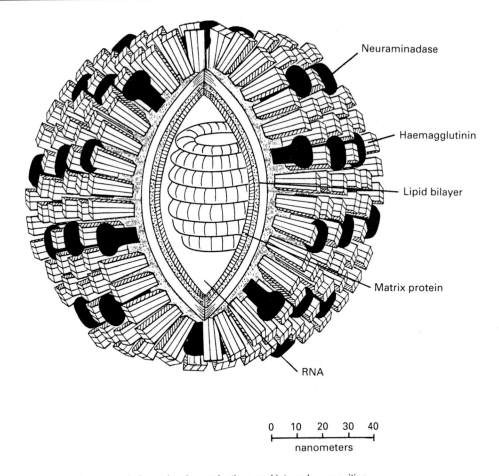

Neuraminadase

Haemagglutinin

Lipid bilayer

Matrix protein

RNA

0   10   20   30   40
nanometers

Fig. 50.2 Influenza in diagrammatic form showing projections and internal composition.

eggs, this method is not usually employed now since cell cultures are generally more convenient. The presence of virus may be detected in baboon kidney cell cultures incubated at 33°C as early as 18 h after inoculation, by haemadsorption using human group O, fowl or guinea-pig red blood cells. Usually, if viable viruses are present in the clinical specimen, isolation is made within 7 d. The virus may then be identified by the fluorescent antibody technique. In the early stages of infection the host cell does not seem to be damaged but a cytopathic effect may develop, which can resemble that associated with adenovirus or enterovirus infection.

Viability

The influenza virus withstands slow drying at room temperature on articles such as blankets and glass: it has been demonstrated in dust after an interval as long as 2 weeks. When contained in allantoic fluid or in infected tissues immersed in glycerol saline it will survive for several weeks at 4°C. Virus can survive in cold sea water for a similar period. It can be preserved for long periods at -70°C and remains viable indefinitely when freeze-dried.

Exposure to heat for 30 min at 56°C is sufficient to inactivate most strains; the few which survive

Table 50.1 Influenza virus proteins

Gene segment	Proteins	Molecular weight ($\times 10^3$)	Location in virion	Function	Comments
1	PB2	87	Internal	RNA	Polymerase proteins
2	PB1	96		transcription	highly conserved
3	PA	85		activity	
4	HA1	47.5	Spikes	Binding to cell	Glycoprotein
	HA2	28.8		receptors	haemagglutinin varies antigenically
5	NA	48–63	Spikes	Neuraminidase	Glycoprotein enzyme activity
6	NP	50–60	Internal	Subunit of nucleocapsid	Nucleoprotein helical arrangement; type-specific
7	M1	28	Beneath lipid bilayer of envelope	Major structural component	Involved in assembly and budding; type-specific
	M2	11–15		Unknown	Non-structural proteins
8	NS1	25	Internal	Unknown	Non-structural
	NS2	13			proteins

this treatment are killed by exposure to the same temperature for 90 min. The viruses are inactivated by a variety of substances such as 20% ether in the cold, phenol, formaldehyde, salts of heavy metals, detergents, soaps, halogens and many others.

Toxicity

Influenza virions are toxic to laboratory animals such as mice and rabbits. After intravenous inoculation of highly purified virus preparations, animals may die in 18–48 h with gastro-intestinal haemorrhages and necrotic lesions in the spleen and liver. Immunized animals do not suffer these effects when given intravenous inoculations of the virus. The ribonucleoprotein (RNP) component present in some whole virus vaccines is the cause of the local and systemic reactions associated with their use.

REPLICATION

Specific attachment of virions to cells depends on interaction between the outer surface of the haemagglutinin trimers with NANA-containing components on the cell surface. Virions are then taken into the cell in vesicles; fusion of the viral envelope with the membrane of the endosome depends on partial unfolding of the haemagglutinin at the low pH found in the endosome. This leads to release of the viral RNP and associated RNA polymerase into the cell cytoplasm. Transcription of the viral RNA molecules produces 10 mRNA species (Table 50.1) as RNA segments 7 and 8 both have two reading frames. mRNA molecules are processed in the cell nucleus where poly (A) sequences are removed from host mRNA molecules and added to the viral transcripts. Unlike most other RNA viruses, assembly of the new viral RNP takes place in the nucleus of the host cell.

The viral matrix (M) proteins migrate to the cell membrane and are joined by the haemagglutinin and neuraminidase glycoproteins. RNP and polymerase locate at the areas of the cell membrane with matrix protein. Release occurs by budding, aided perhaps by the viral neuraminidase. To be infectious the haemagglutinin protein is cleaved into the components HA1 and HA2, which together form the haemagglutinin molecule.

CLINICAL FEATURES

Influenza A

In classical influenza the incubation period is short, 2 d, but it may vary from 1 to 4 d. The illness is characterized by a sudden onset of systemic symptoms such as chills, fever, headache, myalgia and anorexia. Respiratory symptoms are also common but take second place to the systemic effects, especially early in the illness. Many patients have both upper and lower respiratory tract infection, often with a troublesome, dry cough. The main physical finding is pyrexia, which rises rapidly to a peak of 38–41°C within 12 h of onset. Fever usually lasts 3 d but it can be present for 1–5 d. During the 2nd and 3rd day of the illness the systemic effects diminish and by the 4th day the respiratory symptoms and signs are predominant, with pharyngitis, laryngitis and tracheobronchitis. In adults, systemic illness without respiratory symptoms is common, as are febrile convulsions in children. About one-third of patients will suffer only a common cold-like illness and it has been shown that as many as 20% of cases are subclinical. A long convalescence is common, and cough, lassitude and malaise may last for 1–2 weeks after the disappearance of other manifestations. It should be remembered that many other respiratory viruses can cause typical influenza-like illnesses, although the severity of the systemic symptoms is usually greatest with influenza virus. The similarity of the prodromal stages of several infections to influenza has led to the use of the term 'flu-like' to describe these features.

Influenza B

Symptoms closely resemble those associated with influenza A infections, consisting of a 3 d febrile illness with predominantly systemic symptoms. It is generally thought, however, that overall the infection is somewhat milder, and some studies have shown more involvement of the gastro-intestinal tract, with the coining of the term 'gastric flu'.

Influenza C

Infection with this virus is comparatively rare compared with influenza A and B. Clinically, the result is an afebrile upper respiratory tract infection usually confined to young children: outbreaks are not recognized.

Complications of influenza

Primary *influenza pneumonia* may occur especially in young adults during an outbreak and can be fatal after a very short illness of sometimes less than 1 d. A similar rapid illness can occur in the elderly. More commonly a *bacterial pneumonia* caused by *Staphylococcus aureus* or *Streptococcus pneumoniae* may occur late in the course of the illness, often after a period of improvement resulting in a classical biphasic fever pattern. The incidence of chest complications is related to the age of the patient, increasing progressively after the age of 60 years. Severe infections and sudden death can occur, especially if there is some underlying disease, such as cerebrovascular, cardiovascular or chronic respiratory disease.

PATHOGENESIS

Inhaled virus is deposited on the mucous membrane lining the respiratory tract or directly into the alveoli, the level depending on the size of the droplets inhaled. In the former site, it is exposed to mucoproteins containing NANA which can bind to the virus, thus blocking its attachment to respiratory tract epithelial cells.

However, the action of neuraminidase allows the virus to break this bond. Specific local secretory IgA antibodies, if present from a previous infection, may neutralize the virus before attachment occurs, provided the antibody corresponds to the infecting virus type. If not prevented by one of these mechanisms, virus attaches to the surface of a respiratory epithelial cell and the intracellular replication cycle is initiated.

The major site of infection is the ciliated columnar epithelial cell. The first alteration is the disappearance of the elongated form of these cells, which become round and swollen, the nucleus shrinks, becomes pyknotic and fragments. Vacuolization of the cytoplasm may occur. As the nucleus disintegrates, the cytoplasm shows inclusion bodies and the cilia are lost.

Release of the virus from the cells allows it to spread via the mucus blanket to other areas of the respiratory tract. The cell damage initiates an acute inflammatory response with oedema and the attraction of phagocytic cells. The earliest response is the synthesis and release of interferons from the infected cells: these can diffuse to and protect both adjacent and more distant cells before the virus arrives. It appears that interferons released in this way cause many of the systemic features of the 'flu-like' syndrome. While viral components are absorbed and trigger the immune system, the virus itself is confined to the epithelium of the respiratory tract. Specific antibody will help to limit the extracellular spread of the virus, while T cell responses are directed against the viral glycoproteins on the surface of infected cells, leading to their destruction by cytotoxic T cells and also by antibody-dependent cell cytotoxicity.

Immunity

After an attack of influenza the ensuing immunity to the particular subtype of infecting virus is of long duration. It is related to the amount of local antibody (IgA) in the mucous secretions of the respiratory tract together with the specific IgG serum antibody concentration. Immunity to infection, especially with type A, is subtype-specific, giving little or no resistance to subtypes possessing immunologically distinct H or N proteins.

LABORATORY DIAGNOSIS
Virus isolation and detection

As early in the illness as possible, preferably within 3 d of onset, a cotton-budded swab should be vigorously rubbed over the tonsillar region to obtain as many cells as possible. A swab from the nose should also be taken and both cotton ends

broken off into a bottle containing approximately 3 ml of viral transport medium. This should be taken to the laboratory as soon as possible; if delay is inevitable the specimen should be kept at 4°C but it should not be frozen. Appropriate cell cultures are then inoculated for the isolation of virus. Nasopharyngeal aspirates from children are useful specimens, both for the isolation of virus and for fluorescent antibody staining with appropriate tagged monoclonal antibodies to give a rapid diagnosis within a few hours of the specimen being taken.

Serological confirmation of the clinical diagnosis is obtained when a four-fold or greater rise in antibody titre can be shown to any one type of virus. Complement fixation tests (CFTs) are still widely used. They use the 'S' antigens and can distinguish A from B and C infections. Strain differences can be demonstrated by means of haemagglutination inhibition and neutralization assays or strain-specific CFTs. Single, high CFT titres are difficult to interpret in some patients, especially those with chronic respiratory disease since many may exhibit high titres for many years. In patients who are normally healthy a high titre found during an outbreak could, with more assurance, be related to a recent illness.

TREATMENT

After many years of effort there is still no satisfactory anti-influenza drug. Oral *amantadine hydrochloride* was introduced in the early 1980s, followed later by a derivative, *rimantadine*. Unfortunately, these compounds only have activity against influenza virus type A but not B or C. Therefore, it is essential to know the type of virus responsible for the illness or outbreak. A clinical diagnosis can be fairly confidently made in a typical case seen during an epidemic due to a known type, but is impossible in sporadic or milder cases. However, rapid diagnosis by immunofluorescence has proved useful. Amantadine activity has been shown in contacts given the drug prophylactically and also therapeutically in patients treated within 24 h of onset of illness.

Tribavirin given by nebulized aerosol, which has proved useful in the treatment of respiratory

51

Paramyxoviruses

Respiratory infections; mumps; measles

C. R. Madeley and J. S. M. Peiris

The paramyxoviruses are a family of enveloped viruses containing single-stranded RNA as a single piece. They resemble the orthomyxoviruses in both morphology and an affinity for sialic acid receptors on mammalian cells but they are larger and more fragile (Fig. 51.1a).

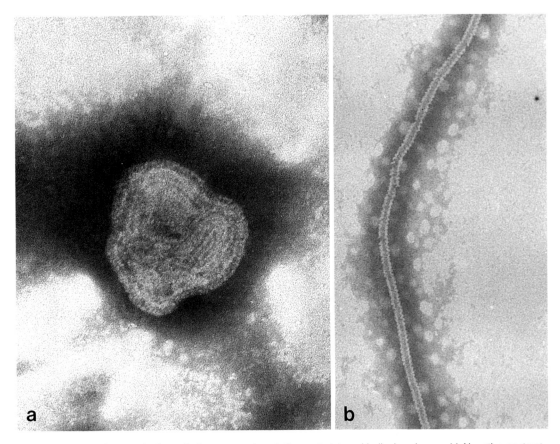

Fig. 51.1 **a** Electron micrograph of a typical paramyxovirus. **b** Separate internal helical nucleocapsid. Negative contrast microscopy × 200 000.

Within the paramyxovirus family there are several genera each with several members: *paramyxovirus* (parainfluenza viruses, mumps virus, Newcastle disease virus (NDV) and simian virus 5 (SV5); *morbillivirus* (measles virus, canine distemper virus and rinderpest virus); and *pneumovirus* (respiratory syncytial (RS) virus). Originally, they were all classified together because they were thought to be similar in structure and function. Neither property is constant throughout the family but there are similarities. For example, parainfluenza, mumps and measles viruses, are identical as seen in the electron microscope (and as described below), while pneumovirus, although very similar, has slightly longer surface spikes and is more difficult to visualize.

Functionally there are other differences. Parainfluenza viruses, NDV, and mumps virus have a surface haemagglutinin and neuraminidase, while measles virus has haemagglutinin but no neuraminidase and pneumovirus has neither. In addition, measles virus has a haemolysin not possessed by the others, while RS virus has a large surface glycoprotein, G, which has a similar cell-attaching function to a haemagglutinin.

PARAINFLUENZA VIRUSES

Description

Parainfluenza viruses, mumps virus, NDV and SV5 are indistinguishable in the electron microscope. Negatively stained virions vary in diameter from 80 to 350 nm; occasionally there are filamentous forms and giant forms up to 800 nm in diameter. The outer surface of the virion is a pleomorphic envelope consisting of a lipoprotein membrane covered by projections 12–14 nm long and 2–4 nm wide. Although generally similar, orthomyxoviruses and paramyxoviruses are morphologically distinct. Paramyxovirus particles are easily deformed by external forces, may assume a variety of shapes and break up more easily than orthomyxoviruses.

The envelope surface projections are of two kinds, the HN and F glycoproteins. The former carries both haemagglutinin (H) and neuraminidase (N) functions, in contrast to orthomyxoviruses, in which these functions are on separate spikes.

The F or fusion protein causes cell membranes to fuse, leading to the formation of syncytia, and is found on all paramyxoviruses. There is also a matrix, protein, M, which lines the inner surface of the envelope. All the paramyxoviruses carry an RNA-dependent RNA polymerase within the virion.

Within the virion there is a nucleocapsid containing a genome of single-stranded negative-sense RNA about 1 μm long with a molecular weight of 7×10^6. Some particles contain multiples of this basic genome. The RNA is complexed with a protein to form a helical ribonucleoprotein. This is contained within the lipid envelope derived from host cell membrane. The envelope ruptures readily when the virus is prepared for electron microscopy, releasing the helical nucleoprotein, which has a herring-bone or 'zipper'-like appearance (Fig. 51.1b). This is more easily recognized in the electron microscope than the complete particle; it is 15–19 nm wide with a pitch of about 6 nm.

Classification

There are four types of parainfluenza viruses which have antigenically distinct epitopes. Nevertheless, there are conserved antigenic sites on the paramyxovirus envelope proteins which are seen as serological cross-reactions between the parainfluenza viruses, mumps virus and SV5. These are particularly close between parainfluenza type 1 and a mouse variant (Sendai) which was used for some time as the antigen in complement fixation tests for antibody to the former. However, it became apparent that there were other cross-reactions which made the results of serological tests virtually uninterpretable. Responses to previously experienced paramyxoviruses as well as the currently infecting virus are found. This phenomenon of response to 'original antigenic sin' has been seen with other viruses such as influenza and coxsackie B viruses. In addition, type 4 has two subtypes 4a and 4b which can be distinguished by neutralization or haemadsorption inhibition.

NDV causes infections in chickens and other domestic birds. Its severity varies considerably from inapparent to fatal. Because some strains can cause major outbreaks with high mortality there is an effective live vaccine. NDV is a typical paramyxovirus, and has been shown to be a rare cause of conjunctivitis in man but only as a result of a laboratory accident. SV5 is often present in monkey kidney cell cultures but there is now some evidence that there may be another human paramyxovirus which is closely related to it or to the pneumonia virus of mice. These findings have yet to be confirmed more widely. Other parainfluenza viruses are natural pathogens for cattle and other domestic species; they are not known to infect man.

Replication

Parainfluenza viruses attach via the haemagglutinin to sialic acid-containing receptors on the cell surface. The F protein then fuses the viral envelope with the cell membrane, releasing the nucleocapsid into the cell. The negative-strand genome cannot act as messenger RNA (mRNA) and the RNA-dependent RNA polymerase carried within the virion is required to produce subgenomic-sized mRNA transcripts, which are translated to produce some of the early virus-specific polypeptides. These include a second RNA polymerase which copies the genome into full-length positive complementary strands which are in turn copied back into negative strands for transcription of later mRNA (coding for structural proteins) and for incorporation into new virions.

The viral components are assembled beneath the cell membrane and the surface HN and F proteins are incorporated into a stretch of membrane, converting it to viral envelope. This evaginates and buds off, enclosing as it does so a nucleocapsid to form a new virion. This is probably released from the host cell by the action of the neuraminidase component of the HN spikes. The incorporation of the HN protein into the cell membrane of infected cells causes red blood cells to adhere to the surface of infected cells—the phenomenon of *haemadsorption*.

Clinical features and pathogenesis

The parainfluenza viruses are mostly associated with *croup*, a harsh brassy cough in children familiar to many mothers as a middle-of-the-night irritant. It is due to a combination of tracheitis and laryngitis, but parainfluenza viruses may also cause minor upper respiratory tract illness, as well as some cases of *bronchiolitis* and 'failure to thrive'. They are responsible for 6–9% of respiratory infections for which a virus cause can be identified. The incubation period is from 3–6 d, during which the virus spreads locally within the respiratory tract.

Many infections occur in infants in the presence of maternal antibody, but it has not been established that this contributes to the severity of the disease.

Laboratory diagnosis

Rapid diagnosis may be made by *immunofluorescent staining* of exfoliated respiratory cells separated from well-taken nasopharyngeal secretions. Preparation of adequately specific polyclonal sera is time-consuming but practicable, although it may not be possible to separate type 4 positives into subtypes. A diagnostic kit in preparation by the World Health Organization for a variety of respiratory viruses includes a reagent (composed of a mixture of monoclonal antibodies) for detecting parainfluenza viruses in general but not for identifying individual types. This reflects the problems of generating and identifying good type-specific monoclonal antibodies against a background of significant antigenic overlap between parainfluenza viruses.

Similar antiviral antibodies may also be used in enzyme immuno-assays to identify viral antigen in specimens from the patient. They have the advantage of requiring only antigen to be present in the specimen while other assays required intact infected cells (for immunofluorescence) or infective virus (for culture). However, enzyme immuno-assays give no information on the quality of the specimen or the extent of infection.

Virus may be isolated in monkey kidney cells. Visible cytopathic effects in the cell sheets are minimal and it will usually be necessary to show infection of the cells by haemadsorption. Guinea-pig red blood cells will adsorb to the haemagglutinin expressed on the surface of infected cells. The infecting virus can be typed (or subtyped) by reacting the cell cultures with type-specific antisera before adding the guinea-pig cells. The appropriate antibody inhibits the haemadsorption. The typing can be confirmed by a neutralization test or by immunofluorescence, but this is not usually necessary.

Serology is not used routinely in diagnosis. Type-specific antibodies may be detected by neutralization or haemadsorption inhibition but these tests are too complex for routine use. Others such as complement fixation are difficult to interpret because of cross-reactions between parainfluenza viruses with mumps virus and, possibly SV5 (see above).

Epidemiology and transmission

Epidemiologically, parainfluenza type 1 infections are more frequent in the winter while type 3 appears to be a summer infection, with small epidemics appearing reliably each year. Type 2 and 4a and b infections are more infrequent, in Newcastle upon Tyne at least, although elsewhere in Britain type 2 may be another summer visitor. Type 4 infections are probably under-diagnosed but reported figures are too low for epidemiological patterns to be clear. The reasons for these variable patterns are unknown.

Numerically, parainfluenza infections are far fewer than those due to RS virus (q.v.) and most diagnosed infections are in pre-school and primary school children. Fatalities are very rare and re-infections occur.

The viruses are present in respiratory secretions and are expelled during coughing and sneezing. Infection is acquired by inhalation and by person-to-person contact.

MUMPS

Description

The mumps virus is a typical paramyxovirus, indistinguishable in appearance from parainfluenza viruses, measles virus and NDV. A similar herring-bone or zipper-like ribonucleoprotein is frequently seen to leak from the virions in preparations examined by electron microscopy and may be the only unequivocally virus-like material seen.

However, if it is found in cerebrospinal fluid it is diagnostic of mumps meningitis because the only other similar virus found in the central nervous system, measles, does not reach levels detectable by electron microscopy in cerebrospinal fluid.

The spikes on the envelope carry either a combined haemagglutinin and neuraminidase (HN) or a fusion (F) protein. The envelope also contains a matrix (M) protein. There is only one serotype, although monoclonal antibodies have shown minor variations in the various surface antigenic epitopes.

Replication

This is indistinguishable from that already described for parainfluenza viruses. Infected cells show haemadsorption but little obvious damage. New virus is released by budding.

Clinical features and pathogenesis

Mumps is something of an 'iceberg' of a disease —it is a common childhood infection but more infections probably occur than are recognized clinically. Although involvement of the *salivary glands* is a frequent feature of the acute disease, inapparent and minor infections are probably much more common. Difficulty in recovering the virus and ambiguity in serology mean that infections can go unconfirmed. The USA was the first country to propose a vaccine to control mumps but elsewhere surprise was expressed that anyone should bother. More complete monitoring of its activity suggests otherwise and it is a full partner in the MMR vaccine (see below), not an afterthought.

Infection is probably by droplet into the respiratory tract. The incubation period is 14–18 d and is followed by a generalized illness with localization in the salivary glands, usually the parotids. The generalized phase is the usual 'flu-like' illness with fever and malaise, followed by developing pain in the parotid glands which then swell rapidly. Much of the swelling is due to blockage of the efferent duct and the sucking of a lemon in front of a sufferer is a refined form of torture!

Neurological involvement is common in mumps (over 50% of infections), though the majority are not clinically apparent. However, clinical *meningitis* remains the most common serious complication of mumps, occurring in 1–10% of patients with mumps parotitis. Meningitis (like any of the other complications of mumps) can occur before, during, after or in the absence of salivary gland involvement. Mumps virus and the enteroviruses (q.v.) account for virtually all the cases of aseptic meningitis in the UK. Of these, the mumps virus is more commonly involved than any other individual virus. Both meningitis and meningo-encephalitis have been described, with the former being very rarely fatal with otherwise complete recovery. The latter is much rarer, carries a poorer prognosis and may result in long term neurological sequelae or in death. Deafness and tinnitus have also been described, but are very rare.

In prepubertal children the acute illness usually subsides in 4–5 d with complete recovery. The best known complication, in post pubertal males, is *orchitis*. This, though painful and causing softening and atrophy of the affected testicle, is usually unilateral and rarely causes sterility. *Oophoritis* also occurs in girls and should be distinguished from a ruptured cyst or acute appendicitis. Both orchitis and oophoritis usually develop as the parotitis resolves and a history of previous parotid pain and swelling will usually provide the clue.

The role of mumps in pancreatitis is difficult to establish. There may be abdominal pain in acute mumps but the levels of serum amylase do not correlate with the clinical picture. High levels may provide supportive evidence are but not diagnostic. Though uncomfortable it is not fatal.

Laboratory diagnosis

Typical mumps does not usually require laboratory confirmation but mild cases with little parotid swelling may not be noticed until complications develop. By this time virus may not be plentiful in the oropharynx. Direct demonstration by immunofluorescence on secretions is very rarely successful and the diagnosis will depend on growing the virus from *throat swabs*, from *saliva* from affected glands or from the *cerebrospinal fluid*. Collection of infected saliva is difficult but throat swabs provide a satisfactory specimen, although

the virus may take up to a week to grow. Virus may be present in urine but not reliably so. The detection of ribonucleoprotein helix in cerebrospinal fluid by electron microscopy is diagnostic but the small quantities of fluid usually taken make this impractical.

Growth of virus in cell cultures (usually monkey kidney or HEp2 cells) produces little cytopathic effect but the virus can be detected by haemadsorption, which can be inhibited by specific antiserum to confirm the presence of mumps virus.

The diagnosis can be made *serologically* by showing a rise in antibody between acute and convalescent specimens. Complement fixation is the usual test, using soluble (S) and viral (V) antigens. Antibodies to the S antigen are said to develop early, within a week of onset, followed by anti-V antibodies, which persist longer. However, these patterns are not invariable and only a rise in titre to both antigens can be relied on. A rise to only one antigen in the absence of typical illness will be difficult to interpret and may reflect infection with other paramyxoviruses. Low rises or low static titres in cases of meningitis should also be interpreted with caution—cross-reactions with other paramyxoviruses provide traps for the unwary and only isolation of the virus provides unequivocal evidence.

Other serological tests have been used, based on enzyme immuno-assays and single radial haemolysis. They have not been used as widely as complement fixation, being more often used in serological surveys or to complement other assays. Neutralization and haemagglutination inhibition tests are more complex to carry out and do not offer any advantages in routine diagnosis.

Epidemiology

Mumps is a world-wide disease, with man the only known reservoir. Most infections are in school-age children, with those in adults being more severe and more likely to develop complications. Although epidemics occur, mumps is less infectious than measles or chickenpox. Infection appears to confer life-long immunity and second infections do not occur.

Control

Some, but not very reliable, protection can be given by passive immunization; it may prevent severe orchitis even when given at the stage of parotitis.

Generally, mumps has not been thought to warrant a vaccine on its own, although one has been available in the USA for several years. This vaccine, based on the Jeryl Lynn or Urabe strains, has now been incorporated into a triple vaccine against measles, mumps and rubella (MMR). All three components are live attenuated viruses and the mumps component induces good antibody levels, lasting long enough to suggest that the recipients will not become susceptible as adults.

MEASLES

Description

Measles virus is morphologically indistinguishable from parainfluenza viruses, mumps virus and NDV, although there are important functional differences. The ribonucleoprotein helix is readily released from the virion and may, as with the others, be the only identifiable virus structure seen in the electron microscope.

The spikes on the measles virus envelope carry a haemagglutinin but not a neuraminidase. There is an F protein which is also a haemolysin. A matrix protein, M, is also present below the envelope lipid bilayer.

There is only one serotype of measles virus and no subtypes have yet been recognized, although monoclonal antibodies show that there may be differences between wild and cultivated strains.

Measles virus is related to two animal viruses– canine distemper virus (CDV) and rinderpest virus in cattle. There is partial cross-protection between measles virus and CDV. Convalescent CDV ferret sera will neutralize measles virus while ferrets inoculated with measles virus are partially protected from CDV. Similar partial cross-reactivity is found with rinderpest virus.

Pathogenesis

Measles is an acute febrile illness, mostly in childhood, after an incubation period of 10–12 d. The onset is flu-like with high fever, cough and conjunctivitis. *Koplik's spots* (red spots with a bluish white centre on the buccal mucosa) may be present at this stage. After 1–2 d the acute symptoms decline with the appearance of a widespread *maculopapular rash*. Viral antigen but not complete virus may be found in the spots. The rash can be inhibited by local injections of immune serum, but will not appear in those who are severely immunocompromised, and this has been thought to point to an immunopathological (T cell-mediated) mechanism.

Over the next 10–14 d recovery is usually complete as the rash fades with considerable desquamation. Complications include a giant cell *pneumonia*, more common in adults, *otitis media* and a post-measles *encephalitis*. The pneumonia is due to direct invasion with virus but the role of virus in the other two is uncertain. Measles encephalitis can cause severe and permanent mental impairment in those it does not kill. It is rare but disastrous.

The mortality of uncomplicated measles in immunocompetent well-nourished children is low but rises rapidly with *malnourishment* (marked in Africa), in the *immunocompromised* and, to a much lesser extent, with age. It has also been devastating in isolated populations into whom it was introduced as a 'new' disease.

One further complication of measles is *subacute sclerosing panencephalitis* (SSPE), which occurs in children or early adolescents who have had measles early in life, usually under 2 years of age. It is a progressive and inevitably fatal degenerative disease. Within infected cells is a defective form of measles virus which, because it is unable to induce the production of a functional M protein, is not released as complete virus from the cells. Patients deteriorate over several years, losing intellectual capacity before motor activities. Oligoclonal antibodies to measles virus proteins appear in the cerebrospinal fluid but the virus cannot be cultivated unless it is 'rescued' by co-cultivating neuronal cells with a susceptible cell type.

The virus has been linked with multiple sclerosis, Paget's disease of bone and Crohn's disease. In each case, tubular structures resembling measles nucleocapsids have been seen and immunofluorescence has been used to demonstrate measles 'antigens' in biopsy material. Serum from about 50% of adults aged over 50 years, however, will fix complement with measles antigen although giving no history suggestive of recent measles and it is possible that auto-antibodies to a measles-like protein can be induced with age. If so, its significance is unknown but would be a factor in assessing measles involvement in older patients with chronic diseases. At present, the evidence linking measles virus in the aetiology of these diseases is less than compelling.

Laboratory diagnosis

Most cases of measles are diagnosed clinically, usually in the patient's home. Virological confirmation is often not attempted and is difficult to do in general practice. In hospital and particularly in immunocompromised patients, in whom the disease will often be rashless, the diagnosis may be made rapidly by *immunofluorescence* on exfoliated respiratory cells in well-taken *nasopharyngeal secretions*. The presence of a large number of giant cells, particularly in patients on cytotoxic drugs, is a bad prognostic sign.

Other immuno-assays have been developed but give no feedback on the extent of the infection. Otherwise the virus may be grown in human fibroblasts, primary monkey cells and vero cells although it does not grow readily.

Measles induces a good antibody response and a rise in complement-fixing antibody is diagnostic. However, complement-fixing antibody in older patients is often detected and its significance is unknown. Other tests for antibody have been developed but are not used widely because diagnosis is usually made clinically.

Epidemiology

Transmission is person to person, probably by respiratory droplets, but the conjunctivitis may also be a source. Despite some anecdotal evidence, there is no good evidence that distemper in dogs can be a source of measles in man.

Measles epidemics occur every 2 years in developed countries with minimal use of vaccine. This periodicity will be absent in isolated populations too small to maintain transmission (<400 000), in poverty and overcrowding and following widespread use of vaccine. The disease is ubiquitous throughout the world and, although a candidate for eradication, this may be difficult to achieve.

In tropical areas, particularly Africa, children become infected under the age of 1 year and the mortality rises in consequence, reaching as high a figure as 42% in children under 4 years of age. Malnutrition is probably one of the main underlying causes of this excess mortality. The attack rate is also very high in isolated populations which have not experienced the disease for some years. In the Faroes in the 1840s, three-quarters of the population were infected although the mortality was low. Most of those who were not infected were aged over 65 years, the interval since the last time the disease had been present in the islands, and confirms that infection gives prolonged immunity.

In the USA, where a serious attempt to eradicate measles has been made, the number of cases was reduced from over 500 000 per year to about 2 000 (a reduction of over 99%) but outbreaks in immigrants and high-school students have recently emphasized the problems of preventing imported cases and of keeping up a high level of immunization.

Control

The first measles vaccine was a formalin-inactivated one. Although inducing circulating antibody, it was found that vaccinees exposed to natural measles were likely to develop atypical disease. The rash was more peripheral, involving palms and soles, and pneumonia was common. It was later recognized that the vaccine had failed to induce adequate levels of antibody to the haemolytic F protein, and the immunity induced did not inhibit cell-to-cell spread of the virus. Consequently it was withdrawn and replaced with a live attenuated one. Early versions of the latter were only partially attenuated and were thought only to offer a choice of when to have measles, but with the added uncertainly over whether the resulting immunity was as long-lasting as that following natural measles. Later versions, containing the Edmonston B or Schwarz strains, have been better attenuated while giving a sero-conversion rate of over 90%. How long this immunity lasts remains to be seen but it appears to be at least 15 years (and may well be life-long).

In Britain, vaccine uptake has been relatively poor at 55–60%, partly because of a reluctance to promote its use enthusiastically. Higher rates have been achieved in some districts but only as a result of promotion campaigns. In contrast, eradication has been attempted in the USA where evidence of vaccination or clinical disease has been a legal requirement for school entry. This has reduced the disease incidence substantially but importation has frustrated any hopes of interrupting transmission completely.

Recently, measles vaccine has been combined with those against mumps and rubella to form the MMR vaccine. This combination of three attenuated viruses has been shown to induce good immunity to all three. Introduced initially in the USA, it is now the preferred vaccine in the UK for administration between 12 and 18 months.

Immunization in the high endemic regions of Africa still presents problems, however. As many infants are infected before their first birthday, the vaccine has to be given under 6 months to have any effect. As passively transferred maternal antibody often interferes with the immune response to a live vaccine, such early immunization does not always produce adequate immunity. A second dose at 12–13 months is then probably necessary but adds to the cost and the logistic difficulties. Solutions to both will have to be found before progress is made towards measles eradication in the developing world.

RESPIRATORY SYNCYTIAL VIRUS

Description

Superficially RS virus resembles other paramyxoviruses, with a similar pleomorphic envelope studded with surface spikes which may be seen more clearly in the electron microscope than those on the parainfluenza viruses, mumps and measles. The spikes may also be slightly longer, but neither the complete virus particles nor the nucleoprotein helix (with a similar diameter to parainfluenza viruses of 17 nm) are easy to visualize in the electron microscope. However, individual particles are generally larger than other paramyxoviruses (Fig 51.2).

RS virus is placed in a separate genus—pneumovirus — because of these minor physical differences and the lack of a haemagglutinin, a haemolysin or a neuraminidase. The nucleic acid is single-stranded RNA of negative sense with a molecular weight of about 5×10^6, coding for both structural and non-structural proteins. RS virus has no haemagglutinin but has a G glycoprotein instead. It is a receptor for cell attachment but not to red blood cells, and differs in chemical composition from the HN protein of other paramyxoviruses. There are fusion (F), matrix (M), polymerase and nucleocapsid proteins. The F protein induces the syncytia in cell cultures from which the virus gets its name, and is probably responsible for both virus penetration and spread in the host.

The virus is relatively fragile and may not survive even snap-freezing to −70°C. Specimens for isolation should not be frozen.

For most purposes there is only one serotype, although the advent of monoclonal antibodies has confirmed that there are two subtypes, A and B. Subtype A may be more virulent than B but this needs to be confirmed. In Newcastle upon Tyne, strains of subgroup A have been prevalent every year since 1974 but subgroup B strains have been more erratic and have not been active in every winter. The reason for this phenomenon is unknown.

RS virus is also a significant pathogen in cattle and infects chimpanzees readily—early isolates were termed chimpanzee coryza agent. Both goats and sheep may be infected naturally and there is evidence that several other domestic and rodent species are susceptible, either naturally or after some adaptation.

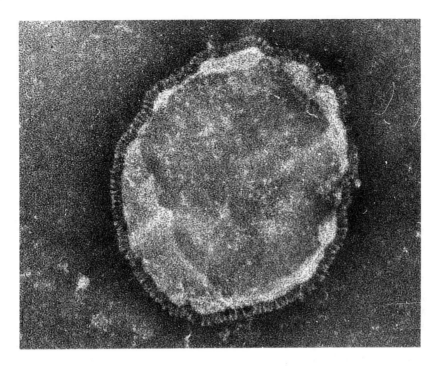

Fig. 51.2 Electron micrograph of respiratory syncytial virus. × 200 000. Phosphotungstic acid stain

Clinical features and pathogenesis

The most serious illness caused by RS virus is *bronchiolitis* in young babies. The peak incidence is in those under 1 year of age and there are (possibly as a consequence) annual winter epidemics. This infection is potentially life-threatening, particularly in those with broncho-pulmonary dysplasia or congenital heart defects. In normal babies it is rarely fatal where medical staff have the experience and facilities for appropriate management. RS virus has been recovered from some victims of sudden infant death syndrome (SIDS). Although it may have contributed to the death it is clear that other factor(s) also contribute.

In older children and adults, the virus causes minor infections, possibly because their air passages are larger. Reinfections are common and in adults may cause no more than a cold. However, the failure of acute infections to immunize, even in the immunocompetent, highlights the difficulty of producing a vaccine. The main clinical feature is bronchiolitis, but the upper respiratory tract remains infected and this makes it possible to confirm the diagnosis. If RS virus is present in the nasopharynx and there is clinical evidence of lower respiratory tract involvement, RS virus is likely to be responsible.

Recovery is apparently complete, although it has been suggested that the infection predisposes to chronic respiratory tract disease (asthma, bronchiectasis, etc.). This has yet to be confirmed although studies are in progress.

The sequelae to the use of an inactivated vaccine (see below) have led to the suggestion that some of the severity of bronchiolitis is due to *hypersensitivity* induced by an earlier infection. Studies in various centres have neither confirmed this theory nor fully excluded it. There is much still to learn about the pathogenesis of RS virus.

There have been reports of severe illness, with some fatalities, in old people's homes. Compared with those associated with influenza, outbreaks of RS virus are reported infrequently, although this may be due to difficulties in diagnosis. A neurological syndrome has also been described, but whether RS virus is the cause is unproven.

Laboratory diagnosis

During the acute phase of illness virus may be readily demonstrated in nasopharyngeal secretions (which are usually copious) by immunofluorescence, enzyme immuno-assays or culture.

Rapid diagnosis in less than 1 h using commercially available conjugated monoclonal antibodies can be made reliably by immunofluorescence, provided an adequate number of desquamated respiratory cells are collected in the secretions. Generally, similar results can be obtained with enzyme immuno-assays. Such assays may be less sensitive when compared to culture, but the virus is slow-growing and positive results will come too late to influence management. This is still true even when the cultured cells are examined by immunofluorescence for the development of virus antigen after a few days' incubation.

Serology is not helpful. Many of the patients are too young to respond reliably and even adults do not always produce a detectable rise in serum antibody levels. Hence, few laboratories offer a serological test. Secretory antibodies may develop more reliably but no routine test is yet available.

Treatment

Appropriate management includes use of oxygen, if indicated, physiotherapy and tube feeding if the baby has difficulty in suckling. Most babies can be managed symptomatically by these measures. The only specific antiviral drug available for chemotherapy is tribavirin. This is a nucleoside analogue with a wide spectrum of activity against a variety of DNA and RNA viruses in vitro. In vivo there is some evidence of efficacy when given as a small-particle aerosol, although it is apparently not effective when given by intravenous infusion. The evidence of efficacy by any route is not overwhelming. This may be because the most affected parts of the lungs are also the least well aerated and therefore least accessible to the aerosolized drug. The drug is expensive and its recommended use is confined to those babies who

are at high risk from RS virus because they have congenital heart or lung abnormalities. Even in these babies the damage may be done by the virus before the drug can be given. This may be an effective drug but proving it remains far from easy.

Epidemiology

In temperate climates in both the northern and southern hemispheres, RS virus causes a substantial winter epidemic every year. In Newcastle upon Tyne (population about 300 000) the number of virologically confirmed diagnoses may reach more than 500 in a more severe epidemic season and rarely falls below 100. Similar figures are obtained elsewhere if adequate facilities for diagnosis exist. Most infected babies reach hospital and the failure to recover it from babies with 'colds' attending well-baby clinics in Newcastle upon Tyne has suggested that comparatively few cases go unrecognized.

Why it induces an epidemic every October/November is unknown. It does not appear to relate to short-term climatic factors (temperature, humidity, etc.) and sporadic cases occur throughout the year. It is probably distributed over all the world but its activities in tropical, overcrowded and poor areas are under-recorded so far.

The significance of subtypes in explaining these RS virus phenomena is not clear so far.

The peak incidence is in those under 1 year of age.

Control

A formalin-inactivated crude whole-virus vaccine was tried in the 1960s. It induced good levels of circulating antibody but failed to protect the recipients, who actually became more ill than placebo controls when subsequently exposed to RSV. A similar situation occurred with measles and, with both vaccines, may have been due to the vaccine failing to induce the right protective antibodies. Subsequently, several live vaccines based on cold adaptation, temperature-sensitive mutants or administration by a different route (intramuscularly) were tried but none has proved satisfactory (through insufficient attenuation or inadequate immunogenicity).

A major obstacle in developing a good vaccine is the fact that the peak of disease occurs within the 1st year of life, and thus a safe vaccine immunogenic to such young and largely immunologically immature recipients is difficult to prepare. In the future, genetic engineering offers new ways to prepare vaccines which contain only the relevant antigens in an appropriate viral or bacterial vector, but at present there is no satisfactory vaccine.

RECOMMENDED READING

Evans A S (ed) Viral Infections of Humans; Epidemiology and Control, 3rd edn. 1989, Plenum Press, New York.

Zuckerman A J, Banatvala J E, Pattison J R (eds) Principles and Practice of Clinical Virology, 2nd edn 1990, Wiley, Chichester.

52

Arboviruses: alphaviruses, flaviviruses (including rubella) and bunyaviruses

Encephalitis; yellow fever; dengue; haemorrhagic fever; miscellaneous tropical fevers; undifferentiated fever; rubella

D. M. McLean and P. Morgan-Capner

The name 'arbo' (arthropod borne) virus has been used for many years to define viruses transmitted by arthropod (mainly insect) vectors. However, it is now recognized that there are many different viruses transmitted by arthropods. Indeed, there are more than 500 individual arbovirus serotypes which are now officially classified in five different virus families. As there are many similarities in their behaviour, they will be considered together in this chapter. Arboviruses were defined by a World Health Organization Scientific Group as 'viruses that are maintained in nature principally, or to an important extent, through biological transmission between susceptible vertebrate hosts by haemotophagous arthropods or through transovarian and possible venereal transmission in arthropods; the viruses multiply and produce viraemia in the vertebrates, multiply in the tissues of arthropods, and are passed on to new vertebrates by the bites of arthropods after a period of extrinsic incubation'.

Additional serotypes within the five taxons are not transmitted by arthropods, but are maintained in nature within rodent reservoirs which may transmit infection directly to humans. They are termed roboviruses. Some of these are discussed in Chapter 53.

signed to the Alphavirus, Flavivirus and Bunyavirus families; some are assigned to the Reovirus (*Orbivirus* such as Colorado tick fever virus) and the Rhabdovirus (*Vesiculovirus* such as vesicular stomatitis virus) families. Within the Alphaviruses, only one genus, *Alphavirus*, contains arthropod-borne serotypes. The Flaviviruses include another genus, *Rubivirus*, which contains rubella virus which is not arthropod-borne. Rubella virus is described in a separate section at the end of this chapter. The hepatitis C virus, one of the main causes of non-A, non-B hepatitis, has features which suggest that it may be a flavivirus. However, until further information is available, hepatitis C is discussed in Chapter 47. The alpha- and flaviviruses were classified as genera within the Togavirus family. However they are now considered as separate families.

Individual serotypes of arboviruses are distinguished from each other by neutralization tests. For arboviruses which multiply in tissue cultures and induce plaques, neutralization tests are performed by plaque reduction, for the remainder, tests are conducted by intracerebral inoculation of suckling mice. Clusters of serotypes which show antigenic overlap are termed serogroups. Table 52.2 lists some of the important members.

DESCRIPTION

Classification

Arboviruses are classified within five families (taxons) (Table 52.1). Most serotypes are as-

Properties

Arboviruses share common biological attributes (Table 52.1):

Table 52.1 Characteristic properties of arboviruses

Property	Arbovirus family				
	Alphavirus	Flavivirus	Bunyavirus	Rhabdovirus[a]	Reovirus[b]
Symmetry[c]	Cubic	Cubic	Helical	Bullet shaped	Cubic
Total diameter (nm)	60–65	40–50	90–100	170×70	60–80
Nucleic acid	(+)ss RNA	(+)ss RNA	(−)ss RNA	(−)ss RNA	ds RNA
Molecular weight ($\times 10^6$)	4.2–4.4	4.2–4.4	0.4–5.0	3.5–4.6	0.2–3.0
No. of molecules	1	1	3	1	10–12
No. of serotypes	29	69	251	50	74
Inactivation by diethyl ether or sodium deoxycholate	+	+	+	+	−

[a] See Chapter 58; [b] see Chapter 54; [c] all have enveloped virions.

1. All induce fatal encephalitis 1–10 d after intracerebral inoculation of suckling mice aged less than 48 h; some also induce fatal encephalitis after intracerebral inoculation of weaned mice aged 3–4 weeks. Encephalitis does not occur after inoculation of virus plus serotype-specific antiserum (neutralization).

2. Haemagglutinin for erythrocytes of geese or newly hatched chicks. Haemagglutination is inhibited by antiserum against virus serotypes within the same serogroup, but not dissimilar serogroups. Antigen can also be detected by enzyme-linked immunosorbent assay (ELISA) and complement fixation tests.

3. Many arboviruses multiply in continuous polyploid tissue cultures of mammalian cells incubated at 37°C.

4. Many arboviruses such as dengue and Ross River viruses multiply in continuous tissue cultures of *Aedes albopictus* mosquito cells when incubated at 28°C or lower temperatures; multiplication is detected by immunofluorescence tests.

5. Mosquito-borne arboviruses multiply after oral feeding or intrathoracic injection of several *Aedes* and *Culex* mosquito species after incubation at 4–28°C (depending on the mosquito species) and mosquitoes transmit virus by biting susceptible vertebrates; virus multiplication in mosquito tissues is revealed by specific immunofluorescence, particularly in salivary glands and in central nervous tissue. Susceptibility of mosquitoes to dengue and California serogroup agents is 10–100 times higher than mammalian tissue cultures or suckling mice.

Some arboviruses, notably bunyaviruses of the California serogroup, phleboviruses and vesiculoviruses of the rhabdovirus family, are also transmitted transovarially.

Mosquito-borne arboviruses are not transmitted by ticks; tick-borne arboviruses are not transmitted by mosquitoes. Sandfly-borne viruses are transmitted only by sandflies (*Phlebotomus* sp., *Lutzomyia* sp.).

6. Tick-borne arboviruses multiply after oral feeding to larval or nymphal ixodid ticks (hard-shelled ticks of the genera *Dermacentor* and *Ixodes*). The virus is transferred trans-stadially to the next development stage of tick (nymph or adult respectively), which then transmits virus by biting susceptible vertebrates.

REPLICATION

The replication of the various arboviruses differs significantly and is one of the features used in their classification.

Alphaviruses

The virus attaches to cellular receptors by means of the envelope glycoproteins E1 and E2, and virus enters the cell by endocytosis. The viral RNA is a linear single-stranded molecule. It is polyadenylated and acts as a messenger molecule.

Table 52.2 Some important arboviruses

Family	Number of members	Some important members	Comments
Alphavirus	27	Western equine encephalitis Eastern equine encephalitis Venezuelan equine encephalitis Chikungunya Ross River	Mosquito-borne Serogroup A
Flavivirus	67	St Louis encephalitis Japanese B encephalitis Murray Valley encephalitis Yellow fever Dengue Ilheus West Nile	Mosquito-borne Serogroup B
		Louping ill Powassan Tick-borne encephalitis Kyasanur Forrest Omsk haemorrhagic fever	Tick-borne Serogroup B

Bunyavirus	187	Bunyaviruses
		  La Crosse
		  Snowshoe hare
		  Oropouche
			California (CAL) serogroup

		Phleboviruses
		  Rift Valley fever
		  Punta Toro
		  Sandfly fever
		  Toscana	

		Nairoviruses Crimean–Congo haemorrhagic fever	
		Hantaviruses Hantaan virus (*not* arthropod-borne)	

Approximately two-thirds of the genome codes for non-structural proteins: the remaining third codes for the capsid and envelope proteins. Viral RNA is replicated from a negative-strand copy catalysed by the viral-specified RNA polymerase. The virus is released by budding from membranes: an essential step in this process is the conversion of a precursor protein to E2.

Flaviviruses

Flaviviruses are similar to alphaviruses in several respects, but they differ in the composition of the envelope glycoprotein and virion RNA. The virions mature in internal vesicles.

Bunyaviruses

The virions of the bunyavirus family are larger than the alpha-and flaviviruses. They differ fundamentally in their nucleic acid, which is present as three molecules (M, S and L strands) of circular single-stranded RNA. The RNA is of negative sense, therefore the virion must contain an RNA polymerase to initiate transcription. The envelope glycoproteins G1 and G2 are derived from the M molecules of RNA: the nucleocapsid protein (N) from the S molecule, which also codes for non-structural protein; the L molecule is presumed to code for the polymerase. Although classified in the same family, there are a number of differences between the phleboviruses and the bunyaviruses.

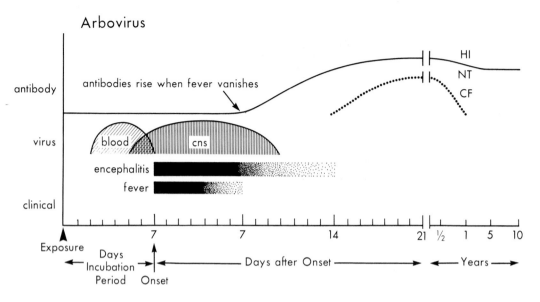

Fig. 52.1   Pathogenesis of arbovirus infection: time course of clinical features, virus detection and antibodies. HI, haemagglutination inhibition; NT, neutralization; CF, complement fixation. Antibodies measured by enzyme immuno-assay (ELISA) parallel the time course for HI and NT antibodies. (Reproduced with permission from McLean D M 1980 *Virology in Health Care*. Williams and Wilkins, Baltimore, p 167.)

PATHOGENESIS

Arboviruses induce high titres of *viraemia* in susceptible vertebrates 1–2 d after parenteral inoculation or following bites by infected arthropods; viraemia persists for several days and serves as a source of infective blood meals for other biting arthropods. The primary site of virus replication is not known but is likely to be in the reticuloendothelial cells in lymph nodes, liver and spleen or endothelial cells of blood vessels. Release of virus from these sites may be associated with non-specific 'flu-like' symptoms. During this period of viraemia, usually at about 5–7 d after exposure, virus enters the target sites of the central nervous system, skin, etc. There may be a brief period of relief after the initial symptoms — before the onset of the specific features. Thus, the presentation is a biphasic illness. Symptoms of encephalitis begin 7–10 d after exposure to infection and persist 1 week or more, followed either by remission or by death. Wild birds and mammals regularly exhibit viraemia without symptoms.

Antibodies are first detected when the fever subsides, usually within 2 d after the onset of en-

cephalitis, and persist for many years (Fig. 52.1). Antibodies are of the IgM class for 1–7 weeks after infection, subsequently they are of the IgG class.

Within the central nervous system, arboviruses multiply in and induce necrosis of neurones, which in turn become surrounded by microglia, forming glial knots (Fig. 52.2). Perivascular cuffing with mononuclear cells affects many cerebral blood vessels. Usually there is concomitant meningitis with accumulation of mononuclear cells in the subarachnoid space and hyperaemia of adjacent capillaries. It is important to note that although many subjects become infected with encephalitis viruses, relatively few develop illness manifested as meningitis or encephalitis. There is little information about the role of the immune system, although it may have a role in the pathogenesis of the dengue haemorrhagic shock syndrome, which is seen in young children who are experiencing a second dengue virus infection. Antigen–antibody complex formation has been thought to underlie the syndrome, which is associated with increased capillary permeability and shock, often with haemorrhage. However, it is known that the uptake of virus into macrophages is enhanced in the presence of antibody as the virus–antibody com-

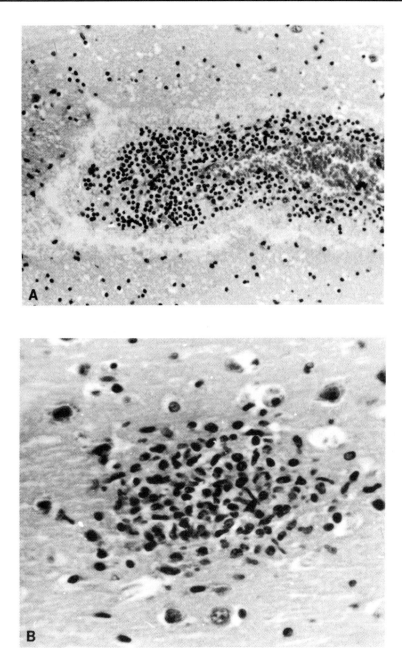

Fig. 52.2 Powassan virus infection in the brain of a fatal case from whom the prototype LB strain was isolated. H & E stain. ×
100. **A** perivascular cuffing of cerebral blood vessel; **B** focus of inflammatory cells around effete neurone (glial knot).
(Reproduced with permission from McLean D M 1980 *Virology in Health Care*. Williams and Wilkins, Baltimore, p 168.)

plexes bind to Fc receptors. In this way there is
likely to be a great increase in the uptake of virus
and hence the release of virus from macrophages.

CLINICAL FEATURES

Arbovirus infections of humans become clinically
manifest according to the target organ principally

Table 52.3 Clinical syndromes associated with selected arboviruses and their geographic distribution

Syndrome	Group	Serogroup (vector)	Causative arbovirus serotype		Geographical distribution
Encephalitis or aseptic meningitis	Alphavirus	A (mosquito)	EEE	eastern equine encephalitis	Eastern Canada, USA, Caribbean
			VEE	Venezuelan equine encephalitis	Central and South America
			WEE	western equine encephalitis	Western Canada and USA, Caribbean
	Flavivirus	B (mosquito)	JBE	Japanese B encephalitis	Orient (Japan to Malaysia)
			MVE	Murray Valley encephalitis	Australia
			SLE	St Louis encephalitis	Canada, USA, Central America
		B (tick)	LI	louping ill	Scotland, Northern Ireland
			POW	Powassan	Canada, Northern USA
			TBE	tick-borne encephalitis complex	Central and northern Europe, Siberia
	Bunyavirus	CAL (mosquito)	LAC	La Crosse	USA
			SSH	snowshoe hare	Canada
Yellow Fever	Flavivirus	B (mosquito)	YF	yellow fever	Tropical Africa, Caribbean, tropical South America
Dengue	Flavivirus	B (mosquito)	DEN	dengue (4 types)	Entire tropical zone
Haemorrhagic fever	Alphavirus	A (mosquito)	CHIK	chikungunya	East Africa, India, Southeast Asia
	Flavivirus	B (mosquito)	DEN	dengue (4 types)	India, Philippines, Southeast Asia, Oceania
		B (tick)	KFD	Kyasanur Forest disease	India
			OMSK	Omsk haemorrhagic fever	Siberia
	Nairovirus	CHF-CON (tick)	CON	Congo haemorrhagic fever	Central and southern Africa
Miscellaneous tropical fevers	Alphavirus	A (mosquito)	CHIK	chikungunya	East Africa, India, South-East Asia
			RR	Ross River[a]	Australia, Oceania
	Flavivirus	B (mosquito)	ILH	Ilheus	Caribbean, South America
			WN	West Nile	Central and northern Africa
	Bunyavirus	SIM (mosquito)	ORO	Oropouche	Caribbean, South America
	Phlebovirus	PHL (mosquito)	RVF	Rift Valley fever	Northern, eastern and southern Africa
		PHL (sandfly)	PT	Punta Toro	Central America
		PHL (sandfly)	SFN	sandfly fever — Naples	Mediterranean
	Vesiculovirus	VS (sandfly)	VSI	vesicular stomatitis — Indiana	USA, Central America[b]
Undifferentiated fever	Orbivirus	CTF (tick)	CTF	Colorado tick fever	Western USA[c]

[a] Ross River virus infections frequently exhibit polyarthralgia.
[b] See Chapter 58.
[c] See Chapter 54.

infected (Table 52.3). These include the following syndromes.

Encephalitis

Encephalitis typically comprises the sudden onset of fever and headache, followed by neck stiffness, nausea or vomiting, drowsiness, and disorientation, frequently advancing into stupor or coma after an incubation period of 4–14 d. Convulsions may be an important feature of the acute illness. Rigidity or weakness of the limbs may occur, together with absent or irregular deep tendon reflexes and upgoing plantar reflexes. Symptoms are most severe 2–5 d after onset, after which the patient may die or the fever and other symptoms may retrogress slowly during the next 2–3 weeks. Characteristically, the cerebrospinal fluid shows pleocytosis with a predominance of leucocytes, but sugar and protein levels remain normal. The peripheral blood leucocyte count usually does not exceed $8000 \times 10^6/l$ and shows a predominance of leucocytes. During most outbreaks of arboviral encephalitis, a proportion of cases develop aseptic meningitis only, without significant neuronal involvement.

Yellow fever

Yellow fever is characterized by the sudden onset of headache and fever with temperatures exceeding 39°C, accompanied by generalized myalgia, nausea and vomiting, after an incubation period of 3–6 d. Jaundice may appear by the 3rd day of illness, but frequently this is mild or absent. Haematemesis and melaena may occur from bleeding into the gastro-intestinal tract and epistaxis and bleeding gums may also be noted. Albuminuria and oliguria may also begin suddenly during the 1st week of illness. In severe cases, death may occur 3 d or more after the onset of illness, and midzonal necrosis is observed in the liver. The case fatality rate is estimated at 20%. Mild cases may develop fever, headache and myalgia only, without gastro-intestinal upsets, jaundice or albuminuria. In such cases, the diagnosis is frequently achieved only by the isolation of virus from the blood or demonstration of rising levels of antibody.

Dengue

This presents as an acute febrile illness with chills, headache, retro-ocular pain, body aches and arthralgia in more than 90% of cases, accompanied by nausea or vomiting and a maculopapular rash resembling measles lasting 2–7 d in about 60% of cases. Illness usually persists for 7 d or longer, with fever remitting after 3–5 d followed by relapse ('saddleback fever'), and pains in the bones, muscles and joints sufficiently severe to earn the epithet 'breakbone fever'. Rash occurs more commonly in patients aged less than 14 years. Complete recovery is the rule. The incubation period is 5–11 d.

Haemorrhagic fever

This is a less common manifestation of dengue, affecting mainly children. It is occasionally accompanied by a shock syndrome with a case fatality rate of 50%. After an acute onset, fever of 40°C, accompanied by vomiting and anorexia, enlarged liver and petechiae persists for 5–10 d. This is followed by a complete recovery unless shock supervenes; this occurs in 7–10% of cases from 2 to 7 d after onset, usually accompanied by haematemesis and melaena. Although dengue haemorrhagic fever with shock syndrome was initially recognized in South-East Asia in 1951, it has since occurred in the south-west Pacific, Puerto Rico and Cuba.

Miscellaneous tropical fevers

These comprise elevation of temperature beyond 39°C, together with any combination of headache, myalgia, malaise, nausea or vomiting, and sometimes accompanied by maculopapular rash or polyarthralgia, i.e. a dengue-like syndrome, but without haemorrhagic manifestations or the shock syndrome. Tropical fevers arise from infection with a wide variety of arboviruses (Table 52.3).

Undifferentiated fever

A US example is Colorado tick fever in which symptoms of chilliness, headaches, retro-orbital pain and generalized aches, especially in the back and limbs, appear 3–6 d after bites by infected *Dermacentor andersoni* ticks in wooded areas of the Rocky Mountain region. Fever with a temperature of 39–40°C often shows a biphasic course, with eventual defervescence within 1 week, followed by complete recovery.

General principles

Certain epidemiological principles apply to human illnesses induced by arboviruses:

1. For each syndrome, several different serogroups may be involved, as in encephalitis due to western equine encephalitis (WEE), Powassan (POW) or La Crosse (LAC) virus infections.

2. There is a high proportion of subclinical infections to clinical illnesses, e.g. 64:1 to 209:1 for St Louis encephalitis (SLE) virus, but this proportion is considerably lower for dengue and miscellaneous tropical fevers.

3. There may be localization of a particular serotype within a particular geographic zone such as: (a) POW virus in forested areas of eastern North America; (b) WEE virus in irrigated farmlands of western North America, where SLE virus is also prevalent; Murray Valley encephalitis (MVE) virus in Australia. However, dengue is distributed widely throughout tropical regions of each continent and in Oceania.

4. Virus transmission by the bite of culicine mosquitoes or ixodid ticks occurs after ingestion of relatively small (0.1–10 plaque forming units) of virus in blood meals from naturally infected viraemic vertebrates after extrinsic incubation periods of 1–3 weeks at usual summertime temperatures.

5. Viraemia develops asymptomatically in birds (alphaviruses and mosquito-borne flaviviruses) and in mammals (bunyaviruses and tick-borne flaviviruses and orbiviruses) at titres sufficient to infect mosquitoes or ticks which imbibe blood meals from them.

LABORATORY DIAGNOSIS

Diagnosis of arbovirus infections depends on the isolation of virus from blood, cerebrospinal fluid or tissues, or on serology. Whenever possible, attempts should be channelled towards virus isolation, especially in febrile illnesses.

Virus isolation

The causative virus can be isolated from blood collected during the initial 3 d febrile illness induced by serotypes such as dengue, Ross River and yellow fever, when viraemia titres are maximum. Collect cerebrospinal fluid or brain biopsy during life, or brain at autopsy of fatal cases of encephalitis. Obtain liver from fatal cases of yellow fever. The isolation procedures are as follows:

1. Inoculate mammalian tissue cultures, e.g. continuous polyploid grivet monkey kidney (Vero) or baby hamster kidney (BHK) and incubate at 37°C under agarose overlay until plaques appear after 7–14 d. Determine the serotype in an extract of an excised plaque by neutralization, immunofluorescence or ELISA tests using appropriate monoclonal antibodies.

2. Inoculate continuous cultures of *A. albopictus* mosquito cells and incubate at 28°C for up to 10 d; examine cells for arbovirus antigen by immunofluorescence.

3. Inoculate acute-phase blood from dengue patients intrathoracically into male mosquitoes and incubate at 30°C for 14 d. Detect viral antigen in head squashes by direct immunofluorescence.

4. Inoculate acute-phase blood, or brain or liver suspensions, intracerebrally into suckling mice aged less than 48 h and examine daily up to 14 d for development of encephalitis (hunching, ruffled fur, convulsions, spasticity and, eventually, death). Remove brains from moribund mice and perform preliminary serogrouping by haemagglutination inhibition tests on sucrose–acetone extracts of brain suspension, followed by final serotypic identification by neutralization tests in suckling mice or by plaque reduction in Vero or BHK tissue cultures.

Serology

Serological tests frequently offer the only available means of laboratory diagnosis of encephalitis. The detection of a four-fold or greater rise of antibody titre by haemagglutinin isolation or ELISA tests on paired sera collected during the initial week and several days later after defervescence provides good evidence of concurrent infection. Antibodies detected by complement fixation first appear 2 or more weeks after onset and become undetectable by 3 years. Serotype-specific IgM antibody may be detected within 1–3 d after onset using an IgM capture ELISA test. IgM antibody wanes 6 weeks after onset and is replaced by IgG antibodies.

TREATMENT

Currently, no specific anti-arboviral therapeutic agent is available. Patients with encephalitis are managed supportively, using anticonvulsants as required, and ice-packs are applied when indicated to reduce hyperthermia. Similarly, in dengue and haemorrhagic fevers supportive nursing measures are employed, including intravenous infusions when indicated to replace fluids and electrolytes.

EPIDEMIOLOGY

Natural cycles

Arboviruses are maintained in nature by one of five natural cycles of infection involving mosquitoes, ticks or sandflies as arthropod vectors and birds or mammals as vertebrate reservoirs, with humans infected tangentially to these cycles (Fig. 52.3). In the arthropod, during the extrinsic incubation period, the virus multiplies initially in gut tissues after an infected blood meal, it then enters the haemocoelic fluid, in which it is carried to the salivary glands where further multiplication occurs, following which it is injected along with saliva into capillaries of new vertebrate hosts through bites. Vertebrates develop viraemia 1–2 d after arthropod bites, and this provides infective blood meals for fresh arthropods. The minimum infective dose of dengue and California serogroup viruses for mosquitoes is 10–100 times smaller than the dose required to infect mice or tissue cultures.

Examples of natural cycles (illustrated in Fig. 52.3) are:

1. Human–mosquito cycle as in dengue and urban yellow fever (Fig. 52.3a). Vectors are typically the highly domesticated *Aedes* mosquito species *A. aegypti*, but peridomestic *A. albopictus* has also been implicated; humans are the sole vertebrate reservoir.

2. Mosquito–bird cycle as in WEE (Fig. 52.3b). Vectors are typically *Culex tarsalis*, which breeds in grass-lined sloughs and irrigation run-offs; reservoirs are typically wild ducks which inhabit these locations; humans are infected tangentially to this rural cycle. Some infected *C. tarsalis* may infect domestic chickens, which in turn may be a source of viraemic blood for domestic *C. pipiens* mosquitoes; these may also transmit infection to humans.

3. Mosquito–mammal cycle, as in California serogroup viruses such as snowshoe hare (SSH) virus in the Canadian Arctic (Fig. 52.3c). Vectors are typically *A. communis*; reservoirs are snowshoe hares or ground squirrels; humans are infected tangentially to this rural cycle. With cool summertime arctic temperatures, mosquitoes transmit SSH virus after extrinsic incubation at 13°C. Virus is maintained from summer to summer by transovarial transmission; mosquitoes are not prevalent during the winter freeze-up. Birds are insusceptible to SSH virus.

Sylvan yellow fever is maintained in the forest canopies of tropical jungles year-round by a cycle involving *Haemagogus* spp. mosquitoes and arboreal primates; humans become infected during tree felling, when these forest canopy mosquitoes are brought to ground level.

4. Tick–mammal cycle as in POW virus (Fig. 52.3d). Vectors are *Ixodes* spp. ticks, reservoirs are groundhogs or tree squirrels; humans are infected tangentially to this cycle. Comparable natural cycles maintain louping ill virus in Scotland and tickborne encephalitis viruses throughout northern Europe.

5. Sandfly–human cycle as in sandfly fever of southern Europe and northern Mediterranean areas (Fig. 52.3e). *Phlebotomus* spp. are the vectors and humans are reservoirs; transovarial transmission maintains virus from one summer to the next. Rodents are reservoirs of some phleboviruses.

Epidemiological aspects of arbovirus infections with major impact on human health are described according to syndrome and infecting serotype (see also Table 52.2).

Alphaviruses

Western equine encephalitis (WEE) virus

This was first isolated from the brain of a horse with fatal encephalitis. WEE is found from the Mississippi Valley to California and northwards to western Canada. The mean incidence of WEE cases throughout the USA between 1966 and 1985 was 17 per year, comprising 7% of the total

a

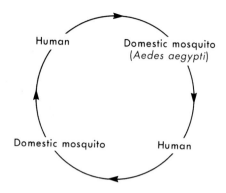

Human-Mosquito Cycle (e.g. dengue virus)

b

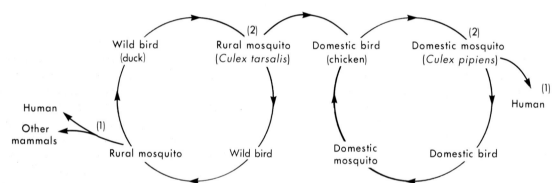

Bird-Mosquito Cycle (e.g. Western equine encephalitis)

c

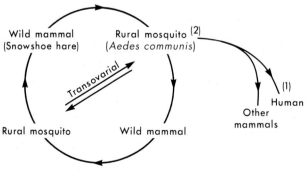

Mammal-Mosquito Cycle (e.g. California encephalitis)

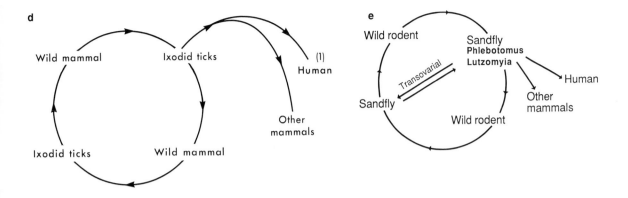

Fig. 52.3   Natural cycles of arbovirus infection. **a** Human–mosquito cycle of infection, e.g. dengue virus. **b** Bird–mosquito cycle of infection, e.g. western equine encephalitis; transmission of infection to humans may be prevented by (1) repellants and protective clothing and (2) mosquito abatement (larviciding, adulticiding). **c** Mammal–mosquito cycle, e.g. California serogroup viruses. **d** Mammal–tick cycle of infection, e.g. Powassan virus. **e** Mammal–sandfly cycle of infection, e.g. Phlebovirus. (Reproduced with permission from McLean D M 1980 *Virology in Health Care.* Williams and Wilkins, Baltimore, pp 170–174 and McLean D M 1988 *Virological Infections.* Thomas, Springfield, Illinois, pp 229–230.)

reported cases of arbovirus encephalitis. Cases occur only during June to September, when mosquitoes are abundant. Outbreaks of infection occur at intervals of a few years and are preceded by epizootic peaks of encephalitis among horses. The principal mosquito vector species in Canada and the western USA is *C. tarsalis*. Ducks and other water birds comprise the principal natural reservoirs.

Although all age groups may be involved, encephalitis due to WEE virus and California serogroup agents commonly affects children in whom the disease is often severe; SLE virus is most often seen in persons aged 55 years or more.

Eastern equine encephalitis (EEE) virus

This was also first isolated from the brain of a horse with fatal encephalitis. Human and horse cases of encephalitis have occurred repeatedly during the summer in Atlantic coastal areas extending from Massachusetts and New Jersey southwards to Florida and Texas. Occasionally, disease extends northwards into the Province of Quebec, Canada. During the 20 year period 1966–85 in the USA, EEE caused a mean of four cases of encephalitis per year, comprising 2% of the total cases of arbovirus encephalitis. Illness affected mainly humans aged under 14 years and

over 55 years, with overall case fatality rates as high as 69%. Most human cases occurred during late August and September, about 3 weeks after the peak of horse cases. Principal mosquito vectors are *Culiseta melanura*, which breeds in freshwater swamps; *Coquillettidia perturbans* and *A. sollicitans* are additional vectors during epidemic periods. Birds such as grackles and pheasants are important vertebrate reservoirs of infection. Human and horse cases of encephalitis due to EEE virus have been identified in Central and South America, but antigenic differences have been demonstrated between North American and South American EEE isolates.

Venezuelan equine encephalitis (VEE) virus

This occurs from Mexico through Central and South America to northern Argentina, including the Caribbean islands. It has also been seen in Texas during a major outbreak in Central America accompanied by neurological disturbances of varying severity, with case fatality rates of 0–33%. Large numbers of horses develop fatal encephalitis before and during the occurrence of human cases. Principal mosquito vectors during recent Central American epidemics were *Psorophora confinnis* and *C. taeniopus*. Vertebrate reservoirs include cotton rats, pigs and horses, but also a variety of birds. There are nine antigenic subtypes of VEE virus which vary in their virulence for humans and horses.

Ross River (RR) virus

This is distributed throughout coastal regions of Queensland and New South Wales, Australia, where it has caused epidemics of fever, maculopapular rash and arthralgia. It is maintained in nature by a cycle involving *C. annulirostris* and *A. vigilax* as the principal mosquito vectors, with flying foxes and marsupial mice as reservoirs; humans are infected tangentially.

Epidemics of polyarthritis with mild fever, sometimes accompanied by rash, have been attributed to RR virus in Fiji and American Samoa, New Caledonia, Wallis Island and also on Rarotonga where *A. polynesiensis* was confirmed virologically as the vector species.

Flaviviruses: mosquito-borne

St Louis encephalitis (SLE) virus

This was first isolated from the brain of a person dying with acute encephalitis in St Louis, Missouri. SLE activity is widely distributed throughout the USA from the Ohio and Mississippi Valleys and extending westwards through Colorado to California and Washington, northwards into the contiguous Canadian Provinces of Ontario, Manitoba and Saskatchewan, eastwards to Ohio and southwards to Florida and Texas. In common with WEE, SLE soon becomes prevalent in arid areas of the north-western and south-western USA which have been opened up for irrigation farming, due to the breeding of massive populations of the principal mosquito vector *C. tarsalis* in semipermanent collections of water in grassy locations. During the largest outbreak of the past quarter-century, in 1975, when 1815 of 2113 (86%) of confirmed cases of arbovirus encephalitis were due to SLE virus, the Chicago metropolitan area was heavily affected for the first time. Substantial SLE outbreaks affected the Houston, Texas, metropolitan area in 1964 and 1986, where attack rates and case fatality rates

were highest among persons over 55 years of age. Metropolitan Los Angeles in coastal southern California was first affected by SLE virus with 26 human cases of encephalitis in 1984. Mosquito vectors in California, the Rocky Mountains and plains states comprise mainly *C. tarsalis*, but *C. pipiens* and *C. quinquefasciatus* are important along the Mississippi Valley and eastwards. The salt marsh mosquitoes *C. restuans* and *A. sollicitans* may be important vectors in some localities.

Japanese B encephalitis (JBE) virus

The virus was first isolated from the brain of a fatal case of encephalitis in Tokyo, Japan. JBE virus continues to cause epidemics of encephalitis, affecting children, particularly in Japan, Korea, China, South-East Asia and Indonesia, with case fatality rates often exceeding 20%. *C. tritaeniorhynchus* mosquitoes are the principal vectors in Japan when maximum virus isolation rates from mosquitoes during late July occur simultaneously with human and equine epidemics. Important vertebrate reservoirs are black-crowned night herons and other water birds, but pigs may also serve as vertebrate reservoirs. In Malaysia, *C. gelidus* is an important vector as well as *C. tritaeniorhynchus*. In northern Thailand about 1500 cases of encephalitis due to JBE virus have been diagnosed each year since the late 1960s with most cases occurring during the rainy season in June, July and August. The case fatality rate of virologically confirmed cases is 33%, and about 1:300 humans infected with JBE virus develops encephalitis.

Murray Valley encephalitis (MVE) virus

This was first isolated from the brain of a fatal case of encephalitis at Mooroopna, Victoria, Australia. MVE caused epidemics of encephalitis in irrigated farming regions of the Murray-Darling River basin of south-eastern Australia during the summer months (January to March) of 1951 and 1974, with case fatality rates approaching 40%. MVE virus was isolated from *C. annulirostris* mosquitoes only during 1974 but not during intervening years, which suggests epidemic introduction of virus into this dry temperate region. In the irrigated Ord River region of Western Australia, encephalitis due to MVE virus has been recognized in 1974, 1978, 1981 and 1986, although the virus is endemic in this tropical region. Another endemic focus exists in the Gulf of Carpentaria region of Queensland. Natural cycles of transmission of MVE virus involve *C. annulirostris* as the principal mosquito vector and water birds as reservoirs.

Yellow fever (YF) virus

This was first isolated in Ghana, West Africa, from the blood of a male patient with fever, headache, backache and prostration. YF virus is prevalent throughout tropical Africa and tropical Central and South America, including the Caribbean islands. There are two epidemiological patterns of YF. In the sylvan cycle, virus is maintained in monkeys by *Haemogogus* mosquitoes. Man is infected tangentially when entering the area, e.g. to work as a forester. In the urban cycle, man-to-man transmission is via *A. aegypti*, which breeds close to human habitation in water, in pits and scrap containers such as oil drums.

In the Americas, a mean of 135 cases of YF were reported each year from Bolivia, Brazil, Columbia, Ecuador and Peru, and from Trinidad–Tobago and Venezuela only between 1978 and 1980. During 1988, 196 cases of YF were reported in Peru with 167 deaths, but no human cases of YF were reported in Trinidad despite deaths of howler monkeys. In South America, most cases occurred in males aged 15–45 years, particularly colonists and temporary workers on agricultural and forestry projects in enzootic areas, as well as residents of those areas. The incidence usually peaks during March and April when populations of *Haemagogus* mosquitoes are highest during the rainy season.

In Africa, YF is endemic throughout West, Central and East Africa, principally between latitudes 15°N and 15°S, extending northwards into Ethiopia and Sudan. Continuing activity has been encountered in Senegal and the Gambia along the west coast and in Upper Volta. Attack rates of 3–4% have been recorded with a case fatality rate of 19% and the ratio of inapparent to apparent infections is about 12:1. In Ethiopia between 1960 and 1962, a major YF epidemic involved about 100 000 cases with a case fatality rate of about 30%. Spread of infection occurred both in irrigated cultivated areas, and in forests and arid areas. Forest mosquito vectors were *A. africanus* but in villages the mosquito vectors were probably *A. simpsoni*, which breeds in peridomestic situations; *Colobus* monkeys served as natural reservoirs.

Dengue (DEN) virus

The infection is endemic in all tropical regions between latitudes 23.5°N and 23.5°S. Typical dengue is induced by any of four serotypes of DEN virus. However, arboviruses from other genera such as the alphavirus serotypes chikungunya (CHIK) and Ross River (RR), bunyavirus serotypes including Oropouche (ORO) and phlebovirus serotypes such as Rift Valley fever (RVF) and Toscana (TOS) have also induced dengue-like disease. These latter agents are differentiated from the dengue virus by elaborate serological procedures.

Dengue is maintained in nature by a cycle involving humans as both reservoirs and definitive hosts, and domestic mosquitoes, principally *A. aegypti*, as vectors. However, the peridomestic mosquito species *A. albopictus* is recognized increasingly as a significant dengue vector in many urban localities.

Dengue has caused numerous outbreaks throughout the south-west Pacific region since it was first encountered among servicemen during the Second World War when the average monthly attack rate of 54 per 1000 peaked to 197 per 1000 during the wet season. Subsequently, in the south-west Pacific, several serotypes of dengue have affected Tahiti with haemorrhagic dengue first encountered in 1971. In addition to *A. aegypti* other species have been implicated as vectors, including *A. scutellaris hebrideus* in New Guinea, *A. polynesiensis* in Tahiti and *A. cooki* in Niue. Cases of imported dengue occurred in Hawaii during 1943 and 1944, probably through the inadvertent transport of dengue-infected mosquitoes on ships returning from dengue-endemic Pacific islands. Currently, with the absence of *A. aegypti*, Hawaii is dengue-free. Also during the Second World War dengue was imported into the Japanese port cities of Kobe, Nagasaki and Osaka.

Dengue activity continues in tropical countries of the Pacific rim, including Australia. Most south-east Asian countries, including Indonesia, Malaysia, Thailand, Vietnam, China, the Philippines and India, experience repeated epidemics of dengue due to all four serotypes, with most cases occurring between June and November. Mostly children are affected, 25% or more of whom may develop haemorrhagic fever. Most epidemics occur in urban areas and villages where *A. aegypti* is abundant, but not in rural environments.

Dengue is endemic throughout tropical Africa, including Nigeria in the west and Mozambique in the east, and also in Middle Eastern countries such as South Yemen.

Caribbean countries have been involved by 10 epidemics waves of dengue between 1827 and 1969, with little evidence of clinical dengue during interepidemic periods. All four dengue serotypes have been implicated in dengue outbreaks affecting residents of Caribbean islands and adjacent portions of Central and South America. There were 43 435 cases reported in the Caribbean region in 1984. Cases of dengue have been frequently imported into the continental USA following visits to dengue-endemic Caribbean countries, including 67 cases during 1984. During 1986, dengue was reported in 233 cases in the USA. Although most infections occurred among travellers returning from the Caribbean, nine cases of indigenous dengue occurred among residents of Texas where *A. aegypti* is prevalent during the nine warmer months each year. Since 1985, *A. albopictus* has been introduced into metropolitan communities of Texas and mid-west, north-east and north-west states along with used motor tyre casings which have been imported for retreading from Japan, South Korea and several South-East Asian countries. The peridomestic mosquito *A. albopictus* was first identified as a dengue vector in Malaysia during the 1960s and it transmits dengue both in the human–mosquito cycle and by transovarial transfer. These factors raise serious concerns that both *A. aegypti* and *A. albopictus* may transmit dengue indigenously in USA, which hitherto has been considered to be dengue-free.

Flaviviruses: tick-borne

Powassan (POW) virus

This, the sole North American tick-borne flavivirus, was first isolated from the brain of a fatal human case of encephalitis in Powassan, Ontario, Canada. To date, POW virus has been recognized as the cause of 19 cases of encephalitis and two deaths among residents of forested areas of Ontario, Quebec and Nova Scotia in Canada, plus New York State and Pennsylvania in the USA. All cases occurred between June and October. Principal tick vector species in Ontario are *Ixodes cookei*, which feeds on groundhogs, and *I. marxi*, which feeds on tree squirrels; both these mammals serve as reservoirs.

Tick-borne encephalitis (TBE) viruses

These agents, related to but distinct from POW virus, have regularly been incriminated as causes of encephalitis or aseptic meningitis from Scotland, Scandinavia, central and northern Europe and Siberia to the Kamchatka Peninsula. Human infections may range in severity from mild biphasic meningo-encephalitis, which is characteristic of the central European TBE viruses and the Scottish louping ill virus (so named because it induces a leaping gait in infected sheep), to a severe form of polio-encephalomyelitis with a case fatality rate of 2–30%, which is characteristic of Far-Eastern Russian spring–summer encephalitis virus. In Scotland and Europe, natural cycles involve *I. ricinus* ticks as vectors and mice, shrews and other small rodents as reservoirs, with infection transferred tangentially to sheep or other farm animals, and also to humans. In Siberia, *I. persulcatus* ticks serve as vectors.

Bunyaviruses: bunyavirus genus

California (CAL) serogroup

There are more than 10 serotypes and the viruses are related antigenically to the prototype California encephalitis virus. In the USA, encephalitis and aseptic meningitis arise commonly from infections with La Crosse virus (LAC), which was first isolated from the brain of a fatal case of encephalitis at La Crosse, Wisconsin. Other serotypes occasionally associated with aseptic meningitis are snowshoe hare (SSH) virus, which was first isolated from the blood of a snowshoe hare in Montana, and Jamestown Canyon (JC) virus, which was first isolated from *Culiseta inornata* mosquitoes collected at Jamestown Canyon, Colorado. In central Europe, febrile illness sometimes associated with aseptic meningitis arises from infection with Tahyna (TAH) virus, which was first isolated from *A. caspius* mosquitoes collected near Tahyna, Czechslovakia.

Currently, CAL serogroup viruses are the commonest arboviruses associated with encephalitis in the USA, during most years, with most cases due to LAC virus. Highest attack rates occur in states adjoining the Great Lakes from Minnesota and Wisconsin through Illinois and Indiana to Ohio, affecting mainly children aged less than 15 years. Abundant tree holes in wooded areas provide optimum breeding sites for the principal mosquito vector *A. triseriatus*, but rainwater collected in disused motor tyres has proved a suitable breeding ground for *A. triseriatus* in suburban locations. Since adult mosquitoes die in winter, CAL serogroup viruses survive through transovarial transmission. Principal vertebrate reservoirs are tree squirrels and chipmunks.

Snowshoe hare (SSH) virus. This CAL serogroup agent is endemic throughout the boreal forest and arctic regions of Canada. Rarely, SSH virus has caused human cases of aseptic meningitis. Principal mosquito vectors are *A. communis* throughout the short arctic summer of June and July, with *Cs. inornata*, an additional springtime vector, and *A. hexodontus*, a late summertime vector. Overwintering of virus is by the transovarial route. Natural vertebrate reservoirs comprise snowshoe hares and arctic ground squirrels.

Oropouche (ORO). This virus was first isolated in Trinidad but is also endemic in tropical forest surrounding the mouth of the Amazon River. Large outbreaks of febrile illness were attributed to ORO virus in Belem during 1961, 1968 and in smaller communities in adjacent areas during 1987–88.

Bunyaviruses: phlebovirus genus

Rift Valley fever (RVF) virus

This virus was first isolated from sheep during an epizootic causing abortion and death in the Rift Valley near Lake Niavasha, Kenya, but is present from South Africa to Egypt. Severe epidemics affected sheep, cattle and humans in South Africa during 1951 when *A. caballus*, *A. circumluteolus* and *Cs. theileri* were found to be vectors, with sheep, cattle, buffaloes and rodents as reservoirs. A large outbreak of RVF occurred in Egypt during 1977, involving about 18 000 humans with a case fatality rate of 3.3%.

Sandfly fever (phlebovirus) group

These viruses are distributed throughout the European and North African countries surrounding the Mediterranean Sea, extending eastward through Israel and Iran to West Pakistan and central India. Sandfly fever — Naples (SFN) virus was first isolated from the sera of US servicemen in Naples during an outbreak during the Second World War. Sandfly fever — Sicilian (SFS) virus was also recovered from US servicemen during a comparable epidemic of fever in Sicily. Epidemics of dengue-like fever occur during the sandfly season (June to September) and affect mainly newcomers rather than long-term residents. Natural vectors are *Phlebotomus papatasi* and other phlebotomine sandflies. Isolation of virus from male sandflies collected during July suggests transovarial transfer of virus. The natural cycle of sandfly fever appears to involve solely man as definitive host and reservoir, with sandflies as vectors.

Toscana (TOS) virus

This virus was first isolated from sandflies collected in Tuscany, Italy. TOS virus is antigenically distinct from SFN and SFS viruses within the phlebovirus antigenic group. It is transmitted by *Phlebotomus perniciosus* sandflies and is transferred transovarially. Natural reservoirs of TOS virus appear to be small rodents (*Apodemus sylvaticus*). Imported infections have been identified in persons returning to Sweden and the USA following visits to TOS-endemic regions.

Bunyaviruses: nairovirus genus

Crimean-Congo haemorrhagic fever (CCHF) virus

There are two antigenically identical arboviruses within the genus *Nairovirus*. Prototype Crimean haemorrhagic fever (CHF) virus was isolated from the serum of a man with fatal haemorrhagic fever in the Samarkand region of Uzbek, USSR; Congo (CON) virus was first isolated from the serum of a child with fever and arthralgia in Zaire. CCHF is distributed widely throughout tropical Africa, from Mauritania and Senegal eastwards through Upper Volta, Nigeria, Congo, Zaire, Uganda, Kenya, the Middle East and West Pakistan, and southwards to South Africa. Haemorrhagic fever due to CCHF virus is also prevalent in Bulgaria and the Soviet Republics adjacent to the Black Sea and Caspian Sea. The geographic distribution of CCHF virus corresponds to that of *Hyalomma* sp. ticks, which have yielded numerous virus isolations from field-collected specimens. Hares are the natural vertebrate reservoirs in Africa and the USSR.

Bunyaviruses: hantavirus genus

Hantaan (HTN) virus. This induces *haemorrhagic fever with renal syndrome* (HFRS) in humans, which is characterized by fever of over 38°C, haemorrhagic manifestations with thrombocytopaenia (petechiae, gastro-intestinal bleeding) and evidence of renal dysfunction. Virologically confirmed haemorrhagic fever due to HTN virus has occurred widely in Japan and Korea. In China, haemorrhagic fever extends southwards to Shanghai, and north of the Himalayas through into Manchuria. Similar haemorrhagic disease has

occurred repeatedly in the USSR. In Scandinavia, HFRS is induced by the serologically related Puumala virus, and serological evidence of hantavirus infection has been demonstrated in patients with HFRS in Scotland, France and Greece. The peak incidence of HFRS in Scandinavia and China is during the winter.

Hantaviruses are typical examples of rodent-borne viruses (roboviruses). Rodents are the principal natural reservoirs, and excrete virus in urine for prolonged periods; virus is transmitted to humans by contact with fomites contaminated by rodent urine.

CONTROL

Strategies for prevention of arbovirus infections depend on either vector control or active immunization with vaccine.

Vector control

This is possible for mosquito-borne viruses in urban and suburban localities; suppression of populations of vector mosquito species can halt virus transmission during epidemics. This can be achieved by:

1. The use of insecticides to kill adult mosquitoes ('adulticiding'), e.g. aerial sprays of Malathion, although this may kill many other species.
2. The elimination of breeding sites of domestic *A. aegypti* by removal of objects such as tin cans and motor tyres that could contain rainwater, both near human habitations and in public parks and drainage systems, has prevented occurrence of dengue in Singapore and urban yellow fever in metropolitan areas in Caribbean countries.
3. The chemical control of larvae, termed 'larviciding', by use of Temephos granules or Malathion in oil for even coverage of small breeding sites, has reduced mosquito vector populations substantially in irrigated localities in California and elsewhere.
4. The biological control of larvae is attempted by microbiological agents such as *Bacillus thuringiensis israeliensis*, larvivorous fish, flatworms or mermethid nematodes, or insect growth regulators such as the juvenile hormone mimic Methoprene.

5. Personal protection against bites by mosquitoes involves a combination of wearing protective clothing, preferably impregnated with permethrin, screening of dwellings to prevent entry of mosquitoes and frequent application of mosquito repellants such as diethyl toluamide to exposed skin areas. For tick-borne viruses, protective clothing should be worn outdoors, followed by rigorous inspection to remove attached ticks from skin.

Vaccines

Prevention of illness following exposure to arbovirus infections is restricted to relatively few serotypes.

Encephalitis viruses

Human and animal infections due to VEE and JBE viruses have been prevented by immunization with live and killed vaccines respectively. Although effective killed vaccines have been developed for prevention of WEE in horses, these are unsatisfactory for administration to humans.

VEE vaccine

This is a live attenuated strain. Widespread vaccination of horses at the advancing edge of epizootics is highly effective in protecting against encephalitis in both horses and humans.

Yellow fever

Prevention against clinical attacks of yellow fever has been outstandingly successful during the past half century through the use of attenuated YF vaccine. The 17D strain, used exclusively in the Americas, and extensively in Africa, was derived from a virulent prototype strain. Each dose of lyophilized vaccine contains 1000 mouse LD_{50} of the 17D virus, which is administered subcutaneously. Vaccine recipients have demonstrated immunity to natural challenge by YF virus commencing 10 d after vaccination and persisting for at least 10 years. The FN strain derived from mouse brain-passaged YF virus has been used

successfully for many years for YF immunization by scarification in certain equatorial regions of Africa. However, adverse reactions, such as fever and occasional encephalopathy, occur more commonly after vaccination with the FN strain than the 17D strain.

Dengue

Administration of the live attenuated MD-1 vaccine strain of DEN-1 virus can produce a three-fold reduction in dengue attack rates among vaccine recipients during an outbreak. Other live attenuated vaccines have induced high rates of seroconversion in human volunteers but dengue-like symptoms are experienced frequently by recipients, thereby rendering these candidate vaccines unsuitable for human use in their present form.

RUBELLA

Rubella (German measles) was first described in the 18th century and was considered a mild illness with only occasional complications until 1941 when the association between maternal rubella in pregnancy and congenital abnormalities in the infant was described by an Australian ophthalmologist, Sir Norman Gregg. He noted an increased incidence of congenital cataracts in children. When questioned the mothers gave a history of having had rubella in early pregnancy when there had been an epidemic in Australia. Since then the importance of maternal rubella for the fetus has been confirmed by many studies.

Description

Rubella virus was first isolated in cell culture in 1962. It is a single-stranded RNA virus with an envelope and is classified as a flavivirus, being the only member of the genus *Rubivirus*. Virions are pleomorphic in appearance and 50–70 nm in diameter with a nucleocapsid of icosahedral symmetry. Rubella is inactivated by many chemical agents. The single-stranded RNA is infective and replication occurs in the cytoplasm of infected cells. Virions acquire the envelope by budding from cell membranes either into intracellular vesicles or to the exterior. There are three major virion polypeptides, C and the envelope glyco-proteins E1 and E2. No major antigenic difference between virus strains has been demonstrated. The virus envelope carries a haemagglutinin (E1), present as 5-6 nm projections, which will agglutinate the erythrocytes of 1-day-old chicks, pigeons, sheep and humans, a characteristic which is utilized in the haemagglutination inhibition test for specific antibodies. Experimentally, infection can be transmitted to rhesus monkeys, rabbits and some other animals, but humans are the only naturally infected species. Virus can be isolated in a range of primary and continuous cell lines, e.g. Vero, RK13 and BHK-21 cells, but in only some cell lines, such as RK13, does a cytopathic effect occur. In other cell lines the presence of virus must be demonstrated by immunofluorescence with specific antibody or by resistance to superinfection with another unrelated virus such as echovirus 11. Only one antigenic type of rubella virus is recognized, although minor differences can be found between strains.

Clinical features and pathogenesis

Postnatal rubella

The incubation period for postnatal primary rubella is 12–21 d, with an average of 16–17 d. Virus may be excreted in the throat for u to a week before and after the rash and this covers the period of infectivity. The characteristic clinical feature is a macular rash which usually appears first on the face and then spreads to the trunk and limbs. Particularly in childhood the rash may be fleeting and perhaps 50% of infections in children are asymptomatic. In adults asymptomatic rubella is less common. General features such as minor pyrexia, malaise and lymphadenopathy also occur, with the suboccipital nodes being those most commonly enlarged and tender.

Arthralgia is uncommon in children but may occur in up to 60% of adult females. The joints commonly involved are the fingers, wrists, ankles and knees and, although arthralgia usually only lasts a few days, it may occasionally persist for some months. Encephalitis and thrombocytopenia are rare complications of rubella and usually re-covery is complete. Unlike a number of other virus infections, rubella appears to present little danger to the immunocompromised patient, in whom the clinical features are similar to those seen in normal individuals.

Rubella reinfection is diagnosed when an antibody response is demonstrated in someone who has either had natural rubella or has been successfully immunized. Such reinfections are seldom clinically apparent and are usually found when someone is investigated after contact with rubella. It is very uncommon for fetal infection and damage to occur in subclinical reinfection. It can be difficult, however, to distinguish serologically between subclinical primary rubella, which is of major risk to the fetus, and re-infection. The rare reinfection which is clinically apparent must be assumed to present a risk to the fetus similar to that of primary rubella.

Rubella is notoriously difficult to diagnose clinically, as other virus infections, such as some enteroviruses and human parvovirus B19, can present with identical clinical features. For correct diagnosis laboratory investigation is essential and a history of rubella is an unreliable indicator of immunity unless it has been serologically confirmed.

Congenital rubella

If the fetus is infected during a primary maternal infection a wide spectrum of abnormalities may occur. The classical congenital rubella syndrome (CRS) triad consists of abnormalities of the eyes, ears and heart. Abnormalities of the eyes, which may be bilateral or unilateral, include cataracts, micro-ophthalmia, glaucoma and pigmentary retinopathy, which may result in blindness. Bilateral or unilateral sensorineural deafness may be present at birth, although it may not be detected until later in life; it may increase in severity as the child gets older. There are many possible heart defects, with patent ductus arteriosus, pulmonary artery and valvular stenosis, and ventricular septal defect being most common.

The baby will often have a low birth weight due to intra-uterine growth retardation. A purpuric rash due to thrombocytopenia may be present at birth but this usually resolves, as does hepatosplenomegaly. Microcephaly, psychomotor retardation and behavioural disorders are manifestations of central nervous system involvement. Rarely, a persistent infection of the central nervous system occurs called *progressive rubella subacute panencephalitis*, which is similar clinically to the *subacute sclerosing panencephalitis* due to measles virus. Other problems which may not be present at birth but which may present later in life include pneumonitis, diabetes mellitus, growth hormone deficiency and abnormalities of thyroid function.

The fetus may be so severely affected that intra-uterine death with abortion or stillbirth occurs. Many infected babies, however, are born with no abnormalities and the risk to the fetus depends on the gestation at which primary rubella occurs. If maternal rubella occurs in the first trimester the risk is considerable, as more than 70% of babies will be affected and have some or many of the abnormalities described above. If rubella occurs in the 4th month of pregnancy the risk reduces to approximately 20% and the only abnormality likely to be seen is sensorineural deafness. Maternal rubella before conception is unlikely to harm the fetus. After the 16th week of pregnancy, although fetal infection still occurs, congenital abnormalities are very infrequent and no more likely to occur than in an apparently uncomplicated pregnancy.

Pathogenesis

Rubella virus is transmitted by the airborne route. Infection is established in the upper respiratory tract and towards the end of the incubation period a viraemia occurs and seeds the target organs such as the skin and joints. Most of the clinical features are probably a consequence of the host's immune response to the virus, e.g. virus can be demonstrated not only in individual lesions of the macular rash but also in unaffected skin. During the viraemia the virus is able to infect the placenta and cross this barrier to infect the differentiating cells of the fetus. If such fetal infection occurs in early pregnancy a persistent infection is likely. The congenital abnormalities arise from a number of effects of the virus infection. Cell division is slowed, cell differentiation is disordered and damage to small blood vessels may occur. Such effects may lead to the abnormalities seen at birth, but the persistence of infection may result in the clinical problems presenting later in life, either due to direct damage, such as late-onset deafness, or due to immunopathological mechanisms, such as pneumonitis. Virus can persist for many years in babies infected during early gestation, but persistent infection is rare in later pregnancy when the babies are not damaged.

Diagnosis

Postnatal rubella

Clinical diagnosis is notoriously unreliable and laboratory investigation is required if a diagnosis of rubella has important implications, such as in the pregnant patient. As subclinical rubella may occur, pregnant women should also be investigated if they are exposed to someone with possible rubella. Investigation by virus isolation is not indicated as it is unreliable and time-consuming. Serological diagnosis is the method of choice, using techniques to detect total rubella antibody or rubella-specific IgG, and rubella-specific IgM. In primary rubella, specific antibody becomes detectable about the time of the rash, although there may be a delay of 7–10 d, and rapidly increases in concentration (Fig. 52.4). Specific IgM usually, but not always, precedes specific IgG by 1–2 d, but unlike specific IgG, which persists for life, specific IgM is usually only detectable for 1–3 months. Thus, seroconversion may be demonstrated if a serum is obtained soon after contact, prior to the illness, and is examined in

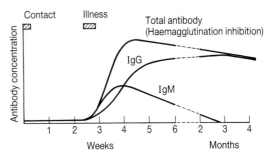

Fig. 52.4 Serological response in primary rubella.

parallel with a sample collected at or soon after the rash; primary infection is confirmed by the development of specific IgM. If serum is collected after the rash or more than 12–14 d after contact, any total rubella antibody or specific IgG may have resulted from recent infection or infection many years previously. Tests for specific IgM must be used to determine if the infection was recent.

Tests for total rubella antibody or rubella-specific IgG are also used for serological screening to ascertain susceptibility and whether rubella immunization is indicated. Many assays of appropriate sensitivity and specificity are available. False-positive results must be avoided as a susceptible woman would not be immunized and may not be investigated if contact or illness occurs.

Congenital rubella

The majority of babies with congenital rubella syndrome excrete large amounts of virus for the first few months of life and, indeed, are highly infectious for their attendants. Thus, virus isolation in cell culture from throat swab or urine is indicated although many laboratories may not have appropriate cell lines readily available. A more sensitive and widely available technique in the first 3–6 months of life is serological testing for specific IgM. Maternal IgM does not cross the placenta so the detection of specific IgM is diagnostic of intra-uterine infection. Specific IgG crosses the placenta from the mother so its detection in the early months of life is no help in diagnosis. Maternal IgG has a half-life in the infant of 3–4 weeks, however, so persistence to the age of 9–12 months is diagnostic of congenital rubella. It is uncommon for the specific IgM to persist to 1 year of age. Occasionally, if an older child presents with deafness, a diagnosis of possible congenital rubella may be suspected. It is impossible, however, to discriminate specific IgG resulting from intra-uterine infection from that persisting after postnatal infection, so the reliable diagnosis of congenital infection in older children is impossible.

Epidemiology

Rubella has a world-wide distribution with infection being endemic in all countries which have not had a highly successful infant immunization policy. Outbreaks usually occur in spring and early summer, with major epidemics occurring every 4–8 years. Infection is common in childhood. Before immunization in the UK, 80–85% of young adults would have had rubella. With rubella vaccine being offered to all adolescent girls in the UK only approximately 2–5% of young adult females are now susceptible, compared with 15% of young adult males.

Control

Passive prophylaxis

There is little evidence that administering normal human immunoglobulin after contact reduces the risk of maternal rubella and fetal infection, although it may attenuate the illness.

Active prophylaxis

Attenuated live rubella virus vaccines have been widely available since the early 1970s. They are safe, although occasional fleeting rashes and arthralgia occur. Seroconversion occurs in over 95% of susceptible vaccinees and protection persists for more than 15 years. Although vaccine virus may be isolated from the throat of vaccinees, there is no evidence of transmission to susceptible contacts. As it is a live virus vaccine, administration in pregnancy is contra-indicated and pregnancy should be avoided for the month following immunization. Although the vaccine virus has been shown to infect the fetus, there is no evidence of teratogenicity, so if a susceptible pregnant woman is inadvertently immunized she should be reassured that the risk to her baby is very remote. It is advisable, however, that all women of child-bearing age are screened for rubella antibody before immunization so that only susceptible women are offered vaccine.

The objective of rubella immunization is to eradicate congenital rubella. Two possible approaches are possible. In the UK it was decided in the early 1970s to target the vaccine at girls aged 11–14 years and susceptible adult women, identified by screening all pregnant women and women attending such facilities as family plan-

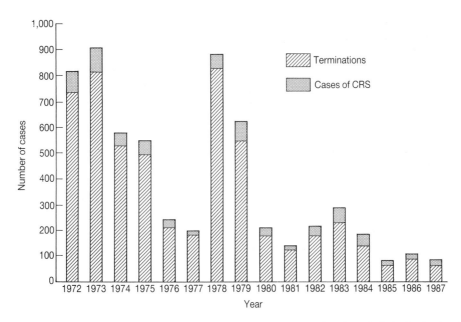

Fig. 52.5 Cases of congenital rubella syndrome and terminations of pregnancy related to rubella in England and Wales. (Courtesy of Dr E Miller, Public Health Laboratory Service, Communicable Disease Surveillance Centre, London.)

ning clinics, occupational health services and on the initiative of general practitioners. Such a policy was adopted because of uncertainties about the duration of protection and the belief that women would have better protection from having had natural rubella; 50% of adolescent girls would have had natural rubella. It was also thought that vaccine-induced protection would be boosted by occasional exposure to natural rubella. It has become apparent over the last few years that such a policy would never achieve eradication as 10–20 cases of congenital rubella and 100–200 terminations of pregnancy still occur each year in the UK (Fig. 52.5). In the second approach, which was adopted in 1988, all children are

immunized in an attempt to eradicate rubella from the community and so avoid exposure of any pregnant woman who is susceptible. Thus, the immunization schedule was augmented by offering rubella vaccine together with mumps and measles vaccine (MMR vaccine) to all children at 15 months of age. For a few years mumps, measles and rubella vaccine will also be offered to children at school entry. Support for such a strategy comes from the success achieved in almost eliminating congenital rubella in the USA by offering rubella vaccine to all children in the 2nd year of life. To achieve such success, however, means that there must be at least a 90% uptake of vaccine in infancy.

RECOMMENDED READING

Best J M, Banatvala J E 1987 Rubella. In: Zuckerman A J, Banatvala J E, Pattison J R (eds) *Principles and Practice of Clinical Virology.* Wiley, Chichester

McLean D M 1988 *Virological Infections.* Thomas, Springfield, Illinois

Miller E, Cradock-Watson J E, Pollock T M 1982 Consequences of confirmed maternal rubella at successive stages of pregnancy. *Lancet* ii: 781–784

Miller C L, Miller E, Waight P A 1987 Rubella susceptibility and the continuing risk of infection in pregnancy. *British*

Medical Journal 294: 1277–1278

Monath T P 1987 Yellow fever: a medically neglected disease. Report on a seminar. *Review of Infectious Diseases* 9: 165–175

Public Health Laboratory Service Working Party 1988 Laboratory diagnosis of rubella. *PHLS Microbiology Digest* 5: 49–52

Report 1985 Arthropod-borne and rodent-borne viral diseases. *WHO Technical Report Series 719.* World Health Organization, Geneva

53

Arenaviruses and filoviruses

Lassa fever; Marburg and Ebola fevers

J. F. Peutherer

Members of these two unrelated RNA virus groups cause severe infections in humans. The clinical features can include fever and haemorrhage and so they are causes of viral haemorrhagic fever. Other viruses associated with a similar presentation are described in Chapter 52 on insect-borne viruses.

ARENAVIRUSES

Properties

In the virions of this family the RNA is single stranded and of negative-sense and exists as two molecules, the L and S segments. The total molecular weight is between 3.2×10^6 and 4.8×10^6 and there is an associated RNA transcriptase. Morphologically the virions consist of an envelope enclosing the helical RNA nucleocapsid; they vary considerably in size, ranging from about 100–150 nm in diameter (Fig. 53.1). The virions usually enclose some cell ribosomes during assembly and thus gain their characteristic grainy appearance in the electron microscope ('arena' is the Latin for sand). There are at least four virion polypeptides, some of which are glycosylated and found in the envelope as short surface projections. The arenaviruses of importance to man are the South American Junin and Machupo viruses; several others are grouped as the African Tacaribe complex. However, Lassa fever virus is the important virus in Africa. Antigenic cross-reactions can be shown between the viruses. Lymphocytic chorio-meningitis (LCM) virus has been much studied in the laboratory because of the effect of the age of the animal and its immune status on the disease presentation after experimental inoculation. It is not a major human pathogen although cases of meningitis have been described. It is world-wide in distribution.

Replication

Viruses can be grown in several mammalian cell cultures, but vero (grivet monkey kidney) and BHK (hamster kidney) are widely used. A minimal cytopathic effect is produced, and cytoplasmic inclusion bodies are formed. A role for the cell nucleus in viral replication has been proposed and nucleocapsids can be detected within the nucleus. The coding on the genome is antisense; this means that genes can be expressed and regulated independently. Thus the expression of the nucleocapsid (N) protein can be separated from that of the envelope glycoprotein (GPC) although both genes are on the S strand of RNA. Hairpin sequences are present in the viral RNA and the complementary strand and these may interrupt the progression of the viral RNA polymerase and thus affect gene expression. It has been shown that during infection RNA molecules consisting of sequences from both the viral RNA and host cell ribosomal RNA (rRNA) are produced. Both the L and S molecules contain sequences which bind the 18S subunit of rRNA.

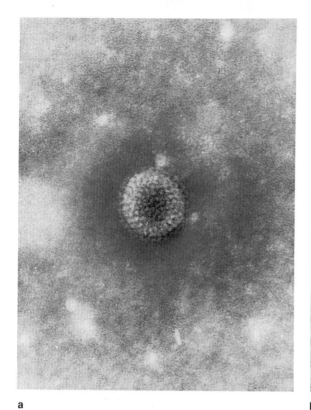

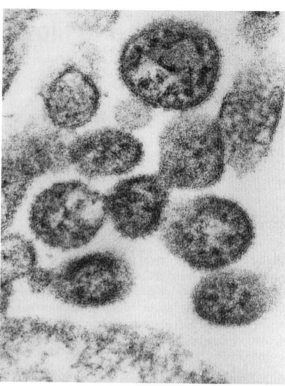

a

b

Fig. 53.1 a Lassa fever virus
b Lassa fever virus cross section showing granular appearance of cell ribosomes.

The N protein is the major component of the virion and of infected cells where it is detectable within a few hours after infection and remains so even after virus synthesis has declined. Viral glycoproteins are detectable on cell membranes also within a few hours of infection. Persistently infected cultures arise readily.

Clinical features and pathogenesis

South American haemorrhagic fevers

Argentinian and Bolivian haemorrhagic fevers are caused by Junin and Machupo viruses, respectively. The incubation period is 1–2 weeks with a 'flu-like' prodromal illness. In serious cases petechiae develop and the patient bleeds from the gastrointestinal tract. Fluid is lost from the circulation and hypotension and oliguria may ensue. Neurological signs occur in many patients. The mortality rate varies in different outbreaks, but is within the range 5–30%, usually with death due to hypovolaemic shock.

The viruses are widespread in the body and at post-mortem there is evidence of lymphadenopathy, lymphocyte loss from the spleen and bone marrow and endothelial damage in small blood vessels. Haemorrhage is related to the capillary damage. During the earlier stages, there is a drop in the number of circulating leucocytes and platelets, resulting from infection of bone marrow precursor cells. About half of those infected have evidence of neurological damage, with tremor as a feature in most cases. There is no clear evidence that the host immune response plays an important role in the pathogenesis of these diseases, although specific antibody appears when the patient is recovering. There is some evidence that there are differences in tissue tropism, in that neurological involvement may be a feature with some virus strains.

Lassa fever

The incubation period is 1–3 weeks, with an insidious onset of fever, headache, muscle and joint pain: pharyngitis is usually present, with an unproductive cough. Electrocardiogram abnormalities are common. Within a few days the fever increases and the patient complains of abdominal and retrosternal pain, diarrhoea and vomiting. The patient is lethargic, with oedema of the face and neck and lymphadenopathy. The blood pressure is often low. Recovery is within 1–3 weeks. In fatal cases the fever is maintained, and deterioration occurs rapidly within the first 2 weeks. This is associated with hypovolaemia, pleural effusion, ascites and anuria. At post-mortem examination there is often liver damage. A poor prognosis is associated with bleeding from the nose, gums, gut and vagina, linked to platelet dysfunction. Neurological complications are also a poor prognostic sign, particularly an encephalopathy rather than the tinnitus and deafness seen in about one-third of patients. The disease is especially severe in the later stages of pregnancy with a mortality rate of 20% which is reduced if the pregnancy terminates.

There is an early drop in the lymphocyte and platelet counts. Endothelial cells are damaged leading to a loss of fluid from the circulation. Specific antibodies are produced to the virus but, unlike the South American fevers, this is not associated with clearance of the virus: neutralizing antibodies are usually absent. It is assumed therefore, that clearance of the virus depends on cell-mediated immune responses. Viraemia can persist for some weeks in those who make a slow recovery and rises to high levels in fatal cases. The level of viraemia is greater in Lassa fever than in South American haemorrhagic fevers: this may be relevant to the observation that Lassa fever virus can transmit man to man whereas the others do not.

Lymphocytic choriomeningitis (LCM) virus

This virus occurs throughout the world in rodents, and most recognized human infections have been acquired from contact with laboratory animals such as mice and hamsters. Clinically apparent infections are rare but may present as a non-specific febrile illness, meningitis or encephalitis. The incubation period is 1–2 weeks and the illness is usually of short duration. Long-term effects have been described and include headache, paralysis and psychological changes. There is little evidence for the involvement of the host immune system in the pathogenesis of the disease and the effects are probably due to virus replication. LCM virus can be isolated directly from the brain at post-mortem.

In contrast, LCM virus infection of mice has been studied extensively due to the importance of the immune response in pathogenesis. Thus, if mice are infected within 24 h of birth they do not develop acute disease but become carriers for the rest of their lives. This reflects the lack of an effective immune response at this stage of development of the mouse. In contrast, inoculation of the adult mouse leads to a fatal choriomeningitis due to the activity of cell-mediated immune responses directed to a region of CP2, one of the envelope glycoproteins expressed on the surface of infected cells. Mice infected early in life do not become tolerant to the virus as specific antibody is produced. However, this may be difficult to detect as it is bound in antigen-antibody complexes in the circulation; some of these are deposited in tissues such as the kidney to cause a chronic nephritis.

Diagnosis

It is important to remember that the viruses of the Tacaribe complex and Lassa fever virus are classified as group 4 pathogens because of the severity of the diseases they cause. This means that they can only be cultured in specially secure laboratories. Suspicion of the diagnosis must depend on the history and clinical features, although these may be difficult to distinguish from those of other infections such as malaria, typhoid fever, *Streptococcus pyogenes* infection, trypanosomiasis, listeriosis and typhus. Laboratory tests to exclude these infections must also be carried out in designated laboratories.

Both virus isolation and serology are useful in establishing the specific diagnosis. Lassa fever virus can be grown in vero cells inoculated with blood and urine, both in the acute stages and for some months thereafter. Viral antigen detection in blood is also possible. The titre of the viraemia is of prognostic significance, as is the level of the aminotransferase enzymes released from the damaged liver. Serological tests show that IgM appears early in the response, to be replaced by IgG; paired sera should be collected for examination.

In human cases of LCM virus infection, the cerebrospinal fluid shows the changes associated with viral meningitis. Virus can be grown from the cerebrospinal fluid, blood and brain.

Treatment

Passive immunization with plasma has been shown to be effective if given within the first few days of infection with Junin virus and in some cases of Lassa fever. Specific therapy with tribavirin can be beneficial. In severe cases it is given intravenously and, if started within 6 d of the fever, the prognosis is improved five-fold.

Epidemiology and transmission

All the arenaviruses infect rodent species. With LCM virus, mice and hamsters are the reservoirs. The route of transmission to man is probably from urine through breaks in the skin or mucous membranes; the oral route is also a possibility.

Field voles are the reservoir of Junin virus, and another species of vole is the host for Machupo virus. Seasonal variations in the incidence of human cases can be related to peaks in the host population numbers. As with LCM virus, the routes of transmission are not established.

Lassa fever was first recognized in 1969 in Nigeria; the initial case, a nurse, may have become infected from a patient, and probably herself infected two of the staff who cared for her. The virus also infected one of the laboratory investigators who made the first isolation. Further outbreaks based on case-to-case transmission in hospitals occurred as well as the detection of cases in which infection was acquired outside of hospitals. Several outbreaks have been recorded with mortality rates in excess of 40% associated with transmission within hospitals, all in West Africa. The natural host is the multimammate rat, *Mastomys natalensis*, which is widely distributed in the region. A persistent infection is established in rats soon after birth and they excrete virus thereafter, especially in the urine. It is now established that infection of man is widespread in endemic areas, with only a 1–2% mortality; however, this will produce many deaths. As described, infection may be acquired directly from patients, probably by contact or by the respiratory route, but perhaps also by inoculation injuries.

Control

Candidate vaccine strains to protect against Junin virus have been produced, but require further development. It is not possible at present to control the natural reservoirs, although the increases in human cases noted when the rodent population increases suggest that it might be a useful approach. The only protection available is against contamination with rodent excreta. This ought to be possible in colonies of laboratory animals to protect handlers against LCM virus infection but is a very difficult task in the endemic areas of Africa and South America for the haemorrhagic fever viruses.

Suspected and confirmed cases must be cared for in strict isolation in designated hospitals to prevent exposure of the attendant staff to the high levels of virus present in acutely ill patients, especially those with Lassa fever.

FILOVIRUSES

Properties

The two members of the filovirus family, Marburg and Ebola viruses, are enveloped, single-stranded negative-sense RNA virions. The RNA is a single molecule with a molecular weight of between 3.5×10^6 and 4.5×10^6, and the helical nucleocapsid is enclosed within an envelope. Overall the virion is tubular in appearance, with a diameter of 80 nm but varying in length from 800 to several thousand nanometres, and may sometimes have a branched or ring structure (Fig. 53.2). The surface spikes are 7 nm high. The nucleocapsid has a dense central core and regular cross striations. There are seven peptides associated with the virion, including nucleoproteins, transcriptase and membrane proteins. There is minor antigenic overlap between Marburg and Ebola viruses.

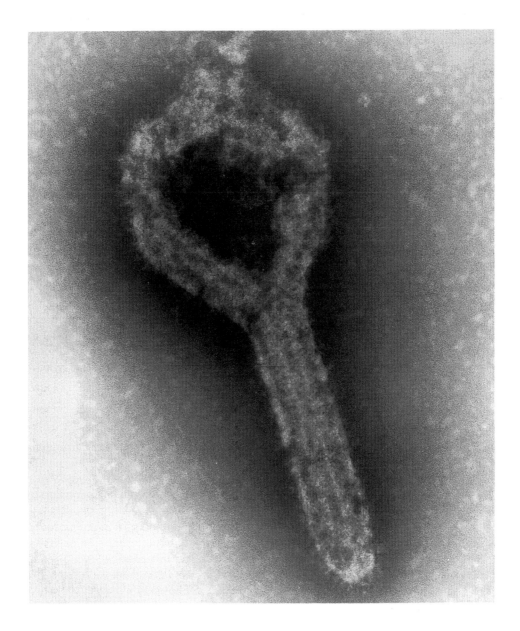

Fig. 53.2 Ebola virus

Replication

Virus can be cultured in the vero cell line, derived from the grivet monkey kidney, and in many other cell types. The strategy of replication is similar to that of the paramyxo- and rhabdoviruses. Nucleocapsids accumulate in the cell cytoplasm to form inclusion bodies; virus matures and is released by budding of the nucleocapsid from the plasma membrane. Large numbers of virions are released from cells which are destroyed in the process.

Clinical features and pathogenesis

The first features of infection are of a non-specific 'flu-like' illness with fever, malaise, muscle aches and headache: conjunctivitis and bradycardia also occur. The onset is rapid, as is the progression with increased myalgia and diarrhoea with abdominal pain: some patients develop a rash. Death can ensue rapidly in 50–80% of cases. The incubation period is 3–7 d.

The liver is a major site of infection, although the virus can infect most tissues in the body, resulting in high levels of virus in the blood. The cause of death is shock associated with fluid or blood loss into the tissues. Petechiae and bleeding are linked to abnormal platelet function and damage to the vascular endothelium. One of the early features is a severe loss of lymphocytes from the circulation while, at the same time, the polymorph count may rise to $20 \times 10^9/1$.

The fatality rate does vary and appears to be greatest in primary cases acquired from animal sources; cases arising from man-to-man transfer do not have such a high mortality.

Circulating antibodies are produced within 10–14 d, but it is difficult to demonstrate neutralizing antibodies in convalescent cases. This implies that cell-mediated immune responses must be important in recovery, although the virus is directly cytotoxic.

In the infected tissues, filamentous structures can be seen in the cytoplasm of cells: the lungs, kidneys and liver show the greatest involvement and virions are present in large numbers in the damaged hepatocytes and in the bile canaliculi.

Diagnosis

Virus isolation from blood samples can be made by inoculation of cell cultures; cytoplasmic inclusion bodies develop in which viral antigen accumulates. Although guinea-pigs are susceptible, vero cells are suitable for virus cultures. The virions can be seen by electron microscopical examination of the blood in the early acute stage of Ebola fever. Antibodies are usually detectable 7–10 d after the onset. As these viruses are group 4 pathogens, virus culture must only be attempted in designated national laboratories.

Treatment

Supportive treatment is all that can be offered to patients as there is no specific therapy. No vaccines are available to give long-term protection. Passive immunization immediately after exposure and interferon therapy have been used, but their value is not established.

Epidemiology and transmission

The routes of transmission of the viruses are unknown, as are their natural hosts. Both occur in Africa. The Marburg virus was isolated from a patient with a severe haemorrhagic illness in 1967. This was one of a number of cases which occurred in Marburg, Germany, and Yugoslavia in persons who had been in contact with the blood and tissues from a batch of African green monkeys from Uganda. Spread to hospital staff occurred and transmission via sexual intercourse was identified in one case 83 d after the initial illness in the index patient. Virus persistence of this duration was also shown in the initial case of another small outbreak in which infection was transmitted to two close contacts who both survived, in contrast to the index case. In the wild, it is possible that Marburg virus may be able to cause a persistent infection of grivet monkeys, although experimental infection is always fatal within 2 weeks and there is no serological evidence of infection in wild monkeys.

Ebola fever was first described in 1977, when an outbreak occurred in Zaire and Sudan. There was a high fatality rate — both in the cases and their hospital contacts who were probably infected by the use of contaminated injection equipment. The animal reservoir is not known, although infection with recovery is implied by the reported finding of antibodies in some human populations.

Control

The only approach to the control of these dangerous infections is by application of strict precautions in patient management, and in the laboratory. The handling of primates and their tissues can be made safe by quarantine of the animals before use. The most difficult decision in the control of hospital acquired infection is when to institute rigorous isolation of a patient who may present with non-specific clinical features and a history of travel to equatorial Africa.

RECOMMENDED READING

Evans A S *Viral Infections of Humans*, 3rd edn. Plenum, New York

Fields B N, Knipe D M (eds) *Virology*, 2nd edn. Raven Press, New York

Table 55.3 Group IV disease (Communicable Disease Surveillance Centre, London)

Not AIDS indicator disease

1. Zoster
2. Oral candidiasis
3. Oral hairy leucoplakia
4. Seborrhoeic dermatitis
5. Other infections — strongyloidiasis, nocardiasis, pulmonary tuberculosis
6. Constitutional symptoms (like wasting disease)
7. Peripheral neuropathy and myelopathy
8. Thrombocytopenia

AIDS indicator disease

1. Bacterial infection, multiple or recurrent in child aged less than 12 years
2. Candidiasis of oesophagus, trachea, bronchi, lungs
3. Coccidioidomycosis
4. Cryptococcosis
5. Cryptosporidiosis
6. Histoplasmosis
7. Isosporiasis
8. Mycobacteriosis — disseminated or extrapulmonary
9. *Pneumocystis carinii* pneumonia
10. Toxoplasmosis of brain
11. Salmonellosis — recurrent septicaemia
12. CMV, e.g. retinitis
13. HSV more than 1 month; or bronchi, lung or oesophagus involved
14. Progressive multifocal leuco-encephalopathy
15. HIV dementia
16. Kaposi's sarcoma
17. Lymphoma — Burkitt's or immunoblastic or primary in brain
18. Lymphoid interstitial pneumonia/pulmonary lymphoid hyperplasia in child aged less than 12 years
19. Wasting syndrome

Kaposi's sarcoma. This was one of the earliest features used to define AIDS. It is seen almost exclusively in homosexual men and is often aggressive and arises in many sites, including the skin, mouth, gut and eye. The tumours arise from endothelial cells of blood vessels causing bluish purple, raised irregular lesions. The aetiology is unknown, but it was seen almost entirely in homosexual men; the incidence has declined since it was first recognized. There is also an increased incidence of B cell lymphomas and other tumours.

HIV dementia. Dementia develops in 25% of patients with AIDS and is marked by a gradual loss of cognitive functions, progressing to overt dementia. In some patients it is the main feature of the disease. Brain scan shows a loss of tissue, with widening of the sulci and ventricles.

Features in developing countries. The features described above are associated with HIV infection in developed countries. In developing countries the clinical presentations may differ in that the types of opportunistic infections reflect those endemic in the region. Many patients show profound weight loss, perhaps accompanied by chronic diarrhoea; the term 'slim disease' is applied to this presentation.

Paediatric AIDS

The features of paediatric AIDS include many of the infections seen in older patients. However, children are also at risk of recurring bacterial infections, lymphoid interstitial pneumonia and pulmonary lymphoid hyperplasia.

PATHOGENESIS OF AIDS

Patients with AIDS are profoundly *immunosuppressed*. It was recognized early that the ratio of T helper to T suppressor (T4:T8 or CD4: CD8) lymphocytes in the blood was upset. In fact, the number of T helper cells declines during the asymptomatic period until it reaches a level where resistance to infection is seriously impaired. This can be demonstrated also by the loss of skin hypersensitivity to various standard test antigens. Monitoring the number of T4 cells is a useful guide to the onset of AIDS; in addition the number of T8 cells increases as disease develops. T4 cells are destroyed when productively infected with HIV and it is likely that factors which activate latent virus are important in determining the rate of progression to AIDS. HIV infects cells expressing CD4 antigen; thus in the circulation the virus is found in T4 cells and also in *monocyte-macrophage* cells, which may act as a reservoir for virus. Macrophages are also important in carrying the virus into the central nervous system across the blood–brain barrier. Only a few T4 cells, perhaps 1 in 10^4, are infected in the asymptomatic patient, but the proportion rises as the infection progresses. Virus is also present in the *plasma* and this increases with time too. Titres rise from 10 to 10^3–10^4 TCD$_{50}$ (median tissue culture dose) per millilitre as the patient becomes symptomatic.

The virus in the plasma is probably derived from the lysis of activated lymphocytes. Activation can be achieved by contact with foreign antigen, as for example during the many infections seen in patients with the virus. In the laboratory, lectins such as phytohaemagglutuin (PHA) are mitogens and can activate latent provirus. There is laboratory evidence too that co-infection or superinfection of cells carrying HIV with other viruses such as CMV and human herpesvirus 6 can lead to HIV replication. This is postulated to be due to trans-activators expressed by these viruses acting on the LTR of HIV. Activation of uninfected T4 cells is also important in increasing their sensitivity to infection.

Destruction of T4 cells is achieved by:

1. Viral replication
2. Syncytium formation via membrane gp120 binding to cell CD4 antigen
3. Cytotoxic T cell lysis of infected cells
4. Cytotoxic T cell lysis of T4 cells carrying gp-120 released from infected cells
5. Natural killer cells
6. Antibody-dependent cell cytotoxicity.

Analysis of the viral genomes from a patient shows that there are several different *variants* present at any time and that these change with time. However isolation of HIV in T4 cell cultures yields virus that may be different from the predominant genomic variants in the blood. Viruses isolated in the later stages of infection have been shown to grow more rapidly and to higher titres and to form syncytia more readily than strains isolated in the early stages: they are described as 'rapid-high' strains. The envelope glycoproteins show most variation and this could affect the ability of neutralizing antibody to react with the variant viruses. While this could be relevant to the progression of the disease, it obviously has implications for the development of vaccines.

Observed immunological changes in HIV infection include:

1. Decreased production of interleukin-2, γ-interferon and other lymphokines
2. Impaired function of lymphocytes and macrophages

3. Reduced natural killer cell activity
4. B cell activation.

HIV infection also has effects on the nervous system. HIV is present in the brain predominantly in macrophages but also in microglial, oligodendroglial and capillary endothelial cells. There is expression of viral antigens in these cells and virus can be isolated from them. Virus from such sources may be more able to infect macrophages in culture than virus recovered from peripheral T cells. Virus in the brain may be an important reservoir.

There may also be host genetic differences in the risk of disease progression, e.g. HLA haplotype A1B8DR3 has been linked to the rapid development of severe disease. There also appears to be an age effect with evidence of faster progression in some infants, the median age at onset being 8 months of age. Table 55.4 lists a number of laboratory markers that are associated with an increased probability of disease progression. The absolute number of CD4-positive cells is the most useful, although it can vary considerably between samples. However, a downward trend in successive samples indicates that the infection is progressing. The presence of p24 antigen in the plasma, the ease of virus culture and the loss of antibody to p24 are all correlated with progression (see also Fig. 55.5) but it must be emphasized that these features are not seen in all patients. The proportion of those infected who will develop AIDS is not known, although the estimates continue to be revised upwards. In the cohorts studied for the longest times, the proportions with AIDS were 5% within

Table 55.4 Laboratory markers associated with progression of HIV infection

1. Number of T4 lymphocytes:
   <200, 80% develop AIDS within 4 years
   200–400, 40–50% develop AIDS within 4 years
2. Increasing proportion of infected T4 cells
3. Increasing titre of virus in plasma
4. p24 antigen in plasma
5. Isolation in culture of virus — rapid growth, high antigen levels
6. Loss of antibody to p24
7. Elevated β_2–microglobulin
8. Elevated serum neopterin
9. Elevated serum soluble interleukin-2 receptors
10. Loss of cutaneous hypersensitivity

3 years, 20–25% at 6–7 years, and more than 50% at 10 years. However, this rate can vary quite widely in different studies. It has been estimated that from 2 years after seroconversion from 5 to 10% of patients will develop AIDS each year.

LABORATORY DIAGNOSIS

HIV infection

A specific virological diagnosis of HIV infection can be achieved by:

1. Isolation of the virus in culture
2. The detection of viral components, e.g. p24 antigen, by direct assay in the plasma or detection of proviral DNA or RNA (after reverse transcription) and amplification by the polymerase chain reaction
3. The presence of antibody to HIV antigens in the serum.

The various tests are used in different circumstances. Thus, to date the main approach to the diagnosis of infection in patients and for screening populations, e.g. blood donors, has been by assaying for anti-HIV.

Tests for anti-HIV

This was the first practical approach and many different assays are now available, most using enzyme tracing of the reaction (enzyme-linked immunosorbent assay or ELISA). Originally, the antigen for these tests was prepared from infected T lymphocyte cultures; however, it was impossible to exclude all lymphocyte-derived material from these preparations and therefore *false-positive* reactions occurred. These were often associated with samples from pregnant women, who had probably been exposed to lymphocyte antigens during pregnancy and patients with auto-immune diseases. The need for confirmation of the results of antibody tests was evident from these findings. In fact, even the early assays were of good specificity, but as a result of the large numbers of tests performed, a significant number of false reactions were bound to occur. Later tests have used antigens prepared by recombinant DNA technology in *Escherichia coli*, or synthetic peptides and monoclonal antibodies. *Western* or *immunoblotting* has been used extensively as a confirmatory assay. In this technique, viral proteins are solubilized, separated by gel electrophoresis and then blotted onto a membrane to which they bind. The patient's sample is allowed to react with the blot, and the human antibody located by an enzyme-linked tracer after washing. The pattern of bands stained should include proteins derived from each of the main viral genes (Fig. 55.2 and 55.3). However, false-positive results are seen with this assay too and care is needed in interpretation. There is extensive cross-reaction in most antibody assays between HIV-1 and HIV-2 antigens so that one test can detect infection with either virus.

As all who are infected with HIV remain so, a positive test for antibody indicates that the patient is infected. Most patients will seroconvert within 2–3 months (Fig. 55.5) but some may take longer.

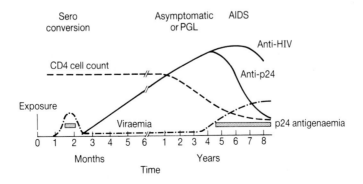

Fig. 55.5 Events in HIV infection.

Thus, there is a gap before antibody tests can detect infection. There have been reports that some patients may remain *seronegative* for much longer periods (6–9 months); transmission from such individuals has been seen. Measurement of the level of antibody to specific viral proteins such as anti-p24 may be of prognostic significance.

Tests for p24 antigen

p24 antigenaemia is usually of short duration at the time of initial infection, and is not always detected (Fig. 55.5). As the antibody response builds up antigen tests become negative. However, late in the infection, p24 antigen may reappear until about half to two-thirds of patients with AIDS give a positive test. At the same time, antibody to p24 declines. Both these events correlate with progression (Table 55.4) and with the level of viraemia.

Virus isolation and detection

Isolation of the virus is a slow process, taking from 3–6 weeks. The usual sample is blood, from which the lymphocytes are separated and co-cultured with donor lymphocytes. Virus presence is detected by assays for reverse transcriptase and p24 antigen in the culture fluids.

Detection of viral nucleic acid in cells and tissues by hybridization is possible, but lacks sensitivity due to the small number of infected cells. However, amplification by the polymerase chain reaction (PCR) can be a useful diagnostic tool in the investigation of patients with indeterminate serological results, and to detect infection in the early stages as in the partners of infected cases. The diagnosis of infection in babies born to infected mothers may require the use of several approaches. All babies will be positive for anti-HIV for up to 18 months until maternal IgG disappears; if antibody persists beyond this time, this indicates infection. However, some babies do not produce anti-HIV. Detection of p24 antigen or a positive culture establishes that the baby is infected, but the PCR may be invaluable in confirming infection.

HTLV-I infection

Assays for the detection of antibody to HTLV-I are available; as with HIV, confirmation by other assays or immunoblot must be attempted, although the interpretation can be difficult with some sera. Current tests do not distinguish between HTLV-I and HTLV-II. Culture and PCR can also be used.

TREATMENT
HTLV-I infection

There is no specific therapy. If T cell leukaemia develops then this is managed by various drug therapies; interferon may have a role in the management.

HIV infection and AIDS

Various approaches have been tried in the hope of halting or at least slowing the progression of HIV infection to AIDS. The most widely used drug is a nucleoside analogue, azidothymidine or *zidovudine*. The drug is inactive until phosphorylated, when it can block the viral reverse transcriptase, although it also has some effect on host DNA polymerase. The initial studies showed that treatment with zidovudine could improve the symptoms and survival of patients with AIDS, although about a quarter of patients developed serious side-effects, in some cases requiring frequent blood transfusions and cessation of therapy. Treated patients usually show initial improvement and the CD4 cell count rises and plasma p24 antigen declines. The patient feels better and may put on weight, but the improvement may not be maintained beyond 6 months. However the use of zidovudine and the prompt, appropriate treatment of infections as they arise can prolong survival of AIDS patients for up to 3 years or more. There is now evidence that the early introduction of zidovudine can delay the development of AIDS. Therapy is started on the basis of their clinical state, CD4 cell count, and other prognostic markers listed in Table 55.4. *Resistance* to zidovudine has been shown to increase during long-term therapy. Other nucleotide analogues, e.g. dideoxycytidine and dideoxyinosine, have shown promise, although toxic effects do occur. A synergistic effect has been claimed between nucleoside analogues and α interferon and various combination therapies are being investigated. Many other approaches are being assessed, including the use of soluble CD4 protein, which can attach to the gp120 of the virus and hence block attachment of the virus, or free gp120, to CD4 positive cells. The role of treatment to improve immune function is not yet clear.

Apart from specific therapy directed against HIV the most important therapy is aimed at controlling or preventing life-threatening opportunistic infections. *Pneumocystis carinii* and *Toxoplasma gondii* are important and suppressive chemotherapy does seem to be effective.

EPIDEMIOLOGY AND TRANSMISSION
HTLV-I and HTLV-II

HTLV-I is endemic in the Southern islands of Japan and around the Caribbean — in the West Indies, the northern countries of South America, Central America and the southern states of the USA. There are varying reports of infection in some tropical countries in Africa. Immigrants from these areas will show a similar prevalence, which can be up to 10–15% in Japan and 5% in Jamaica. The prevalence in some populations of the southern USA is 2–3%. In most studies, the seroprevalence rises with age. Other groups found to carry the virus are parenteral drug misusers and prostitutes in the USA and other areas. In some groups, the prevalence can reach 30–50%, the highest figures being found in drug misusers.

In prostitutes, rates up to 25% have been reported but this varies and is increased in those of African descent, in those who abuse drugs, and with duration of sexual activity. Drug misuse cannot account for all the infections in these studies and transmission by sexual intercourse is the likeliest explanation. As with any venereal infection, the risk rises with the number of sexual partners. This is reflected in the association of infection with other sexually transmitted diseases. HTLV-I can be isolated from semen and the amount of virus may rise with age and, especially, in patients who develop leukaemia and lymphomas. The relative rate of male-to-female transmission is 10 times greater than female-to-male infection. In most population studies therefore, infection is more more frequent in females. The pattern of infection with HTLV-I suggests that transmission is difficult and the evidence indicates that the transfer of infected lymphocytes is the means of infection. Transfusion of infected blood can also lead to infection. Mother-to-child transfer is the other major route, although the exact mechanism is not known. Virus has also been demonstrated in lymphocytes in breast milk and this is a possible source of infection for the child. No evidence of occupational exposure of health workers has been obtained.

HIV-1 and HIV-2

According to the World Health Organization more than 200 000 cases of AIDS had been recorded by the end of 1989 from all parts of the world. Most cases are from the Americas, with the USA accounting for more than half of all notifications. However, it is certain that not all cases are notified and this is probably the case in many areas in Africa where seroprevalence studies indicate that the infection is widespread. It is not known exactly how many people are infected world-wide but the number is estimated to be many millions and still increasing. From this pool AIDS cases will develop in the next decade.

Routes of transmission of HIV

1. By unprotected, penetrative sexual intercourse
2. From mother to child
3. By blood or blood products.

In Africa equal numbers of males and females are infected and so far disease is seen mainly in urban areas. Seroprevalence studies show that 1–20% of some populations are infected, with female prostitutes showing very high rates of infection of up to 80%. Analysed according to age, the peaks of antibody prevalence are in those aged under 1 year and between 16 and 30 years. This is consistent with a sexually transmitted infection. The presence of the virus in the child-bearing age group also suggests that mother-to-child transfer is important. Alternative routes include contaminated blood transfusions, inadequately sterilized syringes and needles used to give vaccines and drug injections. The evidence from the serological studies is that infection built up during the 1970s at much the same time as in the developed world, where infection so far is mainly confined to certain groups of the population. HIV-2 has a more restricted distribution than HIV-1. It is found in West Africa and in some European countries such as Portugal with old colonial links to the area. The routes of transmission appear to be the same as for HIV-1.

In developed countries the same routes of transmission operate but infection and AIDS are associated with certain risk factors related to transmission by sexual intercourse, by blood and from mother to child.

AIDS was first recognized in homosexual men in the USA and, to date, almost two-thirds to three-quarters of notified AIDS cases were infected by homosexual contact. Most studies established that anal intercourse and numerous sexual partners were major risk factors, particularly to the recipient partner in anal intercourse. Among homosexual men, the seroprevalence of HIV reached 60–70% in some groups in San Francisco and New York, while the rate in Europe is lower at 20–40% in Denmark and London. However, the rate of build up of infection indicates that the differences relate to the time of introduction of the virus into each population.

Intravenous drug misuse is a risk factor in about a quarter of AIDS cases. *Heterosexual transmission, paediatric* cases and the use of *contaminated blood* and blood products account for most of the remainder. In Europe the pattern is similar, although about 10% of cases are patients of African origin. In the UK all the major groups are represented, although homosexually acquired cases account for more than 80% of AIDS cases. Haemophiliac patients, heterosexual cases and drug misusers account for 3–6% of cases. However, the

evidence from those identified as infected with the virus is that drug misusers will make up an increasing proportion of AIDS cases. In drug misusers the virus was introduced earlier in the USA, mainly in the east coast cities of New York and New Jersey where up to 60–70% of some groups tested have antibody to HIV. In Europe, drug misusers represent an important group. The virus spread among Swiss, Italian and Spanish drug misusers between 1981 and 1982 while, in the UK, London and other major English cities have shown only a slow increase in prevalence, starting from about 1984–85. As in the USA, there are geographical variations: in Edinburgh the virus was introduced some time in 1983 and spread rapidly thereafter until, by 1984, 40–50% of drug injectors had been infected. This rapid build up reflects the practice of sharing syringes and needles for injection, at a time when there was an 'epidemic' of intravenous drug misuse.

Similar high seroprevalences have been identified in Dublin and Stockholm and may be due to transfer from the foci in southern Europe. In contrast, haemophiliacs in all areas have shown an almost identical pattern of infection from the early 1980s. Heterosexual transmission to partners occurs from infected male and female drug misusers, from bisexual men and from haemophiliacs and others infected through contaminated blood and blood products. A further source in Europe is sexual contact with partners infected in Africa. Transmission rates from both male and female index cases vary from 5 to 25%, but this almost certainly reflects the infectivity of the source at the time of exposure and is likely to increase with time. Although infection has been acquired after a single exposure, there are many instances where frequent contact has not led to transmission.

The other route of infection is from *mother to child*; as described above this is recognized in Africa and other areas where infection is widespread in both sexes. In Europe and North America, paediatric infection is acquired from a mother infected by one of the routes described. Infection occurs in utero, although it could also occur during birth or later through breast feeding. The transmission rate has varied in different studies, ranging from almost 50% to less than 10%. These differences probably reflect the infectivity of the mother and this in turn varies at different stages of the infection. The greatest risk of transmission is seen if the mother has already given birth to an infected child; the lowest rates are seen with mothers who are within a few years of seroconversion.

Virus can be isolated from *blood, semen, cervical and vaginal secretions* and these three sources are important in transmission, although breast milk and donated organs have caused infection. Virus may also be present in cerebrospinal fluid, saliva, tears and urine, but usually to a lower titre than in blood. There is no epidemiological evidence that infection can be acquired from these sources. Free virus is known to increase in the plasma in the later stages of infection and this correlates with the epidemiological evidence of the increased risk of transmission at this time.

Transmission during sexual contact is increased in the presence of *ulcerative genital disease* or other sexually transmitted diseases. Any *trauma* during intercourse will also facilitate spread, although neither factor is essential for infection. The risk of transmission by blood is related to the *volume* transferred. The transmission risk is less than 1% after *needlestick injuries*, but must be considerably higher in drug injectors who share contaminated injection equipment, although the frequency of exposure will also have an effect. Transfusion of blood carries the greatest risk. Factor VIII prepared from large volumes of plasma from many donors is obviously an effective vehicle, as shown by the high rate of infected haemophiliacs.

To date most infected patients can be shown to have been exposed to infection by one of the recognized routes of transmission. There is clear evidence that HIV is *not* spread by casual contact, contamination of intact skin or by inhalation. This is apparent from the lack of transmission in health care staff and family and home contacts who have cared for or shared accommodation with many infected individuals.

CONTROL

The emphasis in control must be on *risk reduction*. For both homosexual men and heterosexuals,

reduction in the number of sexual partners and the use of *condoms*, perhaps supplemented with spermicides such as nonoxynol-9 are important measures. Unfortunately, this advice is difficult to accept when the risk of infection appears to be very low. It has to be emphasized that the only way to slow or stop wide dissemination of the virus is by these means, starting now. Drug injectors of course can remove the risk by not injecting or can reduce the risk by not sharing injecting equipment. Screening of all blood donors for risky behaviour and testing all donations should almost eliminate the possibility of infection. Factor VIII is now heated to inactivate any virus present. All organ donors must be screened before transplantion of tissues.

Cases of occupational infection have been documented. The most frequent means of exposure is by accidental injury with a contaminated needle or sharp object. Blood is the usual inoculum.

Other cases have followed exposure to blood on broken skin or mucous membranes. Overall the risk of transmission from injuries and contamination is estimated as less than 1%. Occupational risk can be controlled by the implementation of straightforward measures to *prevent accidental injury* and contamination with blood. These will include the use of gloves, masks and eye protection if bleeding and spattering are likely and will be difficult to control, as in major surgical procedures, for example. In other situations the risk must be assessed and the appropriate simple precautions taken. *Safe disposal* of needles, blades and other sharp objects is obviously a fundamental requirement. The sensitivity of HIV to heat and various disinfectants has been described on p. 627.

Vaccines

Much effort has been devoted to the development of a vaccine to provide protection. An attenuated virus vaccine is unlikely due to the difficulty of assessing attenuation and the fear of possible interaction with HIV. Killed vaccines, however, are not very effective inducers of cytotoxic T cell responses. By analogy with hepatitis B, the best prospect is the development of vaccines containing the viral *env* proteins gp160, gp120 or gp41 prepared by recombinant DNA cloning and expression, or synthetic peptides identified as being important epitopes for neutralizing antibodies. The presentation of the vaccine components will also be important. Despite the difficulties several vaccines are under trial.

RECOMMENDED READING

Greene W C 1991 The molecular biology of human immunodeficiency virus type 1 infection. *New England Journal of Medicine* 324: 308–316

Lifson A R, Rutherford G W, Jaffe H W 1988 The natural history of human immunodeficiency virus infection. *Journal of Infectious Diseases* 158: 1360–1367

Pinching A J, Weiss R A, Miller D (eds) 1988 AIDS and HIV infection — the wider perspective. *British Medical Bulletin* 44.

Polsky B 1989 Antiviral chemotherapy for infection with human immunodeficiency virus. *Reviews of Infectious Diseases* 11 (suppl 7): S1648–S1663

UK Health Departments 1990 *Guidance for Clinical Health Care Workers: Protection Against Infection with HIV and Hepatitis Viruses.* Her Majesty's Stationery Office, London

Various authors 1988 HIV and AIDS. *Scientific American* 259: 40–134

56

Caliciviruses, 'small round structured' viruses, astroviruses and parvo-like viruses

Diarrhoeal disease

W. D. Cubitt

The introduction of electron microscopy for the examination of faecal samples led, in the 1970s, to the discovery of a number of viruses which cause *diarrhoeal disease* in man and animals. The viruses discussed are Norwalk agent, and morphologically similar agents, collectively referred to as 'small round structured' viruses (SRSVs), parvo-like viruses, astroviruses and human caliciviruses (HCVs). Evidence that they cause diarrhoeal disease has been provided by epidemiological surveys, human volunteer experiments and laboratory investigations.

Diagnosis of these agents is still dependent on the use of electron microscopy, except in a few research laboratories which have developed in-house radio-immuno-assays (RIA) or enzyme linked immuno-assays (ELISA). The application of these techniques is providing increasing evidence that HCVs, SRSVs and astroviruses have a world-wide distribution and that outbreaks of infection involving infants and the elderly are common. The SRSVs are emerging as important causes of food- and water-associated outbreaks of diarrhoea and vomiting, affecting individuals of all age groups. Recently, a calicivirus has been found to be a cause of outbreaks of water-borne non-A, non-B hepatitis (hepatitis E).

DESCRIPTION

The properties of the viruses are shown in Table 56.1.

Morphology

HCVs have a characteristic surface morphology (Fig. 56.1), formed by the 32 cups, 'calices'. Three distinct appearances can be observed depending

Table 56.1 Properties of human caliciviruses, 'small round structured' viruses, astroviruses and parvo-like viruses

	HCV	SRSV	Astrovirus	Parvo-like virus
Nucleic acid[a]	ss RNA	ss RNA	ss RNA	ss DNA
Protein	VP1	VP1	VP1, VP2, VP3, VP4	?
Molecular weight	65 000	60 000–70 000	36 000, 34 000, 33 000, 32 000	?
Lipid	None	None	None	?
Buoyant density (g/cm³)	1.38–1.4	1.38–1.41	1.36–1.38	1.38–1.46
Morphology	See Figs. 56.1, 56.2	See Fig. 56.3	See Fig. 56.4	See Fig. 56.5
Diameter (nm)	28–35	30–38	28–30	20–30
Antigenic strains	5	>12	5	?
Replication	Cytoplasm	?	Cytoplasm	?
Host range	Man	Man	Man	Man
Transmission	Faecal–oral, air-borne, contaminated food, and water			

^a ss, single-stranded.

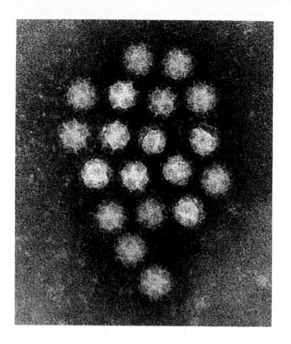

Fig. 56.1 HCVs, displaying characteristic cupped surface morphology. × 270 000. (Reproduced from Cubitt W D et al 1987 *Journal of Infectious Diseases* 156: 806–813, with permission of the editor.)

upon the axis of symmetry along which the particle is aligned (Fig. 56.2). Factors such as freezing and thawing, the presence of proteolytic enzymes, or incorrect staining can affect the appearance of the particles, which may then be indistinguishable from SRSVs. The morphology may be masked also by the presence of antibodies.

SRSVs are the same size as HCVs but particles have an amorphous surface structure and a ragged outline (Fig. 56.3).

Astroviruses can be recognized by a five- or six-pointed star on their surface (Fig. 56.4) but this is generally evident on only a minority of particles in a preparation.

Parvo-like viruses (Fig. 56.5) have no distinctive surface morphology and can be easily confused with bacteriophages, some of which have a similar size and appearance.

Antigenic properties

At present, five strains of HCV have been recognized, four in the UK and a further strain from Japan. The use of hyperimmune guinea-pig anti-

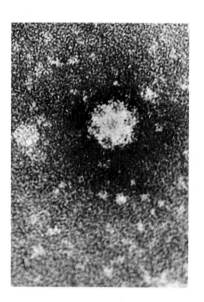
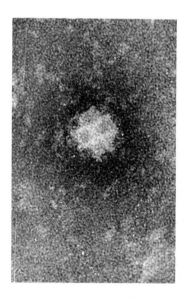
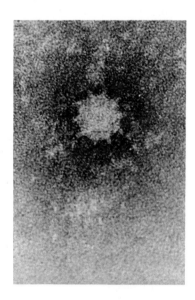

Fig. 56.2 Electron micrograph showing calicivirus morphology when viewed along the two-, five- and three-fold axes of symmetry. × 405 000. (Reproduced from Cubitt W D et al 1979 *Journal of Clinical Pathology* 32: 786–793, with permission of the editor.)

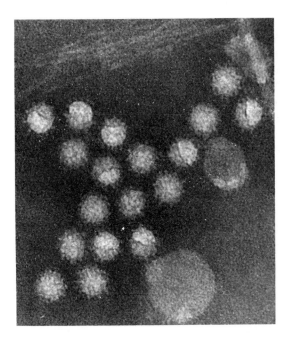

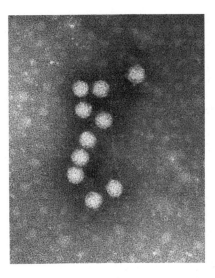

Fig. 56.5 Parvo-like particles. × 200 000. (Courtesy of Dr Hazel Appleton, Virus Reference Laboratory, Colindale,

Fig. 56.3 SRSVs resembling Norwalk agent. × 270 000. (Reproduced from Cubitt W D et al 1987 *Journal of Infectious Diseases* 156: 806–813, with permission of the editor.)

sera raised against HCV (Japan) indicates that at least four of the strains are antigenically related.

The use of immune electron microscopy (IEM) has shown that there are numerous strains of SRSV. Three distinct strains have been recognized in the USA, the Norwalk, Hawaii and Snow Mountain agents. Similar studies performed in

the UK and Japan indicate that there are at least 12 strains.

There are six strains of astrovirus which can be identified with specific antisera. The use of a monoclonal antibody has shown that all six serotypes share a common group antigen. The use of these reagents has recently enabled Marin County agent to be identified as an astrovirus (type 5); previously it had been classified by several authors as an SRSV.

Biochemical and biophysical properties

The biochemical and biophysical properties of the HCVs and the SRSVs (Norwalk and Snow Mountain agents) are compatible with those of the calicivirus family. A major argument for placing Norwalk and Snow Mountain agents in this family is that they possess only a single major structural polypeptide (molecular weight, 60 000–70 000), a feature which is believed to be unique to the caliciviruses. However, because the nature of the nucleic acid and the protein composition of the majority of these agents have yet to be established, they are at present regarded by the International Committee for Taxonomy of Viruses as 'candidate caliciviruses'.

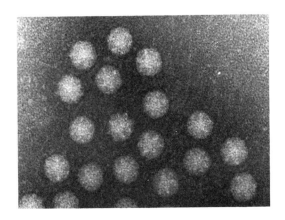

Fig. 56.4 Astroviruses, showing surface star. × 280 000.

The limited amount of biochemical data available on human astroviruses, i.e. positive-sense single-stranded RNA and four viral proteins together with their biophysical properties, suggests that they may be members of the picornavirus family.

Host range

Extensive studies with HCV and Norwalk agent indicate that they are not readily transmitted to other species, although similar viruses have been identified in primates, domestic and farm animals, birds and insects. There are two reports suggesting that primates can undergo subclinical infection when fed with HCV or Norwalk agent. In both these cases animals showed a significant antibody response and were found to be excreting small numbers of virus particles in faeces. Recently, an HCV, which has been shown to be a cause of non-A, non-B hepatitis (hepatitis E), has been serially passaged in marmosets.

Human volunteer studies with HCV, SRSVs (Norwalk, Hawaii and Snow Mountain agents) and astroviruses have shown that adults became infected after they had been challenged with faecal filtrates containing virus.

Replication

Radiolabelling and immunofluorescence studies have shown that HCV can occasionally replicate in the cytoplasm of primary human embryo kidney cells, (HEK).

All attempts to propagate SRSVs in vitro have been unsuccessful.

Astroviruses can be cultured in HEK cells and, once established, passaged in a continuous cell line, LLCMK2, provided trypsin is incorporated in the medium. Immunofluorescence shows that replication occurs within the cytoplasm. Electron microscopical examination of thin sections of infected cells shows the presence of crystalline arrays of particles adjacent to cytoplasmic vacuoles.

PATHOGENESIS AND CLINICAL FEATURES

Human volunteer studies with two SRSVs (Hawaii and Norwalk agents) have shown that replication occurs in the *jejunum*. Light microscopy showed

that the villi in the proximal part of the small intestine were broadened and blunted and the enterocytes covering the damaged villi were cuboidal and vacuolated. At the same time the numbers of intra-epithelial lymphocytes and neutrophils were increased. Electron microscopical studies showed that epithelial cells remained intact but the microvilli were disarranged and reduced in length. A similar histopathological picture has been found in calves experimentally infected with a bovine SRSV, 'Newbury agent 2'.

The only data on astrovirus infection in humans comes from the examination of duodenal biopsies obtained from infants with symptoms of gastroenteritis. Electron microscopical examination of thin sections showed the presence of arrays of virus particles in epithelial cells of the lower third of the villi.

Clinical features

The clinical features of infection with HCV, SRSV and astrovirus are shown in Table 56.2. The symptoms are similar for the three groups of viruses, but vomiting, sometimes projectile, is more frequently reported in HCV and SRSV infections. In some outbreaks of SRSV involving adults the illness resembles 'gastric flu' i.e. *diarrhoea, headache, fever, aching limbs* and *malaise*.

The incubation period for HCVs and SRSVs is between 12 and 72 h, and slightly longer, 3–4 d, for astrovirus. The illness lasts typically for between 1 and 4 d with excretion of detectable numbers of particles for the same period. Occasionally, symptoms may persist for periods of up to 2 weeks.

In patients with severe combined immune deficiency disease, persistent excretion of HCV, SRSV, astrovirus and rotavirus, can occur, either individually or simultaneously; in one report a patient was found to be excreting five different enteric viruses over a period of several weeks, before he eventually died.

Symptoms of illness are generally mild and seldom require hospitalization. However, when outbreaks occur among debilitated elderly patients or infants with other underlying problems, intravenous rehydration may be necessary; fatalities are extremely rare.

Table 56.2 Clinical features recorded in outbreaks

Virus	Number of cases	Cases presenting with symptom (%)						
		V	D	F	AbP	N	AcL	H
Norwalk	30	66	83	47	70	100	73	83
Snow Mountain	59	71	70	32	67	72	NS	68
HCV strain UK4	181	52	66	65	60	NS	56	NS
HCV strain UK1	9	100	22	NS	33	NS	NS	NS
HCV strain Japan	250	42	96	18	77	NS	NS	NS
Astrovirus	14	74	30	30	49	NS	NS	NS

V, vomiting; D, diarrhoea; F, fever; AbP, abdominal pain; N, nausea; AcL, aching limbs; H, headache. NS, not stated.

LABORATORY DIAGNOSIS

Specimens required

Faecal samples should be collected as soon as possible after the onset of symptoms and stored at 4°C. Paired serum samples should be collected, the first taken as soon as possible after onset of symptoms and a further sample 10–14 d later. Blood samples from infants can be obtained by finger or heel pricks and dried on filter papers.

Laboratory tests

The only widely available test for the diagnosis of HCV, SRSV, astroviruses and parvo-like viruses is electron microscopy, which requires skilled operators and expensive capital equipment. All the viruses are small and are often difficult to recognize. The use of solid-phase immune electron microscopy (SPIEM), which relies on particles being captured by antibodies which have been bound to the grid, can increase the sensitivity of electron microscopy and enables virus particles to be more readily recognized. Conventional IEM, in which virus reacts with antibodies in a fluid phase, resulting in aggregates of particles, is also of value, provided particles are not totally masked by excess antibody. IEM can also be used to measure antibody responses.

RIAs and EIAs

Several research laboratories, particularly in the UK, USA and Japan, have developed assays for the detection of the antigens of HCVs and SRSVs and to measure antibody responses to them. However, these tests rely on scarce reagents obtained from well-documented outbreaks or from human volunteer studies. Monoclonal and polyclonal antibodies to HCVs and some SRSVs are being raised and assays should soon become available to diagnostic laboratories.

Tests for astroviruses

Astroviruses can be cultured in HEK cells and replication demonstrated by immunofluorescence 24–48 h post-infection. However, only a few laboratories have access to HEK cells, astrovirus antisera or monoclonal antibodies. Recently, EIAs and RIAs have been developed in the UK and USA which enable antigen and antibodies to astrovirus to be detected.

EPIDEMIOLOGY

Age distribution

Tests for antigen and sero-epidemiological surveys indicate that HCVs, SRSVs and astroviruses have a world-wide distribution. All age groups can be affected but outbreaks of HCV and astrovirus infection most commonly involve infants, schoolchildren and the elderly. In contrast, SRSV outbreaks are more prevalent among adults and the elderly, although there are several reports of episodes in paediatric wards.

Modes of transmission

The various routes of transmission are shown in Fig. 56.6. Epidemiological studies can identify two characteristic epidemic curves for an outbreak. In one (Fig. 56.7), when most cases appear at about the same time, this usually results from a *point source*, e.g. contaminated food or water. In the other (Fig. 56.8) cases occur in smaller numbers over a longer period, often with short intervals between the occurrence of cases. This is characteristic of *person-to-person* spread.

Faecal–oral route

Affected individuals may excrete large numbers of particles in their faeces and/or vomit ($>10^9$ particles per gram). Human volunteer studies indicate that stored viruses can remain viable for several years and that the infectious dose is 10–100 particles. It is therefore important to recognize that even apparently minor contamination of hands, work surfaces, taps, carpets, etc., can be a major source of infection. This is illustrated by the number of people who can become ill when

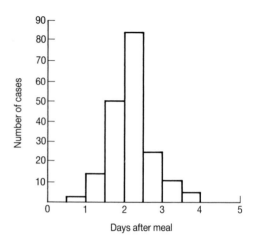

Fig. 56.7 Distribution of cases of SRSV following a meal, indicative of a point source of infection.

food is contaminated by a single handler (Table 56.3).

Respiratory route

There is strong epidemiological evidence that inhalation of aerosols of vomit or faecal material, from bedlinen or nappies, can result in infection. At present, however, there is no evidence that virus replicates in the respiratory tract.

Cold foods

Cold foods which undergo extensive handling during their preparation are a major source of outbreaks of SRSV infection. It is important to note that the foods involved, e.g. sandwiches, iced cakes, melons and salads, are not generally considered as potential causes of food poisoning. It is therefore likely that the true extent of the problem has escaped attention.

Shellfish

Numerous outbreaks of gastro-enteritis due to SRSVs, astroviruses or parvo-like viruses have been caused by the consumption of *bivalve shellfish*, i.e. oysters, clams, mussels, cockles and scallops. The reason for the problem is that they are harvested from estuarine or coastal waters

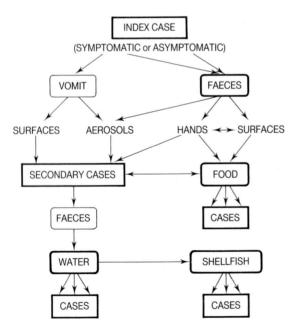

Fig. 56.6 Routes of transmission of viruses associated with gastro-enteritis.

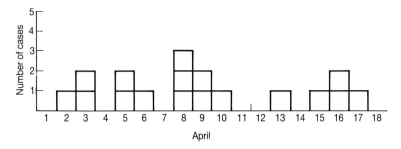

Fig. 56.8 Distribution of cases of astrovirus infection in a geriatric ward indicative of person-to-person spread.

polluted with faecal material which is greatly concentrated by the filter-feeding bivalves. Methods to cleanse them prior to consumption, i.e. holding them in tanks of ultraviolet irradiated, circulating filtered water, although successful in removing bacteria, are ineffective in freeing them of viruses. A further problem is that shellfish are frequently eaten raw or after minimal cooking.

Water

Outbreaks of SRSV and astrovirus infection associated with the consumption of untreated water, contaminated muncipal drinking water or ice have been reported in the USA, UK and Australia. In the developing world where water is often untreated the problem is likely to be far greater. This is emphasized by the recent finding that some large waterborne outbreaks of non-A, non-B hepatitis were due to a calicivirus (hepatitis E).

Asymptomatic excretors

Epidemiological investigation and volunteer trials have shown that *asymptomatic excretion* of SRSVs, HCVs or astroviruses is not uncommon. Such individuals may serve as an important reservoir of infection, particularly in situations such as hospitals or the catering industry.

TREATMENT

At present there is no specific treatment for infections with these agents. Severe *dehydration* in infants or elderly debilitated patients should be managed in hospital with parenteral fluid replacement.

CONTROL
Control of food-borne outbreaks

The following guidelines for the management of an outbreak associated with food have been

Table 56.3 Food- and water-borne infections

Virus	Source	Origin	Attack rate (%)
SRSV	Asymptomatic foodhandler Salads	USA	220/383 (57)
SRSV	Asymptomatic foodhandler Melon	UK	239/280 (85)
SRSV	Caterers Cold foods	Japan	835/3000 (46)
HCV	Oysters	UK	500/1700 (29)
SRSV	Oysters	Japan	63/121 (52)
SRSV	Cockles and mussels	UK	>130/>300
SRSV	Drinking water Secondary home contacts	USA	495/647 (76) 719/1740 (41)

proposed in the UK by The Public Health Laboratory Service, Working Party on Viral Gastroenteritis:

1. Staff who develop or have had symptoms such as diarrhoea and/or vomiting should be excluded from work until 48 h after recovery.

2. If kitchen or adjacent areas have been fouled (e.g. by vomitus) then (a) the area should be thoroughly cleaned and disinfected with a 10 000 p.p.m. hypochlorite solution, and (b) all food to be eaten uncooked should be destroyed.

3. The importance of hygienic practices, particularly hand washing, should be reinforced.

4. High-risk foods such as bivalve shellfish should be excluded from the kitchen, and other foods which require much handling (e.g. salads and sandwiches) should be bought in or obtained from other branches if at all possible.

5. Unnecessary kitchen traffic should be stopped: the kitchen should not be used as a short-cut for other staff, particularly during the period of an outbreak.

Management and prevention of hospital outbreaks

1. Ensure that both bacteriological and virological investigations are instigated at the same time.

2. Whenever possible, affected patients should be isolated and infected nursing, medical and support staff excluded from work.

3. All staff and patients on an affected ward should be screened as asymptomatic infections are not uncommon.

4. Particular attention should be paid to hand washing; 70–90% methanol or ethanol has been shown to be effective against astroviruses and rotaviruses even in the presence of faeces.

5. Bed-pan washers need to be examined to ensure they are working efficiently.

6. In some outbreaks it may be necessary to close wards to new admissions until all patients have stopped excreting virus and no new cases have occurred for a period of 72 h.

7. Staff movement from affected to unaffected wards should be restricted, group activities stopped and visits by children discouraged.

RECOMMENDED READING

Bradley D, Japaridze A, Cook E H et al 1988 Aetiological agent of enterically transmitted non-A, non-B hepatitis. *Journal of General Virology* 69: 731–738

Bock G (ed) 1987 Ciba Symposium. *Novel Diarrhoea Viruses*. Wiley, Chichester, vol 128

Cubitt W D 1989 Diagnosis, occurrence and clinical significance of the human candidate caliciviruses. *Progress in Medical Virology*. S Karger, Basel, vol 36, pp 104–119

PHLS Working Party on Viral Gastroenteritis 1988 Foodborne viral gastroenteritis. *PHLS Microbiology Digest* 5(4): 69–75

57

Coronaviruses   Upper respiratory tract disease

E. O. Caul and J. M. Darville

The relatively short history of the coronaviruses began in the early 1930s when an acute respiratory infection of domesticated chickens was shown to be caused by a virus now known as avian infectious bronchitis virus (IBV). Similarly, in the early 1950s, it was shown that colonies of mice maintained for laboratory research were endemically infected with a virus which in some circumstances caused outbreaks of fatal hepatitis. This virus was termed mouse hepatitis virus (MHV).

In the 1960s, research with human volunteers at the Common Cold Unit near Salisbury showed that colds could be induced by nasal washings that did not contain rhinoviruses. Subsequent in-vitro work using organ cultures revealed the presence of enveloped viruses in these washings. Electron microscopical studies demonstrated a unique morphology for these viruses and comparative studies demonstrated a similarity to IBV and MHV. The term 'coronavirus' was adopted for these agents in 1968, reflecting their morphology in the electron microscope after negative staining. It is now evident that coronaviruses are widespread in nature and infect a range of hosts with variable tissue tropisms. Although in man they appear to be limited to infections of the respiratory and probably the enteric tracts, their involvement in systemic disease in other animals has over the years given rise to the suspicion that they may also cause more severe human disease.

PROPERTIES

Morphology and structure

The most studied coronaviruses are IBV and MHV. The particles are pleomorphic and enveloped, varying between 75 and 160 nm in diameter, although this measurement has been found to be affected by the choice of negative stain used for electron microscopy. Widely spaced club-shaped surface projections or *peplomers* of approximately 20 nm in length give the particles their characteristic *fringed* appearance when negatively stained (Fig. 57.1). It is from this unique appearance that the name of the virus (corona [Latin] = crown) is derived. All species have a single layer of surface projections, with the one exception of the bovine coronavirus, which has distinct long and short peplomers.

The genome is encoded in a single segment of single-stranded positive-sense RNA of between 15 and 20 kilobases. In the virion this is complexed with nucleoprotein (N) in a helical nucleocapsid of 9–11 nm diameter. This is enclosed within a lipoprotein envelope in association with a transmembrane protein (M) to which the peplomers are attached.

Taxonomy

Although originally classified as myxoviruses, coronaviruses are now known to be quite distinct and the genus *Coronavirus* has been allocated to

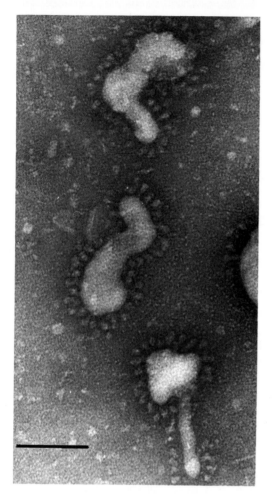

Fig. 57.1 Particles of HCV serogroup 229E grown in human fibroblast cells and stained with 1.5% phosphotungstic acid. The bar represents 100 nm.

its own monogeneric family, the Coronaviruses. Human coronavirus (HCV) is the only human species so far recognized, although human enteric coronavirus (HECV) is a likely second species. Also firmly recognized are coronaviruses of chickens (causing bronchitis), mice (hepatitis, gastro-enteritis and encephalitis), pigs (gastro-enteritis and encephalomyelitis), dogs, turkeys, cattle, horses (all gastro-enteritis), rats (pneumonia and swelling of salivary glands) and cats (peritonitis). In addition, coronavirus-like particles have been demonstrated in the faeces of cats, monkeys and rabbits both with enteritis and in health. In all

probability they infect all or most higher-animal species.

The 11 confirmed species of coronavirus may readily be distinguished from each other by their limited host range. Serological studies of the N, M and peplomer proteins (see below) have revealed antigenic relationships, allowing classification into four groups with a tentative fifth (Table 57.1).

Cultivation

Some avian and mammalian coronaviruses can be cultivated in fertile eggs or in cell culture with relative ease. The study of many coronaviruses, including HCV, has, however, been hampered by a relative difficulty in cultivation.

The traditional method of cultivating HCV has been in fetal tracheal organ culture. However, HCV strains related to 229E may be isolated more readily in human diploid cells and strains related to OC43 may be adapted to grow in them after initial isolation in organ culture.

REPLICATION

Coronaviruses replicate in the *cytoplasm* with a growth cycle of 10–12 h. They do not bud from the plasma membrane but from the endoplasmic reticulum into *intracytoplasmic* vesicles and leave

Table 57.1 Antigenic relationships of coronaviruses

Group 1	Avian infectious bronchitis virus (IBV)
Group 2	Turkey coronavirus (TCV)
Group 3	Human coronavirus (HCV) 229E Porcine transmissible gastro-enteritis virus (TGEV) Canine coronavirus (CCV)
Group 4	Feline infectious peritonitis virus (FIPV) Human coronavirus (HCV) OC43 Rat coronavirus (RCV) Rat sialodacro-adenitis virus (RSDV) Porcine haemagglutinating encephalomyelitis virus (HEV) Bovine coronavirus (BCV)
Group 5	Porcine epidemic diarrhoea

the cell by fusion of these with the plasma membrane. Viral infection may result in cell lysis but fusion of adjacent cells leading to the formation of *syncytia* can also occur and the virus may have a potential for persistence.

The optimum temperature for the replication of HCV is 33°C, reflecting the usual habitat in the upper respiratory tract.

CLINICAL FEATURES AND PATHOGENESIS

Human coronavirus

The only significant condition known to follow HCV infection is upper respiratory tract disease and it is estimated that up to 30% of '*common colds*' are caused by coronaviruses. Statistically, these viruses cause more coryza and discharge than do rhinoviruses, which in turn cause pharyngitis more frequently. However, individual cases cannot be attributed to either virus group on clinical grounds.

In some cases infection is mild or even *subclinical*. In contrast, there is some suspicion that coronaviruses may cause severe lower respiratory tract infection in the very young and the very old. However, although coronaviruses have been detected in such cases they have also been detected in control groups and so at present the association remains tentative.

Although the morbidity caused by HCV infection is trivial to the individual, it is economically important in that illness is so widespread in the community that the virus is a major contributor to time lost from work and from academic studies.

The incubation period is from 2 to 4 d and virus is detectable at the onset of symptoms and for 1–4 d thereafter. Symptoms outlast virus shedding and typically persist for a week.

After infection, humoral and local serological responses are detectable and cellular immune responses are presumed to develop. Despite this, however, *reinfection* commonly occurs, and this can happen as little as 4 months after infection with the same serotype.

Non-human coronaviruses

In other animals coronaviruses regularly infect and cause disease beyond the mucosal surfaces. In infected adult mice, for example, hepatitis is sometimes a consequence of reactivation and it is tempting to speculate that in man a form of non-A, non-B hepatitis might be associated with a coronavirus infection. However, there is, so far, no evidence to support this idea.

In rats and mice, MHV strain JHM has been shown to cause demyelinating disease via an auto-immune mechanism. Thus, the coronaviruses too have been added to the list of agents, viral and otherwise, which have been implicated in the aetiology of human multiple sclerosis, none with any substantial supporting evidence.

Again, the cause of encephalomyelitis in pigs has been shown to be a coronavirus, *haemagglutinating encephalomyelitis virus* (HEC). We may thus speculate, if only most tentatively, on the possible involvement of coronaviruses in some unexplained cases of human encephal(omyel)itis. *Feline infectious peritonitis virus* (FIPV) frequently infects feline populations of most species and all ages. Although usually asymptomatic the infection may cause severe peritonitis, which appears to be immune-mediated and is usually fatal. This condition has no obvious parallel in human disease.

Pathogenesis

It is presumed that the major pathogenic process, at least in human coronavirus infection, is the direct cytolysis of infected cells as a result of viral replication. However, the ciliostasis observed in organ culture may also be a contributory factor in vivo. Since HCV can cause disease on reinfection soon after primary infection, it cannot be excluded that humoral antibody or some other component of the immune system has some role in causing or aggravating acute disease. That coronaviruses have the potential to cause disease by immunopathological mechanisms is shown in the examples already given of central nervous system disease in mice and rats and of peritoneal disease in cats.

LABORATORY DIAGNOSIS

There is no clinical requirement for laboratory diagnosis since human respiratory tract infections with coronaviruses are known to be mild. At present, therefore, laboratory diagnosis has essentially research and epidemiological applications. This position would change should suspicions of a role in more severe human disease prove to be well founded.

Virus isolation

Members of the OC43 group of HCV will only grow on primary inoculation in *organ culture* (hence the designation). Virus growth may be detected by indirect means, such as passage to suckling mouse brain (resulting in fatal encephalitis and yielding a complement-fixing antigen from brain tissue) or by the demonstration of a haemagglutinin. Passage to diploid cell cultures may result in a cytopathic effect while infection of human volunteers may result in clinically apparent respiratory disease. Premature inhibition of ciliary motion in organ cultures, i.e. *ciliostasis* can be seen and, furthermore, characteristic particles can be demonstrated by electron microscopy.

In contrast to the OC43 group, the 229E group can be cultivated directly in human diploid cells such as WI38 or human embryo kidney (HEK). The cytopathic effect, often described as 'tatty', resembles the non-specific degeneration of aged cultures with individual cells rounding and detaching from the cell monolayer. However, overlays such as agarose or methylcellulose may reveal the development of plaques by some strains while others produce syncytia.

Serology

Antibodies to HCV have been detected by complement fixation, by haemagglutination inhibition (some strains) and by neutralization. The last is always a complex procedure and is especially so with these viruses. More recently, reliable enzyme-linked immunosorbent assay (ELISA) tests for detecting anti-HCV antibody have been developed although their use is still limited to research and epidemiology.

Antibody is a marker of past infection but, as reinfections are well documented, such antibody cannot be regarded as reflecting immunity.

Rapid techniques

Although not yet of any practical value in monitoring HCV disease the methods developed for the rapid diagnosis of other agents have been applied to HCV. For example, ELISAs have been used to detect antigens in respiratory secretions. Since coronavirus antigens are associated with cell membranes the virus should be as easy to detect using techniques based on monoclonal antibody immunofluorescence, as are other respiratory viruses. Rapid diagnostic assays of this type have been described.

Finally, as with most if not all human viruses, we can confidently expect techniques based on nucleic acid technology, such as the polymerase chain reaction and probes, to be developed for the detection and diagnosis of coronavirus infections.

TREATMENT AND PREVENTION

The treatment of coronavirus infections, in common with most viral infections, remains *symptomatic* only. Indeed, since disease in man is almost invariably mild, coronavirus infection ranks low on the list of candidates for specific antiviral chemotherapy. Although tribavirin has an in vitro effect against coronaviruses there is no record of this drug being used in vivo. Recombinant α-interferon has been used to prevent infection in volunteers in experimental studies.

EPIDEMIOLOGY

Studies using both virus isolation and serology have shown that HCV infections occur wherever in the world they have been sought. Similarly, HCV activity can be widespread in the community and in widely separated areas. Rates of infection are similar in all age groups and there are no other factors, e.g. sex or socio-economic status, known to influence the frequency of infection. Given the above, coronaviruses behave in the same way as other human respiratory viruses.

Infection with HCV is markedly *seasonal*, with peaks of disease usually occurring late in winter or early spring. However, the exact timing of the peak can vary within the season, as it does with respiratory syncytial virus, and occasionally peaks of infection have been observed outside the usual season.

The two HCV serogroups 229E and OC43 display an unusual periodicity. Each group becomes prevalent every 2–3 years with only sporadic isolates being made of the non-dominant type within the same community. However, the cycles do overlap so that in a single season 229E might predominate in one region and OC43 in another. This short-term cycling indicates that despite the diversity which exists within the OC43 serogroups at least, there are functionally few serotypes of HCV. Were it not for the ease with which reinfection occurs, this might be thought to indicate the feasibility of control by vaccination.

Transmission

HCV infects the respiratory tract by the *airborne* route, i.e. by the inhalation of droplets or aerosols generated by the coughs and sneezes of infected individuals. There is some evidence that fomites are a secondary factor in transmission.

HUMAN ENTERIC CORONAVIRUS (HECV)

In 1975 simultaneous reports of the discovery of coronavirus-like particles in human faeces by electron microscopy were made in Bristol, UK, and in southern India. It was at first suggested that these particles were derived from host cells or mycoplasmas.

However, it was soon shown that they could be propagated in human fetal intestinal organ cultures with cytoplasmic replication and 'budding' from the smooth endoplasmic reticulum, indistinguishable from that which occurs with HCV. More recently, unconfirmed reports have been made of the serial propagation of these agents in intestinal organ culture and of their detailed biochemical analysis. Although a causative association of HECV with human enteric disease has yet to be proven, there is no doubt that coronaviruses are significant agents of *enteritis* in other animal species. Recent studies indicate the existence of two serotypes of HECV, one of which is reported to cross-react serologically with HCV strain OC43.

Other than the labour-intensive organ culture method described above, the only means of detecting HECV is by electron microscopy. The introduction of other techniques awaits the confirmation and upgrading of the virus as a pathogen.

HECV appears to be endemic throughout the world with a high prevalence in the developing countries, in which there may be some seasonal variation.

In western countries the prevalence is high in travellers from third-world countries and in low socio-economic groups and is markedly higher in male homosexuals than in the normal population.

Although it has not been proved that HECV is spread by the enteric or faecal–oral route there is strong circumstantial evidence that this is so; transmission by contaminated water may also be possible. The observed high prevalence among western male homosexuals may be explained by oral–anal–genital contact.

CONTROL

Given the economic impact of the common cold, HCV infections, like those with rhinoviruses, are obvious targets for control. However, the ease of reinfection suggests that the development of conventional vaccines would be an unrewarding approach. Nevertheless, in the veterinary field, effective vaccines have been developed to protect animals of economic importance, e.g. chickens, from outbreaks of infection in which flocks or herds can be devastated.

RECOMMENDED READING

Ashley C, Caul E O 1989 Human enteric coronaviruses. In: Farthing M J G (eds) *Viruses and the gut* (*Proceedings of the ninth BSG: SK & F International Workshop 1988*). Smith, Kline and French Laboratories, Welwyn Garden City, pp 91–95

Monto A S Coronaviruses. In: Evans A S (ed) *Viral Infections of Humans: Epidemiology and Control.* 3rd edn. 1989 Plenum Press, New York pp 153–167

Resta S, Luby J P, Rosenfield C R, Seigel J D 1985 Isolation and propagation of a human enteric coronavirus. *Science* 229: 978–981

Siddel S, Wege H, ter Muelen V 1983 The biology of coronaviruses. *The Journal of General Virology* 64: 761–776

Sturman L S, Holmes K V 1983 The molecular biology of coronaviruses. *Advances in Virus Research* 28: 35–112

Tyrrell D A J, Alexander D J, Almeida J D et al 1978 Coronaviridae: second report. *Intervirology* 10: 321–328

Table 58.1 Lyssaviruses

Species	Serotype	Source	Occurrence
Rabies (prototype)	1	Carnivores, cattle, man, bats (warm-blooded animals)	World-wide
Lagos bat (rabies-like)	2	Fruit-eating bats, cat	West Africa
Mokola (rabies-like)	3	Shrews, man, cats, dogs, rodents	Africa
Duvenhage (rabies-like)	4	Man, bat (insectivorous)	South Africa, Europe
Kotonkan (rabies-like)	No type allotted	*Culicoides* (midges)	West Africa
Obodhiang (rabies-like)	No type allotted	Mosquitoes	East Africa

periods when stored as infected brain tissue suspended in 50% glycerol at 4°C and indefinitely when stored at or below $-70°C$ or in a freeze-dried state. It is sensitive to lipid solvents, β-propiolactone, detergents and proteolytic enzymes.

REPLICATION

Virus replication will occur in all warm-blooded animals, of which rabbits, guinea-pigs, rats and

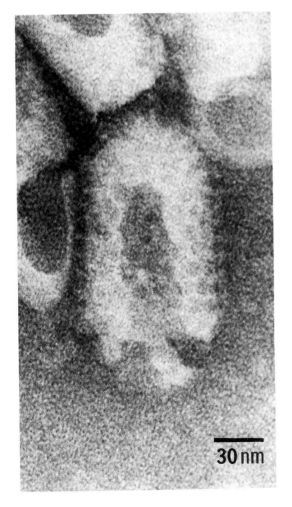

Fig. 58.2 Rabies virus particle. (Courtesy of Dr Joan Crick, Animal Virus Research Institute, Pirbright, UK.)

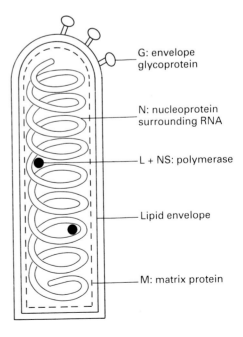

G: envelope glycoprotein

N: nucleoprotein surrounding RNA

L + NS: polymerase

Lipid envelope

M: matrix protein

Fig. 58.3 Diagram of rabies virus.

mice are useful for primary isolation. Growth also occurs in the chick or duck embryo and in a range of cell cultures, including baby hamster kidney and mouse neuroblastoma cells, human diploid lung fibroblasts, chick embryo fibroblasts and Vero monkey kidney cells, though with minimal cytopathic effects. The last three are among cells used in vaccine production.

Virus attaches via the glycoprotein of the envelope. In neural tissue virus attachment occurs at neuromuscular junctions via the acetylcholine receptors. However, while this may account for the localization and spread of the virus within the nervous tissue, there must be other receptors since the host cell range is broad and not confined to the central nervous system. Entry is by endocytosis; transcription of five messenger RNA species is catalysed by the virion RNA polymerase. The corresponding viral proteins are: N, the nucleoprotein; L and NS, together forming the polymerase; M, the internal membrane protein; and G, the protein which is glycosylated and inserted into the viral envelope (Fig. 58.3). Viral RNA is replicated on a positive-strand template by a viral polymerase. Only negative strands are enclosed in new virions. The M protein appears to be important in packaging the RNA and protein N and linking it to the envelope. Virions are formed by budding in association with the endoplasmic reticulum of the cell. The virus affects cell protein synthesis and the cell will die but, before this stage, it is possible to detect viral antigens by immunofluorescence or immunoprecipitation tests. Accumulation of cytoplasmic viral protein inclusions (*Negri bodies*) may be visible by light microscopy after appropriate staining. This has long been a useful diagnostic feature.

In the laboratory, rhabdoviruses produce *defective interfering* (DI) particles which lack part of the RNA and can only form in association with the replication of complete virus. However, as their name implies, they can interfere with the replication of the parental virus. It is not known if they have a role in the pathogenesis of infection.

Newly recovered strains from animals are capable of killing laboratory animals such as mice within 10–20 d after intracerebral inoculation. The appearance of eosinophilic inclusions or Negri bodies, particularly in nerve cells of the hippocampus, brain stem or cerebellum, and specific rabies immunofluorescence confirm the diagnosis. Such strains, stemming from Pasteur, are called 'wild' or 'street' viruses. Serial animal passage may select out attenuated strains of lesser virulence called 'fixed' viruses. They are usually no longer able to multiply when injected extraneurally, but reversion to greater virulence is possible by the use of an alternative host.

CLINICAL FEATURES AND PATHOGENESIS

The incubation period in man, mostly pinpointed from the time of a bite, can be very variable. It may range from less than a week after head and neck wounds, when the virus site of entry is close to the brain, to up to a year or more from distal sites. On average it may range between 1 and 3 months; the duration is shorter in children than adults. Initial virus replication is considered to occur in the tissues at the point of entry, persisting there for 48–72 h. The virus then spreads to gain access to the nerves via the motor end plates. Once within the nerve fibres it is out of reach of any circulating antibody as it travels along the axons towards the central nervous system. To early manifestations of illness, *fever, malaise* and *headache,* may be added symptoms related to the wound site, e.g. *tingling, pain,* lumbar weakness and ascending *paralysis* after leg bites, and *numbness, hyperaesthesia,* pain with increasing shoulder weakness after hand or arm bites. The predominantly neurological mode of spread has had experimental support in that section of the main nerve trunk proximal to the inoculation site can prolong the incubation period, as can the use of drugs which inhibit axonal flow such as colchicine. The variation of the incubation period could be influenced by a latent phase after the initial introduction of virus or by a block from the presence of defective interfering virus particles at the site of inoculation.

Despite an inflammatory reaction from the developing encephalomyelitis accompanied by considerable virus multiplication, observable damage to the nerve cells in the brain appears minimal, though if survival is sufficiently prolonged, specific cytoplasmic eosinophilic inclusions (Negri bodies) will appear. Non-specific changes include a parenchymal microglial response and perivascular cuffing with lymphocyte and plasma cell infiltration in the grey matter of the brain stem and spinal cord. From the brain the virus spreads via efferent nerves to most body tissues, including: salivary glands, with multiplication in the acinar cells and extrusion into the saliva; conjunctival cells with release into tears and exudates; the kidneys with excretion in the urine; and lactating glands and milk after pregnancy. Virus has also been found in the suprarenal glands, pancreas, myocardium and at the base of hair follicles, as in the neck. Study of saliva, corneal impression smears, conjunctival exudate or hair follicle biopsy from the nape of the neck, all by immunofluorescence, may provide an initial diagnosis. As the disease progresses, changes in the cerebrospinal fluid, increasing pressure, lymphocyte cells and extracellular virus are present. When survival is prolonged some antibody may appear though this does not affect the outcome.

The prodromal symptoms include malaise, headache, fever, a profound sense of apprehension and feelings of irritation with paraesthesia at the wound sites. There are complaints of dry throat, cough and thirst but patients will not drink. High fever, rigors, difficulty in swallowing and *revulsion of water* predominate, followed by bizarre behaviour, *excitement, agitation, hallucinatory seizures, laryngeal spasms*, choking and gagging, intermingled with lucid intervals. This state, the *furious* form of rabies, gradually subsides into delirium, convulsions, coma and death. Sometimes only the *dumb* form is seen, with symmetrical ascending paralysis followed by coma and death. The illness lasts from 4 to 14 d unless prolonged by intensive treatment. The disease, once developed, is almost always fatal, reports of patient survival being rare.

Clinically, the disease may resemble other types of acute encephalomyelitis although there will usually be a history of exposure to, or an unprovoked attack by, a deranged animal. Tetanus with its severe spasms may confuse but it does not induce cerebrospinal fluid changes.

LABORATORY DIAGNOSIS

The history may be so characteristic that early laboratory confirmation of rabies, often a problem in itself, is not necessarily requested. Difficulties can arise when information about exposure to a rabid animal is not elicited, as shown in the USA where more than a fifth of deaths due to rabies are in this category. It is worth remembering that when any visits, particularly to known rabies endemic areas, have been made up to a year or more before a death which is ascribed to encephalitis, post-mortem examination of brain and cord tissue should include a search for rabies virus.

Because of risks from contact and handling, the British Advisory Committee on Dangerous Pathogens, in line with World Health Organization (WHO) safety recommendations, has classed rabies virus as a hazard group 4 pathogen on the basis that it can cause severe human disease and is dangerous for any person in contact, but effective prophylaxis is available. Regulations provide that high-risk diseases such as rabies and viral haemorrhagic fevers should be treated in secure isolation units and the virological investigation of specimens from such patients is permitted only in specially designated laboratories. Similarly, for suspect rabid animals there is a designated veterinary laboratory. Stringent government regulations allow propagation of rabies virus only in designated category 4 laboratories.

Where rabies is endemic, wild animals or bats captured after biting incidents should be immediately sent for laboratory confirmation of rabies but post-exposure treatment of persons bitten should not be delayed pending a laboratory diagnosis. Domesticated dogs and cats, particularly if previously vaccinated against rabies, may be observed in isolation for up to 10–14 d. If they survive for that time it is unlikely they were incubating rabies at the time of the incident but, if they succumb quickly, antirabies treatment of persons bitten should be started without waiting for laboratory confirmation. Britain, being free from indigenous rabies, usually offers vaccine only to persons bitten while abroad but may make an exception for anyone bitten by a bat.

Diagnostic methods

1. Identification of rabies antigen by specific immunofluorescence:
   a. Ante-mortem — in salivary, corneal or conjunctival smears or skin biopsy from the nape of the neck. Negative results, which are frequent, do not exclude rabies.
   b. Post-mortem — in impression smears of the cut surface of the salivary gland, hippocampus, brain stem or cerebellum.
2. Virus isolation:
   a. Ante-mortem — from saliva or cerebrospinal fluid.
   b. Post-mortem — from salivary gland or brain tissue extract by mouse intracerebral inoculation. Cell culture inoculation may be used but cytopathic changes are minimal and viral antigen must be looked for by specific immunofluorescence.
3. Histological examination of fixed brain tissues by staining or immunofluorescence, including a search for Negri inclusions.
4. Fluorescent or enzyme-linked immunosorbent assay (ELISA) tests on serum or cerebrospinal fluid for evidence of specific antibody. This would not, however, be present until 7–10 d or more had elapsed since the onset of illness.

TREATMENT AND PROPHYLAXIS

It is essential that the risk of infection is assessed, to take account of the type of exposure, the animal involved and whether rabies is known to be present in that species in the geographical area where the injury occurred.

As yet, no specific antiviral therapy has emerged nor has human interferon been found effective. Supportive post-exposure treatment entails:

1. Prompt cleansing of wounds with plenty of soap and water or solutions of quaternary ammonium compounds
2. Stimulating immunity by vaccination as soon as possible after contact with a rabid animal
3. Initiating intensive ventilation therapy to offset muscle spasms or paralysis.

The main aim of vaccination is to stimulate the formation of specific neutralizing antibody, with the object of suppressing introduced virus before it can multiply and spread. The antibody resides mainly in the IgG fraction, which can diffuse into the tissues. It is persistent and responds quickly to a fresh stimulus. There is, however, a time lapse of 1–2 weeks before it can be detected after the start of active immunization. Because of this, human rabies immune globulin (HRIG) is injected as a passive measure at the start of the post-exposure vaccination.

Vaccination

Vaccination after exposure to rabies was introduced by Pasteur in 1885 on the basis that a long incubation period should allow time for immunity to develop before the onset of symptoms. His vaccine was a crude extract of rabbit spinal cord containing virus 'fixed' as a result of serial passage. A well-publicized early success established the procedure, still in use despite various vicissitudes. Whether there was live virus in the original vaccine is uncertain but increasing demand together with the use of larger animals such as sheep or goats for its preparation led to steps to inactivate residual virus without destroying antigenicity. A substance widely used was dilute phenol. A phenolized brain suspension formed the basis of the Semple vaccine used in the UK from 1919 until 1966. Its drawbacks included a variable but generally low potency, which necessitated a considerable number of daily, often painful, injections with an antibody response mainly of the IgM class. There was also the disadvantage that the amount of myelin in its nervous tissue content sensitized a proportion of those being immunized, estimated to range from 1 in 500 upwards, so that many went on to develop an allergic type of encephalomyelitis. When the risk of a possible exposure to a rabid animal was assessed as only marginal, it was a matter of whether the risk of rabies was greater than the risk of allergic encephalomyelitis.

A suckling mouse brain vaccine (SMBV) containing much less myelin and with a claimed five-fold reduction or more in the incidence of allergic encephalomyelitis has been developed and is widely used in Latin American countries.

A non-neurogenic duck embryo vaccine (DEV) was used in the UK from 1966–1976. Still of marginal potency it required a similar regimen of daily injections as the brain tissue vaccine. The neurological complications were minimal though it did carry a risk of sensitization to avian tissue. It was, however, deemed safe to use for pre-exposure vaccination of persons at special risk. By 1976 it was superseded in the UK by *human diploid cell vaccine* (HDCV), which originated in the USA and was further developed in France. It is prepared from virus grown in cell culture and is the only rabies vaccine licensed in the UK and the USA for both pre- and post-exposure treatment. Having greater potency, i.e. more than 2.5 IU per dose, it needs fewer injections. Severe reactions are rare after use, though up to 20% may report minor local effects, and a smaller proportion systemic, influenza-like or sensitization effects.

In the UK stocks of vaccine and of HRIG are held and distributed mainly through the Public Health Laboratory Service in England and Wales and from designated centres in Scotland and Northern Ireland.

The post-exposure regimen in the UK consists of thorough washing of all wounds, the intra-muscular injection of HRIG, 20 IU per kilogram of body weight, with half the dose infiltrated around the wounds and a course consisting of 1 ml vaccine injected into the deltoid muscle of the arm on days 0, 3, 7, 14, 30 and 90. Because of the considerable cost of vaccine, the alternative of giving a reduced amount intradermally has been investigated and claimed to be as effective as the standard regimen. Whether this could be adopted as a standard procedure is under discussion. In the search for cheaper and even more potent vaccines Vero cell and chick embryo cell vaccines have been tested in a number of countries and there is the possibility of recombinant vaccines being available in the future.

EPIDEMIOLOGY

During the period 1946–89 there were 19 human cases of rabies in the UK. All were infected in other countries, 18 the result of *dog bites* and one from cat scratches and bites. Of the 11 cases since 1975 none had received any post-exposure treatment. In Europe, between 1977 and 1988, 38 human cases were reported but 15 of them had been infected elsewhere. World surveys of rabies report about 25 000 cases annually, but this is thought to be an underestimate.

Among animals the disease may spread via two intercommunicating pathways, urban and sylvatic. The *urban* mode, more immediately dangerous for man, diffuses among domestic or scavenger dogs and cats, a situation prevailing in Third-World countries. The *sylvatic* mode, as it affects small carnivores and mustelids, provides less opportunity for contact with man. Its main focus in different regions may be confined to separate species, e.g. *foxes* in continental Europe, Canada and northern parts of the USA, *racoons* along the eastern seaboard and skunks in the mid-western USA and the *mongoose* in the West Indies. Spread to other species or to man, though a potential threat, appears unusual. Perpetuation of the disease comes particularly from salivary excretion of the virus during the early stages of illness combined with the biting tendencies of carnivores. Despite some evidence of the presence of circulating anti-body in animals, the absence of major antigenic variation in virus strains together with the slow rippling type of spread of the disease in affected species during epizootics does not support the existence of a large animal reservoir of carriers.

Dogs, and to a lesser extent cats, are the main sources of human infection so that control of such animals by surveillance, with elimination of strays and the initiation of vaccination programmes, as has occurred in the USA and many European countries has considerably reduced the incidence of human rabies in these countries. In other areas without the benefit of these programmes the incidence of both human and animal disease is much greater.

As well as the involvement of terrestrial animals there is widespread rabies infection in numerous species of *bats*. This was first noted in Brazil about 1916 when it was realized that both cattle and man could develop rabies after being bitten by blood-sucking vampire bats. A similar situation was then found to exist in many Central and South American countries and also in the West

Indies with considerable mortality in cattle. Some human and animal infections may have followed the eating of infected carcasses.

From 1953, reports, initially from the USA, have shown that many species of insectivorous and fruit-eating bats may also harbour rabies viruses with excretion and transfer of infection when they are sick. It is now believed that affected vampire bats, although thought to be mostly carriers, do ultimately succumb to the disease. Spread can readily occur in some bat colonies from the close contact among large numbers congregating together.

Most viruses isolated from bats in the western hemisphere resemble the classic serotype 1 rabies virus, though in cross-protection and neutralization tests, as would be expected, minor antigenic differences are found. Bites by bats form the usual mode of transmission to man, though in two reported fatal cases in the USA in 1956 and 1958 direct inhalation of virus while working in bat-infested caves in Texas led to the disease. Later studies showed that certain susceptible animal species could be similarly infected. For this to occur, however, an extremely high virus concentration in the atmosphere was necessary.

In continental Europe the fox provides the main animal reservoir but rabies-like viruses have also been recovered in a small number of instances from some bat species in Germany since 1954. Infected bats have also been identified in Yugoslavia, the USSR, Poland and Turkey and, more recently, in Denmark, Holland and Spain. No interchange of viruses between bats and animals such as foxes has so far been observed. The European bat viruses more closely resemble the serotype 4 Duvenhage virus than the serotype 1 prototype rabies virus. Three persons are known to have died after being bitten by bats though the incidents were widely separate.

In the UK the system of 6 months' quarantine for imported canines and felines was introduced in 1886, together with measures for the muzzling of dogs. By 1902 this step had succeeded in freeing the country from rabies. The disease was reintroduced in 1918 via a dog brought back illegally from Europe. The disease was again eliminated from animals by 1922. Since that time the UK has been free from indigenous rabies despite two incidents in 1969 and 1970 when dogs released from quarantine developed rabies but, fortunately, there was no further spread. The quarantine barrier, still in force, has been extended to include most other imported animals with an additional proviso that quarantined dogs and cats must be injected, under veterinary supervision, with an acceptable animal rabies vaccine on entry to quarantine and again after one month. In Britain foxes do not appear to have been involved, and laboratory studies of bat species have not shown the presence of rabies or rabies-like viruses so far. Whether the increasingly close links with Europe now occurring will alter the situation remains to be seen.

Transmission

Rabies virus does not penetrate intact skin and, if deposited on it from saliva, would become inactivated through such factors as temperature, time and the process of drying. The portal of entry from the infected saliva of a rabid animal is via abrasions or scratches on the skin, or mucous membranes exposed to saliva from licks, but more frequently via *deep penetrating bite wounds*. The amount of virus excreted in saliva is variable and bites through clothing by absorption of the saliva may reduce the amount so that not every person bitten by a rabid animal necessarily develops the disease. Uncommon routes include inhalation while in bat-infested caves, or from aerosols released during centrifugation of infected materials in the laboratory, or from ingestion of the flesh of rabid animals. High doses of virus would be necessary in such instances.

Despite the excretion of virus in the saliva and conjunctival exudates and occasional misguided attempts at mouth-to-mouth resuscitation man does not figure as a spreader of rabies. Transfer via infected *corneal transplants* has, however, been reported on at least four occasions.

CONTROL

Because rabies has a world-wide distribution its complete elimination would need the eradication of infection from all susceptible animal species. The current more limited drive for protection, aimed mainly at human beings, consists of vaccination — *post-exposure* for those exposed in specific incidents to suspect rabid animals and *pre-exposure* for those who may come in contact with such animals in the course of their work.

Immunization requires two injections of 1 ml of vaccine, given into the deltoid muscle 4 weeks apart. A test for neutralizing antibody is advised 4 weeks later. A reinforcing dose is given at 12 months, followed by boosters every 2–3 years. A booster can be given after any potential exposure.

Human exposure has arisen mostly from contact with infected dogs and cats and it seems logical, therefore, to vaccinate domestic pets to block this route. The evidence is that this approach can almost completely prevent human infection, even in enzootic areas.

Clear signs of case reduction have come from the developed countries which have applied this scheme and now the need is to extend the procedure to other, particularly enzootic, regions.

Past attempts to control wild-life rabies by such draconian measures as shooting and gassing have had short-lived effects. More recently, feeding live virus vaccine in bait has had greater success among foxes, particularly in continental Europe, and among skunks and racoons in the USA. Extension to canine and other species may become feasible. *Recombinant vaccinia virus* expressing the rabies glycoprotein has been used in this way but caution in its handling and distribution is needed.

Other types of information leading to greater understanding of the disease come from ecological studies and studies of virus properties. From environmental investigations in the USA it appears that there are at least partial restrictions on viral spread. Once the infection is established in one animal species dispersal is by no means a random process, being confined for the most part to the same species. In part this reflects some selective adaptation of viral strains. Supportive evidence of strain variation within the main serotype came from studying strains from a number of animal sources with a panel of monoclonal antibodies against viral nucleocapsid proteins. Separation of strains into several antigenic subgroups provided a means of identifying the origins of epizootics and following their spread. Again, distinctive antigenic patterns were found in strains of virus from bats, but there was no suggestion that the bat strains could be correlated with animal epizootics, though occasional transfer from bat to an individual animal might occur. Like human infection it appeared to be a dead-end phenomenon.

An increasing number of European and African bats have been found to harbour rabies-like viruses rather than serotype 1 rabies virus. Human disease, clinically rabies, has been reported, so far rarely, after biting incidents. Post-exposure treatment is advisable, even though it is uncertain whether the current vaccine will protect.

RECOMMENDED READING

Editorial 1989 Bat rabies in Europe. *Journal of Infection* 18: 205–208

Gardner S D 1986 In pursuit of the perfect rabies vaccine. *British Medical Journal* 293: 516–517

Porterfield J S 1989 Rhabdoviridae. *Viruses of Vertebrates*, 5th edn. Ballière Tindall, London, pp 214–229

Smith JS 1989 Rabies virus epitopic variation: use in ecologic studies. *Advances in Virus Research* 36: 215–253

Supplement 1988 Research towards rabies prevention. *Reviews of Infectious Diseases* 10: S573–S815

Warrell M J, White N J, Looareesuwan S et al 1989 Failure of interferon alfa and tribavirin in rabies encephalitis. *British Medical Journal* 299: 830–833.

59

Slow and atypical agents

Scrapie; kuru; Creutzfeldt–Jakob disease

R. H. Kimberlin

Scrapie is a very old disease, easily recognizable from the accurate clinical descriptions made by 18th century European observers. It is the first, and best understood, member of a group of atypical slow infections that occur in animals and man. At present, seven other diseases are known which share the same diagnostic features as scrapie (see Table 59.1). Three of these diseases occur in man, and two of them, *Creutzfeldt–Jakob disease* (CJD) and *Gerstmann–Straussler syndrome* (GSS) are the only known transmissible human dementias.

All the diseases that have been tested are experimentally transmissible, by injection, to a variety of laboratory mammals. Incubation periods range from 60 d, in the fastest scrapie model, to more than the natural lifespan, which, in mice and hamsters, is about 2 years. With the naturally occurring human diseases, the incubation time can be decades. Host genetic factors control the incubation period (susceptibility) of some of these diseases, but not others (Table 59.2).

These diseases affect the central nervous system (CNS) and they are invariably fatal after a chronic, progressive clinical course lasting weeks to months. They are characterized by a non-inflammatory vacuolar degeneration of CNS grey matter, affecting neurone cell bodies and the neuropil (hence the generic term 'the *spongiform encephalopathies*'). The non-inflammatory nature of the lesions is in keeping with another characteristic feature, namely that these infections neither induce an immune response nor impair the immunological responsiveness of the host to other infections. This is one reason why there are no laboratory diagnostic tests for infection with any of the atypical agents, and why vaccination is not an appropriate strategy for the prevention or cure of these diseases at the moment. No other kinds of treatment are available either.

A new diagnostic criterion for these diseases became established in the 1980s. Extracts of affected brain contain abnormal *scrapie-associated fibrils* (SAFs), readily identified by electron microscopy (Fig. 59.1). SAFs are amyloid fibrils which are derived from a normal glycoprotein (PrP; apparent molecular weight of 33 000–35 000) that is present in many uninfected tissues. During the course of scrapie infection, this protein undergoes subtle, but unknown post-translational modification(s). The result is that it accumulates in the brain, becomes relatively resistant to digestion with proteinase K and acquires the ability to form SAFs. Labelled antibodies readily stain modified PrP (SAF protein) in sections of brain, particularly when it is deposited to form the cores of extracellular amyloid plaques as occurs with some, but not all, of these diseases.

Histologically these amyloid plaques resemble those which are characteristic of Alzheimer's disease, the commonest human dementia. However, it is emphasized that the Alzheimer amyloid is derived from a different host protein than the amyloid of scrapie and CJD. Also, there is no firm evidence that Alzheimer's disease is transmissible.

Table 59.1 Diseases caused by scrapie and the related agents in the order of the demonstration of transmissibility or discovery

	Disease and occurrence	Natural hosts (captive species)	Date[a]
1.	Scrapie Common in several countries throughout the world	Sheep Goats	1936
2.	Transmissible mink encephalopathy (TME) Very rare, but mortality has been 100% in some outbreaks	(Mink)	1965
3.	Kuru Once common among the Fore-speaking people of Papua New Guinea, now rare	Man	1966
4.	Creutzfeldt–Jakob disease (CJD) Uniform world wide incidence of 1 in 10^6 per annum	Man	1968
5.	Gerstmann–Straussler syndrome (GSS) A familial form of CJD; less than 1 in 10^7 per annum	Man	1981
6.	Chronic wasting disease (CWD) Isolated foci in Colorado and Wyoming	(Mule deer) (Rocky Mountain elk)	1983 [b]
7.	Un-named spongiform encephalopathy Isolated cases in zoos and wild-life parks in the UK	(Nyala) (Gemsbok) (Greater kudu) (Arabian oryx) (Eland)	[b] [b] [b] [b] [b]
8.	Bovine spongiform encephalopathy (BSE) Widespread throughout the UK	Domestic cattle	1988

[a] Date when experimental transmissibility was reported.
[b] Experimental transmission not completed or not attempted.

Table 59.2 Summary of the diseases in which there is host genetic control of incubation period (susceptibility).

Disease	Host species	Genetic control[a]
Scrapie (natural)	Sheep	Yes (*Sip* gene)
Scrapie (experimental)	Sheep Goats Mice Hamsters	Yes (*Sip* gene) No Yes (*Sinc* gene) No
TME	Mink	No
Kuru	Man	No
CJD	Man	Yes (in 5–10% of cases)
GSS	Man	Yes

[a] It is not known whether genetic factors play a role in the other diseases listed in Table 59.1 which are not included here.

PROPERTIES

Scrapie is the best understood of these agents. The disease can be passaged experimentally in animals, including mice and hamsters. The agent is small enough to pass through bacteriological filters, making it virus-like or subviral in size. However, infectivity is notoriously *resistant* to many physicochemical treatments such as heat and exposure to ionizing or ultraviolet radiation. The unusual stability and the immunological neutrality of these agents are the basis for their description as the '*unconventional slow viruses*'.

Strains of scrapie can be identified by their incubation periods under standard conditions of infection and by the type, severity and distribution of histological lesions in the CNS. For example, some strains produce large amounts of

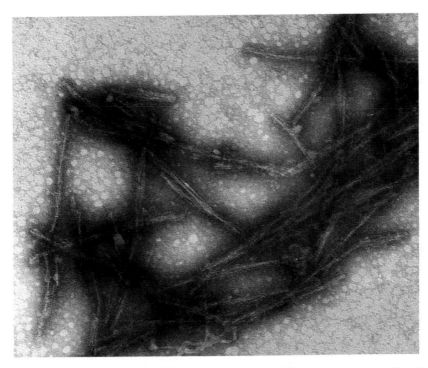

Fig. 59.1 Scrapie-associated fibrils (SAFs) purified from scrapie-affected (ME7 strain) mouse brain (*Sinc* s7s7). Negative staining with phosphotungstic acid. × 115 000. (Courtesy of Dr P. H. Gibson.)

extracellular cerebral amyloid plaques in the brain whereas others produce none. About 10 different strains of scrapie are easily recognizable by their biological properties in mice. Mutation has been well documented in both hamsters and mice, and is clearly not a rare event. Therefore, scrapie resembles other microbial infections in exhibiting strain variation and mutation. This means that the infectious agent has a strain-specific genome. On a priori grounds alone, the genome is likely to be nucleic acid, although it has not yet been identified.

The ultraviolet irradiation properties of the scrapie agent indicate that the putative nucleic acid genome is very small. Its estimated target size to ionizing radiation is less than a molecular weight of 100 000, which may be too small for it to code for the protein, which studies with proteases show is a necessary component of the infectious agent. This gave rise to the 'virino' hypothesis which proposes that the protein is host coded (Fig. 59.2). The lack of an immune response to scrapie and the related agents could

then be explained simply by the absence of foreign antigens. Taxonomically this puts 'virinos' between the true viruses and viroids, which neither need nor code for proteins.

The 'stickiness' of the scrapie agent has bedevilled attempts at purification and impeded con-

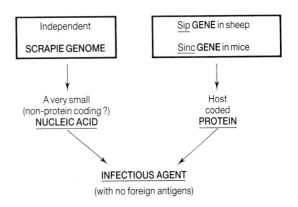

Fig. 59.2 The virino hypothesis of the composition of the scrapie agent.

firmation of this or any other hypothesis. The purification of SAFs (also known as *'prion rods'*) is associated with the partial co-purification of infectivity. However, a large amount of modified PrP accumulates in clinically affected brains and it is not easy to prove that the association of infectivity with purified SAFs is other than fortuitous. Indeed, there is clear evidence that even if some modified PrP is a component of the infectious agent, much of it is not.

Nevertheless, the association between infectivity and modified PrP has sparked off further speculations. One possibility is that modified PrP may be the host protein, which, according to the 'virino' hypothesis, protects the putative nucleic acid genome. Disease could then be a consequence of either the modification of normal PrP or of the genome interfering with the function of host nucleic acids.

Because modified PrP is the only molecule to have been identified in preparations containing high infectivity, another possibility, the *'prion'* hypothesis, is that modified PrP is itself the infectious agent. However, it is difficult to account for scrapie strain variation and mutation on the basis of what is essentially a normal protein.

PATHOGENESIS

Scrapie

In natural scrapie, there is early replication and life-time persistence of infection in certain tissues of the lymphoreticular system (LRS), notably Peyer's patches, spleen and lymph nodes. Disease occurs only if infection spreads to the CNS. Studies of experimental scrapie in hamsters and mice revealed the spread of infection along sympathetic nerve fibres which connect with the mid-thoracic spinal cord as part of the splanchnic nerve complex. If the spleen is removed, a similar pathway operates from the visceral lymph nodes. After intragastric inoculation, which approximates a natural route, infection probably spreads from Peyer's patches to the mid-thoracic spinal cord via the enteric and sympathetic nervous systems.

Once in the thoracic spinal cord, infection then spreads at a maximum rate of about 1 mm per day to the rest of the CNS. There is good evidence that infection is transported within neurones. Scrapie replication in certain specific, but unknown, 'clinical target areas' then drives the production of cellular lesions (dysfunction and perhaps cell death) which lead eventually to overt clinical disease. The nature of the primary lesions is not known.

The basis of the long incubation period

The slowness of scrapie may seem paradoxical given the absence of any induced immune responses to slow it down. However, there appears to be only a limited number of intracellular 'replication' sites in a finite number of non-replaceable, permissive cells. In the LRS these cells are among the radiation-resistant, non-circulating populations, and in the CNS, neurones are the most likely candidates. There is also evidence for restrictions on the cell-to-cell spread of scrapie infection at two specific control points in scrapie pathogenesis. The first is at the cellular interface between the LRS and the peripheral nervous system. This restriction on neuro-invasion is easily bypassed experimentally by infecting the mice intracerebrally. The second control is exerted in the CNS where the rate of replication and spread of infection to the clinical target areas varies, thus determining the incubation period.

Genetic control of disease

It appears that all strains of mice are susceptible to scrapie, but the incubation period is controlled by the *Sinc* gene (also known as the *Prn-i* gene). The *Sinc* gene has little effect on scrapie replication in the LRS but it may influence the initiation of neuro-invasion, acting on the neural side of the interface with the LRS. It certainly has a major effect on either the rate of replication within infected cells (neurones) or the rate of spread to other permissive cells.

There is a close linkage between the gene coding for the normal protein, PrP, and the *Sinc* gene. Recent evidence suggests that the two genes are one and the same; in other words, normal PrP may be the *Sinc* gene product. The open-reading frame of the *PrP* gene has a highly conserved sequence in mammals, which implies an important physiological function for normal PrP. The messenger RNA is found in several cell types, including CNS neurones, and the mature protein seems to be anchored to the cell surface by covalent linkage through phosphatidylinositol. It is therefore possible that PrP could be a receptor which, in either its native or modified form, may serve as a binding site in the cell-to-cell spread of scrapie infection in vivo. However, there are other ways in which this protein could mediate the genetic control of scrapie neuropathogenesis.

It has already been mentioned that some modified PrP may also be a component of the infectious agent. This is an attractive idea because there is no simpler way in which a host gene could influence the replication of the scrapie agent than by coding for the precursor protein needed to make the genome infectious. Such a close interaction between a host gene and the scrapie genome could explain the phenomenal predictability of incubation period in some experimental scrapie models.

Sheep genetics

Sheep carry a single gene (*Sip*) which is linked to the *PrP* gene and has two alleles, sA and pA. The sA allele confers susceptibility to the experimental disease but the heterozygotes tend to have a longer incubation period than the homozygotes. However, the occurrence of natural scrapie is largely confined to sheep of the sAsA genotype. The relative insusceptibility of the heterozygotes to natural scrapie suggests that the natural disease might be controlled by the use of *Sip* pApA sires, which can be identified by differences in nucleotide sequence associated with the *PrP* gene. But the reliability of the allelic markers and the success of this strategy have yet to be established.

If the *Sip* gene in sheep controls the neuropathogenesis of scrapie in the way that the *Sinc* gene does in mice, then sheep of a genotype which would not develop natural scrapie could be carriers of infection in the LRS and, as such, be sources of infection to other sheep. Nevertheless, the genetic control of natural scrapie could still be of considerable practical value in reducing the incidence of clinical cases.

EPIDEMIOLOGY

Scrapie

Infection is endemic in sheep and goats in many parts of the world. It is transmitted from the mother at parturition or beforehand, and also afterwards, because the incidence of scrapie in progeny increases with the time that ewes and lambs run together. Selective culling in the female line is, therefore, a useful way of controlling the natural disease.

There is also good evidence for the contagious spread of scrapie between unrelated adult sheep. Infection by the oral (alimentary) route and by scarification have been shown experimentally, and these are likely routes of natural infection. The placenta from an infected ewe is one known source of infection and the physicochemical stability of the agent allows contamination to build up in the farm environment.

Other animal diseases

In the last 40 years, scrapie-like diseases have appeared in nine species of captive or domesticated animals (Table 59.1). Transmissible mink encephalopathy (TME) was the first to be recognized. It is a rare disease but, in some outbreaks, the mortality among adult breeding mink was close to 100% with no evidence of any host genetic factors. Bovine spongiform encephalopathy (BSE) is the most recent and by far the most important because of the size of the outbreak in the UK, which, in 1989, affected 0.1% of the adult cattle population.

Scrapie is unique among the animal diseases as it is the only one that has been firmly established as an endemic infection of its natural hosts. Although little is known about some of the other diseases, it is possible that the sole cause of all of them is scrapie infection getting into animals as a result of human intervention (Fig. 59.3). Exogenous sources of infection are certainly responsible for both TME and BSE. The inadvertent feeding of scrapie-infected sheep carcasses, or offal, is believed to have caused rare outbreaks of TME; and scrapie-contaminated meat and bone meal supplements to concentrated feedstuffs are strongly implicated in the current outbreak of BSE in the UK.

Epidemiological and pathogenesis studies of TME show that infection is not transmitted from mink to mink except by cannibalism; in other words, mink are dead-end hosts, incapable of maintaining the infection in the population. If the same is true for BSE, then the ban on the feeding of animal protein to ruminants, introduced in the UK in 1988, should lead to the eventual disappearance of BSE, but not until the mid-1990s because of the long incubation period.

Kuru

This disease occurs uniquely among the Fore-speaking people of Papua New Guinea, and at the height of the epidemic in the 1950s, it was the biggest single cause of death. Like TME, there is no evidence that host genetic factors are important. Kuru also resembles TME in being essentially a dead-end infection that was effectively passaged within a small, isolated human population by cannibalism of dead relatives (Fig.

59.3). The brain was the probable source of infection, and the most likely routes were by ingestion and scarification. Unlike scrapie, there is no evidence for maternal transmission of infection, and in the absence of other mechanisms of contagion, cessation of cannibalism in the late 1950s has led to the gradual disappearance of kuru. A few well-documented cases occurring in the 1980s indicate incubation periods of 30 years or so. It is not known how the kuru epidemic started but it could have been due to an isolated case of CJD.

Creutzfeldt–Jakob disease (CJD)

Clinically, CJD presents as a *progressive dementia* often accompanied by myoclonus and characteristic changes in the electro-encephalogram (EEG) pattern. CJD is typically sporadic with a remarkably uniform rate of occurrence worldwide of about 1 case in 10^6 per year. Unlike TME and BSE, there is no evidence that CJD is caused by an exogenously acquired infection; sheep have been excluded as a major zoonotic source of infection and no other animal reservoir of CJD infection has been identified.

Therefore, CJD seems to be an *endemic infection* of man but epidemiological studies in many

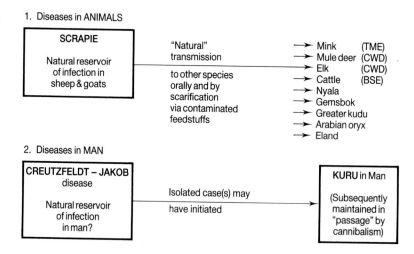

Fig. 59.3 Possible relationships between animal (1) and human (2) spongiform encephalopathies.

60

Fungi   Thrush; ringworm; subcutaneous and systemic mycoses

E. G. V. Evans

Fungi constitute a large, diverse group of hetero-trophic organisms which exist as saprophytes, parasites or commensals. Most are found as saprophytes in the soil and on decaying plant material. Fungi are eukaryotic, with a range of internal membrane systems, membrane-bound organelles, and a well-defined cell wall which is composed largely of polysaccharides and chitin. They show considerable variation in size and form, but can be divided into two main groups: *moulds* and *yeasts*.

Moulds. Moulds, also known as *filamentous* or *mycelial* fungi, are composed of branching filaments called *hyphae* which grow by apical extension, forming an interwoven mass, the *mycelium*; in most fungi the hyphae have regular cross-walls (*septa*) but in lower fungi these are usually absent (Fig. 60.1). In some higher fungi the hyphae may be compacted together to form a fungal tissue from which macroscopic structures such as mushrooms and toadstools are formed.

Moulds reproduce by means of *spores* which are produced, often in large numbers, by asexual cell division or as a result of sexual reproduction. Many fungi can produce more than one type of spore, depending on the growth conditions. The precise method of spore production and the type(s) of spore produced are unique to each individual fungal species. In laboratory cultures, moulds mainly produce asexual spores; examples of the different types of spores and methods of spore production are shown in Fig. 60.2.

Yeasts. Yeasts are predominantly unicellular. Most reproduce by an asexual process called

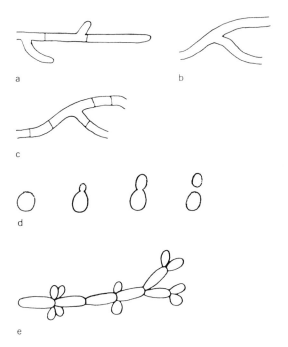

Fig. 60.1   Diagrammatic representation of vegetative forms of fungi: **a** hyphal tip with lateral branching; **b** aseptate (coenocytic) hypha; **c** septate hypha; **d** yeast cells showing stages in budding; **e** yeast pseudomycelium (pseudohypha). (From Evans E G V, Gentles J C 1985 *Essentials of Medical Mycology*. Churchill Livingstone, Edinburgh.)

budding in which the cell develops a protuberance which enlarges and eventually separates from the parent cell. Some yeasts produce chains of elongated cells (*pseudomycelium*) that resemble

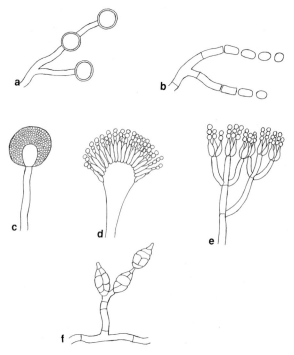

Fig. 60.2 Types of asexual spores produced by moulds: **a** chlamydoconidia; **b** arthroconidia; **c** sporangium of *Mucor* species, containing sporangiospores; **d** and **e** sporing heads of *Aspergillus* and *Penicillium* species, respectively, with unicellular conidiospores; **f** multicelled conidia of *Alternaria* species.

the mycelium of moulds; some species also produce true mycelium (Fig. 60.1).

Dimorphic fungi. Fungi that are capable of changing their growth to either a mycelial or yeast phase, depending on the growth conditions, are called *dimorphic fungi*. Many of the fungi pathogenic for man are dimorphic.

Identification. The identification of moulds is based on a detailed study of their macroscopic and microscopic morphology and, in particular, the type of spores they produce. Yeasts are primarily identified according to their ability to ferment sugars and to assimilate carbon and nitrogen compounds.

Classification. The classification of fungi is based primarily on the method of sexual reproduction, although morphology and the method of asexual reproduction are also important. Moulds and yeasts are organized into five subdivisions of

the Eumycetes, one of which is an artificial group which contains fungi with no known sexual phase.

FUNGAL DISEASES OF MAN
Fungal pathogens

About 180 of the 250 000 known fungal species are recognized as capable of causing disease (*mycosis*) in man and animals. Most of these are moulds but there are number of pathogenic yeasts and many are dimorphic. Dimorphic fungi usually assume the mould form when growing as saprophytes in nature and the yeast form when causing infection; in the laboratory, the tissue form can be induced by culture at 37°C on rich media such as blood agar, whereas the mould form develops when incubated at a lower temperature (22–27°C) on a less rich medium such as Sabouraud's agar.

Some fungi are highly pathogenic and are capable of establishing an infection in all exposed individuals, e.g. the systemic pathogens *Histoplasma capsulatum* and *Coccidioides immitis*. Others, such as *Candida* and *Aspergillus* species, are opportunist pathogens, which ordinarily cause disease only in a compromised host. In some mycoses the form and the severity of the infection depend on the degree of exposure to the fungus, the site and method of entry into the body, and the level of immunocompetence of the host.

Some fungi may cause serious, occasionally fatal toxic effects in man, either following ingestion of poisonous toadstools or consumption of mouldy food that contains toxic secondary metabolites (*mycotoxins*). Allergic disease of the airways may result from inhalation of fungal spores.

Epidemiology

Most fungal infections are caused by fungi which grow as saprophytes in the environment. Some yeasts are commensals of man and cause endogenous infections when there is some imbalance in the host. Only ringworm infections are truly contagious.

Many fungal diseases have a world-wide distribution but some are endemic to specific geographical regions, usually because the causal agents are saprophytes which are restricted in their distribution by soil and climatic conditions.

Types of infection

Superficial mycoses

Diseases of the skin, hair, nail and mucous membranes are the most common of all fungal infections and have a world-wide distribution.

Ringworm. This is a complex of diseases which affects the keratinous tissues of hair, nail and the horny layer of the skin; it is caused by a group of closely related mould fungi called *dermatophytes* which have the ability to colonize and digest keratin. Ringworm infections occur in both humans and animals.

Yeast infections. These affect the skin, nail and mucous membranes of the mouth and vagina, and are usually caused by *Candida* species, notably *C. albicans*, which are found as commensals of man. Yeast infections are generally endogenous in origin but can be transmitted sexually. The yeast *Malassezia furfur* causes an infection of the skin called *pityriasis versicolor*.

Subcutaneous mycoses

Mycoses of the skin, subcutaneous tissues and bone, which show slow localized spread, occur mainly in the tropics and subtropics; they result from the inoculation of saprophytic fungi from soil or decaying vegetation into the subcutaneous tissue. The principal subcutaneous mycoses are mycetoma, chromomycosis and sporotrichosis.

Systemic mycoses

Disseminated fungal infections generally result from the inhalation of airborne spores produced by the causal moulds, which are present as saprophytes in soil and on plant material. They are mostly caused by dimorphic fungi and occur mainly in the Americas. The principal diseases are coccidioidomycosis (caused by *C. immitis*), blastomycosis (*Blastomyces dermatitidis*), histoplasmosis (*H. capsulatum*) and paracoccidioidomycosis (*Paracoccidioides brasiliensis*).

Systemic mycoses due to opportunistic pathogens such as *Aspergillus*, *Candida* and *Cryptococcus* species have a more widespread distribution. These infections are being seen with increasing frequency in patients compromised by disease or drug treatment. In transplant patients these fungi are among the most frequent causes of mortality due to infection.

Incidence

The incidence of all the mycoses is related directly to factors which affect the degree of exposure to the causal fungi, e.g. living conditions, occupation and leisure activities. Ringworm of the foot (*athlete's foot*), with associated infections of nails and groin, occurs most commonly in competitive swimmers, sportsmen and industrial workers who use communal bathing facilities. Animal ringworm is an occupational hazard for farmers, veterinarians and others closely associated with animals. Field workers in warm climates who wear little protective clothing frequently contract subcutaneous infections following minor injuries from thorny vegetation. Systemic mycoses occur most frequently in workers in agriculture or the construction industry and following disturbance of soils containing the causal agents. The incidence of infections due to opportunistic systemic pathogens has increased with developments in medical and surgical practice.

Pathogenesis and immunity

Relatively little is known about the pathogenesis of fungal infections or the mechanisms of immunity to fungal disease, but it is clear that infection often arises due to deficiencies in the host rather than because of any inherent pathogenic properties of the fungus.

Antigenic variation on the surface of *Candida* cells may help the organism to avoid host defences. Furthermore, mannan, a cell wall polysaccharide of *Candida* species, and the capsular mucopolysaccharide of *Cryptococcus neoformans* have been shown to suppress cellular immunity. However, the importance of various fungal antigens in the disease process has yet to be elucidated fully; since anergy is a feature of serious disseminated mycotic disease, it is possible that some antigens, depending perhaps on their mode of presentation, may be inducing this anergic state.

Diagnosis

Diagnosis of fungal infections is based on a combination of clinical observation and laboratory investigation. Laboratory diagnosis depends on recognition of the pathogen in tissue by microscopy, isolation of the causal fungus in culture, and the use of serological tests.

Clinical diagnosis

Superficial and subcutaneous mycoses often produce characteristic lesions which strongly suggest a fungal aetiology but they may also closely resemble other diseases. Also, the appearance of lesions may be modified beyond recognition by previous therapy, e.g. with topical steroids.

The first indication that a patient may have a systemic mycosis is often their failure to respond to antibacterial antibiotics. Since early diagnosis considerably increases the chances of successful treatment, it is important that the possibility of fungal involvement should be considered from the outset.

Laboratory diagnosis

It is important that the correct type of specimen together with adequate clinical data is sent to the laboratory so that the appropriate investigations can be carried out. Information on factors such as travel or residence abroad, animal contacts and the occupation of the patient will enable the laboratory staff to direct their investigations towards a particular fungus or group of fungi when appropriate.

Types of specimen. Skin scales, nail clippings and scrapings of the scalp which include hair stubs and skin scales are the most suitable specimens for the diagnosis of ringworm; these are collected into folded paper squares for transport to the laboratory. Swabs should be taken from suspected *Candida* infections of the mucous membranes and preferably sent to the laboratory in transport medium. For subcutaneous infections the most suitable specimens are scrapings and crusts, aspirated pus and biopsies. In suspected systemic infection, specimens should be taken from as many sites as possible.

Direct microscopy. Most specimens can be examined satisfactorily in wet mounts after partial digestion of the tissue with 10–20% potassium hydroxide. Gram films may also be used for the diagnosis of yeast infections of mucous membranes. Giemsa staining of smears is advised for detection of the yeast cells of *H. capsulatum* because of their small size. Fluorescent antibody staining can be used to demonstrate fungi in tissues and smears but this requires specific antisera which are not widely available.

Histology. Invasive procedures are required to obtain specimens for histological examination and, while sometimes necessary to provide firm evidence of invasive disease, such procedures are often impracticable on patients who are already seriously ill. Haematoxylin and eosin staining is seldom of value for demonstrating fungi in tissue and specific fungal stains such as periodic acid–Schiff (PAS) and Grocott–Gomori methenamine–silver are widely used.

Culture. Most pathogenic fungi are easy to grow in culture. The agar media most commonly used are Sabouraud's glucose agar and 4% malt extract agar. These may be supplemented with chloramphenicol (50 mg/l) to minimize bacterial contamination and cycloheximide (500 mg/l) to reduce contamination with saprophytic fungi. Many fungal pathogens have an optimum growth temperature below 37°C. Consequently, cultures are incubated at 25–30°C and 37°C. With some of the dimorphic pathogens, enriched media such as brain–heart infusion or blood agar are used to promote growth of the yeast phase.

Many fungi develop relatively slowly and cultures should be retained for at least 2–3 weeks and in some cases up to 6 weeks before being discarded; yeasts usually grow within 1–5 d. Moulds are identified by their macroscopic and microscopic morphology; yeasts are identified by sugar fermentation and other biochemical tests. Commercial kits are available for this purpose.

Culture may provide unequivocal evidence of fungal infection when established pathogens are isolated or fungi are recovered from normally sterile sites. However, when commensals such as *Candida* species are isolated, results must be interpreted according to the quantity of the fungus isolated, the source and clinical evidence.

Serology. Serological tests for the detection of fungal antigens or specific antibodies to pathogenic fungi are used mainly in the diagnosis of systemic fungal infections. Many tests lack sensitivity or specificity and their precise value varies from disease to disease.

The most common tests for fungal antibodies are: immunodiffusion (ID), countercurrent immuno-electrophoresis (CIE), whole cell agglutination (WCA), complement fixation (CF) and enzyme-linked immunosorbent assay (ELISA). For antigen detection, latex particle agglutination (LPA), ELISA and radio-immunoassay (RIA) are used.

Treatment of mycoses

There are relatively few therapeutically useful antifungal agents compared to the large number of antibacterial agents that are available (see Chapters 6 and 65). This is due mainly to the fact that fungi and man are both eukaryotes and most substances that kill or inhibit fungal pathogens are also toxic to the host. Most antifungal agents exploit differences in the sterol composition of the fungal cell membrane.

Antifungal agents vary considerably in their spectrum of activity (see Table 6.7, p. 75). Primary or acquired resistance is not a major problem, although resistance to azole antifungals is occasionally encountered. About 12% of clinical isolates of yeasts are resistant to flucytosine and resistance may also develop during therapy. Except for flucytosine, sensitivity testing is not carried out routinely unless a drug is failing to produce the expected therapeutic response.

Most antifungal agents are available only for topical use and relatively few can be administered systemically. Some such as ketoconazole and terbinafine are usually administered orally; others like amphotericin B and miconazole are given parenterally because of poor absorption from the gastro-intestinal tract; flucytosine, fluconazole and itraconazole are available for oral or parenteral administration.

Combinations of antifungal agents may be useful in some systemic infections. A combination of amphotericin B and flucytosine allows amphotericin B, a toxic drug, to be used at a lower dose and reduces the likelihood of the emergence of resistance to flucytosine. Azole drugs and amphotericin B are antagonistic, at least in vitro, and such combinations are not recommended for therapeutic use.

Antifungal prophylaxis may be used for the prevention of opportunistic *Candida* infections in patients undergoing transplants or cardiac surgery and those with haematological malignancies. Oral or topical antifungals are also used to prevent recurrent vaginal candidosis and the acquisition of foot ringworm.

SUPERFICIAL INFECTIONS

Ringworm

Ringworm infections are common diseases of the stratum corneum of the skin, hair and nail; they are also referred to as *dermatophytosis* or *tinea*, a name which is qualified by the site affected, e.g. *tinea pedis* or *tinea capitis* for infections of the feet or scalp, respectively.

Ringworm infections are caused by about 20 species of dermatophyte fungi which are grouped into three genera, *Trichophyton*, *Microsporum* and *Epidermophyton* (Tables 60.1 and 60.2), some of which are restricted to certain parts of the world. Most ringworm infections in Europe are caused by *Trichophyton rubrum*, *T. mentagrophytes*, *T. verrucosum*, *Epidermophyton floccosum*, and *Microsporum canis*.

Some dermatophytes are primarily animal pathogens which may also infect man (Table 60.2); a few species are saprophytes of keratinous material in soil, but these only occasionally infect man and animals.

Table 60.1 Common dermatophyte pathogens of man

Species	Common site(s) of infection[a]	Chief area of distribution
Epidermophyton floccosum	Groin, feet, (nail)	World-wide
Microsporum audouinii	Scalp, (body)	Africa, America and Europe
M. ferrugineum	Scalp, (body)	Africa, Balkans and Asia
Trichophyton mentagrophytes ssp. interdigitale	Feet, (nail, groin)	World-wide
T. concentricum	Body	South Pacific
T. rubrum	Feet, nail, groin, body	World-wide
T. schoenleinii	Scalp, (body, nail)	Eurasia and North Africa
T. soudanense	Scalp, (body)	Africa
T. tonsurans	Scalp, body, (nail)	Europe and America
T. violaceum	Scalp, body, (nail)	Africa and Eurasia

[a] Parentheses indicate secondary sites of infection.

Ringworm infections are spread by direct or indirect contact with an infected individual or animal. The infective particle is usually a fragment of keratin containing viable fungus. Indirect transfer may occur via the floors of swimming pools and showers or on brushes, combs, towels and animal grooming implements. Dermatophytes can remain viable for long periods of time and the interval between deposition and transfer may be considerable. In addition to exposure to the fungus, some abnormality of the epidermis, such as slight peeling or minor trauma, is probably necessary for the establishment of infection.

In the industrialized countries, ringworm of the scalp accounts for only a small proportion of infection, and is mostly caused by dermatophytes of animal origin. However, the use of communal bathing facilities has resulted in a considerable increase in the incidence of foot ringworm and associated nail and groin infections. These now comprise about 75% of all ringworm infections diagnosed in temperate zones.

Table 60.2 Common dermatophyte species of animals

Species	Animals commonly affected	Chief area of distribution
Microsporum canis	Cat, dog	World-wide
M. distortum	Cat, dog	Australasia, USA
M. nanum	Pig	World-wide
M. persicolor	Bank field voles	Europe
Trichophyton mentagrophytes ssp. mentagrophytes	Rodents (horse, cat, dog)	World-wide
T. equinum	Horse	World-wide
T. erinacei	Hedgehog	UK, New Zealand
T. quinckeanum	Mice	Europe, North America
T. simii	Monkey, chicken	India
T. verrucosum	Cattle	World-wide

There is no evidence of natural immunity to ringworm. Scalp ringworm is predominantly a disease of children and foot ringworm a disease of adults, particularly adult males. Resistance to infection is partly determined by the production of inhibitory fatty acids and the rate of epithelial cell turnover, but the development of active T cell-mediated immunity and, in follicular infections, phagocytosis by neutrophils, also play a part.

Dermatophytes invade keratin by enzymic digestion and mechanical pressure; the hyphae grow into newly differentiated keratin as it is formed, keeping pace with the keratin growth. In tissue the dermatophytes take the form of branching hyphae, which may eventually break up into arthroconidia, particularly in infected hair.

Many dermatophyte species produce two types of asexual spore: *macroconidia* and *microconidia* (Fig. 60.3). Classification into the three genera *Trichophyton*, *Microsporum* and *Epidermophyton* is based on the morphology of the macroconidia, although the identification of species is also based on the shape and disposition of the microconidia and the macroscopic appearance of the colony. Biochemical tests can also be used to differentiate some species.

Pathogenesis

Ringworm lesions vary considerably according to the site of the infection and the species of fungus involved. Sometimes there is only dry scaling or hyperkeratosis, but more commonly there is irritation, erythema, oedema and some vesiculation. More inflammatory lesions with weeping vesicles, pustules and ulceration are usually caused by zoophilic species of dermatophyte.

In skin infections of the body, face and scalp, spreading annular lesions with a raised, inflammatory border are produced. Lesions in body folds, such as the groins, tend to spread outwards

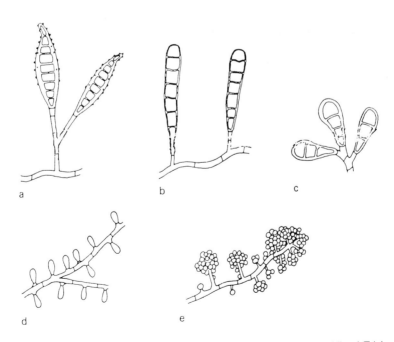

Fig. 60.3   Dermatophyte spore forms: **a** macroconidia of *Microsporum* species **b** macroconidia of *Trichophyton* species; **c** macroconidia of *Epidermophyton* species; **d** microconidia along sides of vegetative hyphae (*en thyrses*); **e** microconidia in grape-like bunches (*en grappe*). (From Evans E G V, Gentles J C 1985 *Essentials of Medical Mycology*. Churchill Livingstone, Edinburgh.)

from the flexures. In foot ringworm, infection is often confined to the toe clefts, but it can spread to the sole; sometimes painful secondary bacterial infection occurs in the toe clefts.

In nail infection, the nail becomes discoloured, thickened, raised and friable; most nail infections are due to *T. rubrum*.

In scalp infections there is scaling and hair loss, the extent of which depends on the causal fungus. Some zoophilic species give rise to a highly inflammatory, raised suppurating lesion called a *kerion*; kerions may also occur in the beard area of adults. It is important that scalp ringworm is recognized and treated promptly since it can lead to scarring and permanent hair loss.

In scalp infection the fungus surrounds and invades the hair shaft, where the hyphae break up into chains of arthroconidia. In some species (e.g. *T. tonsurans, T. violaceum*) the spores are retained within the hair shaft (*endothrix* invasion), whereas in others (e.g. *Microsporum* species, *T. verrucosum*) they are produced in a sheath surrounding the hair shaft (*ectothrix* invasion) (Fig. 60.4). The pattern of hair invasion affects the clinical appearance of the lesion: in endothrix infection the hair breaks off at, or just below, the mouth of the follicle, which then becomes plugged with dirt and sebum to give what is described as *black dot* ringworm, but in ectothrix infection the hair usually breaks off 2–3 mm above the mouth of the follicle, leaving short stumps of hair. In the condition called *favus*, caused by *T. schoenleinii*, fungal growth within the hair is minimal and the hair remains intact but intense fungal growth within and around the hair follicle produces a waxy, honeycomb-like crust on the scalp.

Infections of the groins, hands and nails are nearly always secondary to infection of the feet and are usually caused by *T. rubrum, T. mentagrophytes* or *E. floccosum* (mixed infections may also occur).

Occasionally, patients with chronic ringworm infections develop a secondary rash known as an *id* reaction, which is thought to be an immunological reaction to the fungus. In patients with foot ringworm this takes the form of a vascular eczema of the hands or feet, whereas patients with scalp or body ringworm develop a rash which probably

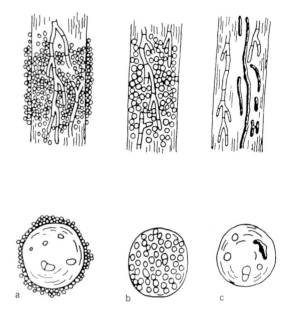

Fig. 60.4 Diagrammatic representation of various forms of hair invasion by dermatophytes as seen in longitudinal and transverse sections of hair shaft: **a** ectothrix (e.g. *M. audouinii, M. canis, T. mentagrophytes*) with hyphae sparsely distributed within hair shaft and a sheath of arthrospores on the outside; **b** endothrix (e.g. *T. tonsurans, T. violaceum*) with heavy arthrospore formation completely filling hair shaft; **c** favus (*T. schoenleinii*) showing sparse hyphal growth and formation of air spaces. (From Evans E G V, Gentles J C 1985 *Essentials of Medical Mycology.* Churchill Livingstone, Edinburgh.)

represents a form of cutaneous vasculitis. None of these secondary lesions contain any viable fungus.

Laboratory diagnosis

Ringworm infections may be reliably diagnosed in the laboratory by direct microscopical examination and culture of skin, crusts, hair and nail.

Collection of samples. The site should be cleaned with surgical spirit before taking the specimen, especially if greasy ointments or powders have been applied. Skin, hair and nail samples are best collected into folded squares of black paper, which can be fastened with a paper clip. The use of paper allows the specimen to dry out, which helps reduce bacterial contamination and provides conditions under which specimens can be stored for 12 months or more without loss in viability of the fungus.

Nail samples should be collected by taking clippings from any discoloured, dystrophic or brittle parts of the nail. The clippings should be taken from as far back as possible from the free edge of the nail and include its full thickness.

Scales from skin lesions should be collected by scraping outwards with a blunt scalpel from the edges of the lesions where most viable fungus is likely to be. If there is only minimal scaling, Sellotape can be used to remove material adequate for examination. The Sellotape strips are pressed against the lesion, peeled off and placed sticky-side down on a glass microscope slide. Specimens from the scalp should include hair stubs, the contents of plugged follicles and skin scales. Infected hairs are usually easy to pluck from the scalp with forceps. Cut hairs are unsatisfactory since the focus of infection is usually below or near the surface of the scalp.

Wood's lamp. This is a source of long-wave ultraviolet light that can be used to detect fluorescence in infected hair. It is especially useful for the detection of inconspicuous scalp lesions, and to select infected hairs for laboratory investigation.

Hairbrush sampling technique. Adequate material from minimal lesions may be obtained by brushing the scalp with a sterilized plastic hairbrush or scalp massage pad; this is then used to inoculate an appropriate culture medium by pressing the brush or pad spines into the agar.

Processing of specimens. If there is insufficient material for both microscopy and culture, the sample should be used for culture, since this is generally the more sensitive procedure.

The specimen should first be examined macroscopically; hair samples are examined under a Wood's lamp. Material from representative parts, and any fluorescent hairs, are divided up into 1–2 mm fragments with a sterile scalpel blade before microscopical examination and culture.

Direct microscopy. Microscopy of potassium hydroxide mounts of keratinous material is simple and reliable. The preparation should be allowed to stand for 15–20 min to allow digestion and 'clearing' of the keratin.

Dermatophytes are seen in skin and nail as branching hyphae which often appear slightly greenish in colour and run across the outlines of the colourless host cells.

Culture. Small fragments of keratinous material are planted or scattered on Sabouraud's glucose or 4% malt extract agar and incubated at 27–30°C for up to 3 weeks; room temperature is adequate but the dermatophytes grow more slowly. Only *T. verrucosum* grows well at 37°C.

Identification of dermatophytes is based on colonial appearance and colour, pigment production, and the micromorphology of any spores produced. Special tests exist for differentiating certain morphologically similar species. Thus, the ability of *T. mentagrophytes* to produce urease within 2–4 d distinguishes it from *T. rubrum*, and the ability to grow on rice grains distinguishes *M. canis* from *M. audouinii*.

Treatment and prevention

Topical therapy is satisfactory for most dermatophyte infections of skin. However, oral antifungals are required to treat infections of the nail and scalp, and severe skin infections. Some chronic infections require prolonged oral and topical therapy.

Topical agents such as Whitfield's ointment and tolnaftate have largely been superseded by azole compounds. Oral griseofulvin is useful but the cure rates for nail infections are poor; up to 18 months' treatment is required for toenail infections and the cure rate is only 30–40%. Newer oral agents such as terbinafine and itraconazole achieve better cure rates with shorter periods of treatment and have lower relapse rates.

Relatively little has been done to control the spread of ringworm, although improved living conditions and standards of hygiene, and better diagnosis have led to a reduction in the incidence of scalp ringworm. The prophylactic use of antifungal foot powder after bathing has been shown to be beneficial in reducing the spread of infection among swimmers; the foot-baths containing antiseptic solutions which are commonplace in swimming pools are of no value and only serve to concentrate infected skin material in one area where everyone is expected to walk.

Superficial candidosis

Superficial *Candida* infections are very common throughout the world. They may involve the skin, nails and mucous membranes of the mouth and vagina; infection of the mucous membranes is commonly referred to as *thrush*.

Candida albicans accounts for 80–90% of cases, but other species, notably *C. tropicalis*, *C. lusitaniae*, *C. (Torulopsis) glabrata*, *C. parapsilosis* and *C. guilliermondii* may occur.

Candida species, usually *C. albicans*, are found in small numbers in the commensal flora of about 20% of the normal population. The carriage rate tends to increase with age and is higher in the vagina during pregnancy. Commensal yeasts are more prevalent among hospitalized patients. Yeast overgrowth and infection occur when the normal microbial flora of the body is altered or when host resistance to infection is lowered by disease. Infection is most likely when several factors operate together to compound their effects, and in some cases deep-seated candidosis may result (see p. 694).

Immunity to *Candida* species depends on a combination of non-specific and immunological defences. In superficial infections the non-specific inhibitory factors include inhibitors in serum such as unsaturated transferrin and epithelial proliferation. Specific immunity largely depends on the appearance of sensitized T lymphocytes and phagocytes, particularly neutrophils.

On Sabouraud's glucose agar *Candida* species grow predominantly in the yeast phase as round or oval cells, 3–8 μm in diameter. A mixture of yeast cells, pseudomycelium and true mycelium is found in vivo and under micro-aerophilic growth conditions on nutritionally poor media. *C. glabrata* never forms either mycelium or pseudomycelium.

Pathogenesis

Mucosal infections. These are the commonest forms of superficial candidosis; they are characterized by the development of discrete white patches on the mucosal surface which may eventually become confluent and form a curd-like pseudo- membrane.

In oral candidosis white flecks appear on the buccal mucosa and the hard palate and although these are adherent, they can be removed; the surrounding mucosa is red and sore. Infection may spread to the tongue. This form of oral candidosis occurs most frequently in infancy and old age, or in severely immunocompromised patients, including those with acquired immune deficiency syndrome (AIDS). Other forms of oral candidosis occur: in those who wear dentures, lesions often appear in the occluded area under the denture, and in some individuals antibiotic therapy may result in a painful *Candida* infection of the tongue. Chronic oral candidosis may also occur with extensive leucoplakia and infection of the angles of the mouth (*angular cheilitis*).

In vaginal candidosis, typical white lesions on the epithelial surfaces of the vulva, vagina and cervix are accompanied by itching, soreness and a non-homogenous white discharge. Sometimes the mucosa simply appears inflamed and friable. The perivulval skin may become sore and small satellite pustules may appear around the perineum and natal cleft.

Vaginal candidosis is common, especially during pregnancy; most women will have at least one episode during their lifetime and some suffer recurrent attacks.

Skin and nail infections. *Candida* infections of the skin almost invariably occur at moist sites such as the axillae, groins, perineum, submammary folds and occasionally the toe clefts. In infants, *Candida* species are frequently involved in napkin dermatitis. Infection of the finger webs, nail folds and nails is associated with frequent immersion of the hands in water and is an occupational disease among housewives, nurses and barmaids. Secondary invasion and discoloration of the lateral border of the nail may develop. Superficial *Candida* infections occasionally occur on the penis after intercourse with females with vaginal thrush. The yeast may also infect the outer ear.

Chronic mucocutaneous candidosis. This is a rare form of candidosis which usually becomes apparent in childhood and takes the form of a persistent, sometimes granulomatous infection of the mouth, skin and nails. Some of those who develop this condition have subtle defects in lymphocyte or neutrophil function.

Laboratory diagnosis

Specimens of skin and nail are collected in the same way as for suspected ringworm. For infections of the mouth or vagina, scrapings taken with a blunt scalpel or a spatula from areas with erythema or white plaques are better than swabs, if the material is to be processed immediately. However, swabs are more convenient for transport to the laboratory, and they are better for collecting vaginal discharge.

Swabs should be moistened with sterile water or saline before taking the sample and sent to the laboratory in transport medium.

In Gram-stained smears of mucous membrane samples the fungus is seen as budding Gram-positive yeast cells; mycelium is usually present except in the case of *C. glabrata*. Contrary to popular belief, the presence of *Candida* mycelium in clinical material does not confirm invasive infection with the organism, particularly as the mycelium may have developed in the period between collection and processing of the sample.

Candida species grow well on Sabouraud's medium or on bacteriological media such as blood agar at 25–37°C, and typical yeast colonies appear within 1–2 d. *C. albicans* isolates can be identified by the germ tube test; the yeast is incubated at 37°C in serum for 1.5–2 h and under these conditions *C. albicans* produces hyphae known as *germ tubes*. Other yeasts may be identified with one of the commercial kits or by fermentation and assimilation tests.

It is useful for culture results to be quantified, especially in the case of vulvovaginal samples, since this may help the clinician to distinguish between commensal carriage and infection.

Treatment and prevention

Most superficial *Candida* infections respond well to topical therapy with nystatin, amphotericin B, or an azole. In addition to treating the *Candida* infection it is important, if possible, to identify and correct any predisposing factor.

In oral candidosis, nystatin, amphotericin B and miconazole may be effective in lozenge or gel form. Most cases of vaginal candidosis can be treated successfully with a single application of an azole derivative or with oral therapy with fluconazole or itraconazole for 1 d. Intermittent prophylaxis with azole vaginal pessaries is of benefit in controlling recurrent vaginal candidosis.

Treatment of chronic paronychia involves a combination of antifungal therapy, nail care and avoidance of prolonged exposure to water by use of protective gloves; patients should dry their hands carefully after washing. Regular application of an azole lotion is the most appropriate therapy but it may take several months to cure the condition; antifungal creams or ointments are less effective.

Oral therapy is essential for the treatment of intractable chronic *Candida* infections; treatment is given until remission is achieved but relapse is common and intermittent therapy may be required.

Pityriasis versicolor

Pityriasis versicolor is a mild, chronic infection of the stratum corneum which produces a patchy discoloration of the skin caused by the lipophilic yeast *Malassezia furfur*.

M. furfur is a common member of the normal skin flora and most infections are thought to be endogenous. The disease is probably related to host or environmental factors. It is very common in the tropics and, although it occurs in all age groups, it is most prevalent in young adults.

M. furfur requires lipids for growth and media containing Tween and lipid supplements have been developed specifically to grow the organism. On skin and in conditions such as dandruff and seborrhoeic dermatitis (in which its precise role is uncertain) *M. furfur* is present as an oval or bottle-shaped yeast (2–3 × 4–5μm), which characteristically produces buds on a broad base; in this form the organism is known as *Pityrosporum ovale*. In pityriasis versicolor the organism produces predominantly round yeast cells and short hyphae, the *P. orbiculare* form. The optimum growth temperature is about 30°C but in culture the colonial morphology and growth rate vary with the strain and the medium. All forms of *M. furfur* are Gram-positive.

Pathogenesis

Small, well-demarcated, non-inflammatory, scaling macules are usually present on the upper trunk or neck; these may appear hypo- or hyperpigmented, depending on the degree of pigmentation of the surrounding skin. The lesions tend to spread and coalesce, and occasionally they spread to other sites.

Laboratory diagnosis

The diagnosis can be confirmed reliably by demonstration of the organism in skin scales by direct microscopy and culture is unnecessary. Clusters of characteristic round yeast cells (5–8 μm in diameter) are seen together with short, stout hyphae, which may be curved and occasionally branched.

Treatment

Pityriasis versicolor responds well to topical therapy with 1% selenium sulphide or azoles in cream, lotion or shampoo. Oral azole therapy is sometimes used for recalcitrant infections. Relapse is common, particularly in hot climates.

Other superficial infections

Skin and nail

Certain non-dermatophyte moulds may cause infection of skin and nail. It is important that these are recognized since they are often resistant to the agents used to treat ringworm and superficial candidosis.

In the UK, about 5% of fungal nail infections are caused by non-dermatophytes, most commonly *Scopulariopsis brevicaulis*, an ubiquitous saprophyte of soil. Other saprophytic moulds such as *Fusarium*, *Aspergillus* and *Penicillium* species are also occasionally implicated. Two other moulds, *Nattrassia mangiferae*, a pathogen of fruit trees, and *Scytalidium hyalinum*, a soil fungus, occasionally cause an infection of nails and sometimes skin in the tropics. These infections are diagnosed by microscopy and culture, as for ringworm infections. However, *N. mangiferae* and *S. hyalinum* are both sensitive to cycloheximide and will not grow if this antibiotic is included in the medium.

Non-dermatophyte mould infections do not respond to existing antifungal agents. Attempts may be made to remove the nail with topical 40% urea paste.

Tinea nigra. This is a superficial, asymptomatic skin disease characterized by pigmented macules of variable size, usually on the palms and soles. It is caused by a black mould, *Phaeoannellomyces* (*Cladosporium*) *werneckii*, and occurs mainly in the tropics. Tinea nigra is not contagious but is contracted by contact with the fungus in soil.

Diagnosis is made easily by recognition of the dark-coloured hyphal elements on microscopical examination of skin scrapings in potassium hydroxide. On Sabouraud's agar the fungus develops as grey, yeast-like colonies which gradually become more mycelial and darker coloured with age.

Tinea nigra responds well to treatment with keratolytic agents such as Whitfield's ointment.

Hair

White piedra. This disease, caused by the yeast *Trichosporon beigelii*, results in soft, white, greyish or light-brown nodules on the hair shafts, mainly in the axillae. The hair often breaks at the point of infection, leaving hairs with a clubbed or swollen end. Shaving of the affected area is usually sufficient to effect a cure.

Black piedra. This condition, caused by *Piedraia hortae*, is characterized by the presence of black, hard nodules up to 1 mm in diameter, mainly on the hairs of the scalp. It occurs in humid, tropical climates. Crushing the nodules reveals the sexual reproductive phase, club-shaped asci, each with eight ascospores. Culture is not necessary. Shaving to remove infected hairs is a satisfactory treatment.

Otomycosis

About 10–20% of chronic ear infections are due to fungi. The commonest causes are species of *Aspergillus*, in particular *A. niger*. The fungi are easy to see in material from swabs or scrapings and grow readily in culture.

Treatment with topical antifungals is usually successful, although relapse is common. Any concurrent bacterial infection or other underlying abnormality should also be treated.

Mycotic keratitis

Fungal infections of the cornea are secondary to injury, bacterial infection and treatment with antibacterial agents and steroids. They are caused by moulds which occur commonly as saprophytes in nature, in particular species of *Aspergillus* and *Fusarium*. Culture results should be interpreted with care since these opportunist pathogens are also encountered as contaminants. Superficial swabs are of no value for laboratory investigation and scrapings should be taken from the base or edge of the ulcer. The branched, septate hyphae may be rather sparse in potassium hydroxide mounts and some of the material should also be stained with PAS or methenamine–silver techniques.

Treatment is with topical antifungal agents, in particular natamycin.

SUBCUTANEOUS INFECTIONS

Mycetoma

Mycetoma is a chronic, granulomatous infection of the skin, subcutaneous tissues, fascia and bone, which most often affects the foot or the hand. It may be caused by one of a number of different actinomycetes (*actinomycetoma*) (see Chapter 21) or moulds (*eumycetoma*). The disease is most prevalent in tropical and subtropical regions of Africa, Asia and central America. Infection follows traumatic inoculation of the organism into the subcutaneous tissue from soil or vegetable sources, usually on thorns or splinters. Consequently, the disease occurs most frequently in male agricultural workers, in whom minor skin injuries are common.

A large number of organisms have been implicated in this disease, including species of *Madurella, Exophiala, Acremonium, Actinomadura, Nocardia* and *Streptomyces*. Within host tissues the organisms develop to form compacted colonies (grains), 0.5–2 mm in diameter, whose colour depends on the organism responsible; for example, *Madurella* grains are black.

Pathogenesis

Localized swollen lesions, which develop multiple draining sinuses, are usually found on the limbs, although infections occur on other parts of the body. There is often a long period between the initial infection and formation of the characteristic lesions; spread from the site of origin is unusual but may occur.

Laboratory diagnosis

The presence of grains in pus collected from draining sinuses or in biopsy material is diagnostic. The grains are visible to the naked eye and their colour may help to identify the causal agent. Grains should be crushed in potassium hydroxide and examined microscopically to differentiate between actinomycetoma and eumycetoma; material from actinomycetoma grains may be Gram stained to demonstrate the Gram-positive filaments. Samples should also be cultured, at both 25–30°C and 37°C, on brain–heart infusion agar or blood agar for actinomycetes and on Sabouraud's agar (without cycloheximide) for fungi. The fungi that cause eumycetoma are all septate moulds which appear in culture within 1–4 weeks, but their identification requires expert knowledge. Serological tests for precipitins have been used to differentiate between eumycetoma and actinomycetoma and to identify specific causal agents, but they are not in routine use.

Treatment

The prognosis varies according to the causal agent, so it is important that its identity is established. Actinomycetoma responds well to rifampicin in combination with sulphonamides or co-trimoxazole but an average of 9 months of therapy is required. In eumycetoma, chemotherapy is ineffective and radical surgery is usually necessary. However, some of the newer antifungals have yet to be properly evaluated in this condition.

Chromoblastomycosis

This disease, also known as *chromomycosis*, is a chronic, localized disease of the skin and subcutaneous tissues, characterized by crusted, warty lesions usually involving the limbs. The disease is mainly encountered in the tropics. The principal causes are *Fonsecaea pedrosoi*, *F. compacta*, *Phialophora verrucosa*, *Exophiala dermatitidis* and *Cladosporium carrionii*. Like mycetoma, the disease is seen most often among males in rural areas.

Laboratory diagnosis

The dark-coloured fungal elements are relatively easy to see on microscopical examination of skin scrapings, crusts and pus.

Culture on Sabouraud's agar at 25–30°C yields slow-growing, greenish grey to black, compact, folded colonies. Cultures should be incubated for 4–6 weeks. Specific identification of these closely related fungi is usually left to a reference laboratory.

Serological tests are not used routinely.

Treatment

Treatment is unsatisfactory but itraconazole either alone or in combination with flucytosine may be useful. Early, solitary lesions may be excised.

Phaeohyphomycosis

This is a general term given to non-specific solitary subcutaneous lesions caused by any black fungus. Diagnosis is often made at surgery, and treatment is by excision. These fungi may also cause opportunistic, deep-seated infections, such as brain abscesses, which require therapy with amphotericin B and flucytosine.

Sporotrichosis

Sporotrichosis is a chronic, pyogenic granulomatous infection of the skin and subcutaneous tissues which may remain localized or show lymphatic spread. It is caused by *Sporothrix schenckii*, a saprophyte in nature. The disease occurs mainly in Central and South America, parts of the USA and Africa, and Australia; it is rare in Europe.

S. schenckii is a dimorphic fungus. In nature and in culture at 25–30°C, it develops as a mould with thin (1–2 μm) septate hyphae; spore-bearing hyphae carry clusters of oval spores. The yeast phase is formed in tissue and in culture at 37°C, and is composed of spherical or cigar-shaped cells (1–3 × 3–10 μm).

Pathogenesis

Sporotrichosis most frequently presents as a nodular, ulcerating disease of the skin and subcutaneous tissues, with spread along local lymphatic channels. Typically, the primary lesion is on the hand with secondary lesions extending up the arm. The primary lesion may remain localized or disseminate to involve the bones, joints, lungs and, in rare cases, the central nervous system. Disseminated disease usually occurs in debilitated or immunosuppressed individuals.

Laboratory diagnosis

Diagnosis is confirmed by isolation of the causative organism by culture of swabs from moist, ulcerated lesions or pus aspirated from subcutaneous nodules; biopsy specimens may be necessary in some cases. Direct microscopy is of little value since so few of the small *S. schenckii* yeast cells are present in diseased tissue. The mycelial phase develops within 7–10 d on Sabouraud's agar or blood agar at 25–30°C and the yeast phase develops in 2 d at 37°C.

Identification depends on the micromorphology of the mould phase and the conversion to the yeast phase at 37°C.

An LPA test is of value for the diagnosis of the extracutaneous forms of sporotrichosis. The test has poor prognostic value since titres change little after successful therapy. A skin test with sporotrichin antigen is positive in almost all patients with cutaneous sporotrichosis.

Treatment

For the cutaneous form, treatment with potassium iodide or itraconazole is satisfactory. In disseminated disease, intravenous amphotericin B is required.

Rhinosporidiosis

This is a chronic, granulomatous disease of the mucocutaneous tissues, caused by *Rhinosporidium seeberi*, which results in the production of large polyps or wart-like lesions in the nose or conjunctiva. More than 80% of reported cases have been from India and Sri Lanka, although the disease is also seen in South America.

All attempts to isolate *R. seeberi* from clinical material have failed but the morphology of the organism suggests that it is related to aquatic fungi.

Laboratory diagnosis depends on the demonstration of sporangia, which may be visible to the naked eye.

Treatment is by surgical excision.

Other subcutaneous mycoses

Several other fungi, including *Loboa loboi*, *Basidiobolus haptosporus* and *Conidiobolus coronatus*, occasionally cause subcutaneous infections, usually in the tropics. Surgical excision is often curative in *L. loboi* infections; antifungal therapy may be of use for the other infections, but the newer drugs have not been properly evaluated.

SYSTEMIC MYCOSES
Coccidioidomycosis

Coccidioidomycosis is primarily an infection of the lungs caused by *Coccidioides immitis*, a dimorphic fungus found in the soil of semi-arid areas, mainly in the south-west USA and northern Mexico. Agricultural workers with a higher exposure risk and dark-skinned people are especially prone to the disease. In endemic regions over 90% of inhabitants may exhibit positive skin tests and infection rates of 20% or higher have been recorded among newcomers to the areas in their first year of residence. Recovery from coccidioidomycosis usually confers lifetime immunity.

In culture and in soil *C. immitis* grows as a mould, producing large numbers of barrel-shaped arthroconidia ($4 \times 6 \mu m$ diameter), which are easily dispersed in wind currents. In the lungs the arthroconidia form spherules (30–60 μm diameter) which contain numerous endospores (2–5 μm diameter). Endospores are released by rupture of the spherule wall and develop to form new spherules in adjacent tissue or, following dissemination, in other organs of the body. In culture the mycelial colony is initially moist and white but changes within 5–12 d to become pale grey or brown.

Pathogenesis

C. immitis usually causes an asymptomatic or self-limiting pulmonary illness but a progressive and sometimes fatal secondary disease occasionally develops. Primary pulmonary coccidioidomycosis develops 7–28 d after infection. Skin rashes develop in up to 20% of those with the primary disease and indicate a good prognosis. In some cases primary infection may result in a chronic, cavitating, pulmonary infection which may resolve after several years, or may progress to the disseminated form. Localized subcutaneous infection may result from direct inoculation of the fungus through the skin or may be secondary to pulmonary disease.

Disseminated infection occurs in about 1% of those who contract the primary pulmonary disease; it is more common in immunocompromised individuals, and in Filipinos, Negroes and American Indians. When dissemination occurs, it involves virtually every tissue of the body, including the central nervous system, skin and joints. The prognosis for disseminated coccidioidomycosis is generally poor, particularly in immunosuppressed individuals and those with meningeal involvement.

Laboratory diagnosis

Microscopical examination of sputum, pus and biopsy material is helpful since the relatively large size and numbers of mature spherules present makes their detection and identification comparatively straightforward. Material for culture should be inoculated onto test-tube slopes of Sabouraud's agar and incubated at 25–30°C for at least 3 weeks. The fungus can be identified by its colonial morphology and the presence of numerous thick-walled arthroconidia formed in chains from alternate cells of the fine, septate hyphae.

The arthroconidia are highly infectious and are a serious danger to laboratory staff. Consequently, Petri dishes should *never* be used for isolation of the organism and all procedures should be carried out in a safety cabinet. Preparations for microscopy should be made only after wetting the colony to reduce spore dispersal.

Skin tests and serological tests are useful although cross-reactions may occur in patients with histoplasmosis and blastomycosis. The tests use either coccidioidin, a culture filtrate antigen from the mycelial phase of *C. immitis*, or spherulin, an extract of the spherules.

The skin test does not distinguish present from past infection and a negative skin test does not preclude infection with *C. immitis*.

Serological tests play an important part in diagnosis. The precipitin test is most useful for detection of early, primary infection or exacerbation of existing disease; precipitins appear 1–3 weeks after infection but are seldom detectable after 2–6 months, or in patients with disseminated coccidioidomycosis. The LPA test gives similar results to the precipitin test, but is not as specific. The CF test is most useful for detecting disseminated disease: CF antibodies appear 2–3

months after infection and persist until death or recovery.

Treatment

Intravenous amphotericin B is indicated and concomitant intrathecal therapy is required in the meningeal form. Ketoconazole and itraconazole are also useful.

Histoplasmosis

Histoplasmosis, caused by *Histoplasma capsulatum*, is ordinarily an asymptomatic or relatively mild, self-limiting pulmonary infection, although chronic or acute disseminated disease may also occur. *H. capsulatum* is unique among pathogenic fungi in that it is an intracellular parasite.

H. capsulatum is found in soil enriched with the droppings of birds and bats, and infection results from the inhalation of spores. The major endemic areas for histoplasmosis are the Mississippi and Ohio river valleys of the eastern USA, where the prevalence of infection may be as high as 95%. It also occurs in other parts of the USA and many other temperate and tropical areas.

H. capsulatum grows in soil and in culture at 25–30°C as a mould and as an intracellular yeast in animal tissues. The yeast phase cells (2–3 × 3–4 μm) can also be produced in vitro by culture at 37°C on blood agar or other enriched media containing cysteine. In culture the mould colonies are fluffy, white or buff-brown; the mycelium is septate and two types of unicellular asexual spores are usually produced: large round, tuberculate macroconidia (8–14 μm in diameter) are most prominent and are diagnostic, but smaller broadly elliptical, smooth-walled microconidia (2–4 μm in diameter) are also present in primary isolates.

Pathogenesis

Most infections are asymptomatic and are detected only when individuals develop a positive skin test reaction. Sometimes an acute influenza-like illness develops with fever and a non-productive cough. These infections are usually self-limiting, but patients are frequently left with discrete, calcified lesions in the lung.

A chronic form of histoplasmosis occurs mainly in adults; large cavities develop directly from primary lesions in the lung or by reactivation of old lesions. The clinical picture closely resembles tuberculosis; in some cases the infection may disseminate to give acute generalized disease.

Occasionally, patients develop an acute progressive form of the disease, with widespread infection of the reticulo-endothelial system and dissemination to other organs of the body. The rate of progression of the disease varies considerably, but generally the prognosis is poor.

Disseminated infection occurs most often in old age, infancy, or in individuals with impaired immune responses.

Laboratory diagnosis

Microscopy of smears of sputum or pus should be stained by the Wright or Giemsa procedure. Blood smears may be positive for *H. capsulatum*, especially in patients with AIDS. Liver or lung biopsies stained with PAS, or methenamine–silver may provide a rapid diagnosis of disseminated histoplasmosis in some patients. *H. capsulatum* is seen as small, oval yeast cells, typically packed within macrophages or monocytes.

Specimens should be cultured on Sabouraud's agar at 25–30°C to obtain the mycelial phase. Mycelial colonies develop within 1–4 weeks but cultures should be retained for 6 weeks before discarding. The fungus is identified by its colonial morphology and the presence of the characteristic macro- and microconidia. Culture at 37°C for the yeast phase is not used for primary isolation but conversion from the mould to yeast phase is useful to confirm the identity of isolates. Mould cultures of *H. capsulatum* are a hazard to laboratory staff and consequently test-tube slopes rather than Petri dishes should be used for isolation.

A histoplasmin skin test has been used, but a positive result does not differentiate between active and past infection, and false-positive reactions can occur in patients with other fungal infections; furthermore, skin testing induces humoral antibodies which complicate the interpretation of subsequent serodiagnostic tests.

Serological tests are useful, but cross-reactions can occur, mainly with *C. immitis*. CF, precipitin and LPA tests are commonly used in combination. The CF test, with histoplasmin or killed whole yeast cells as antigen, is positive in up to 96% of culturally proven cases. Generally, titres of 8 are regarded as presumptive evidence of infection, and titres of 32 or above indicate active disease. Low titres or negative results do not exclude infection. The precipitin test gives positive results in up to 85% of infected patients; there are few problems with cross-reactions but positive results should be confirmed by a CF test. The LPA test is useful for detection of acute histoplasmosis but is of less value than CF and precipitin tests.

Antibody tests fail to detect antibodies in up to 50% of immunosuppressed individuals although more sensitive techniques such as ELISA have given improved results. Detection of *H. capsulatum* polysaccharide antigen in blood and urine by sensitive techniques such as RIA may prove to be a useful diagnostic method.

Treatment

Intravenous amphotericin B is the treatment of choice for histoplasmosis. Azole antifungal agents have given promising results in a few cases.

African histoplasmosis

This disease, caused by *Histoplasma duboisii*, is mainly restricted to the continent of Africa. It is primarily a disease of the cutaneous and subcutaneous tissues with little evidence of pulmonary involvement. *H. duboisii* is morphologically identical to *H. capsulatum* in its mycelial phase but differs in that the yeast phase, both in vivo and in vitro, has larger cells (12–15 µm in diameter); some consider *H. duboisii* to be a variety of *H. capsulatum*. Treatment is as for histoplasmosis.

Blastomycosis

Blastomycosis is a chronic infection of the lungs which may spread to other tissues, particularly skin and bone. It is caused by *Blastomyces dermatitidis* and occurs mainly in the central and mid-western states of the USA and eastern Canada. The disease is slowly progressive and if left untreated has a poor prognosis.

B. *dermatitidis* has been isolated from the environment on only a few occasions and its exact ecological niche has yet to be established. Infection results from inhalation of spores and most infections appear to be contracted sporadically in cool, wet climatic conditions. The disease is seen most often among males in the 30–50 year age group. A subclinical pulmonary form of the disease, similar to that seen in coccidioidomycosis and histoplasmosis, probably exists.

B. *dermatitidis* is a dimorphic fungus. In culture at 25–30°C it grows as a mould with a septate mycelium. The colony varies in texture from floccose to smooth and from white to brown in colour. Asexual conidia are produced on lateral hyphal branches of variable length; the conidia range in size from 2 to 10 μm in diameter and some may be dumb-bell shaped. In tissue and in culture at 37°C the fungus grows as a yeast (8–15 μm in diameter) which characteristically produces broad-based buds from a single pole on the mother cell.

Pathogenesis

Primary pulmonary disease is usually relatively mild, but within a few weeks the disease may disseminate to other tissues. The chest radiograph can resemble that of tuberculosis or carcinoma. In disseminated infection the chronic pulmonary disease persists and abscesses and granulomatous lesions are found in most organs and body tissues including bone. Disseminated blastomycosis has been described in immunosuppressed patients including those with AIDS. Chronic cutaneous lesions occur in about 80% of patients with pulmonary infection; the characteristic secondary skin lesions are typically raised with a well-demarcated edge. It is from these skin lesions that the diagnosis is most often made. Primary cutaneous infection resulting from the introduction of the fungus to the skin is rare and produces a localized, self-limiting lesion.

Laboratory diagnosis

Direct microscopy of pus, scrapings from skin lesions, or sputum usually shows thick-walled yeast cells (8–15 μm in diameter) which characteristically produce buds on a broad base (4–5 μm); the buds remaining attached until they are almost the size of the parent cell, often forming chains of three or four cells. In biopsy material the yeasts are best seen in sections stained with PAS or methenamine–silver.

B. *dermatitidis* will grow in culture on Sabouraud's agar or blood agar, but since it is sensitive to cycloheximide this must not be used in isolation media. The mycelial phase develops slowly at 25–30°C and cultures must be retained for 6 weeks before discarding. Test-tube slopes rather than Petri dishes are used for culture. Identification is usually confirmed by subculturing at 37°C to convert it to the yeast phase.

Most skin and serological tests are unreliable because of poor sensitivity and cross-reaction with histoplasmosis and coccidioidomycosis. However, an ELISA test has been developed that appears to be more than 90% specific.

Treatment

Intravenous amphotericin B is used to treat all forms of blastomycosis. Hydroxystilbamidine has been used in localized disease or when amphotericin B fails or proves too toxic. Azole antifungals have given promising results in some cases.

Paracoccidioidomycosis

This is a chronic, granulomatous infection, caused by *Paracoccidioides brasiliensis*, which may involve the lungs, mucosa, skin and lymphatic system. The disease is fatal if untreated.

P. *brasiliensis* enters the body via the lungs; it grows as a saprophyte in nature but the precise reservoir is unknown. The disease occurs most frequently in humid mountain forests of South and Central America. Most infections are seen in rural workers 20–40 years of age.

P. brasiliensis grows in the mycelial phase in culture at 25–30°C, and in the yeast phase in tissue or at 37°C on brain–heart infusion or blood agar. The mould colonies are slow-growing with a variable colonial morphology, although most are white and velvety to floccose in texture with a pale brown reverse. Spore production is usually sparse and best seen in 8–10 week cultures. Asexual conidia may be produced but are not characteristic and the identification of *P. brasiliensis* depends on its conversion from the mycelial to the yeast phase. The yeast phase consists of oval or globose cells 2–30 μm in diameter with small buds attached by a narrow neck, encircling the parent cell.

Pathogenesis

Paracoccidioidomycosis usually presents as an ulcerative, granulomatous infection of the oral and nasal mucosa and the adjacent skin. The lymphatic system, spleen, intestines, adrenals and liver are also often involved. Primary skin lesions are rare. There is evidence of prolonged latent infection before overt disease develops, and a mild, self-limiting pulmonary form of paracoccidioidomycosis probably exists.

Laboratory diagnosis

Microscopy of sputum or pus, crusts and biopsies from granulomatous lesions usually reveals numerous yeast cells of *P. brasiliensis*. Yeasts showing the characteristic multipolar budding are diagnostic. Tissue sections should be stained with PAS or methenamine–silver. In culture the mycelial and yeast phases both develop slowly and cultures must be retained for 6 weeks before discarding. The mould phase can be isolated on Sabouraud's agar supplemented with yeast extract at 25–30°C, but colonies may take 15–25 d to appear. Blood agar (without cycloheximide) and incubation at 37°C is recommended for isolation of the yeast phase.

Skin tests for paracoccidioidomycosis are of limited diagnostic value because of poor sensitivity and cross-reactivity with other systemic mycoses. Serological tests are of value for diagnosis and for monitoring the response to therapy. Precipitin tests and CF tests, when used together, detect about 98% of infections. Cross-reactions are rare, particularly with the precipitin test.

Treatment

Intravenous amphotericin B or sulphonamides, or both, have been used to treat paracoccidioidomycosis. The choice of therapy depends on the site of infection and its severity. Ketoconazole and itraconazole have given promising results.

Cryptococcosis

Cryptococcosis, caused by the capsulate yeast *Cryptococcus neoformans*, is most frequently recognized as a disease of the central nervous system, although the primary site of infection is the lungs. Cryptococcosis occurs sporadically throughout the world but it is now seen most often in patients with AIDS.

There are four serotypes of *C. neoformans* (A, B, C, D). Most infections are caused by serotypes A and D, which are commonly found in the excreta of wild and domesticated birds throughout the world. Pigeons carry *C. neoformans* in their crops and counts of up to 5×10^7 cells per gram of pigeon faeces have been found. The birds themselves do not appear to become infected, probably because of their high body temperature. Serotypes B and C are associated with the flowers of *Eucalyptus camaldulensis* and the distribution of this tree coincides with the occurrence of infections due to the B and C serotypes of *C. neoformans*.

Pathogenesis

Infection follows inhalation of the cells of *C. neoformans* which, in nature, are thought to be small, allowing the organism to enter deep into the lung.

The disease is more common in males than females. The meningeal form of cryptococcosis can occur in individuals who appear otherwise healthy but occurs most frequently in patients with abnormalities of T lymphocyte function, including those with Hodgkin's disease, sarcoidosis, collagen disease and neoplasms. However, most cryptococcal infections are now seen in individuals with AIDS, about 10% of whom develop cryptococcosis.

A mild, self-limiting pulmonary infection is believed to be the commonest form of cryptococcosis. In symptomatic pulmonary infection there are no clear diagnostic features. Lesions may take the form of small discrete nodules which may heal with a residual scar or may become enlarged, encapsulated and chronic (*cryptococcoma* form). An acute pneumonic type of disease has also been described.

Chronic meningitis or meningo-encephalitis develops insidiously with headaches and low-grade pyrexia, followed by changes in mental state, anorexia, visual disturbances and eventually coma. The disease may last from a few months to several years, but the outcome is always fatal unless it is treated. AIDS patients with cryptococcosis generally develop a chronic meningeal form with milder symptoms.

Although predominantly a disease of the central nervous system, lesions of the skin, mucosa, viscera and bones may also occur; in its disseminated form, the disease may resemble tuberculosis. Rarely, lesions of skin and bones may occur without any evidence of infection elsewhere.

Laboratory diagnosis

C. neoformans is readily demonstrated in cerebrospinal fluid (CSF) or other material by direct microscopy, culture or serological tests for capsular antigen. The yeast load is generally higher in patients with AIDS. The cellular reaction and chemical changes in CSF usually resemble those seen in tuberculous meningitis. The yeast cells of *C. neoformans* are round (4–10 µm in diameter) and are surrounded by a mucopolysaccharide capsule. The width of the capsule varies and is greatest in vivo and on rich media in vitro.

In unstained, wet preparations of CSF mixed with a drop of India ink or nigrosine, the capsule of *C. neoformans* can be seen as a clear halo around the yeast cells. Capsulated yeasts are seen in the CSF of about 60% of patients with cryptococcosis, but the capsule may be difficult to visualize in some cases. Sputum, pus or brain tissue should be examined after digestion in potassium hydroxide and here the capsulated yeasts are often delineated by the cellular debris. For examination of tissue sections it is best to use a specific fungal stain such as PAS; alcian blue and mucicarmine stain the capsular material, enabling the organisms to be differentiated from *H. capsulatum* and *B. dermatitidis*.

The yeast is easily cultured from CSF although large volumes or multiple samples may be required in some cases. On Sabouraud's agar (without cycloheximide) cultured at 25–30°C and 37°C, colonies normally appear within 2–3 d, but cultures should not be discarded for 3 weeks. In culture, *C. neoformans* appears as creamy-white to yellow-brown colonies, which are mucoid in appearance in well-capsulated strains and dry in poorly encapsulated strains. The cells of *C. neoformans* produce buds at any point on the cell surface but mycelium or pseudomycelium are not normally produced. Preliminary identification depends on demonstration of the capsule but this may be absent or difficult to see. *C. neoformans* is distinguished from other yeasts by its lack of fermentative ability, its ability to produce urease, to grow at 37°C and to assimilate inositol.

The most useful serological test is the LPA test for the detection of cryptococcal polysaccharide antigen. This test is highly sensitive and specific for the diagnosis of cryptococcal meningitis and disseminated forms of the disease and gives better results than microscopy and culture. With CSF samples the LPA test is positive in well over 90% of infected patients. In patients with AIDS titres of over 1×10^6 may be detected. Antigen may also be detected by ELISA.

Tests for serum antibody (WCA) are positive in less than 50% of proven cases of cryptococcal meningitis, since antibodies are rapidly neutralized by the large amounts of capsular antigen released during evolution of the infection. Antibodies may subsequently reappear in patients after successful treatment. Consequently, the progress of the disease and the response to therapy can be monitored by using antigen and antibody tests in combination.

Treatment

Intravenous amphotericin B in combination with flucytosine is the treatment of choice for cryptococcosis. Intrathecal amphotericin B may also be used in severe meningeal disease. Patients with AIDS commonly relapse after the initial course of therapy and many react badly to the drugs. Fluconazole can be administered orally and is useful if amphotericin B proves too toxic; it is also used as a maintenance therapy to control cryptococcosis in AIDS patients.

Individuals at risk of developing cryptococcosis should avoid contact with bird droppings.

Aspergillosis

There are more than 100 species of *Aspergillus* but only a few have been implicated in human disease: the most important are *A. fumigatus, A. niger, A. flavus, A. terreus* and *A. nidulans*. All grow in nature and in culture as mycelial fungi with septate hyphae and distinctive sporing structures; the spore-bearing hypha (conidiophore) terminates in a swollen cell (vesicle) surrounded by one or two rows of cells (sterigmata) from which chains of asexual conidia are produced (Fig. 60.2).

Aspergillosis most frequently affects the lungs, but infections at other sites such as the nasal sinuses and superficial tissues may also occur. The disease is usually caused by *A. fumigatus*. Inhalation of *Aspergillus* spores may lead to colonization of existing lung cavities (*aspergilloma* form) or a hypersensitivity reaction (*allergic aspergillosis*). Rarely, *Aspergillus* may cause invasive disease of the lung and may disseminate to other organs; this form is seen in severely immunocompromised patients.

Aspergillus spores are ubiquitous and in winter months counts may reach 600 spores/m³ of air in the UK. The fungus is particularly prevalent in decaying vegetation, such as mouldy hay, and counts as high as 2.1×10^7 spores/m³ of air have been recorded inside farm buildings.

Pathogenesis

Allergic aspergillosis. Allergy to *Aspergillus* species is usually seen in atopic individuals with elevated IgE levels; about 10–20% of asthmatics react to *A. fumigatus*. Asthma with eosinophilia is a more chronic form, which manifests as episodes of lung consolidation and fleeting shadows on chest radiography; the fungus grows in the airways to produce plugs of fungal mycelium which may block off segments of lung tissue and which, when coughed up, are a diagnostic feature. Allergic alveolitis follows particularly heavy and repeated exposure to large numbers of spores. Breathlessness, fever and malaise appear some hours after exposure, and repeated attacks result in progressive lung damage. A well-known example of this form of the disease is *Maltster's lung*, which occurs in workers who handle barley on which *A. clavatus* has sporulated during the malting process.

Aspergilloma. In this form of aspergillosis, also referred to as *fungus ball*, the fungus colonizes pre-existing (often tuberculous) cavities in the lung and forms a compact ball of mycelium, eventually surrounded by a dense fibrous wall.

Aspergillomas are usually solitary. Patients are either asymptomatic or have only a moderate cough and sputum production. Occasional haemoptysis may occur, especially when the fungus is actively growing, and haemorrhage following invasion of a blood vessel is one of the complications of this condition. Surgical resection is most often used to treat this condition.

Invasive aspergillosis. This form occurs in severely immunocompromised individuals who have a serious underlying illness. *A. fumigatus* is the species most frequently involved.

The lung is the sole site of infection in 70% of patients, but dissemination of infection to other organs occurs in many cases. There is widespread destructive growth of *Aspergillus* species in lung tissue and the fungus invades blood vessels, causing thrombosis; septic emboli may spread the infection to other organs, especially the kidneys, heart and brain. Invasive aspergillosis has a poor prognosis and is often diagnosed post-mortem.

Endocarditis. *Aspergillus* species may rarely cause endocarditis in immunosuppressed patients and those who have undergone open-heart surgery. The condition has a poor prognosis and successful therapy depends on a combination of antifungal treatment and surgical removal of infected tissue.

Paranasal granuloma. *A. flavus* and *A. fumigatus* may colonize and invade the paranasal sinuses and the infection may spread through the bone to the orbit of the eye and brain. This condition is seen most often in warm dry climates and is common in parts of the Sudan.

Laboratory diagnosis

The value of the laboratory in diagnosis varies according to the clinical form of aspergillosis; the diagnosis of invasive disease is particularly difficult.

Direct microscopy. In sputum the fungus appears as non-pigmented septate mycelium (3–5 μm in diameter) with characteristic dichotomous branching and an irregular outline; rarely the characteristic sporing heads of *Aspergillus* species are present.

In allergic aspergillosis there is usually abundant fungus in the sputum and mycelial plugs may also be present. In aspergilloma, fungus may be difficult to find on microscopy. In invasive aspergillosis, microscopy is usually negative and biopsy may be the only reliable method of making a definitive diagnosis, although this is a procedure many clinicians are reluctant to undertake because of the associated risk.

In tissue sections *Aspergillus* species are best seen after staining with PAS or methenamine–silver.

Culture. Aspergilli grow readily at 25–37°C on Sabouraud's agar without cycloheximide; colonies appear after incubation for 1–2 d. Isolates can be identified by their colonial appearance and micromorphology. The ability of *A. fumigatus* to grow well at 45°C can be used to help identify this species or to selectively isolate it.

Since aspergilli are among the commonest contaminants in the laboratory, quantification of the amount of fungus in sputum helps to confirm the relevance of a positive culture.

Large quantities of fungus are usually recovered from the sputum of patients with allergic aspergillosis but cultures from those with aspergilloma or invasive disease are commonly negative or yield only a few colonies.

Skin tests. Skin tests with *A. fumigatus* antigen are useful for the diagnosis of allergic aspergillosis. All patients give an immediate type I reaction and 70% of those with pulmonary eosinophilia also give a delayed type III arthus reaction.

Serological tests. Immunodiffusion and immuno-electrophoresis are widely used for the detection of precipitins in the diagnosis of all forms of aspergillosis, particularly aspergilloma.

Antigen detection has also been used successfully for diagnosis of invasive aspergillosis by techniques such as LPA, RIA and ELISA. However, currently available tests generally lack sensitivity.

Treatment

Allergic forms of aspergillosis are treated with corticosteroids. Aspergilloma is treated by surgical excision or sometimes with antifungal agents. In invasive aspergillosis, the treatment of choice is intravenous amphotericin B; itraconazole has given good results in some cases but has yet to be fully evaluated.

Systemic candidosis

Systemic forms of candidosis may be localized, e.g. in the urinary tract, liver, heart valves (endocarditis), meninges or peritoneal cavity, or the infection may be widely disseminated and associated with a septicaemia (*candidaemia*). *Candida albicans* is most frequently involved. Deep-seated candidosis is difficult to diagnose and treat, and the prognosis is generally poor.

Systemic candidosis usually follows overgrowth of commensal yeasts in association with serious abnormality of the host. It is generally an iatrogenic infection encountered among certain groups of hospitalized patients who are known to carry more yeasts in the mouth and gastro-intestinal tract than the normal population. Several factors are known to predispose to yeast overgrowth (Table 60.3). but the highest numbers of yeasts occur in patients treated with antibiotics or steroids, in immunosuppressed patients, and after surgical procedures such as organ transplants or heart surgery.

Candidaemia is seen mainly in postoperative or immunosuppressed patients; in some patients the candidaemia clears spontaneously, or disappears when contaminated intravenous catheters are removed. However, some patients with candidaemia, notably those treated with cytotoxic drugs or corticosteroids, develop generalized or localized, deep-seated infection.

Common sites of involvement in disseminated infection include the kidney, liver, brain and gastro-intestinal tract; pulmonary infections are rare. One common sign of deep-seated candidosis is the presence of white candidal lesions within the eye (*Candida* endophthalmitis). *Candida* endocarditis usually follows surgery for valve replacement, but also occurs in drug addicts and occasionally in patients on immunosuppressive therapy.

Infection of the kidney is usually blood-borne and ascending infection is thought to be rare. Bladder infections are usually associated with the presence of an indwelling urinary catheter; the infection often clears when the underlying cause is corrected.

Table 60.3 Factors associated with yeast overgrowth and candidosis

1. Natural receptive states (infancy, old age, pregnancy)
2. Changes in local bacterial flora (e.g. secondary to antibiotics)
3. Changes to epithelial surfaces (e.g. due to moisture, local occlusion, trauma)
4. T lymphocyte defects (primary or secondary to disease, e.g. AIDS or immunosuppression)
5. Neutropenia (primary or secondary to disease or immunosuppression)
6. Endocrine disease (e.g. diabetes mellitus)
7. Miscellaneous conditions (e.g. zinc or iron deficiency)

C. albicans accounts for most cases of systemic candidosis, but *C. tropicalis* and *C. lusitaniae* are also frequently implicated, and *C. parapsilosis* is responsible for about 25% of cases of yeast endocarditis; *C. glabrata* is often involved in infections of the urinary tract. The mycological features of these organisms have been outlined in the section on superficial candidosis (p. 682).

Laboratory diagnosis

Diagnosis of deep-seated candidosis is difficult and many cases are revealed post-mortem. There are no distinctive clinical signs to indicate *Candida* infection, unless endophthalmitis is present. Laboratory diagnosis of candidosis is complicated by the fact that *Candida* species may be present as commensals in the absence of infection. Isolation of *Candida* species from clinical material, except from sites that are normally sterile, is therefore of little significance. Similarly, antibodies to *Candida* species can be detected in uninfected individuals because of their exposure to commensal yeasts, although a change in antibody titre may be of diagnostic significance. In suspected systemic candidosis, samples from as many sources as possible should be examined by direct microscopy and culture and results should always be interpreted in the light of clinical findings.

Direct microscopy. Appropriate samples are examined microscopically in potassium hydroxide or after Gram staining. In tissue sections, the fungus is seen best if stained with PAS or methenamine–silver. Mycelium is often abundant but the presence of mycelium in sputum or urine does not confirm that the yeast is present as a pathogen.

Culture. *Candida* species grow readily in culture at 37°C on common isolation media, such as Sabouraud's agar (see p. 683). Blood cultures provide the most reliable evidence of systemic infection, although repeated attempts to isolate the organism may be necessary. However, transient candidaemia is not uncommon, especially in patients with indwelling intravenous catheters. Isolation of the yeast from otherwise sterile sites provides reliable evidence for the diagnosis but cultures obtained from urine, faeces and sputum are of value only if done quantitatively over a period of time. Cell counts of the yeast in urine in excess of 10^4 per millilitre are usually taken to indicate urinary tract infection, except in patients with indwelling urinary catheters.

Since *Candida* species multiply rapidly in clinical material it is important that specimens are processed as soon as possible after collection.

Serological tests. Currently available tests lack specificity and sensitivity and the results must be interpreted with care. The most widely used tests are ID and CIE for detection of precipitins to somatic extracts of *C. albicans* and *C. parapsilosis*. A positive test does not necessarily indicate infection since the antigens used are unable to differentiate antibodies formed during mucosal colonization from those produced during deep infection. Similarly, a negative antibody test does not necessarily rule out the possibility of deep-seated candidosis in immunocompromised patients who are incapable of mounting an adequate antibody response; in such cases a more sensitive assay system such as ELISA gives better results.

Antigen tests based on ELISA, RIA, PHA and LPA, to detect either cell wall mannan or cytoplasmic components, are being developed and antigen detection is likely to become the main method for serodiagnosis of systemic candidosis.

Treatment

Intravenous amphotericin B in combination with flucytosine is the treatment of choice for most forms of systemic candidosis. Flucytosine is not used on its own due to problems of resistance. Fluconazole, ketoconazole and itraconazole have also been used successfully.

Zygomycosis

Zygomycosis, also referred to as *mucormycosis* or *phycomycosis*, is a relatively rare, opportunistic infection caused by saprophytic mould fungi, notably species of *Mucor, Absidia* and *Rhizopus*. The best known form of the disease is rhino-cerebral zygomycosis, a rapidly fulminating infection which is almost invariably associated with either acute diabetes mellitus, or with debilitating diseases such as leukaemia or lymphoma. There is extensive cellulitis with rapid tissue destruction, most commonly spreading from the nasal mucosa to the turbinate bone, paranasal sinuses, orbit and brain. Rhinocerebral zygomycosis is rapidly fatal if untreated and although the prognosis of this infection has improved over recent years, most diagnoses are still made at necropsy. Primary cutaneous infections have also been reported but these are extremely rare and usually occur in patients with severe burns. Subcutaneous forms of zygomycosis are less serious.

The fungi responsible for zygomycosis are characterized by having broad, aseptate mycelium, with large numbers of asexual spores inside a sporangium which develops at the end of an aerial hypha.

Laboratory diagnosis

Recognition of the fungus in tissue by microscopy is considerably more reliable than culture but material such as nasal discharge or sputum seldom contains much fungal material and examination of a biopsy is usually necessary for a firm diagnosis. Direct examination of curetted or biopsy material in potassium hydroxide may reveal the characteristic broad, aseptate, branched mycelium and sometimes distorted hyphae. However, they are seen much more clearly when stained with methenamine–silver; the hyphae of these fungi do not stain with PAS.

The fungi are readily isolated on Sabouraud's agar at 37°C but isolation of the causal agents is of little diagnostic significance in the absence of strong supporting clinical evidence of infection.

There are no established serological tests for the diagnosis of zygomycosis.

Treatment

Successful treatment depends on early diagnosis of the infection, allowing prompt therapy with intravenous amphotericin B and aggressive surgical intervention.

Other opportunist systemic pathogens

Almost any fungus may invade a severely immunocompromised host and infections with many common fungi including *Fusarium* species, *Penicillium* species. *Trichosporon beigelii* and *Pseudallescheria boydii* have been reported.

Diagnosis is made by culture of the causative organism from clinical specimens and serological tests play little part. Tissue sections are often not very helpful since the causal fungi either have no special features to enable identification, or they resemble other fungal pathogens.

Infections are usually treated speculatively, and sometimes successfully, with amphotericin B.

RECOMMENDED READING

Chandler F W, Kaplan W, Ajello L 1980 *Histopathology of Mycotic Diseases. A Colour Atlas and Textbook*. Wolfe, London

Clayton Y, Midgley G 1985 *Medical Mycology. Pocket Picture Guide Series*. Gower, London

Evans E G V, Gentles J C 1985 *Essentials of Medical Mycology*. Churchill Livingstone, Edinburgh

Evans E G V, Richardson M D (eds) 1989 *Medical Mycology. A Practical Approach*. Oxford University Press, Oxford

Koneman E W, Roberts G D 1985 *Practical Laboratory Mycology*, 3rd edn. Williams and Wilkins, Baltimore

McGinnis M R 1980 *Laboratory Handbook of Medical Mycology*. Academic Press, New York

Odds F C 1988 *Candida and Candidosis*, 2nd edn. Baillière Tindall, London

Rippon J W 1988 *Medical Mycology. The Pathogenic Fungi and the Pathogenic Actinomycetes*, 3rd edn. W B Saunders, Philadelphia

Roberts S O B, Hay R J, Mackenzie D W R 1984 *A Clinician's Guide to Fungal Disease*. Marcel Dekker, New York

Ryley J F 1990 *Chemotherapy of Fungal Diseases*. Springer–Verlag, Berlin

Warnock D W, Richardson M D (eds) 1991 *Fungal Infection in the Compromised Patient*, 2nd edn. Wiley, Chichester

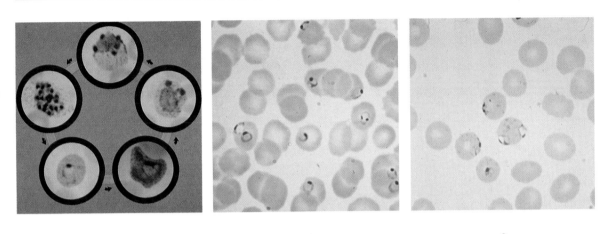

| 1 | 2 | 3 |

Plate 1 Stages in the erythrocytic cycle of *Plasmodium vivax*.

Plate 2 Ring form trophozoites of *P. falciparum*.

Plate 3 Trophozoites of *P. falciparum*. Note peripheral location of the parasites (*appliqué* or *accolé* forms) and light stippling of the red cells (*Maurer's spots*).

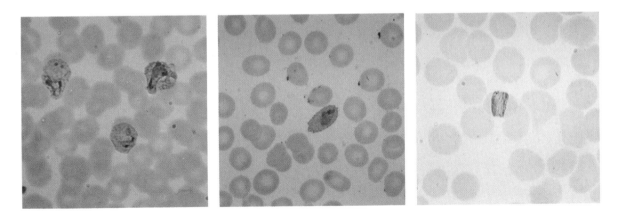

| 4 | 5 | 6 |

Plate 4 Amoeboid trophozoites of *P. vivax*. Note the marked enlargement of the parasitized red cells and the intense stippling (*Schüffner's dots*).

Plate 5 Trophozoite of *P. ovale*. Note the fimbriate, oval-shaped red cell and marked stippling (*James' stippling*).

Plate 6 Band-form trophozoite of *P. malariae*.

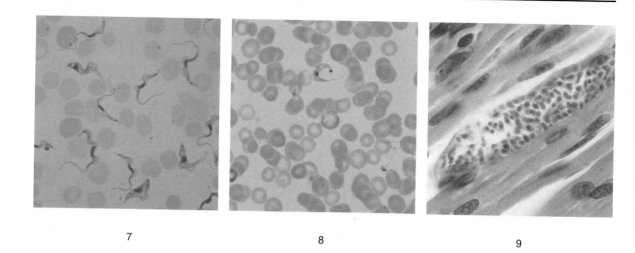

7 8 9

Plate 7 Trypomastigotes of *Trypanosoma brucei rhodesiense* in mouse blood.

Plate 8 Trypomastigote of *T. cruzi* in blood. Note the prominent kinetoplast and the 'C' shape adopted by the parasite.

Plate 9 Amastigotes of *T. cruzi* in heart muscle.

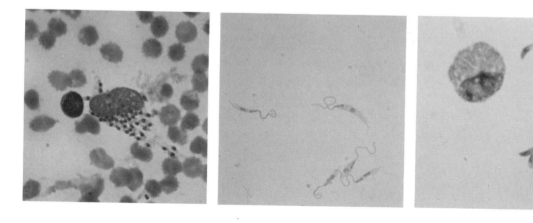

10 11 12

Plate 10 Amastigotes of *Leishmania tropica* in a ruptured macrophage from a cutaneous lesion (*Oriental sore*).

Plate 11 Promastigotes of *L. tropica* from laboratory culture in Novy, MacNeal and Nicolle's (NNN) medium.

Plate 12 Tachyzoites of *Toxoplasma gondii* in a macrophage (top left) and lying free (bottom right).

61

Protozoa

Malaria: toxoplasmosis; amoebic dysentery; sleeping sickness; Chagas' disease; leishmaniasis

D. Greenwood

Infection with pathogenic protozoa exacts an enormous toll of human suffering, notably, but not exclusively, in the tropics. Numerically the most important of the life-threatening protozoan diseases is malaria, which is responsible for at least 1 million deaths a year, mostly in young children in tropical countries.

Pathogenic protozoan parasites are conveniently dealt with under four headings: *sporozoa, amoebae, flagellates* and a miscellaneous group of other protozoa that may cause human disease (Table 61.1).

Table 61.1 Principal protozoan pathogens of man

Group	Species	Disease
Sporozoa	*Plasmodium falciparum*	Malignant tertian malaria
	P. vivax	Benign tertian malaria
	P. ovale	Benign tertian malaria
	P. malariae	Quartan malaria
	Toxoplasma gondii	Toxoplasmosis
	Isospora belli	Diarrhoea
	Cryptosporidium parvum	Diarrhoea
Amoebae	*Entamoeba histolytica*	Amoebic dysentery
	Naegleria fowleri[a]	Meningo-encephalitis
	Acanthamoeba spp.[a]	Keratitis
Flagellates	*Giardia lamblia*	Diarrhoea, malabsorption
	Trichomonas vaginalis	Vaginitis, urethritis
	Trypanosoma brucei gambiense	Sleeping sickness
	T. brucei rhodesiense	Sleeping sickness
	T. cruzi	Chagas' disease
	Leishmania spp.	See Table 61.4
Others	*Babesia microti*[a]	Babesiosis
	B. divergens[a]	Babesiosis
	Balantidium coli[a]	Balantidial dysentery
	Encephalitozoon cuniculi[a]	Microsporidiosis
	Enterocytozoon bieneusi[a]	Microsporidiosis
	Nosema connori[a]	Microsporidiosis
	Blastocystis hominis[b]	Pathogenicity doubtful
	Pneumocystis carinii[b]	Pneumonia

[a] These organisms are rarely encountered in human disease.
[b] Organisms of uncertain taxonomic status.

SPOROZOA

This group includes the malaria parasites and related coccidia. These parasites exhibit a complex life-cycle involving alternating cycles of asexual division (schizogony) and sexual development (sporogony). In malaria parasites, the sexual cycle takes place in the female anopheline mosquito (Fig. 61.1).

Malaria parasites

Description

Four species of malaria parasite are encountered in human disease: *Plasmodium falciparum*, which is responsible for most fatalities; *P. vivax* and *P. ovale*, both of which cause *benign tertian malaria* (febrile episodes typically occurring at 48h intervals); and *P. malariae*, which causes *quartan malaria* (febrile episodes typically occurring at 72 h intervals). The typical appearances of trophozoites of the four species are illustrated in the colour plate section (facing p.699).

Life cycle. When an infected mosquito bites, *sporozoites* present in the salivary glands enter the bloodstream and are carried to the liver, where they invade liver parenchyma cells. They undergo a process of multiple nuclear division, followed by cytoplasmic division (*schizogony*) and, when this is complete, the liver cell ruptures, releasing hundreds of individual parasites (*merozoites*) into the bloodstream. The merozoites penetrate red blood cells and adopt a typical 'signet-ring' morphology.

In the case of *P. vivax* and *P. ovale* some parasites in the liver remain dormant and the cycle of pre-erythrocytic schizogony is completed only after a long delay. Such parasites are responsible for the relapses of tertian malaria that may occur up to 2 years after the initial infection.

In the bloodstream, the young ring forms (*trophozoites*) develop and start to undergo nuclear division (*erythrocytic schizogony*). Depending on the species, about 8–24 nuclei are produced before cytoplasmic division occurs and the red cell ruptures to release the individual merozoites, which then infect fresh red blood cells.

Instead of entering the cycle of erythrocytic schizogony, some merozoites develop within red cells into male or female *gametocytes*. These do not develop further in the human host, but when the blood is ingested by the insect vector, the nuclear material and cytoplasm of the male gametocytes differentiate to produce several individual *gametes*, which give the gametocyte the appearance of a flagellate body (*exflagellating male gametocyte*). The gametes become detached and penetrate the female gametocyte, which elongates into a zygotic form, the *ookinete*. This penetrates the mid-gut wall of the mosquito and settles on the body cavity side as an *oocyst*, which is yet another multiplicatory phase within which numerous *sporozoites* are formed. When mature, the oocyst ruptures, releasing the sporozoites into the body cavity, from where some find their way to the salivary glands.

Erythrocytic cycle of P. falciparum. *P. falciparum* differs from the other forms of malaria parasite in that developing erythrocytic schizonts form aggregates in the capillaries of the brain and other internal organs, so that only relatively young ring forms are found in peripheral blood.

The cycle of erythrocytic schizogony takes 48 h, except in the case of *P. malariae*, in which the cycle occupies 72 h. Since febrile episodes occur shortly after red cell rupture, this explains the characteristic periodic fevers. However, with *P. falciparum*, the cycles of different broods of parasite do not become synchronized as they do in other forms of malaria and typical tertian fevers are not usual in falciparum malaria.

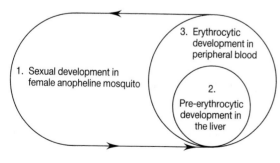

Fig. 61.1 Schematic representation of the life cycle of malaria parasites.

Laboratory diagnosis

Acute falciparum malaria is a medical emergency that demands immediate diagnosis and treatment. To establish the diagnosis, a drop of peripheral blood is spread over a 2 cm area on a glass slide. The smear should not be too thick; a useful criterion is that print should be just visible through it. The smear is allowed to dry thoroughly and stained by Field's method. This is an aqueous Romanowsky stain which stains the parasites very rapidly and haemolyses the red cells, so that the parasites are easy to detect despite the thickness of the film.

With experience, the species of malaria can usually be determined from a thick blood film, but some of the characteristic features that assist in establishing the identity of the parasites, such as the typical stippling of the red cell that accompanies infection with *P. vivax* or *P. ovale*, are better observed in a conventional thin blood film. This is stained by one of the many modifications of Giemsa's or Leishman's stain, but the water used to dilute the stain should be of pH 7.2 (not 6.8 as used for haematological purposes) in order optimally to demonstrate parasite morphology and associated red cell changes. The chief morphological features used in differentiating the four kinds of human malaria are shown in Table 61.2. Several serodiagnostic tests for malaria have been devised, notably the indirect immunofluorescence test, but these are of limited value.

Treatment

For many years the standard treatment for acute malaria was chloroquine. However, resistance to that drug in *P. falciparum* (but not other species) is now widespread and alternative agents often have to be used. The most reliable alternative to chloroquine is quinine, the traditional remedy that has been available for centuries in the form of cinchona bark.

Newer antimalarials include mefloquine and halofantrine. Although these compounds are active against chloroquine-resistant strains, resistance to them has already been described and there are fears that this will become widespread with indiscriminate use.

Treatment of acute malaria with chloroquine, quinine or other antimalarials will not eliminate exo-erythrocytic parasites in the liver. For this purpose the 8-aminoquinoline drug primaquine must be used. This agent carries the risk of precipitating haemolysis in individuals who are deficient in the enzyme glucose-6-phosphate dehydrogenase.

Table 61.2 Differential characteristics of human malaria parasites as seen in Romanowsky-stained thin films of peripheral blood (see also colour plates 1–6)

Species	Morphology of trophozoite	Morphology of red cell	Stippling of red cell	Morphology of gametocyte	No. of merozoites in mature schizont
P. falciparum	Ring forms only	Normal	Maurer's spots[a]	Crescentic	(16–24)[b]
P. vivax	Rings, becoming amoeboid during development	Enlarged	Schüffner's dots	Large, round	16–24
P. ovale	Rings, becoming compact during development	Slightly enlarged; sometimes oval with fimbriate edge	James' stippling[c]	Round	8–12
P. malariae	Rings, becoming compact in form of band across red cell	Normal or slightly shrunken	(Ziemann's dots)[d]	Small, round	8–12

[a] Maurer's spots (or clefts) are relatively scanty and accompany more mature ring forms.
[b] Mature schizonts of *P. falciparum* are rarely seen in peripheral blood.
[c] James' stippling is similar to the intense stippling of Schüffner's dots.
[d] Ziemann's dots are rarely seen, except in intensely stained preparations.

Prophylaxis

Chloroquine and the antifolate drugs pyrimethamine (often combined with sulfadoxine or dapsone) and proguanil have been widely used for antimalarial prophylaxis, but the development of resistance to these agents has made it difficult to offer definitive advice to travellers, particularly those going to regions where chloroquine-resistant *P. falciparum* is prevalent. One solution has been to suggest a combination of pyrimethamine and sulfadoxine with either chloroquine or mefloquine. Such cumbersome regimens invite lapses in compliance and increase the risk of side-effects; moreover, they are not completely protective. For these reasons some authorities prefer to recommend a simple prophylactic regimen such as daily proguanil, or weekly mefloquine, together with advice to bring any fever to medical attention. The combination of daily proguanil and weekly chloroquine is also widely recommended. Whatever prophylactic advice is given, it should be combined with recommendations to avoid exposure to mosquito bites: wearing long clothing in the evening when the insects are most active; use of insect repellants; and sleeping under mosquito netting.

Because parasites in the pre-erythrocytic stage of development escape the action of prophylactic drugs, prophylaxis should continue for at least 4 weeks after leaving a malarious area. This will effectively prevent the development of falciparum malaria, although long-term relapses of other types may occur up to 2 years after exposure.

Other sporozoa

Toxoplasma gondii

This is a coccidian parasite of the intestinal tract of the cat but is transmissible to many other mammals. Serological evidence suggests that human infection commonly occurs, presumably as a transient febrile illness or a subclinical attack. Occasionally, more severe infection occurs: intra-uterine toxoplasmosis is an important cause of stillbirth and congenital abnormality, and cerebral toxoplasmosis sometimes occurs as a life-threatening complication of generalized infection in severely immunocompromised patients, such as those suffering from acquired immune deficiency syndrome (AIDS).

The parasites develop intracellularly in macrophages (see colour plate 12), but it is not usually possible to demonstrate them in clinical material. Laboratory diagnosis can be made by demonstration of a rising titre of serum antibodies to *T. gondii* by the Sabin-Feldman dye exclusion test, which recognizes the ability of serum antibody to kill viable toxoplasmas. An immunofluorescence test and an enzyme-linked immunosorbent assay (ELISA) are also available; they are now preferred to the dye test because they avoid the risk of the use of live toxoplasmas.

The combination of pyrimethamine and a sulphonamide is generally considered as the treatment of choice for toxoplasmosis, but clindamycin and spiramycin are also said to be effective and may be preferred, especially during pregnancy.

Isospora belli

This coccidian parasite may cause a mild self-limiting diarrhoea in man. It occasionally causes a more severe infection in immunocompromised patients.

Sarcocystis species

The animal parasites *Sarcocystis bovihominis* and *S. suihominis* occasionally invade the intestinal tract or muscle of man. Infection is usually subclinical and discovered accidentally.

Cryptosporidium species

Cryptosporidia have long been recognized as animal parasites; it is now clear that some species, notably *Cryptosporidium parvum*, are a common cause of human diarrhoeal disease. Large numbers of oocysts are often present in faeces; they are partially acid-fast and can be demonstrated by modifications of the Ziehl–Neelsen method with carbol–fuchsin or auramine as the primary stain.

No specific treatment has been found that is unequivocally effective, but the infection usually responds to symptomatic treatment, with fluid replacement if necessary. In severely immunocompromised patients, cryptosporidia may cause a severe life-threatening diarrhoea for which spiramycin has been used with modest success.

AMOEBAE

Entamoeba histolytica

This is much the most important amoebic parasite of man. The amoebae invade the colonic mucosa, producing characteristic ulcerative lesions and a profuse bloody diarrhoea (*amoebic dysentery*). Systemic infection may arise, leading to abscess formation in internal organs, notably the liver. Such disease may arise in the absence of frank dysentery.

Laboratory diagnosis

In acute amoebiasis, blood-stained mucus, or colonic scrapings from ulcerated areas, are examined by direct microscopy. The material should be examined within 2 h of collection, but it is not necessary to use a warm-stage microscope. *E. histolytica* may be recognized by its active movement pushing out finger-like pseudopodia and sometimes progressing across the microscope field. If mucosal invasion has occurred, the amoebae usually contain ingested red blood cells, but these may be absent if infection is confined to the gut lumen. The nucleus is not usually visible in unstained 'wet' preparations, but in fixed smears stained with haematoxylin, the nucleus is seen as a delicate ring of chromatin with a central karyosome (Fig. 61.2).

Typical amoebic trophozoites may also be seen in aspirates of liver abscess. The pus often has a distinctive red-brown 'anchovy sauce' appearance. Since the amoebae actively multiply in the walls of the abscess, the last few drops of pus drained from the lesion are most likely to yield recognizable forms of the parasite.

In the intestinal carrier state, active amoebae are usually absent, but amoebic cysts (which, conversely, are normally absent in acute amoebiasis) may be found. The cysts are the form by which infection is spread. They are spherical, about 10–15 μm in diameter, and contain one to four of the nuclei typical of *Entamoeba* species: a circular ring with a central dot. Young, uninucleate cysts may also contain a large glycogen vacuole and, in fresh specimens, cysts of all stages of development may exhibit one or more thick, blunt-ended *chromatoidal bars* (Fig. 61.2).

Serology. Demonstration of active amoebae or cysts is the best way to make a definitive diagnosis, but serology is also sometimes helpful, particularly in systemic disease. Various immunodiagnostic tests have been described, but they are usually performed only in reference centres.

Culture. Culture of *E. histolytica* is unhelpful as a diagnostic procedure.

Treatment

Not all strains of *E. histolytica* are invasive and some never cause disease. Nevertheless, it is not possible readily to distinguish pathogenic from non-pathogenic strains in asymptomatic cyst excreters and, at least in areas of the world in which amoebiasis is uncommon, it is prudent to treat all excreters, particularly if they are food handlers. For this purpose, diloxanide furoate is often used.

Acute amoebiasis is usually effectively treated with 5-nitroimidazole derivatives, such as metronidazole or tinidazole. Chloroquine is also useful in amoebic liver abscess. Older drugs, including emetine and dehydroemetine, are effective, but more toxic.

Non-pathogenic intestinal amoebae

Although there are occasional reports of diarrhoea associated with other intestinal amoebae, notably *Dientamoeba fragilis* (an amoeba flagellate), most occur as commensals and are important only because of potential confusion with *E. histolytica*. The greatest opportunity for confusion arises with the other intestinal *Entamoeba* species, *E. hartmanni* and *E. coli* (Fig. 61.2). *E. hartmanni* is morphologically identical to *E. histolytica*, but is smaller and the trophozoite never contains ingested red blood cells. *E. coli* is somewhat larger than *E. histolytica*, particularly in the cyst form. The trophozoites are more sluggish than those of *E. histolytica* and mature cysts contain up to eight

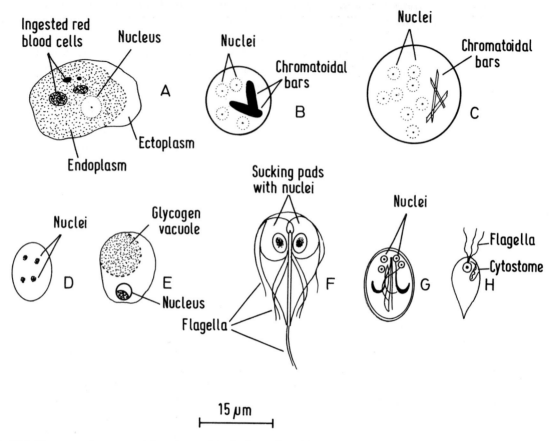

Fig. 61.2 Diagrammatic representation of some intestinal parasites: **A** *Entamoeba histolytica*, trophozoite with ingested red blood cells; **B** *E. histolytica*, mature cyst; **C** *E. coli*, mature cyst; **D** *Endolimax nana*, mature cyst; **E** *Iodamoeba buetschlii*, mature cyst; **F** *Giardia lamblia*, trophozoite; **G** *G. lamblia*, mature cyst; **H** *Chilomastix mesnili*, trophozoite.

nuclei; chromatoidal bars, if present, are fine and pointed, rather like slivers of broken glass.

The differential characteristics of these and other non-pathogenic intestinal amoebae are compared with those of *E. histolytica* in Table 61.3.

Free-living amoebae

Environmental amoebae belonging to *Naegleria* species (usually *N. fowleri*) have occasionally been implicated in meningo-encephalitis. The outcome is ordinarily fatal, although amphotericin B has been successfully used. *Acanthamoeba* species sometimes cause keratitis; the condition has sometimes been associated with contaminated cleaning fluids for soft contact lenses. Optimal antimicrobial

chemotherapy remains to be defined, but topical propamidine in combination with neomycin or other agents has been used.

FLAGELLATES

Giardia lamblia (syn.: *G. intestinalis*)

This intestinal parasite lives attached to the mucosal surface of the small intestine, notably in the duodenum. Vast numbers may be present and their presence may lead to malabsorption of fat and a chronic bulky diarrhoea.

The trophozoite form is kite shaped, with two nucleated sucking pads, and four pairs of flagella (Fig. 61.2). Trophozoites may be found in duodenal

Table 61.3 Differential characteristics of intestinal amoebae

Species	Trophozoites		Cysts			
	Size (μm)	Ingested RBCs[a]	Size (μm)	No. of nuclei[b]	Chromatoidal bars	Nuclear morphology[c]
Entamoeba histolytica	10–40	+	10–15	4	Solid, blunt-ended	Fine ring of chromatin with central karyosome
E. hartmanni	4–10	–	6–10	4	As above	As above
E. coli	10–40	–	15–25	8	Slender, pointed	As above, but karyosome sometimes eccentric
E. gingivalis[d]	10–25	–	No cyst stage			
Iodamoeba buetschlii	10–20	–	10–15	1	None	'Basket' shaped: chromatin massed at one end of ring
Endolimax nana	5–12	–	5–8	4	None	Small shadowy masses of chromatin
Dientamoeba fragilis	5–10	–	No cyst stage			Ring containing several chromatin granules

[a] RBCs, red blood cells.
[b] Refers to mature cyst.
[c] Refers to the trophozoite or cyst.
[d] E. gingivalis is a commensal of the mouth.

aspirate, but examination of faeces usually reveals the cyst form by which the disease is transmitted. This is oval about 10 × 8 μm, and contains up to four nuclei as well as the remains of the skeletal structure of the trophozoite (Fig. 61.2).

Cysts of other, non-pathogenic, intestinal protozoa, including *Chilomastix mesnili*, *Enteromonas hominis* and *Retortomonas intestinalis*, may be mistaken for *G. lamblia*, but they are usually smaller and lack the regular oval shape and characteristic internal morphology. These non-pathogenic protozoa may also be found as trophozoites during microscopy of diarrhoeic faeces, but the most common intestinal flagellate is *Trichomonas hominis*, which is recognizable by its undulating membrane. There is no cyst form.

Giardiasis can be treated with 5-nitroimidazoles such as metronidazole, or, on the rare occasions when this fails, with mepacrine.

Trichomonas vaginalis

T. vaginalis is a flagellate protozoon with four anterior flagella and one lateral flagellum which is attached to the surface of the parasite to form an undulating membrane. As with *T. hominis* there

is no cyst form; the parasite is transmitted by sexual intercourse.

As the name suggests, *T. vaginalis* is predominantly a vaginal parasite, although urethritis may occur in the male consorts of infected women. The organism is responsible for a mild vaginitis, with discharge, which ordinarily responds to treatment with metronidazole or tinidazole.

T. vaginalis is readily identified by its characteristic motility in untreated 'wet' films of vaginal discharge and can be cultivated in appropriate culture media.

Trypanosomes

In contrast to the flagellates already described, trypanosomes have a complex life-cycle involving an insect vector. The diseases that are caused in man, African trypanosomiasis (*sleeping sickness*) and South American trypanosomiasis (*Chagas' disease*) are restricted in distribution according to the habitat of the insect host.

African trypanosomiasis

African sleeping sickness is caused by trypanosomes that are now considered to be subspecies of *Trypanosoma brucei*, an important aetiological agent of *nagana* in cattle in tropical Africa. The human parasites are: *T. brucei gambiense*, which occurs in west and central Africa, where it is transmitted by riverine tsetse flies, notably *Glossina palpalis*; and *T. brucei rhodesiense*, a parasite transmitted by *G. morsitans* in the savannah plains of east Africa, where cattle and wild antelope act as reservoirs of infection.

Pathogenesis

Following the bite of an infected tsetse fly, a localized *trypanosomal chancre* may appear transiently, but invasion of the bloodstream rapidly occurs. The parasites multiply in blood, but parasitaemia may be accompanied only by non-specific symptoms with occasional febrile episodes and some lymphadenitis. Swollen lymph glands in the posterior triangle of the neck (*Winterbottom's sign*) are often present in *T. brucei gambiense* infection. If untreated, the disease inexorably progresses to involve the central nervous system with the classic signs of sleeping sickness and, ultimately, death.

Infection with *T. brucei rhodesiense* tends to follow a more acute, fulminating course over a period of a few months, whereas *T. brucei gambiense* infection usually progresses slowly, sometimes over several years.

Laboratory diagnosis

During the parasitaemic stage, scanty trypanosomes can be detected in peripheral blood in unstained 'wet' mounts or in smears stained by the Giemsa or Leishman methods. Examination of lymph node exudate may also be helpful.

Once the disease has progressed to involve the central nervous system, examination of cerebrospinal fluid reveals a lymphocytic exudate, often with *morula cells* (plasma cells) and scanty motile trypanosomes.

The parasites have a characteristic morphology: they are elongated, about 20–30 μm in length, with a single anterior flagellum arising via an undulating membrane from a basal body situated near a posteriorly placed kinetoplast (Fig. 61.3 and colour plate 7).

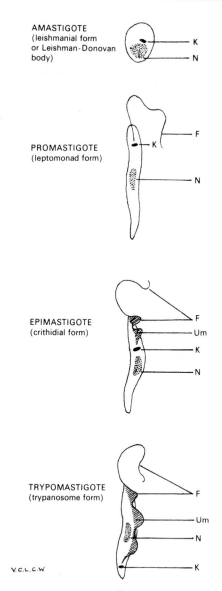

Fig. 61.3 Forms which may be adopted by *Leishmania* and *Trypanosoma* spp. In brackets are given the terms for the forms under the old nomenclature now superseded. F—flagellum; K—kinetoplast; N—nucleus; Um—undulating membrane.

In-vitro cultivation is unreliable, but animal inoculation is sometimes useful, particularly with *T. brucei rhodesiense*, which infects laboratory mice more readily than *T. brucei gambiense*.

Various immunodiagnostic tests have been described, but they are not as reliable as direct microscopy in establishing a definitive diagnosis.

Treatment

In the early, parasitaemic stage the infection is amenable to treatment with suramin or pentamidine, but if the disease has progressed to sleeping sickness, the trivalent arsenicals melarsoprol or tryparsamide must be used. Less toxic alternatives are clearly required; very encouraging results have been obtained in *T. brucei gambiense* infections in field trials of eflornithine, but surprisingly the drug does not appear to be effective in disease caused by *T. brucei rhodesiense*.

South American trypanosomiasis

Chagas' disease is caused by *T. cruzi* and is quite different from African trypanosomiasis. The insect vectors are various species of reduviid bugs, often called *kissing bugs* because of their predilection for feeding round the mouths of sleeping individuals. The trypanosomes are not transmitted by the bite, but are present in the bug's faeces, which the unwitting sleeper rubs into the irritating bite wound. The trypanosomes enter the bloodstream, but do not multiply there; instead, they invade cells of the reticulo-endothelial system and muscle, where they lose their flagellum and associated undulating membrane and adopt a more rounded shape (Fig. 61.3). This morphological form is called an *amastigote* and suggests a phylogenetic relationship with *Leishmania* species (see below). The amastigotes multiply in muscle and are liberated from ruptured cells as trypanosomal forms (*trypomastigotes*) to disseminate the infection and to provide the parasitaemia needed to infected fresh reduviid bugs when they next feed.

Pathogenesis

Chagas' disease is a chronic condition, characterized by extensive cardiomyopathy, sometimes with gross distension of other organs (e.g. megaoesophagus and megacolon) and, ultimately, death, usually from heart failure.

Laboratory diagnosis

Trypomastigotes of *T. cruzi* may be seen in peripheral blood, although they are often extremely scanty. They are shorter than those of the *T. brucei* group and have a characteristically large kinetoplast (colour plate 8). Unlike the African trypanosomes, *T. cruzi* can be grown in vitro in the rich blood agar medium also used to isolate leishmania (see below). Biopsy of skeletal muscle is sometimes performed but is usually of little value. The appearance of amastigotes in heart muscle is shown in colour plate 9.

T cruzi is infective to laboratory mice. Alternatively, a procedure known as *xenodiagnosis* may be used: uninfected reduviid bugs are allowed to feed on the patient and after about 3–4 weeks the gut contents of the bug are examined for trypanosomes.

Immunofluorescence tests, ELISA and complement-fixation tests may be used for presumptive serological diagnosis.

Treatment

There is no reliable antimicrobial chemotherapy for Chagas' disease, but the nitrofuran derivative nifurtimox and the imidazole compound benznidazole have been used with modest success.

Leishmania species

Leishmania are intracellular parasites of the reticulo-endothelial system. They are related to trypanosomes, but exist in only two morphological forms: *amastigotes* (non-flagellate forms), which occur in the infected lesion; and *promastigotes* (flagellate forms that lack an undulating membrane), which occur in the insect vector, or in laboratory culture (Fig. 61.3 and colour plates 10 and 11).

The parasites are transmitted by sandflies (*Phlebotomus* or *Lutzomyia* species) in various parts of the world, including the Middle East, India, South America, the Mediterranean littoral and parts of Africa.

Pathogenesis

Several distinct types of disease are recognized (Table 61.4), although they are caused by morphologically identical parasites. The taxonomic

Table 61.4 *Leishmania* species involved in human disease

Species	Form of disease	Common names	Main geographical distribution
Leishmania tropica	Cutaneous	Oriental sore,	Mediterranean coast,
L. major	Cutaneous	Delhi boil,	Middle East, Africa,
		Baghdad boil,	Indian sub-continent
		Aleppo button, etc.	
L. aethiopica	Cutaneous, DCL		Ethiopia, Kenya
L. donovani	Visceral	Kala azar,	Mediterranean coast,
L. infantum[a]	Visceral	Dum-dum fever	Middle East, Africa,
			Indian sub-continent
L. chagasi	Visceral		Tropical South America
L. mexicana[b]	Cutaneous, DCL	Chiclero's ulcer	Central America, Amazon basin
L braziliensis[b]	Mucocutaneous	Espundia	Tropical South America
L. peruviana	Cutaneous	Uta	Western Peru

DCL = disseminated cutaneous leishmaniasis.
[a] *L. infantum* may be a subspecies of *L. donovani*.
[b] These species may represent groups of closely related organisms.

relationships between the various forms have still not been entirely clarified. *Cutaneous leishmaniasis (oriental sore)* is the least troublesome, causing a boil-like swelling on the face or other exposed part of the body. The central part of the lesion may become secondarily infected with bacteria, but the leishmania reside in the raised, indurated edge of the lesion. The sore usually heals spontaneously, leaving a scar, but with some species a more severe *disseminated cutaneous leishmaniasis* may occur. Parasites of the *Leishmania mexicana* complex may cause a destructive lesion of the outer ear (*Chiclero's ulcer*).

In *mucocutaneous leishmaniasis (espundia)*, which is associated with the *L. braziliensis* complex, disfiguring lesions of the mouth and nose may be caused. However, the most serious form of leishmaniasis is *visceral leishmaniasis (kala azar)*, which is a life-threatening disease involving the whole of the reticulo-endothelial system.

Laboratory diagnosis

In the cutaneous or mucocutaneous form of the disease, typical intracellular amastigotes may be recognized in Giemsa-stained smears of material obtained from tissues at the margin of the lesion (see colour plate 10). Free amastigotes are commonly seen because of rupture of the macrophage host cell. Material should also be cultured in a modification of Novy, MacNeal and Nicolle's

(NNN) medium. This is a rabbit blood agar containing antibiotic to prevent bacterial contamination and a buffered salt overlay solution in which the parasites grow as promastigotes. (see colour plate 11). Incubation is maintained for up to 3 weeks at room temperature (*not* 37°C).

In kala azar, spleen puncture is the most reliable method of diagnosis, but sternal marrow aspirate (a safer procedure) is usually preferred. Smears and cultures are made and examined as for cutaneous leishmaniasis.

Various serological tests have been designed. A haemagglutination test and an indirect fluorescent antibody test have been successfully used in the diagnosis of kala azar, but demonstration of the parasite by microscopy or culture is preferable whenever possible.

Treatment

The pentavalent antimony compounds sodium stibogluconate and meglumine antimoniate offer the most reliable therapy for leishmaniasis. In intractable cases, pentamidine and the antifungal agent amphotericin B have also been used.

OTHER PATHOGENIC PROTOZOA
Babesia species

These are predominantly animal parasites related to the piroplasmas that cause theileriasis in wild and domestic animals in many parts of the world.

Babesiae are transmitted by arthropod vectors, usually ixodid ticks, and human infection is uncommon. Cases that have been described in Europe have all been in patients whose resistance was impaired by lack of a functioning spleen; the causative parasite was usually considered to be *Babesia divergens*. In contrast, babesiosis caused by *B. microti* has been reported in otherwise healthy persons in parts of the east coast of North America.

Babesiae are intracellular parasites living within red blood cells; they superficially resemble young ring forms of plasmodia. The disease in immuno-competent individuals is usually self-limiting, so that specific treatment is not required. Optimal treatment for more serious cases has not been properly defined. Chloroquine has sometimes been used, following a mistaken diagnosis of malaria, but is clearly not effective. Primaquine, quinine and clindamycin, alone or in combination, have been suggested to have some therapeutic value.

Balantidium coli

B. coli is the only representative of the ciliates to exhibit pathogenicity to man. It is a common parasite of the pig, and human infections have usually been traced to contact with these animals. The infective form is a large (about 50 μm in diameter), thick-walled cyst. The trophozoite inhabits the lumen of the gut and may attack the colonic mucosa in much the same way as *E. histolytica*, to cause balantidial dysentery.

Many highly motile ciliate trophozoites are readily seen in untreated 'wet' films of diarrhoeic faeces.

Treatment has not been fully defined, but tetracyclines and 5-nitroimidazoles, such as metronidazole, are said to be effective.

Microsporidia

These animal parasites are represented by several genera, including *Encephalitozoon*, *Enterocytozoon* and *Nosema*, which have, on rare occasions, been implicated in opportunistic infections of immuno-compromised patients. Infections of the eye, meninges and other organs have been reported. The most suitable antimicrobial treatment is unknown.

ORGANISMS OF UNCERTAIN TAXONOMIC STATUS

Blastocystis hominis

This organism, which has been variously described as a yeast or a protozoon, is commonly found in faeces. Any pathogenic role is the subject of dispute, but there are claims that it may be associated with diarrhoea in the absence of other known pathogens. Metronidazole is said to be useful if true infection is suspected.

Pneumocystis carinii

There is evidence that this organism may be a fungus, but its morphology, behaviour and response to antimicrobial agents are more typical of a protozoon. It was originally recognized as an uncommon cause of atypical pneumonia in mal-nourished infants, but has sprung to prominence more recently as a common cause of pneumonia in patients with AIDS.

Diagnosis depends on the identification of typical octonucleate 'cysts' in material obtained from the lung, since serology is unreliable. Simple expectorated sputum commonly fails to reveal evidence of the organism, and broncho-alveolar lavage or biopsy may be needed to establish the diagnosis.

The organisms are sensitive to co-trimoxazole, which is the treatment of choice, but patients with AIDS often suffer unacceptable side-effects. Consequently, pentamidine has been widely used in AIDS patients; the drug may be instilled into the lungs by nebulizer to minimize the risks of toxic side-effects. Several investigational drugs are also under trial; these include trimetrexate, piritrexim (both antifolate compounds) and eflornithine.

RECOMMENDED READING

Crewe W, Haddock D R W 1985 *Parasites and Human Disease*. Edward Arnold, London

Fleck S L, Moody A H 1988 *Diagnostic Techniques in Medical Parasitology*. Wright, London

James D M, Gilles H M 1985 *Human Antiparasitic Drugs*. Wiley, Chichester

Maegraith B 1989 *Adams and Maegraith's Clinical Tropical Diseases*, 9th edn. Blackwell, Oxford

Manson-Bahr P E C, Bell D H 1987 *Manson's Tropical Diseases*, 19th edn. Baillière Tindall, London

Muller R, Baker J H 1990 *Medical Parasitology*. Gower, London

Peters W, Gilles H M 1989 *A Colour Atlas of Tropical Medicine and Parasitology*, 3rd edn. Wolfe, London

Report 1989 Prophylaxis against malaria for travellers from the United Kingdom. *British Medical Journal* 299: 1087–1089

World Health Organization 1991 *Basic Laboratory Methods in Medical Parasitology*. WHO, Geneva

62

Helminths

D. Greenwood

Medical helminthology is concerned with the study of parasitic worms. These creatures are responsible for an enormous burden of infection throughout the world and, although few helminth infections are life-threatening, their impact on human health is incalculable. Most helminths have no independent existence outside the host and are therefore truly parasitic. Since they rely on the host for sustenance, it is not in their interest to cause the host harm; consequently they do not usually exhibit great virulence and are characterized more by the novel methods that they have evolved to prevent rejection by the host defences. The pathogenic manifestations of helminthic disease, which can nonetheless be considerable, are ordinarily due to physical factors related to the location of the worms, their lifestyle or their size.

There are two major groups of helminths: *nematodes*, or roundworms, and *platyhelminths*, or flatworms. Flatworms are, in their turn, represented by two classes: *trematodes* (flukes) and *cestodes* (tapeworms).

NEMATODES

The principal nematode parasites of man are conveniently considered under two headings: intestinal nematodes and tissue nematodes.

Intestinal nematodes

Infection with intestinal roundworms (Table 62.1) is generally associated with conditions of poor hygiene. Such infections are extremely common, particularly throughout the tropics and subtropics, although a number are also found in temperate regions.

Table 62.1 Principal intestinal helminths of man

Species	Common name	Relevant examination
Ancylostoma duodenale	Hookworm	Stool concentration (ova)
Ascaris lumbricoides	Common roundworm	Stool concentration (ova)
Enterobius vermicularis	Threadworm	Perianal swab (ova), adult worms on stool
Necator americanus	Hookworm	Stool concentration (ova)
Strongyloides stercoralis	—	Stool concentration or culture (larvae)
Toxocara canis[a]	Dog roundworm	Serology
Trichostrongylus spp.	Hookworm	Stool concentration (ova)
Trichuris trichiura	Whipworm	Stool concentration (ova)

[a] Not an intestinal parasite of man; causes visceral larva migrans (see text).

Ascaris lumbricoides

This is the common roundworm which probably infects over a 1000 million people in the world. The adults are large and fleshy, rather like a garden worm, and as with many nematodes (other than the hookworm group), the smaller male can be recognized by his characteristically crooked tail. The eggs (ova) are produced in huge numbers; they are thick walled, bile stained and typically exhibit a corrugated albuminous coat (Fig. 62.1a). In the absence of a male worm, the female will produce infertile eggs, which tend to be more elongated and irregular than the fertile variety (Fig. 62.1b).

In warm, moist conditions, infective larvae quickly form within fertile eggs, but do not hatch. Such eggs can survive for long periods in soil. If ingested, the eggs hatch in the duodenum and the larvae penetrate the gut mucosa to reach the bloodstream. They are carried to the pulmonary circulation, where they gain access to the lung and undergo two moults before migrating via the trachea to the intestinal tract. Having completed their round-trip, they mature in the gut lumen and live for several years.

A. lumbricoides is a well-adapted parasite that is not usually pathogenic in the ordinary sense. However, pneumonic symptoms may accompany the migratory phase and the adult worms may invade the biliary and pancreatic ducts. Moreover, heavy infection with these large worms can cause intestinal obstruction. Allergy is also sometimes a problem.

The dog ascarid, *Toxocara canis*, may accidentally infect humans. Larvae hatch in the small intestine and penetrate the gut wall, but they are unable to complete their migratory phase. Instead, they find their way to remote parts of the body, a condition known as *visceral larva migrans*. Occasionally the larvae reach the eye and cause serious retinal lesions.

Trichuris trichiura

This is the common whipworm, often found together with ascaris. The adults live with the head (the 'whip' end of the worm) embedded in the colonic mucosa. Each female lays thousands of characteristic 'tea-tray' eggs (Fig. 62.1c) every day. Like those of ascaris, they develop infective larvae in warm, moist conditions, but the ova do not hatch outside the body. However, after ingestion and hatching, there is no migratory phase and adult worms develop directly in the large intestine.

Infection is usually trivial, though massive infections can cause rectal prolapse in young children.

Hookworm

The two human hookworms, *Ancylostoma duodenale* and *Necator americanus*, are widely distributed throughout the tropics and subtropics. The two species produce indistinguishable thin-walled eggs (Fig. 62.1 d) which hatch in soil. The larvae undergo several moults before infective larvae are produced. These are capable of penetrating unbroken skin, and in this way they gain access to the bloodstream to begin a migratory phase similar to that of ascaris. When they reach the gut they attach by their mouthparts to the mucosa of the small intestine.

Hookworms ingest blood and, moreover, move from site to site in the gut mucosa, leaving behind small bleeding lesions. These two facts are responsible for the chief pathological manifestation of heavy infection with hookworms: iron-deficiency anaemia.

Larvae of animal hookworms, notably the dog hookworm, *A. caninum*, may penetrate human skin, but do not migrate further. They do, however, cause irritation by wandering locally through subcutaneous tissue to cause *cutaneous larva migrans*.

Trichostrongylus species

Various species of *Trichostrongylus* have been associated with human disease, particularly in the Middle East. The eggs are similar to those of hookworm, but are more elongated.

Strongyloides stercoralis

This parasite is also related to the hookworms, but differs in several important respects. There is

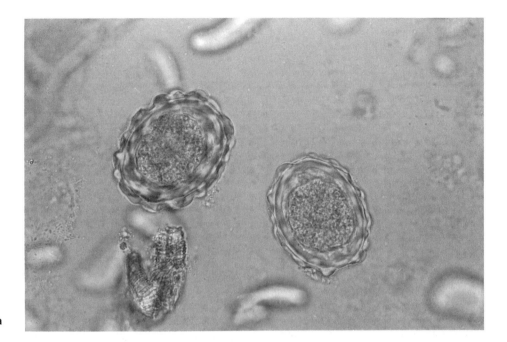

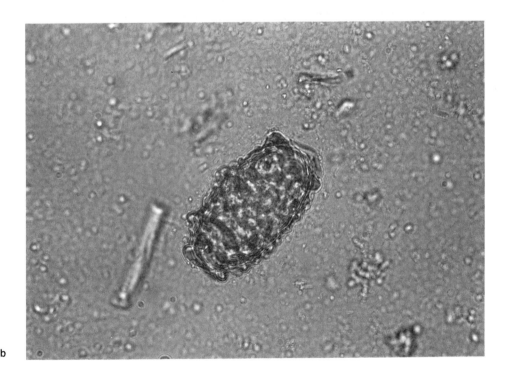

Fig. 62.1 Eggs of intestinal helminths: **a** *Ascaris lumbricoides* (fertile eggs); **b** *A. lumbricoides* (infertile egg).

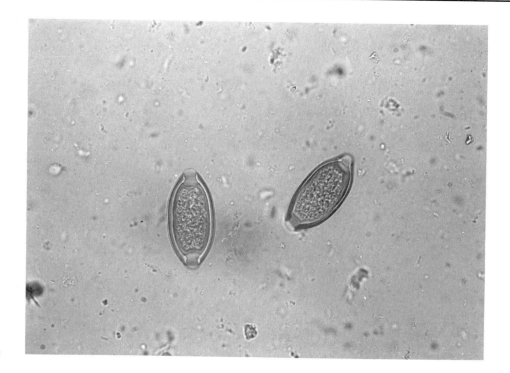

c

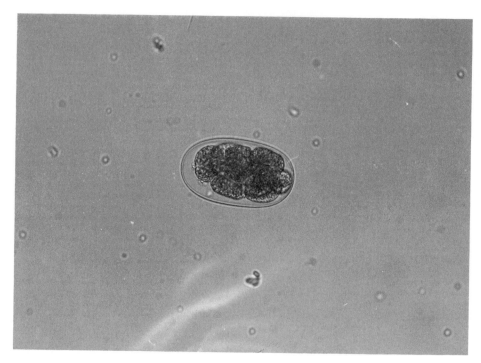

d

Fig. 62.1 c *Trichuris trichiura;* **d** hookworm.

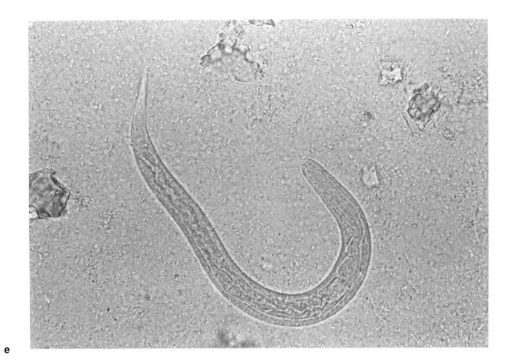

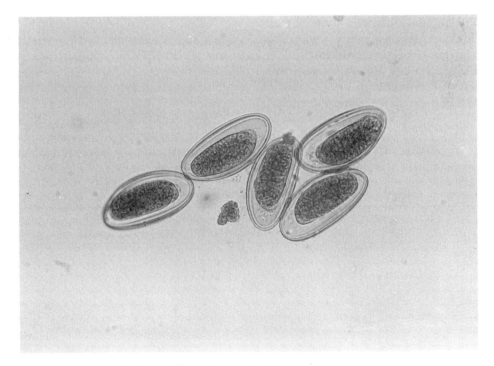

Fig. 62.1 e *Strongyloides stercoralis* (larva); **f** *Enterobius vermicularis.*

a distinct free-living phase in the life-cycle, during which males and females reproduce. Human infections arise after penetration of infective larvae through skin and there is a migratory phase involving the lungs. However, human infection appears to be restricted to female worms, which reproduce parthenogenetically after attaching to the gut mucosa. Eggs contain fully developed larvae when laid and these hatch within the intestinal lumen so that larvae, not eggs, are found in faecal samples (Fig. 62.1e). Infection can persist for many years, probably because some larvae can develop sufficiently within the body to initiate a fresh cycle of development and cause auto-infection.

Symptoms are usually benign, but in immuno-compromised individuals larvae may be activated to penetrate the gut wall and invade other organs, a serious condition known as *hyperinfection*.

Enterobius vermicularis

This is the common threadworm, which infects children throughout the world. It has the simplest life cycle of all intestinal worms. Adults live in the large intestine and are occasionally found in the appendix. Mature, gravid females crawl through the anus at night and lay their eggs in the perianal area. The eggs are characteristically flattened on one side (Fig. 62.1f) and usually contain fully developed larvae. Ingestion of these eggs initiates a fresh infection. Symptoms are restricted to itching (*pruritus ani*) associated with the deposition of eggs.

Since eggs are not discharged by the worm into faeces, faecal examination is not appropriate in the laboratory diagnosis of threadworm infection. The diagnosis is established by finding the characteristic threadworms on the surface of formed stools, or by examination of swabs, or Sellotape impressions, of unwashed peri-anal skin.

Treatment of intestinal nematode infections

In endemic areas, the need to treat intestinal worm infections has to be balanced against the severity of symptoms (if any), the inevitability of reinfection, and the use of scarce medical resources. In the industrially developed world, where the infections are less common and mostly imported, a more liberal approach to treatment can be adopted.

The range of options is listed in Table 62.2. Most effective (and expensive) are the benzimidazole derivatives mebendazole and thiabendazole. Evidence is accumulating that the related imidazole compound albendazole, which is widely used in veterinary practice, is equally effective.

Tissue nematodes

This group includes the filarial worms, the Guinea worm (*Dracunculus medinensis*) and *Trichinella spiralis* (Table 62.3).

Filarial worms have a complex life-cycle involving developmental stages in an insect vector. They vary considerably in their pathogenic effects, but some are responsible for disabling diseases that have a major impact on communities living in endemic areas.

Table 62.2 Spectrum of activity of drugs used in the treatment of intestinal helminthiasis

Drug	Ancylostoma duodenale	Necator americanus	Ascaris lumbricoides	Strongyloides stercoralis	Trichuris trichiura	Enterobius vermicularis
Tetrachloroethylene	+	+++	–	–	–	–
Piperazine	–	–	+++	–	–	+++
Bephenium	+++	+	+	–	–	–
Levamisole	++	++	+++	–	–	–
Pyrantel pamoate	++	++	+++	+	++	+++
Thiabendazole	++	++	+++	++	–	++
Mebendazole	++	++	+++	+	++	+++

+++, highly effective; +, poorly effective; –, no useful activity.
(From Greenwood D (ed) *Antimicrobial Chemotherapy*, 2nd edn. Oxford University Press, Oxford.)

Table 62.3 Principal tissue nematodes of man

Species	Intermediate host	Geographical distribution	Relevant examination
Wuchereria bancrofti	Mosquitoes	Tropical belt	Night blood
Loa loa	*Chrysops* spp.	West and Central Africa	Day blood
Brugia malayi	Mosquitoes	South-East Asia	Night blood
Mansonella perstans	*Culicoides* spp.	Tropical Africa, South America	Blood
M. ozzardi	*Culicoides* spp.	West Indies, South America	Blood
Onchocerca volvulus	*Simulium* spp.	Tropical Africa, Central America	Skin shavings
M. streptocerca	*Culicoides* spp.	West and Central Africa	Skin shavings
Dracunculus medinensis	Water fleas	Africa, Indian sub-continent	Adult worm when mature
Trichinella spiralis	None[a]	World-wide	Muscle biopsy, serology

[a] Pork forms the chief reservoir.

Wuchereria bancrofti

This filarial worm is transmitted by the bite of various species of mosquito throughout the tropical belt of the world. It is believed that over 100 million people may be infected. The larvae invade the lymphatics, usually of the lower limbs, where they develop into adult worms. Presence of the adult worms causes lymphatic blockage and gross lymphoedema, which sometimes leads to the bizarre deformations associated with bancroftian filariasis, *elephantiasis*.

Embryonic forms (*microfilariae*) are liberated into the bloodstream. They retain the elastic egg membrane as a sheath, which covers the whole larva (Fig. 62.2 a). Microfilariae remain in the pulmonary circulation during the day, emerging into the peripheral circulation only at night, to coincide with the biting habits of the insect vector. The physiological basis of this nocturnal periodicity is not understood, but it can be reversed by altering sleep patterns in, for example, night-shift workers. Moreover, strains of *W. bancrofti* encountered in some Pacific islands do not exhibit a noctural periodicity. Aside from these exceptions, blood for examination for *W. bancrofti* must be taken during the night, optimally between midnight and 2 a.m.

Loa loa

This worm is restricted in distribution to central and western parts of tropical Africa, where it is transmitted by the mango fly (*Chrysops* species). The adult worms live in subcutaneous tissue and wander round the body, provoking localized reactions known as *Calabar swellings* and sometimes migrating across the front of the eye.

The sheathed microfilariae of *Loa loa* (Fig. 62.2b) exhibit diurnal periodicity, so that, unlike those of *W. bancrofti*, they appear in peripheral blood only during the day.

Brugia malayi

This parasite is probably related to *W. bancrofti*. It is transmitted by mosquitoes in parts of India, the Far-East and South-East Asia. Adult worms inhabit the lymphatics and, like *W. bancrofti*, can cause elephantiasis. Microfilaraemia usually shows a nocturnal periodicity.

Onchocerca volvulus

This filarial worm is common in parts of tropical Africa and central America. It is transmitted by *Simulium damnosum*, and related species of blackfly, which breed in vegetation on the banks of rivers. Adult worms develop in subcutaneous and connective tissue and often become encapsulated in nodules which form on bony parts of the body, such as the hip, elbow and (particularly in central America) the head. The microfilariae are not found in blood, but live in the superficial layers of the skin causing itching and, in heavy, chronic infections, gross thickening of the skin. The eye is commonly invaded by microfilariae, which may cause corneal and retinal lesions that lead to

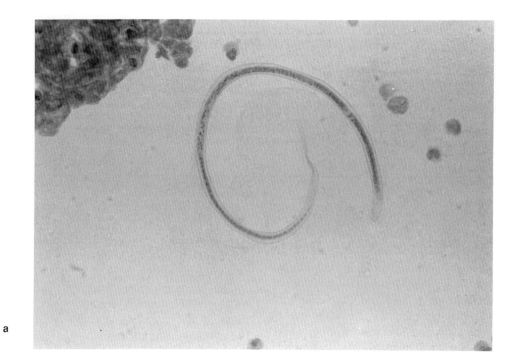

Fig. 62.2 Sheathed microfilariae of **a** *Wuchereria bancrofti* and **b** *Loa loa*.

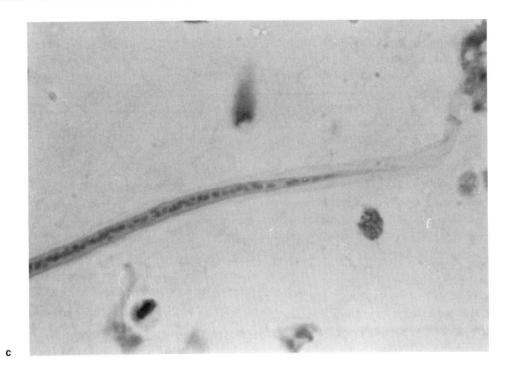

c

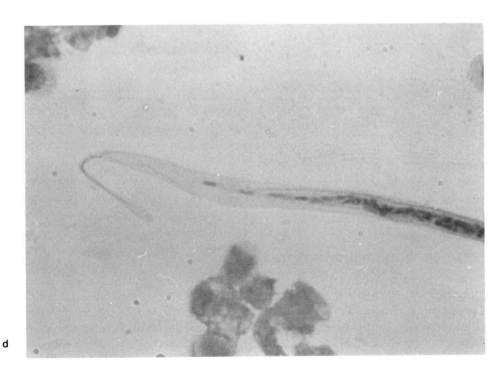

d

Fig. 62.2 c Tail of microfilaria of *W. bancrofti* showing tip devoid of somatic nucleic; **d** tail of microfilaria of *L. loa* showing nuclei extending to tip of tail.

blindness. Because of the association of the vector with rivers, the condition is known as *river blindness*.

If nodules are present, diagnosis can be made by finding macroscopic worms within an excised nodule. Otherwise, superficial slivers of skin, taken from calves, buttocks and shoulders, are suspended in a drop of saline and examined microscopically for motile microfilariae.

Mansonella species

Mansonella perstans (formerly *Acanthocheilonema perstans* or *Dipetalonema perstans*) is widespread throughout tropical Africa and parts of South America; the related *M. ozzardi* is restricted to parts of the West Indies and South America. They are transmitted by biting midges (*Culicoides* species). The unsheathed microfilariae appear in the bloodstream and exhibit no periodicity. They are generally regarded as being non-pathogenic.

M. streptocerca (formerly *A. streptocerca*) causes skin infections similar to those of *O. volvulus*, although the symptoms are usually milder. It is restricted to parts of western and central Africa.

Differential characteristics of microfilariae

The microfilariae of filarial worms can be differentiated in stained preparations of clinical material by various criteria, the most useful of which are the presence or absence of a sheath and the disposition of the somatic nuclei in the tip of the tail (Table 62.4 and Fig. 62.2 c and d). Giemsa stain is suitable for the demonstration of somatic nuclei, but hot (60°C) haematoxylin is necessary to stain the sheath.

Treatment of filariasis

Diethylcarbamazine (DEC) has been used for many years for the treatment of all forms of filariasis. It effectively kills microfilariae, but is not reliably lethal to adult worms. It is relatively non-toxic, but death of the microfilariae is often accompanied by a severe allergic reaction, especially in onchocerciasis. Suramin kills the adult worms, but is much more toxic than DEC.

The treatment of onchocerciasis and, probably, other forms of filariasis, has been revolutionized by use of the veterinary anthelminthic *ivermectin*. This drug appears to be highly effective in a single oral dose and is less likely than DEC to elicit a severe reaction. The infection can be controlled in endemic areas by administering ivermectin at yearly intervals.

Dracunculus medinensis

This is the *Guinea worm*. The infective larvae develop within water fleas of the genus *Cyclops* and human infection is normally acquired through infected drinking water. The larvae penetrate the gut mucosa and grow to maturity in connective tissue, usually of the lower limbs. The male is small and insignificant, but the female may reach a length of 1 m. After fertilization, the female worm incubates the larvae to maturity and, when ready to give birth, emerges to the skin surface to provoke an intensely irritating blister. When the sufferer immerses the blister in water, the uterus of the female worms bursts, liberating up to 1 million larvae, which are ingested by water fleas to continue the cycle.

Attempts can be made to wind out the dead worm over several days, but breakage of the worm often occurs, and pyogenic cocci may be carried into the tissues to cause a cellulitis. Prevention is the best approach and campaigns for the provision of safe water should help to eradicate this disease.

Trichinella spiralis

Unlike most parasitic worms, *T. spiralis* has an extremely wide host range. Man is infected accidentally, usually by eating undercooked pork products, although other meat, including bear and walrus meat, has been incriminated. The infected larvae lie dormant in skeletal muscle (Fig. 62.3) and are released when the meat is digested. Male and female worms develop to maturity attached to the mucosa of the small intestine. The female is viviparous, producing numerous larvae during a life-span of only a few weeks. The

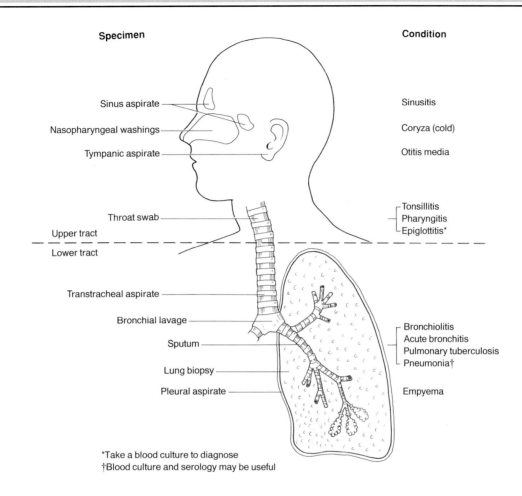

Specimen

Sinus aspirate

Nasopharyngeal washings

Tympanic aspirate

Throat swab

Upper tract

Lower tract

Transtracheal aspirate

Bronchial lavage

Sputum

Lung biopsy

Pleural aspirate

*Take a blood culture to diagnose
†Blood culture and serology may be useful

Condition

Sinusitis

Coryza (cold)

Otitis media

Tonsillitis
Pharyngitis
Epiglottitis*

Bronchiolitis
Acute bronchitis
Pulmonary tuberculosis
Pneumonia†

Empyema

Fig. 63.2 Microbial infections of the respiratory tract and the appropriate specimens for laboratory investigation.

to medical service and pharmacies. However, these improvements have occurred in concert with better housing and social conditions.

There is little need to make a virological diagnosis as specific therapy is not available. However, epidemiological studies of patients with throat symptoms have revealed how common and varied are the viruses in the respiratory tract.

In the severely ill child with toxaemia and a membrane, diphtheria must be considered and treatment should not await laboratory confirmation. Moreover, the laboratory needs to do special tests to isolate and identify *Corynebacterium diphtheriae*, and communication (by telephone, if possible) between the clinician and laboratory is

essential. Other corynebacteria such as *C. ulcerans* and *C. haemolyticum* may rarely cause ulcerated sore throats. In the sexually active, gonococcal pharyngitis should not be missed and again the laboratory needs to be told as they will use special selective media for *Neisseria gonorrhoeae*.

Common cold (coryza)

This common complaint, characterized by a nasal discharge (acute rhinitis) which is usually watery with scanty cells, afflicts humans of all ages who congregate together. Since there are many types of rhinoviruses, coronaviruses, adenoviruses, etc. and since immunity may be short lived, individuals in a crowded environment, such as at school and university or travelling on public transport, may suffer three or four clinical infections a year. Most of these do not seek medical help knowing that there is little to offer. This is a condition for which many 'alternative' remedies are tried from garlic to peppermint and vitamin supplements.

Bacterial superinfection with pneumococci and *H. influenzae* can occur in the nasopharynx but is only symptomatic when the sinuses or middle ear are involved. Pharyngitis and, occasionally, tracheobronchitis may occur with a cold or develop in more susceptible individuals. Respiratory syncytial virus (RSV) may cause upper respiratory symptoms in children and adults but in those contracting the virus for the first time (usually infants under 1 year of age) acute bronchiolitis is common.

Sinusitis and otitis media

Direct extension of a viral or bacterial infection from the nasopharynx into frontal and maxillary sinuses in adults and into the middle ear in children is not uncommon. Obtaining adequate material for microbiology is difficult and requires the expertise of ear, nose and throat specialists. In most cases of acute sinusitis or otitis media the microbial cause is not found. It is assumed that severe pain and discharge of pus from the nose or ear is suggestive of bacterial infection and antibiotics are usually given to cover streptococci (mainly *Str. pneumoniae*) and *H. influenzae*. In adults with recurrent or chronic sinusitis, anaerobes (peptostreptococci or bacteroides) are often found in sinus washings.

Lower respiratory tract

Epiglottitis

Although situated in the upper part of the respiratory tract, *epiglottitis* behaves like a serious systemic infection which requires urgent admission to hospital and treatment. The diagnosis should be made clinically in a toxic child (usually under 5 years old) with respiratory obstruction and stridor. The most useful investigation is blood culture, which invariably grows *H. influenzae* type b unless antibiotics have been given. The epiglottis, which is swollen and cherry-red in appearance, should only be examined by skilled paediatricians prepared for a respiratory arrest. A lateral X-ray shows a soft tissue swelling in the throat.

Laryngotracheobronchitis

In adults, some viral infections cause acute laryngitis with voice loss or tracheitis with a dry cough. Respiratory tract infection in children is usually generalized and presents as *croup*. This may lead to respiratory obstruction and, as with haemophilus epiglottitis, urgent admission to hospital is necessary. The condition may be caused by a variety of respiratory viruses with parainfluenza, adeno- and enteroviruses the most common. RSV can also cause croup but more commonly this virus attacks infants in the first few months of life. In the UK there are winter epidemics of *acute bronchiolitis* due to RSV. This clinical syndrome starts as a cold which is followed by wheezing. In older children, asthmatic attacks are often precipitated by viral respiratory infections.

Whooping cough

Pertussis may be confused with croup and, as special specimens need to be taken, the laboratory must be informed. A pernasal swab in special transport medium is required and *Bordetella pertussis* will only grow on enriched culture media in conditions of high humidity.

Acute bronchitis

Acute exacerbations of chronic obstructive airways disease (COAD) is the commonest adult lower respiratory infection. It is invariably due to pneumococci, non-encapsulated haemophili, or both. Sometimes, acute bronchitis follows a viral infection. Although often examined, expectorated sputum from ambulatory patients with COAD is almost always a waste of effort.

Cystic fibrosis patients have frequent exacerbations and, in those situations, sputum examination is valuable because the causative bacteria

(*Staphylococcus aureus*, *H. influenzae* and *Pseudomonas aeruginosa*) may show variable antimicrobial resistance and appropriate therapy is essential.

Acute pneumonias

It is sometimes possible on clinical and radiological grounds to distinguish between *lobar pneumonia* (pneumococcal), *bronchopneumonia* (staphylococcal, klebsiellal) and '*atypical' pneumonias* (mycoplasmal, chlamydial). This division is of importance in guiding primary treatment but should not give the clinician a blinkered view in investigation as some cases will invariably not follow a text book! Expectorated sputum is often poorly collected and may not yield the pathogen. Blood cultures should always be taken from pneumonia patients but may not yield an organism, especially if antibiotics have been started. *Antigen detection* in urine or sputum by fluorescent antibodies, immuno-electrophoresis, latex agglutination or enzyme-linked immunosorbent assay (ELISA) is a promising method for rapid diagnosis but may lack sensitivity. Most cases of 'atypical' pneumonia are diagnosed by obtaining acute and convalescent sera and finding a significant titre or a rising titre of antibodies. *Legionnaires' disease* may be diagnosed by culture of *Legionella pneumophila* from sputum or a biopsy, but this has too low a sensitivity and treatment must often be given on the grounds of serological evidence or clinical suspicion.

Chronic chest disease

Tuberculosis must always be considered in any patient with fever, cough and weight loss. Again, a request for examination for mycobacteria must be included on the request card.

In the immunocompromised, various opportunist pathogens may give rise to respiratory infection. *Pneumocystis carinii* is demonstrated by fluorescent antibody staining of bronchial lavage. Fungal infections are diagnosed by growth of the pathogen or by serology. Special investigations are required for all these situations and unless the diagnosis is considered the laboratory cannot assist the clinician.

Gastro-intestinal infection

Acute diarrhoea with or without vomiting is a common complaint. Microbial causes, either by multiplication in the intestine or from the effects of preformed toxin, are the most important reasons for acute gastro-intestinal upset in an otherwise healthy individual. Non-infective causes of diarrhoea, such as ulcerative colitis, may present similarly but usually the natural history and chronicity of the condition makes the distinction obvious.

Although many new causes of bowel infection have been discovered in the past 15 years the majority of food-related and short-lived episodes do not yield a microbial cause. In part this is due to the wide range of viruses, bacteria and protozoa which may be sought (Table 63.1). A search for all causes involves extensive and expensive laboratory effort and this is often considered unnecessary for a condition which is usually self-limiting and relatively harmless.

Toxin-mediated disease of microbial origin ranges in severity from relatively trivial episodes of food poisoning caused by enterotoxin-producing strains of *Staph. aureus*, *Clostridium perfringens* and *Bacillus cereus*, to the life-threatening systemic disease (*botulism*) caused by *Cl. botulinum*, and the severe *pseudomembranous colitis* caused by *Cl. difficile*, which occasionally follows depletion of the gut flora by antibiotic treatment. There are, in addition, many non-microbial causes of

Table 63.1 Common microbial causes of gastro-intestinal illness

Viruses	Rotavirus
	Astrovirus
	Calicivirus
Bacteria	*Salmonella* spp.
	Campylobacter spp.
	Shigella spp.
	Escherichia coli (ETEC, EIEC, EPEC, EHEC)
	Vibrio cholerae
	V. parahaemolyticus
	Yersinia enterocolitica
Protozoa	*Cryptosporidium parvum*
	Entamoeba histolytica
	Giardia lamblia

ETEC, enterotoxigenic *Esch. coli*; EIEC, entero-invasive *Esch. coli*; EPEC, enteropathogenic *Esch. coli*; EHEC, enterohaemorrhagic *Esch. coli*.

food poisoning, such as that due to the ingestion of certain toadstools, undercooked red kidney beans or various types of fish (*ciguatera toxin, scombrotoxin*); most notorious is the puffer fish which, during part of its reproductive cycle, produces a neurotoxin that is responsible for more than 100 deaths a year in Japan where the delicacy *fugu* is enjoyed.

It may be possible on clinical grounds to distinguish between patients with dysentery, in which bloody diarrhoea and mucus are found, and those with watery diarrhoea, due to the toxic effects of the pathogen on the small intestinal mucosa, leading to accumulation of fluid in the bowel. Some conditions such as staphylococcal food poisoning and some viral illnesses present largely with vomiting. A specific cause is also suspected if there is a history of foreign travel, if the case forms part of an outbreak which is food or water associated, or if the individual has a relevant food history.

Travellers' diarrhoea encompasses many clinical and microbial causes but the commonest organisms implicated are enterotoxigenic strains of *Escherichia coli* (ETEC). However, a host of microbes must be considered. Some, such as salmonellae, are found world-wide; others, such as vibrios, have a more limited distribution.

More chronic intestinal infections contracted in warmer climates usually do not present with diarrhoea but with vague abdominal symptoms. Many helminths and protozoa are found on screening faeces for other pathogens.

Urinary tract infections

The diagnosis of urinary tract infection cannot be made without bacteriological examination of the urine because many patients with the frequency-dysuria syndrome have sterile urine and, conversely, asymptomatic bacteriuria is a common condition. Infection is most commonly caused by members of the Enterobacteriaceae (Table 63.2), but there are great variations in antimicrobial susceptibility and control of chemotherapy requires laboratory examination. Occasionally, *Mycobacterium tuberculosis* invades the kidney and appropriate tests must be carried out if this is suspected.

Table 63.2 Common causes of urinary tract infection (approximate percentages)

Organism	Domiciliary	Hospital
Escherichia coli	70–80	50
Proteus mirabilis	10	1–5
Klebsiella spp.	1–5	5–10
Staphylococcus saprophyticus	10–15	0
Staph. epidermidis	1–5	10–20
Enterococci	1–5	10–20
Other coliforms	<1	5–10
Pseudomonas aeruginosa	1–2	5–10

Infection in the urinary tract may be confined to particular anatomical sites, e.g. urethritis or renal abscess. Alternatively, the urine may become infected and, in cases of obstruction or reflux, bacteria may ascend from the bladder to give rise to kidney infections. *Urethritis* is really a genital infection and is most commonly due to sexually transmitted organisms such as chlamydiae or *N. gonorrhoeae*. Confirmation depends on obtaining, by swabbing or scraping, a sample of urethral discharge for microscopy and culture. *Metastatic abscesses* in the kidney and *perinephric abscesses* cannot usually be diagnosed by urine examination, although pyuria may be present. Specific radiological or surgical exploration is necessary, as with any localized infection.

Throughout most of their life-span women suffer far more attacks of urinary tract infection than men. In young adult women who become sexually active, frequency and dysuria are common reasons to seek medical attention. Only about one-half of these yield an organism in 'significant' numbers, usually defined as $>10^7$ organisms per litre. The commonest cause by far is *Esch. coli* (Table 63.2), some strains of which possess specific uropathogenic determinants. It has been suggested that many of the culture-negative infections are due to coliforms which are present in small numbers in urine. Infection of the urine is common and may be asymptomatic in up to 20% of elderly patients.

Infections of the central nervous system

Meningitis

Meningeal irritation may occur in association with other acute infections (*meningism*) or with non-infective conditions such as subarachnoid haemorrhage. Infarcts may have meningitis without tell-tale signs and with a vague history. In the early stages of meningococcal disease, signs of meningitis may be absent yet examination of the cerebrospinal fluid (CSF) yields *N. meningitidis*. Thus, CSF and blood cultures should be examined from all suspected cases. There are contra-indications to performing a lumbar puncture in any patient with raised intracranial pressure because of the danger of herniation through the foramen magnum (*coning*). Thus, lumbar puncture should only be carried out in hospital. In fulminating disease, especially if it is meningococcal, it is prudent to give penicillin as soon as the diagnosis is suspected and before admission.

It is often possible to consider the likely pathogen on clinical and epidemiological grounds. *H. influenzae* type b occurs almost always in infants from 6 to 24 months of age. *Str. pneumoniae* is seen generally in the very young and the elderly. *Meningococcal meningitis* is characteristically a disease of children and young adults. In the neonate, coliforms (mainly *Esch. coli K1*), *Listeria monocytogenes*, group B streptococci and pneumococci may be found. In infants a few months old, salmonella meningitis is an important condition in some warm-climate countries.

If no readily cultivated organism is found, but the CSF shows an increase in cells, the syndrome of *aseptic meningitis* is present. Table 63.3 shows

some of the causes of this condition. If the symptoms are short in duration, viruses are most likely. If the child has been unwell for more than 1 week *tuberculous meningitis* must be considered. This is one of the most difficult and important microbiological diagnoses to make.

In the immunocompromised, listeria meningitis may be seen in the adult and *Cryptococcus neoformans* in all age groups but particularly those with human immunodeficiency virus (HIV) infection. Central nervous system disease in patients with acquired immune deficiency syndrome (AIDS) is a very complicated differential diagnosis (Table 63.4).

Cerebral infections

Encephalitis may extend into the meninges with signs and CSF findings of an aseptic meningitis. Many viral infections may, however, only infect the brain cortex and clinical symptoms may be vague: loss of consciousness, fits, localized paralysis. This can also occur in toxaemia, cerebral malaria, electrolyte disturbances or vascular accidents.

In western Europe, herpes simplex or varicella-zoster viruses are the most common causes of encephalitis but in many parts of the world arboviruses such as Japanese B encephalitis virus are important.

Abscesses in the brain or subdural space may arise from haematogenous spread during bacteraemia or by direct extension, either through the cribriform

Table 63.3 Causes of aseptic meningitis

Viruses	Enteroviruses (Echo–, polio–, coxsackie viruses) Mumps (including post-immunization) Herpes (herpes simplex and varicella–zoster) Arboviruses
Spiral bacteria	Syphilis (*Treponema pallidum*) Leptospira (*Leptospira canicola*)
Other bacteria	Partially treated with antibiotics Tuberculous (*Mycobacterium tuberculosis*) Brain abscess
Fungi	*Cryptococcus neoformans*
Protozoa	*Acanthamoeba, Naegleria* *Toxoplasma gondii*
Non-infective	Lymphomas, leukaemias Metastatic and primary neoplasms Collagen–vascular diseases

Table 63.4 Causes of neurological damage in HIV-infected patients

Direct HIV Infection	Subacute encephalomyelitis (AIDS–dementia complex)
Opportunist infections Viruses	 Cytomegalovirus Herpes simplex Varicella–zoster Papovavirus
Bacteria	*Treponema pallidum* (syphilis)
Fungi	*Cryptococcus neoformans*
Protozoa	*Toxoplasma gondii*
Malignancy	
Primary	Brain lymphoma
Secondary	Kaposi's sarcoma Systemic lymphoma

plate from the nasopharynx or from sinuses or the middle ear. They may be clinically silent or present as a space-occupying lesion accompanied by fever and systemic upset. Skilled radiological scanning by computerized axial tomography (CAT) or magnetic resonance imaging (MRI), if available, and early neurosurgical intervention will reduce complications and, if appropriate systemic antibiotics are given for a prolonged period, the success rate is nowadays good.

Skin and soft-tissue infections

Human skin acts as an excellent barrier to infection. Some parasites, such as hookworm larvae and schistosome cercariae can penetrate skin to initiate infection. This may also be true of some bacteria, notably *Treponema pallidum*, although in primary syphilis the spirochaete probably enters through minute abrasions which are present even in healthy skin. Primary skin infection such as *impetigo* is due to *Staph. aureus* or *Str. pyogenes*, or both, gaining access to abrasions, usually in children. *Dermatophyte* fungi are specialized to grow well in keratinized tissue.

Skin lesions are a feature of some virus infections, such as warts, herpes simplex and molluscum contagiosum. In other virus diseases, including rubella, measles, chickenpox (and, before its eradication, smallpox) a characteristic rash follows the viraemic phase of the illness. *Wound infections* may be accidental or postoperative and many organisms can cause sepsis. Even after surgery many wounds are infected with the endogenous flora of the patient. Swabs, or preferably pus, obtained directly from the wound or abscess, is adequate to find the causative organisms. *Anaerobic* sepsis most commonly occurs following amputations or in contaminated traumatic wounds, particularly if the blood supply has been compromised or the bowel perforated. In classic *gas gangrene*, bubbles of gas may be felt in the wound and surrounding tissues and the muscle and fascia have a black necrotic appearance. Less florid examples of anaerobes causing extensive cellulitis are more commonly seen and the laboratory should be requested to look carefully for anaerobes in all situations where deep wounds may be contaminated with endogenous flora.

Genital tract infections

In the male, acute urethritis is a common condition which is usually due to a sexually transmitted microbe such as *N. gonorrhoeae*, *Chlamydia trachomatis* or *Ureaplasma*. If untreated these organisms can cause prostatitis or epididymitis, and gonorrhoea may produce unpleasant consequences such as urethral stricture or sterility. Genital ulcers in both sexes may be due to herpes simplex virus, syphilis or chancroid (*H. ducreyi*).

The more complicated female reproductive organs are subjected to many more infections with a greater scope for sequelae. Vaginitis may present as vaginal discharge or irritation and often these are due to infections that are not always exogenously acquired. *Trichomonas vaginalis* is the most common sexually acquired microbe, although both *N. gonorrhoeae* and chlamydia may also present as discharge. Thrush due to *Candida* species is especially common in pregnancy and in diabetics. It is usually an endogenous condition due to disturbances in the normal commensal flora. Another cause of vaginal discharge, but usually without inflammatory cells and irritation, is associated with an alteration of local pH with proliferation of *Gardnerella vaginalis* and anaerobic spiral bacteria, now termed *Mobiluncus* species. The alkaline conditions and characteristic amines found in *bacterial vaginosis* allow a diagnosis to be easily made on examination of the patient. This condition, which used to be called non-specific vaginitis, is a common condition in sexually active women, although probably not a venereal disease in the usual sense.

The endocervical canal is the site of infection with *N. gonorrhoeae* and *C. trachomatis* in the sexually mature woman. During parturition both organisms may be passed to the baby's eyes to give rise to *ophthalmia neonatorum*. The cervix may also be infected with human papillomavirus (HPV) and this is associated with a high risk of cervical cancer. HPV commonly causes warts on the external genitalia, peri-anally as well as in the vagina and cervix. Herpes, chancroid and syphilis may cause ulcers in parts of the genital tract which are not visible without a speculum.

Ascending genital infection due to gonococci or chlamydia is a common sequela. In cases of *acute gonococcal salpingitis* there is usually fever and pelvic pain. On vaginal examination, there is referred lower abdominal pain on moving the cervix (*cervical excitation*) and tenderness in the iliac fossae on abdominal palpation. Signs and symptoms in cases due to *C. trachomatis* are much less pronounced and some women develop chronic *pelvic inflammatory disease* (PID) without having suffered a recognizable acute episode. PID, although most often initiated by these two common sexually transmitted pathogens, is usually a polymicrobial infection, in which endogenous commensals, particularly anaerobes, play an important role.

Infection may progress outside the fallopian tubes to give rise to *pelvic abscesses*, especially in the pouch of Douglas, and peritonitis. Spread across the peritoneal cavity may give rise to *perihepatitis*, which was first described in gonorrhoea as the Fitz-Hugh–Curtis syndrome, but also occurs in chlamydial disease.

Eye infections

Various microbes may cause acute conjunctivitis. Ophthalmia neonatorum may be due to gonococci or chlamydia. In the newborn, *Staph. aureus* is commonly found in 'sticky eyes', either as a primary cause of conjunctivitis or after infection with another pathogen. In older infants and children, *H. influenzae* and *Str. pneumoniae* are common. Chlamydia give rise to *trachoma*, the commonest cause of blindness in the world, and to a milder form of inclusion blennorrhoea in sexually active individuals.

Primary viral conjunctivitis often occurs in epidemics when certain types of adenovirus are implicated. This is usually a mild condition with few sequelae compared with the keratitis due to herpes simplex virus or in shingles when the ophthalmic division of the trigeminal nerve is infected with varicella–zoster virus.

Corneal damage due to fungi as well as herpesviruses is seen in immunosuppressed patients, and keratitis caused by free-living amoebae (*Acanthamoeba* species), though rare, is becoming more common, particularly in wearers of contact lenses.

Penetrating injuries of the eye and ophthalmic surgery may introduce a wide range of bacteria and fungi into the chambers of the eye which may give rise to *hypopyon* (pus in the eye). This condition requires prompt surgical drainage and instillation of appropriate antibiotics such as gentamicin. *Ps. aeruginosa* and *Proteus* species are among the more common organisms isolated.

Infections of the back of the eye (choroidoretinitis) are seen in many diverse infectious diseases (see Table 63.5).

SYSTEMIC AND GENERAL SYNDROMES

Pyrexia of unknown origin (PUO)

PUO may be defined as a significant fever (greater than 38°C) for a few days without an obvious cause, i.e. no apparent infection of an organ or system. In the classic studies of PUO only patients with persistent fever for at least 3 weeks were included. These chronic cases are often due to non-infective causes such as malignancy (especially lymphomas) or auto-immune and connective tissue diseases (such as systemic lupus erythematosus).

In determining an infective aetiology some of the most important questions to be asked of the patient are:

1. Have you been abroad recently?
2. What is your occupation (especially, is animal contact involved)?
3. What immunizations have you had — in particular have you had BCG?
4. Have you or your family ever had tuberculosis?

Table 63.5 Causes of choroidoretinitis

Viruses	Cytomegalovirus, rubella
Bacteria	*Treponema pallidum*
Protozoa	*Toxoplasma gondii*
Helminths	*Toxocara canis, Onchocerca volvulus*

5. Are you taking or have you recently had any drugs (especially antibiotics)?

Character of fever

The individual with suspected PUO should be admitted to hospital so that measurements can be made regularly by skilled staff. Rarely, malingerers may be found out and drug reactions discovered by controlling intake. Rhythmical fevers such as the quartan fever (every 72 h) of *Plasmodium malariae* or undulant fever of *Brucella melitensis* may be rarely found and point to the aetiology. More commonly, fevers are intermittent with rises at the end of the day and falls after rigors or extensive sweating.

The degree of temperature depends also on the host response as well as the pyrogens produced by microbes. Generally, the older the patient the less able they are to mount a pyrexia. Many elderly patients with septicaemia may have normal or subnormal temperatures whereas infants can have fevers of 40°C and febrile convulsions with otherwise mild respiratory viral infections.

Endocarditis

Infections of the tissue of the heart usually involve damaged valves, either post-rheumatic fever or with atheroma. Another important group of patients are those who have had heart surgery, in particular prosthetic valve replacements. In addition, intravenous drug addicts or patients who have had indwelling vascular devices are liable to bacteraemia and, occasionally, endocarditis may follow. The most common causative organisms are listed in Table 63.6.

Septicaemia

It is not clinically useful to distinguish between *bacteraemia*, organisms isolated from the bloodstream, *septicaemia*, which is a clinical syndrome, and *endotoxaemia*, which is circulating bacterial endotoxin. The spectrum of clinical disease ranges from hypotensive shock and disseminated intravascular coagulation (DIC) with a high mortality, to transient bacteraemia, which may occur in healthy individuals during dental manipulations.

The vascular compartment is sterile and usually intact. Microbes gain entry from breakages of blood vessels adjacent to skin or mucosal surfaces or by phagocytic cells carrying organisms into capillaries or the lymphatic system. Active multiplication within the bloodstream probably only occurs terminally, but in many cases of septicaemia there are high numbers of bacteria recovered from blood cultures, which often only sample 10 ml at a time. This occurs from a heavily contaminated site such as an indwelling urinary

Table 63.6 Common causes of infective endocarditis (approximate percentages)

Organism	Non-operative	IVDA/surgery
Viridans group of streptococci	70	35
Enterococci	5	3
Other streptococci (group G, F)	10	<1
Staphylococcus epidermidis	10	25
Staph. aureus	5	25
Gram-positive rods (diphtheroids)	<1	5
Haemophilus spp. and other fastidious Gram-negative organisms[a]	<1[b]	<1
Gram-negative bacilli (coliforms, *Pseudomonas* spp.)	0	5
Coxiella burnetii (Q fever)	<1[b]	0
Chlamydia psittaci	<1	0
Fungi (*Candida* sp.)	<1	2

IVDA, intravenous drug abusers.
[a] *Neisseria, Brucella, Cardiobacterium, Streptobacillus* spp.
[b] These are rough UK figures; in some parts of the Middle East, brucellae and Q fever cause significant numbers of infective endocarditides.

catheter which releases bacteria into veins on movement. Septic shock may be due to Gram-negative lipids (endotoxins) or Gram-positive toxins (e.g. staphylococcal enterotoxin), which are usually proteins. The end result of both is to initiate a cascade of events involving cytokines, especially tumour necrosis factor and interleukin-2, vascular mediators and platelets, which combined lead to DIC and hypotension. This process becomes irreversible and produces failure of all major organs. Patients die from a variety of terminal events which make up the syndrome of *septic shock*. The main microbial causes are listed with approximate frequency in Table 63.7.

Clinical features may occasionally suggest the aetiological agent, e.g. the characteristic purpuric rash of meningococcal disease and the black lesions (*ecthyma gangrenosum*) seen on the skin of compromised patients with pseudomonas septicaemia, but in the majority of bacteraemias the agent can only be determined after blood culture. Sometimes, prior antibiotic therapy may render cultures negative and new methods of antigen detection or gene probes may be useful. Non-specific investigations such as those shown in Fig. 63.1 may offer some help that the cause of the illness is infective. C-reactive protein (CRP), an acute-phase protein which is often greatly elevated in the serum during bacterial infections, may be the most useful of these but, as with peripheral leucocyte counts, there are a signficant number of errant results.

Imported fevers

An important group of patients with fever are those who have recently returned from abroad. In whichever country a doctor may practice he will encounter travellers with unfamiliar diseases. A knowledge of medical geography is useful but conditions vary greatly within one country and with time. Up-to-date information is held, often on computer, by communicable disease centres and tropical disease hospitals and schools. The World Health Organization and the Centers for Disease Control, Atlanta, publish international notification data and maps. Undoubtedly, the most important condition to diagnose is malaria due to *Plasmodium falciparum*, which may be rapidly fatal without appropriate treatment in the non-immune subject. The wide distribution of drug resistance in *P. falciparum* has led to difficulties in giving adequate prophylaxis and in treating an acute attack. Other common febrile illnesses which are imported into northern countries are typhoid and paratyphoid. These do not usually present with diarrhoea so the possibility of an enteric fever may not be considered. It is also obvious, but sometimes overlooked, that the fever may not be related to the travel history and

Table 63.7 Major causes of septicaemia (approximate percentages)

Organism	Community acquired	Hospital acquired	Sources and comments
Escherichia coli	35	30	UTI (catheters), biliary tract
Other enterobacteria	5	10	UTI, chest
Pseudomonas spp.	5	5	UTI, immunocompromised
Other Gram-negative rods	2	5	Ventilator pneumonia
Neisseria meningitidis	3	0	Characteristic skin rash
Staphylococcus aureus	30	25	Vascular, postoperative
Staph. epidermidis	<1	20	Vascular devices
Streptococcus pneumoniae	10	0	Pneumonia
Str. pyogenes	5	2	Skin, soft tissue
Other Gram-positive cocci	2	0	Skin
Listeria monocytogenes	<1	0	Bowel, foods
Clostridium spp.	<1	0	Bowel, gangrenous wounds
Bacteroides spp.	3	1	Bowel, pelvis, wounds
Mixed infection	10	7	Bowel, intensive care

UTI, urinary tract infection.
Data from Dr P. Ispahani, Nottingham Public Health Laboratory UK.

Table 63.8 Some important infective conditions imported to temperate regions from the tropics

Causative organism	Tourists[a]	Expatriates[a]	Immigrants[a]
Viruses	Hepatitis A Influenza	HIV Yellow fever (Other arboviruses)	Hepatitis B Haemorrhagic fever
Rickettsiae and chlamydiae Bacteria	Tick typhus Typhoid Toxigenic *Escherichia coli*	Q fever Brucellosis Shigellosis	Trachoma Tuberculosis, leprosy Cholera
Protozoa	Cryptosporidiosis Falciparum malaria Cutaneous leishmaniasis	Giardiasis Malaria (all) Schistosomiasis	Amoebiasis Vivax malaria Kala-azar (visceral leishmaniasis)
Helminths	—	Tapeworm Stronglyloidiasis Filariasis	Roundworm Hookworm
Ectoparasites (ticks, mites and insects)	—	Myiasis Jigger flea	Scabies
Fungi	—	Dermatophytosis Histoplasmosis	Mycetoma

[a] These categories are not mutually exclusive.

that the cause is a microbe which could have been caught at home.

Imported infections

Table 63.8 lists some of the more common causes of infectious diseases imported from tropical countries into temperate regions where the diseases are not normally transmitted. There are three groups of patients who are considered separately but the separation of diseases and microbes is not exclusive:

1. Short-term travellers or *tourists* who usually visit major cities or special holiday areas and stay in good accommodation and have minimal contact with the indigenous population.

2. Long-term visitors who may be engaged in lengthy overland trips or be working abroad as *expatriates*.

3. *Immigrants* who were brought up abroad and visit or have residence in the host country; also settled immigrants who pay short-term visits to their country of origin.

Individuals who travel abroad vary in their risk behaviour and their exposure to potential pathogens. Generally, advice given by travel operators, tourist offices, embassies and medical sources

has greatly improved in the past few years. Companies sending out expatriate workers tend to look after their staff well. Nevertheless, many tourists (up to 50% in some studies) have episodes of travellers' diarrhoea, which in some cases results in admission to hospital. The major groups

Table 63.9 Some common sites of infection in PUO.

Abdomen	Subphrenic abscess Appendix abscess Ileal tuberculosis Pelvic abscess
Liver and biliary tract	Intrahepatic abscess Empyema of gallbladder Ascending cholangitis Cholecystitis Viral hepatitis
Kidney and urinary tract	Perinephric abscess Renal tuberculosis Pyelonephritis (especially children)
Bones	Vertebral osteomyelitis Tuberculosis Prosthetic infections
Cardiovascular	Endocarditis Graft infections
Respiratory	Tuberculosis Empyema and lung abscess
Nervous system	Cryptococcal or tuberculous meningitis Brain or spinal abscess

who are missed in preventative programmes are overland travellers and immigrants returning to their homeland, often with young families who have never been exposed to the infectious risks of their parents' home. Immigrants returning for visits to malarious areas seldom take prophylactic advice, believing themselves to be immune, but protective immunity wanes with prolonged absence.

Cryptogenic infections

Some of the commonly encountered sites of infection which may give rise to fever, and must be considered in the differential diagnosis of PUO, are listed in Table 63.9.

RECOMMENDED READING

Christie A B 1987 *Infectious Diseases: Epidemiology and Clinical Practice*, 4th edn. Churchill Livingstone, Edinburgh, vols 1 and 2
Emond R T D, Rowland H A K 1987 *A Colour Atlas of Infectious Diseases*, 2nd edn. Wolfe, London
Grist N R, Ho-Yen D O, Walker E, Williams G R 1987 *Diseases of Infection*. Oxford University Press, Oxford

Lambert H P, Farrar W E 1982 *Infectious Diseases Illustrated*. Pergamon, Oxford
Mandell G L, Douglas R G, Bennett J E 1990 *Principles and Practice of Infectious Diseases*, 3rd edn. Churchill Livingstone, New York
Shanson D C 1989 *Microbiology in Clinical Practice*, 3rd edn. Wright, London

Diagnostic procedures

R. C. B. Slack

The role of the laboratory in assisting clinicians in the diagnosis of infection is illustrated in the specimen flow diagram shown in Fig. 64.1. The choice of specimen depends on following the principles outlined in Chapter 63. The micro-biology laboratory requires enough information on the request card accompanying the specimen to use the optimal methods necessary for identification of potential pathogens in particular infective syndromes. At the most basic level, it is obvious that when a swab is received in the laboratory, it is necessary to know if it comes from the throat or the vagina! But additional information is also essential: is the patient being investigated for pharyngitis or diphtheria; for vaginal discharge or septic abortion? Furthermore, the specimen must be obtained with care and transported to the laboratory without delay in an appropriate manner. The value of the result is in direct proportion to the attention given to these details, as well as to the skill and efficiency of the laboratory. For further details of laboratory methods, including specimen containers and culture media used, the reader is encouraged to consult the companion volume *Practical Medical Microbiology* listed in the recommended reading section.

COLLECTION OF SPECIMENS

Samples for microbiological examination need to be carefully collected, if possible without contamination with commensals or from external sources. Some points to remember with specimens from

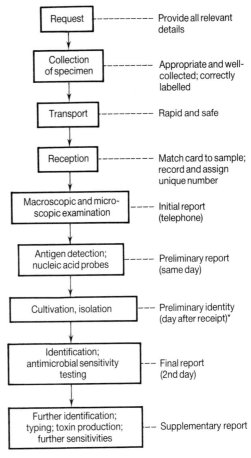

Fig. 64.1 Steps in the isolation and identification of pathogens from an infected patient.

Table 64.1 Some important points to remember in the collection of specimens for microbiological examination

Respiratory secretions

Nasal swab (anterior)	Only for carriage of staphylococci and streptococci
Nasopharyngeal swab	For pertussis and meningococci
External ear swab	Wide range of microbes including fungi
Myringotomy and sinus samples	As for abscesses — including anaerobes
Throat (pharyngeal) swab	Specify if only for streptococci; mention if diphtheria possible; use special transport media for virology
Saliva	Used for antibody detection; otherwise discard
Laryngeal swab	Specify for mycobacteria
Expectorated sputum	Often poorly collected; specify mycobacteria, legionellae, pneumocystis
Transtracheal aspirate, bronchoscopy specimens, lung biopsy	Specify likely diagnosis; ask for specific tests
Pleural fluid	Treat as pus; always look for mycobacteria

Gastro-intestinal specimens

Vomitus	Only for virology
Gastric washings	For mycobacteria (particularly in children)
Gastric biopsy	For *Helicobacter pylori*
Duodenal/jejunal aspirates	Protozoa (*Giardia lamblia*, microsporidia, etc.)
Liver aspirates	As for pus (anaerobes); consider amoebae
Spleen puncture	For *Leishmania* spp.
Rectal biopsy	Schistosomiasis
Rectal swab	Only for gonococci and chlamydia
Colonic biopsy	Histopathological diagnosis of amoebiasis, pseudomembranous colitis (*Clostridium difficile*)
Colonic scrapings	Protozoa; amoebic trophozoites (deliver to laboratory immediately)
Faeces	Specify possible diagnosis; ask for clostridial toxins, parasite examination if suspected
Peri-anal swab	For eggs of threadworm

Urine

Mid-stream (MSU)	Suitable for most patients
Clean catch	Infants and elderly — increased contamination
Suprapubic aspirate	Infants and neonates
Ureteric/bladder washout	To localize infection
Prostatic massage	Collect samples before, during and at end of micturition
Terminal urine	Schistosome ova
Complete early morning or 24 h urine	Mycobacteria (tubercle)

Central nervous system

Cerebrospinal fluid by spinal tap	For meningitis collect sample for protein and glucose — test blood sugar simultaneously, specify virology, fungi or syphilis serology.
Ventricular tap	Specify if through an indwelling shunt or catheter
Brain abscess	As for pus (include anaerobes)

Table 64.1 (cont'd)

Skin and soft tissue

Skin scraping/nail clipping	Dermatophyte fungi
Skin swab	Rarely valuable without pus
Skin snips	Onchocerciasis — seek advice
Vesicle fluid	Suitable for electron microscopy for viruses
Wound swab	Obtain pus if possible; record site
Pus, tissues, aspirates	Describe site and any relevant operative details

Genital

Urethral swab	Pus for gonococci, scrape for chlamydia
Vaginal swab (adult)	Only for candida, trichomonas and bacterial vaginosis
Vaginal swab (prepubertal)	State age; caution required if abuse possible
Cervical swab	Separate media for chlamydia
Ulcer scrape	Immediate dark-ground microscopy; separate media for virology or chancroid
Uterine secretions	Specify puerperium or post-abortion
Pelvic aspirates	As for pus
Laparoscopy specimens	Include chlamydia specimen

Eye

Conjunctival swab	Separate virology; scrape for chlamydia
Aspirates	As for pus

Blood

Culture	Strict aseptic technique; take large sample in special media before antibiotics
Bone marrow	Valuable for leishmania, mycobacteria, brucella
Film	Malaria (thick and thin), filaria, borrelia, trypanosomes
Whole blood	Filaria (day or night samples as appropriate)
Serum antigen	Rapid diagnosis of many microbial diseases (e.g. hepatitis B)
Serum antibody	Retrospective diagnosis of common viral diseases, syphilis and other selected infections; need rising titre or specific IgM.

individual sources are shown in Table 64.1. It is essential to use sterile containers which are leak-proof and able to withstand transportation through the post if necessary. It is more convenient for both the clinician and microbiologist if the laboratory provides request cards, containers and an efficient transport system. There is a need for staff to be aware of safety regulations and for all parties to understand who has responsibility for each step of the process and how to minimize handling by untrained people. Special precautions required for 'high-risk' specimens need to be defined by the laboratory and hospital management. Storage of clinical material must be separate from food and drugs and this may necessitate provision of additional refrigerator space and transport facilities.

Food and water

The examination of non-clinical specimens is beyond the scope of this book and readers are referred to appropriate reading. However, an outbreak of gastro-intestinal disease inevitably leads to the question of identifying the source. When disease is due to preformed toxins, as with staphylococcal food poisoning, faecal examination is unhelpful and the diagnosis can only be made by testing the food. Frequently, the offending item has been discarded and the examination of food and water related to specific patients is often unrewarding. Routine sampling of water sources and potentially contaminated food such as poultry at various critical points of production is essential in maintaining good public health.

TRANSPORT

Many microbes may perish on transit from the host's body to a laboratory incubator. Some contaminants, especially coliforms, may overgrow the pathogen and so mask its presence. These two constraints make it essential that any material for cultivation of microbes is transported as quickly as possible to the laboratory in a manner expected to protect the viability of any pathogens. Such problems may be minimized by the use of antigen or gene probe detection because of the relative stability of the chemical structures identified.

The ideal situation is to bring the patient to the laboratory for specimen collection or take the laboratory to the clinic. Both approaches are used for special purposes but are obviously inconvenient for many patients and inappropriate and costly for complicated techniques like virus isolation which need specialized (and safe) facilities.

To overcome any drawbacks due to delay in reaching the microbiology department the following methods may be used:

1. *Transport media* (Table 64.2).
2. *Boric acid* added to urine at a concentration of 1.8% (v/w) will stop bacterial multiplication but lower concentrations are ineffective and higher ones may kill the pathogen.

3. *Dip slides.* These provide a convenient way of inoculating urines at the clinic. They comprise small plastic spoons or strips holding a thin layer of agar which is dipped into the urine and then put in a screw-topped bottle for transport. The agar adsorbs a fixed volume of urine and, after incubation, colony counts of bacteria give a semi-quantitative estimation of numbers.

4. *Refrigeration.* Storage at $4^{\circ}C$ before processing will prevent multiplication of most bacteria. However, delicate microbes like neisseriae may not survive whereas certain organisms, notably listeriae, flourish at low temperatures.

5. *Freezing.* Temperatures of $-70^{\circ}C$ or below which can be achieved in liquid nitrogen or special deep freezes will preserve many microbes, providing they are protected by a stabilizing fluid such as serum or glycerol.

RECEPTION

The importance of good documentation cannot be overstressed. No matter how well the specimen was taken, transported and processed in the laboratory, the end result depends on communication between people. The clinician making the request must give complete details on the request card and specimen to reduce errors. Staff receiving specimens in the laboratory must match them with the cards and record them into a book or computer. This is usually done by assigning a unique number to each specimen and labelling both the specimen and the request. When parts of the specimen are separated from the original bottle, e.g. after centrifugation of serum, the

Table 64.2 Types of transport medium

Type of organism	Medium	Comments
Bacteria	Stuart's semi-solid agar	Contains charcoal to inactivate toxic material
Anaerobic bacteria	Various systems, including gassed-out tubes and anaerobic bags	Not widely used, but essential for some strict anaerobes
Viruses	Buffered salts solution containing serum	Contains antibiotics to control bacteria and fungi
Chlamydiae	Similar to viral transport medium, but without agents that inhibit chlamydiae	Chlamydial antigen media contain detergent to lyse infected cells
Protozoa, helminths	Merthiolate–iodine–formalin	Kills active protozoa, but preserves cysts and ova in a form suitable for concentration and microscopy

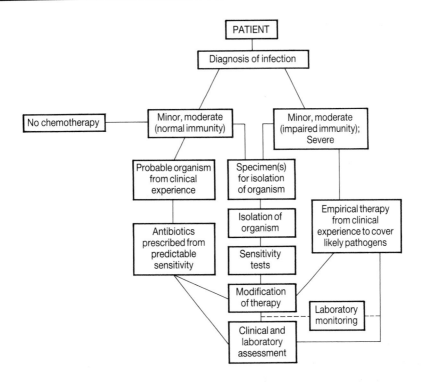

Fig. 65.2   *General strategy of chemotherapy.*

multiple antibiotics. In such cases, the power of the body fluid to inhibit or kill the infecting organism in vitro may be a more useful measurement of adequate dosage; for example, in bacterial endocarditis, the patient's serum should kill the causative organism at a dilution of 1 in 4 or more.

It is important to know the relationship of the sample being assayed to the time of dosage: maximum or *peak* levels are usually measured in serum 0.5–1 h following a dose; minimum or *trough* levels are from a sample taken shortly before the next dose.

Assays should always be carried out in close collaboration with the microbiologist to ensure the correct timing of samples and to avoid errors of interpretation.

Assay of urine

Urine samples may be screened for antibacterial activity. This can be of value in determining patient compliance with treatment and also in interpreting the culture result in relation to possible inhibition by residual antibiotic.

Clinical correlation of laboratory tests

The epithet *sensitive* or *resistant* is a clinical description; in laboratory tests it is usual to select a concentration of the agent which is known to approximate to the level attained in serum, other body fluids or tissue after normal recommended dosage. Organisms susceptible to this, or lower concentrations, are regarded as sensitive; those growing at higher concentrations are resistant. The correlation between this interpretation and clinical results is generally good, but not perfect. Discrepancies may be due to a failure to attain adequate concentrations at the site of infection, resulting in clinical failure. However, there are many factors on which the outcome of the host–parasite relationship in infection depends, and it would be surprising if a complete correlation between in vitro sensitivity tests and the results of chemotherapy was observed.

PREDICTABLE SENSITIVITY

Once the identity of an infecting organism is known, the sensitivity pattern is often predictable with a fair degree of accuracy. Not surprisingly, however, the susceptibility of common pathogens may change with time. Thus, predictable sensitivity of micro-organisms, while useful, is a changing concept and will have local variations, so that the advice of local microbiologists should be sought.

Organisms with predictable sensitivity patterns

Streptococcus pyogenes is a good example of an organism that has retained a sensitivity pattern that has changed little in 50 years. Thus, penicillin is always the drug of choice for the treatment of haemolytic streptococcal infections. Erythromycin is an alternative if the patient cannot be given penicillin because of allergy, but an increasing number of strains in some areas show some resistance to this antibiotic in vitro. Other β-lactam antibiotics are also uniformly active against *Str. pyogenes*. Similarly, most strains of *Str. pneumoniae* are highly sensitive to β-lactam agents, including penicillin, although some resistant strains have been described.

Reproducible patterns of sensitivity to antimicrobial drugs can be shown for many other groups of bacteria and offer a useful guide to the choice of chemotherapy (Table 65.1). However, exceptions to these patterns occur and resistant variants may become prevalent in some localities, particularly under the pressure of intensive antibiotic usage.

In the same way that organisms may exhibit predictable sensitivity to some agents, they may be predictably resistant. Some examples are shown in Table 65.2.

Organisms of variable sensitivity

Many groups of pathogenic bacteria, notably staphylococci and enterobacteria, vary unpredict-

Table 65.1 Examples of organisms and antimicrobial agents for which susceptibility is *usually* predictable

Organism	Antimicrobial agents normally active
Streptococci	Penicillin, erythromycin, vancomycin
Enterococci	Ampicillin, vancomycin
Anaerobic cocci	Penicillin, erythromycin, metronidazole
Staphylococci	Flucloxacillin, clindamycin, fusidic acid, gentamicin, vancomycin
Haemophilus	Amoxycillin, co-trimoxazole, tetracycline, chloramphenicol, erythromycin
Escherichia	Gentamicin, trimethoprim, co-amoxiclav, ciprofloxacin
Proteus	
Pseudomonas	Gentamicin, ceftazidime, azlocillin, ciprofloxacin
Bacteroides	Metronidazole, cefoxitin, co-amoxiclav
Rickettsia	Tetracyclines, chloramphenicol, rifampicin
Chlamydia	
Mycoplasma	Tetracyclines, erythromycin
Candida	Nystatin, amphotericin B, miconazole
Herpes simplex	Acyclovir

ably in their sensitivity to antimicrobial drugs. With these organisms there is a greater need to carry out sensitivity tests on individual isolates.

Staphylococci

Four kinds of staphylococci may be encountered:

1. Penicillin-sensitive strains. These are almost invariably sensitive to all antistaphyloco-

Table 65.2 Examples of organisms and antimicrobial agents for which resistance is usually predictable

Organism	Antimicrobial agents not normally active
Streptococci	Aminoglycosides, nalidixic acid, aztreonam
Enterococci	
Staphylococci	Most penicillins[a], nalidixic acid, aztreonam
Esch. coli	Penicillin, vancomycin, erythromycin, clindamycin
Klebsiella	Most penicillins, erythromycin, clindamycin
Pseudomonas	Penicillin, ampicillin, amoxycillin, most cephalosporins, erythromycin, clindamycin
Anaerobes	Aminoglycosides, aztreonam, nalidixic acid

[a] Except methicillin and isoxazolylpenicillins

ccal antibiotics, including other penicillins and cephalosporins, erythromycin, lincosamides and fusidic acid. Penicillin-sensitive strains now account for less than 10% of isolates of staphylococci.

2. β-Lactamase (penicillinase)-producing strains. These strains are resistant to all penicillins, except methicillin, the isoxazolyl group (flucloxacillin, etc.) and nafcillin; they usually retain susceptibility to cephalosporins and other antistaphylococcal agents. Most strains of *Staphylococcus aureus* isolated from patients belong to this group.

3. Antibiotic-resistant strains. All these strains produce β-lactamase and are additionally resistant to one or more of the antistaphylococcal antibiotics, most frequently to tetracyclines and erythromycin; less commonly to lincosamides, fusidic acid and the aminoglycosides. Resistant strains of this kind are in a minority and are almost always isolated from hospital-contracted infections, where they may occur in small epidemics as a result of cross-infection.

4. Methicillin-resistant strains. Although these strains are usually detected in tests of methicillin, they are also resistant to flucloxacillin and, indeed, virtually all β-lactam agents. They are believed to have epidemiological significance as a group and have been isolated from a number of hospital outbreaks in different countries. Some strains are also highly resistant to aminoglycosides and other antistaphylococcal agents (multiresistant strains) and may require treatment with vancomycin or teicoplanin.

Enterobacteria

Escherichia coli includes many strains of variable sensitivity, but among the general population most strains (about 60%) are sensitive to ampicillin and amoxycillin and an even higher proportion are sensitive to cephalosporins, co-amoxiclav (the combination of amoxycillin and clavulanic acid) and trimethoprim.

Variable sensitivity is also a feature of other enterobacteria. If there is doubt about the clinical response, or the sensitivity of the strain, laboratory tests should be carried out.

ANTIBIOTIC POLICIES AND THE CONTROL OF RESISTANCE

The widespread benefits from the use of antibiotics, not only in medicine but also in animal husbandry, must be taken into account in considering the merits of restrictive policies ostensibly undertaken to control antibiotic resistance.

There is, without doubt, a problem of resistance among many commonly occurring microorganisms. The possibility of rapid spread of multiresistant bacteria means that difficulties might arise in the future with infections highly refractory to therapy with available agents. However, most of the problems of resistance occur among patients susceptible to colonization by resistant strains within closed communities such as hospitals. This is most marked in areas of intensive care, where large amounts of antibiotics are used in highly susceptible patients with low immunity to infection. In the general community and in most small hospitals, multiple resistance to antibiotics is not a major problem.

Accordingly, attention should be directed to those hospital units in which the problem of resistance is significant and which may be the most important source of spread to the general community. As resistance in bacteria has many of the features of an epidemic disease, the application of classic rules for the prevention of infection may prevent the spread of antibiotic-resistant organisms from such units.

Restrictive policies

The use of antibiotics by general practitioners and clinicians must be influenced by the use of antibiotics by other medical colleagues in the area. Thus, an ordered and systematic use of antimicrobial drugs might be of benefit in the general strategy of chemotherapy. Since the use of antibiotics acts as a powerful selective factor in the emergence and spread of resistant micro-organisms, a restriction of use should have the opposite effect and reduce the proportion of resistant organisms in a community. The acceptance of this thesis has encouraged restrictive policies involving temporary bans on the use of certain antibiotics. Such policies may also lead to a reduced chance of prescription error and some cost benefits.

Rotational policies

Periodic changes of antibiotics used in treatment might also help to avoid the emergence of resistant strains by altering the selective pressures and discouraging opportunistic pathogens such as *Pseudomonas* and *Acinetobacter* species. Such a rotational policy might help to retain the therapeutic value of antibiotics over a longer period. The availability of a large range of clinically useful antibacterial substances (Table 65.3) makes this kind of policy more practicable.

PROPHYLACTIC USE OF ANTIBIOTICS

The unnecessary prophylactic use of antibiotics should be discouraged since this may result in increased selection of resistant variants or super-infection with resistant flora. However, there are several circumstances in which chemoprophylaxis is clearly beneficial.

A widely accepted use of antimicrobial agents for the prevention of infection is in patients who have suffered from rheumatic fever, or are thought otherwise to be at risk of rheumatic carditis. In these patients long-term treatment with penicillin or other suitable antibiotics is justified to prevent further streptococcal infection. It has also become routine to give patients undergoing hip joint replacement peri-operatively, and sometimes postoperative antibiotics to reduce the chance of potentially disastrous infection. Similarly, patients undergoing lower bowel resection receive peri-operative treatment with combinations of agents intended to suppress the lower bowel flora. The clinical and laboratory evidence for the benefit of these kinds of prophylaxis is now well established.

Table 65.3 Main groups of antibiotics available for clinical use

Antibacterial agent	Route of administration	Antibacterial spectrum[a]	Some indications for therapy
Penicillins	O P	+	Streptococcal, pneumococcal, meningococcal infections
Ampicillin } Amoxycillin	O P	+ −	Respiratory, urinary, hepatic, biliary infections
Flucloxacillin	O P	+	Staphylococcal infections
Amoxycillin + clavulanic acid	O P	+ −	Infections due to β-lactamase-producing organisms
Ticarcillin + clavulanic acid	P	+ −	Serious infections with mixed organisms
Cephalosporins	O P	+ −	Respiratory and urinary infections; staphylococcal infections
Aminoglycosides	P	−	Gram-negative coliform infections; endocarditis; pseudomonas infections
Macrolides } Lincosamides	O P	+	Streptococcal and staphylococcal infections and those due to legionellae, campylobacters, chlamydiae and coxiellae
Tetracyclines	O P	+ −	Respiratory infections and those due to chlamydiae, mycoplasmas and rickettsiae
Chloramphenicol	O P	+ −	Serious infections due to *Haemophilus influenzae*, salmonellae and rickettsiae
Fusidic acid	O T	+	Staphylococcal infections
Glycopeptides	O P	+	Resistant staphylococcal infections; *Clostridium difficile* enteritis
Trimethoprim } Co-trimoxazole	O P	+ −	Urinary and respiratory infections; salmonellosis
Imidazoles	O P	+ −	Anaerobic infections
Sulphonamides	O T	+ −	Intestinal and eye infections
Fluoroquinolones	O P	−	Urinary infections; pseudomonal infections

O, oral; P, parenteral; T, topical. +, mainly active against Gram-positive bacteria; −, mainly active against Gram-negative bacteria. [a] See also Table 6.1, p. 68.

The long-term treatment of chronic infection, though not strictly prophylaxis, may be of great value in the management of conditions such as chronic pyelonephritis, prostatitis and chronic bronchitis.

HOST FACTORS INFLUENCING RESPONSE

In most individuals with normal immune systems the antimicrobial drug assists in a more rapid recovery from the infection, but the choice of agent is often not critical providing it has some effect on the causative organisms (Fig. 65.1). In very serious infections, or when the patient is at a disadvantage because of impaired or absent immunity, the role of the antibiotic becomes more important and more care should be taken in its selection, dosage and administration.

Problems of toxicity

The final choice of the most appropriate antimicrobial drug may be influenced by the history and responses of the patient. Known hypersensitivity to a drug such as penicillin means that neither this antibiotic nor other penicillins can be safely given and alternatives must be used. Side-effects such as nausea, vomiting, diarrhoea or pruritis may be severe enough to warrant a change in treatment. Some antibiotics have potentially serious side-effects, such as the ototoxicity of the aminoglycosides, and care must be taken to avoid these by laboratory monitoring of drug levels, since such toxicity is usually dose related. Intercurrent disease may require modification of the dosage of certain antibiotics because of specific organ deficiency, e.g. liver failure or impaired renal function. Ototoxicity of the aminoglycosides must always be borne in mind in patients who have poor renal function.

Failure to reach the site of infection

The absorption of oral antibiotics varies widely from patient to patient and, if poor, may be a cause of treatment failure. Alternatively, infection may be localized within a large collection of pus or at an anatomical site that is penetrated by antibiotics with difficulty. Obstruction to the flow of body fluids may likewise militate against success; this is important in infections of the urinary tract, biliary system and the central nervous system. In some of these cases more radical interference may be indicated to relieve the obstruction.

Alteration of normal flora

Antibiotic therapy may upset the ecology of the microflora of the patient's surfaces and result not only in the selection of resistant strains of commensals, such as staphylococci on the skin, or *Esch. coli* in the intestinal tract, but also colonization with species not normally present. This can lead to antibiotic-induced infection, such as candidosis. Diarrhoea is frequently associated with antibiotic therapy and reflects disturbance of the normal bowel flora. In a few patients the clinical condition can be severe and proceed to pseudomembranous colitis associated with the toxins of *Clostridium difficile* (see Chapter 23).

Intravenous administration

When antibiotics are given intravenously, they should normally be administered directly into the vein and not added to other infusion fluids; otherwise adequate blood levels of the drug may not be attained owing to excretion outpacing administration. There is also the possibility of incompatibility between the antibiotic and the contents of the fluid. In all cases, the manufacturer's instructions and recommendations about the administration of the drug should be closely followed.

COMBINATIONS OF ANTIBIOTICS

The clinical benefits of the use of combinations of antibacterial agents tend to be exaggerated. The combination of two or more agents has been long accepted in the treatment of tuberculosis, so limiting the selection of mutants resistant to the individual components. The use of β-lactam antibiotics with an aminoglycoside in the treatment of streptococcal endocarditis is also accepted, since the mixture is more bactericidal than the individual components.

A combination of a β-lactam antibiotic with a β-lactamase inhibitor may prevent destruction of the antibiotic. Thus, the enzyme inhibitor clavulanic acid in combination with amoxycillin (co-amoxiclav) restores the activity of the antibiotic against many β-lactamase-producing bacteria.

Potentiation of the antibacterial effect by combinations is referred to as *synergy*; some combinations exhibit a lesser effect than the individual components and this is called *antagonism*. These interactions are generally displayed in vitro and it is difficult to establish evidence of advantages or disadvantages in the patient. Thus, the combination of trimethoprim and sulphamethoxazole (co-trimoxazole) can be shown to be synergistic in the test-tube, but it has been difficult to demonstrate any clinical benefit, and trimethoprim is now used on its own by many clinicians to avoid the chance of toxic reactions to sulphonamides.

ANTIVIRAL THERAPY

Only a few agents have as yet found a place in the prophylaxis or treatment of viral infections (see Chapter 6; Table 6.8).

Acyclovir is most widely used at present and is prescribed for the treatment of herpes simplex and herpes zoster. This drug can be given orally, but in severely ill patients it is administered intravenously, for example in treating herpes encephalitis. Acyclovir is also used in the prophylaxis and treatment of varicella, particularly in immunocompromised patients. The related compound ganciclovir is available for the treatment of cytomegalovirus infection, but is associated with considerable toxicity.

Amantadine is active against influenza A virus, but not against influenza B virus. This drug, and the related rimantadine, have been chiefly used for the prophylaxis of influenza.

Tribavirin (ribavirin) is useful in the treatment of respiratory syncytial virus infections in children and is possibly also effective against the para-influenza group and some haemorrhagic fever viruses, such as Lassa fever virus.

Zidovudine (azidothymidine) is an inhibitor of human immunodeficiency virus and is used in the management of patients with acquired immune deficiency syndrome (AIDS).

ANTIFUNGAL THERAPY

Superficial fungal infections are very common. Systemic fungal disease is relatively rare in the UK, except in patients who are immunosuppressed or otherwise compromised. There is only a limited number of clinically effective antifungal agents (see Chapter 6; Table 6.7) and some have considerable toxicity.

For many years the chemotherapy of superficial fungal infections depended on preparations of benzoic, salicylic or undecanoic acids. More effective is griseofulvin, given orally, sometimes over long periods, for the treatment of dermatophytoses; the new allylamine, terbinafine promises to be at least as effective in these conditions. Nystatin and other polyenes are used for the topical treatment of superficial candidosis (thrush). Imidazoles such as clotrimazole are also used in the treatment of vaginal yeast infections.

Amphotericin B is used parenterally for the treatment of systemic candidosis, cryptococcal infections and aspergillosis. Flucytosine is also active against yeasts and has been used in combination with amphotericin B. Amphotericin B is toxic and treatment has to be carefully monitored in specialist units accustomed to its use to obtain the most satisfactory clinical results.

Ketoconazole, and triazoles such as itraconazole and fluconazole, also have a fairly wide range of antifungal activity and are being used more widely in the treatment of systemic fungal disease because of their relative lack of toxicity.

CHEMOTHERAPY OF SYSTEMIC INFECTIONS
Serious generalized infection

Patients with serious and often overwhelming generalized infection include those with *bacterial shock syndrome* and others with the symptomatology of acute infection without localizing signs. These syndromes may be related to postoperative infection, to instrumentation, or to the aggravation of a previously mild infection (e.g. extension of a middle ear infection to the brain). Generalized infection may also follow a reduction in the natural resistance of the patient. Such a situation may arise in renal failure, immune deficiency states, in blood dyscrasias and in neoplastic disease. Specific measures used in the treatment of these diseases may further reduce resistance to infection and the clinical features characteristic of infection may be muted or absent.

Appropriate specimens should be submitted to the laboratory before treatment is begun, in an effort to isolate the causative organisms. However, these patients may require immediate treatment and often there will be little indication of the nature of the infecting organism; more than one species may be involved, especially when the source of the infection is within the abdomen. Empirical chemotherapy must therefore cover Gram-positive cocci, Gram-negative bacilli and anaerobes such as bacteroides. A combination of amoxycillin, an aminoglycoside and metronidazole is suitable. Co-amoxiclav improves the spectrum of amoxycillin and allows omission of the metronidazole. Alternatively, an expanded-spectrum cephalosporin such as cefotaxime can be used. Therapy may be subsequently changed according to the results of laboratory tests. If the patient fails to respond after treatment for 3 d, the use of alternative agents should be considered.

In some patients in intensive care, and in the immunocompromised, the possibility of systemic fungal infection or activation of dormant viruses, such as cytomegalovirus, must be considered.

It must always be remembered that bacterial toxins are unaffected by antibacterial therapy. Supportive treatment will include correction of fluid and electrolyte imbalance and appropriate treatment of any coexisting organ failure. In future, immunotherapy such as the use of anti-endotoxin preparations may find a place in treatment.

Infective endocarditis

Whenever possible, treatment of endocarditis should be related to the results of sensitivity tests made on the organism isolated from the blood.

Formerly, viridans streptococci were the most common isolates and penicillin was the drug of choice. Viridans streptococci are now isolated from only about one-third of patients and the organisms from the remainder are usually relatively resistant to penicillin. In a proportion of cases believed to be infective on clinical evidence, no organism can be isolated and treatment must be empirical.

It seems to be important to kill all the organisms growing in heart valve tissue since the normal body defences find it difficult to penetrate this site to assist the antibiotic. Bactericidal therapy with a penicillin in combination with an aminoglycoside is usually indicated. It is sometimes helpful to carry out bactericidal tests against the causative organism and it may also be useful to monitor the progress of the patient by assays of the bactericidal activity of the serum against the causative organism.

After operations for the replacement of heart valves it may be difficult to isolate an organism and there may be doubt as to whether or not infection has become superimposed. The risk of withholding treatment, however, is so great that empirical treatment may be indicated, and as staphylococcal infection may occur in such circumstances, it is best to include an antistaphylococcal antibiotic.

For the prevention of bacterial endocarditis in patients at risk following dental extraction, 3 g of amoxycillin, given orally 1 h before surgery is recommended.

Rare causes of infective endocarditis in which blood cultures are negative include infections with *Coxiella burnetii* or certain chlamydiae. The diagnosis of these conditions depends largely upon serological evidence as it is difficult to isolate the organisms. An aetiological diagnosis is important as treatment with an appropriate antibiotic, usually tetracycline, may be life-saving.

Urinary tract infections

Uncomplicated cystitis

Uncomplicated urinary infections and asymptomatic bacteriuria are common in adolescent and adult women seen in general practice and maternity clinics. Most infections are due to *Esch. coli* and most are sensitive to a wide range of drugs. In about three-quarters of the cases, eradication of the organism is achieved after a short course of therapy with an oral agent such as amoxycillin or trimethoprim. The remainder will often respond to a second course of treatment, but if the bacteriuria still persists, fuller urological investigation is required since failure of treatment is more usually related to an abnormality of the urinary system than to resistance of the organism.

Recurrence of bacteriuria within weeks of a short course of treatment is quite common and patients should have their urine bacteriologically examined 3–7 d after the cessation of any antibacterial treatment and again after 1 month.

Infections following catheterization

Infection of the urinary tract sometimes occurs after instrumentation such as catheterization or cystoscopy; it is almost unavoidable if indwelling catheters are used. Often the strains causing these infections are derived from the hospital environment and include resistant strains of Gram-negative bacilli, sometimes in mixed culture. Frequently, the patient is not greatly inconvenienced by such infection and chemotherapy is not indicated in most cases. If therapy is required, elimination of the organisms can be difficult, particularly if there is residual pathology or a degree of urinary obstruction. Sensitivity tests must be carried out to assist in the choice of therapy. The most useful agents are cephalosporins, trimethoprim and ciprofloxacin; for more serious or refractory cases, in which there is the hazard of systemic spread of the infection, parenteral treatment with an aminoglycoside or an expanded-spectrum cephalosporin must be considered.

Recurrent infection

In chronic pyelonephritis and recurrent bacteriuria it may be important to control infection by continuous treatment with antibiotics such as trimethoprim. Unfortunately, some patients may become reinfected with resistant species so that alternative drugs must be used. Thus, long-term therapy may require periodic bacteriological reassessment and sensitivity tests on the flora isolated to indicate when changes in therapy are required.

Prostatitis

Prostatitis is common in men over a wide age range and it is often difficult to obtain categorical evidence of bacterial infection; examination of seminal fluid, prostatic secretions and urine specimens may help. Treatment with trimethoprim, ciprofloxacin or erythromycin is sometimes beneficial as these drugs penetrate well into the prostate, but short-term use is rarely curative. Prophylaxis during prostatectomy is now well established; cephalosporins such as cephradine or cefotaxime have been used for this purpose.

Respiratory infections

Respiratory tract infections are extremely common and although many are primary virus infections, those that are more severe and prolonged usually indicate secondary bacterial invasion. Laboratory diagnosis of these conditions is important since effective treatment depends on use of an antibiotic specifically active against the causative organisms.

Upper respiratory tract infections

A number of bacteria may be associated with sore throat, pharyngitis and sinusitis, including *Str. pyogenes*, *Str. pneumoniae*, *Haemophilus influenzae* and Vincent's organisms. The most important infections from the point of view of the development of sequelae are those due to *Str. pyogenes*, for which the treatment of choice is penicillin given for at least 7 d to ensure eradication of the organism. All the other important bacterial pathogens will also respond to this treatment, with the exception of *H. influenzae*, for which treatment with amoxycillin, tetracycline, co-trimoxazole or erythromycin is appropriate.

If for some reason penicillin cannot be prescribed, the antibiotic of choice is erythromycin or co-trimoxazole. Ampicillin and amoxycillin should be avoided if there is any likelihood of glandular fever because these antibiotics tend to cause a rash and prolong the disease. Tetracyclines should be avoided in young children because of the risk of discoloration of developing teeth.

Lower respiratory tract infections

Lobar pneumonia is most frequently caused by pneumococci and penicillin is the drug of choice; erythromycin or cefotaxime are good alternatives. Infection due to klebsiellae or other organisms will require treatment with antibiotics according to the results of sensitivity tests; cefotaxime or cefuroxime are usually effective if laboratory confirmation is not available. Other coliform bacilli are rarely involved in pulmonary infections although they often colonize the upper respiratory tract; they seldom require specific treatment.

Among atypical pneumonias, mycoplasma infections respond best to a tetracycline or erythromycin; legionella infections to erythromycin, alone or combined with rifampicin.

Bronchopneumonia is most frequently associated with pneumococci or haemophilus, so that amoxycillin, tetracycline or co-trimoxazole should be effective. More rarely, bronchopneumonia is caused by *Staph. aureus* and flucloxacillin, fusidic acid or clindamycin is urgently required for treatment.

Acute exacerbations of chronic bronchitis are almost invariably associated with either *Str. pneumoniae* or *H. influenzae*. Amoxycillin, tetracycline or co-trimoxazole are usually effective.

In bronchiectasis, lung abscess or cystic fibrosis, antimicrobial treatment should be prescribed according to laboratory culture and sensitivity test results. Combinations of antibiotics may be effective in some of these patients. In pulmonary tuberculosis, combination treatment, usually with rifampicin, isoniazid and pyrazinamide, is mandatory.

Meningitis

A Gram film and cell count of cerebrospinal fluid (CSF) will usually differentiate viral from bacterial meningitis. If bacteria cannot be seen, initial treatment with a combination of penicillin or ampicillin with chloramphenicol is indicated; this combination ensures adequate treatment of infections with Gram-negative bacilli (most common in neonates) and of infections with *Neisseria meningitidis*, *H. influenzae* and *Str. pneumoniae*, which are the most common causes of meningitis in young children. Cefotaxime will also cover for these pathogens. Care must be taken to differentiate *Listeria monocytogenes* infection, as this organism is less sensitive to penicillin and cefotaxime, and treatment is best with a combination of amoxycillin and gentamicin.

When the causative organism is isolated, combination therapy may be discontinued: chloramphenicol or cefotaxime are the drugs of choice for haemophilus infections; penicillin for meningococcal or pneumococcal infections. *Pseudomonas aeruginosa* meningitis may occasionally occur as a nosocomial infection and should be treated with full doses of gentamicin plus a β-lactam agent such as azlocillin. It is rarely necessary to give intrathecal antibiotics.

Where there is increased CSF pressure, as in spina bifida, shunts are inserted to facilitate the circulation of fluid. These often become contaminated, usually with staphylococci, probably derived from the skin. Antistaphylococcal antibiotics are used to control the growth of the infecting organism in anticipation of replacement of the prosthesis.

Intestinal infections

The consensus of medical opinion is that mild bacillary dysentery, salmonella food poisoning and other forms of bacterial diarrhoea do not ordinarily require chemotherapy. Indeed, such therapy may make intestinal carriage more likely and increase the risk of the selection of antibiotic-resistant strains. The most important treatment is correction of fluid balance.

Patients with invasive infection (e.g. typhoid and paratyphoid fever) and those with severe bacillary dysentery or cholera may warrant treatment (see appropriate chapters).

Many intestinal infections are due to viruses, for which there is presently no specific chemotherapy. Cryptosporidiosis is now being diagnosed more frequently, but again there is no specific antibiotic treatment. Infection with other protozoa, such as *Giardia lamblia* or *Entamoeba histolytica*, requires treatment with metronidazole.

Spread of infection from the bowel may give rise to serious infections and associated toxaemia. If subphrenic, retrocolic or pelvic abscesses form, drainage is the most important aspect of treatment, but antibiotics can assist recovery of the patient. Cephalosporins or an aminoglycoside plus ampicillin are useful in empirical treatment and metronidazole should be added if bacteroides is likely to be present. Acute peritonitis after non-specific inflammation of the bowel, such as appendicitis, is usually effectively treated with amoxycillin (with or without clavulanate) or cefotaxime combined with metronidazole.

Liver infections

Bacterial infections of the liver and portal pyaemia are best treated with large doses of cefuroxime, cefotaxime, or an antibiotic chosen on the basis of laboratory findings (e.g. ampicillin against enterococci). Liver abscesses occur most frequently by spread via the portal tract of intestinal Gram-negative bacilli, or to retrograde spread in the biliary passages of streptococci (especially *Str. milleri*) and anaerobes from the gall bladder. Ampicillin is selectively concentrated in the bile and is often useful in treatment of cholecystitis. Amoebic abscess requires prompt and specific treatment and its possibility should always be kept in mind, particularly in a patient who has been abroad.

Liver infection may cause severe impairment of function of the organ with secondary effects on other organs such as the heart and kidneys. Treatment must involve correction of these effects.

Bone and joint infections

Most infections of bones and joints are due to *Staph. aureus*. Large doses of flucloxacillin should be given in combination with either fusidic acid or clindamycin.

Streptococci are responsible for many cases of septic arthritis and penicillin is the drug of choice, given in prolonged high dosage. Where other organisms, such as *H. influenzae*, neisseriae or Gram-negative rods are involved in bone and joint infections, specifically directed therapy is required.

Genital tract infections

Venereal infections such as syphilis and gonorrhoea are traditionally treated with penicillin, but a proportion of isolates of gonococci are now resistant to this agent, in which case cefotaxime, co-amoxiclav or ciprofloxacin should be used.

Non-specific infections of the genital tract are common in women; aerobic and anaerobic bacteria, Candida species, or *Trichomonas vaginalis*, may be involved. Frequently, an abnormal flora is isolated in the absence of an inflammatory exudate and it may be difficult to decide on the necessity for chemotherapy. Vaginal candidiasis is usually treated topically with nystatin or an antifungal imidazole. In trichomoniasis, metronidazole is indicated.

More serious pelvic infection in women is often associated with chlamydiae, and tetracycline or erythromycin is the drug of choice. Anaerobic bacteria may be involved and metronidazole or co-amoxiclav may be prescribed.

Surgical wound infections

Most surgical infections are caused by the patient's own organisms, but some arise exogenously, often by cross-infection. In orthopaedic units most exogenous infections are due to staphylococci, but in gastro-intestinal units, Gram-negative bacilli and anaerobes are more common. The situation may change from time to time as a result of ecological movements in the microbial flora within the unit, associated with selective pressures of antibiotic use.

Specimens from infected lesions should always be sent to the laboratory, since the identity of the isolate may have epidemiological significance as well as being of importance in the management of the patient. The microbiologist should always be informed of any therapy as this may affect the interpretation of bacteriological tests.

Superficial infections

Skin and soft-tissue infections are common in general practice. The majority are of bacterial origin, although some have a fungal or viral aetiology.

Common lesions such as boils, carbuncles, impetigo and infected wounds are associated with *Staph. aureus* and *Str. pyogenes*. Systemic treatment with appropriate antibiotics may be indicated in some patients, but topical treatment is often effective. The use of antibiotics commonly prescribed for systemic infections should be avoided in favour of topical antiseptics or topical antibiotics such as mupirocin.

RECOMMENDED READING

Christie A B 1987 *Infectious Diseases*, 4th edn. Churchill Livingstone, Edinburgh

Greenwood D (ed) 1989 *Antimicrobial Chemotherapy*, 2nd edn. Oxford University Press, Oxford

Kucers A, Bennett N Mck 1987 *The Use of Antibiotics*, 4th edn. Heinemann, London

Lambert H P, O'Grady F 1992 *Antibiotic and Chemotherapy*, 6th edn. Churchill Livingstone, Edinburgh

Mandell G L, Douglas R G, Bennett J E (eds) 1990 *Principles and Practice of Infectious Disease*, 3rd edn. Wiley, New York

66

Epidemiology and control of community infections

D. Reid

When you can measure what you are speaking about and express it in numbers, you know something about it; when you cannot express it in numbers, your knowledge is of a meagre and unsatisfactory kind.

William Thomson, Lord Kelvin
(*Popular Lectures and Addresses*, 1891)

Good surveillance does not necessarily mean the making of right decisions but it reduces the chances of wrong ones.

Alexander Langmuir, 1963

Once is happenstance, twice is coincidence, the third time it's enemy action.

Ian Fleming
(*Goldfinger*, Jonathan Cape, 1959)

Attempts to observe and record diseases in order to devise means of determining their cause and control have a long history. Hippocrates (460–361 BC) 'the father of medical science' and Herodotus (484–425 BC) 'the father of history' both related environmental factors to health. Hippocrates when writing of the occurrence of diseases distinguished between the 'steady state', the 'endemic state' and the abrupt change in incidence, the 'epidemic'.

Probably the first public health measures based on case reports of infectious diseases taken by a European government occurred in 1348 when the Republic of Venice excluded ships with affected people on board in order to control outbreaks of pneumonic plague (the *black death*). Fifty years later, again in Venice, the concept of *quarantine* was introduced when ships from plague-stricken areas had to stay outside the harbours for 40 days (*quaranta giorni*).

Also because of the fear of a plague epidemic, the first of the *Bills of Mortality*, in which causes of death were recorded, was published in London in 1532. In 1662 John Graunt (1620–74) in his book *Natural and Political Observations made upon the Bills of Mortality* was the first to count the number of persons dying in London from specific illnesses and to advocate the value of obtaining numerical data on a population in order to study the causes of disease (Table 66.1). In 1837 the office of the Registrar General was established to develop the work started by John Graunt; the English physician William Farr (1807–83) added reports to those of the Registrar General which dealt with infectious diseases, occupational diseases, accidents or hazardous work conditions.

The importance of keen observation of disease in order to deduce the likely cause has been demonstrated on many occasions. In 1849, 34 years before the identification of *Vibrio cholerae*

Table 66.1 Selection of causes of death in London taken from the Bills of Mortality, 1632

Causes of death	Numbers
Chrisomes[a] and infancy	2268
Consumption[b]	1797
Fever	1108
Aged	628
Smallpox	531
Teeth	470
Abortive and stillborn	445
Bloody flux,[c] scouring[d] and flux	348
Dropsy[e] and swelling	267
Convulsions	241
Childbed	171
Measles	80
Ague[f]	43
King's evil[g]	38

[a] A child who died during the first month of life or a child who died unbaptized. [b] Usually pulmonary tuberculosis.
[c] Dysentery. [d] Diarrhoea. [e] Oedema. [f] Malaria.
[g] Tuberculosis of the skin.

by Robert Koch (1843–1910), John Snow (1813–58), a London physician, proved by epidemiological observation that cholera is mainly spread by drinking infected water and not through the air in the form of miasmas as was commonly thought at the time. Similarly, William Budd (1811–80), a general practitioner from Devon, showed in 1873 how typhoid was caused, even though it was not until 1885 that *Salmonella typhi* was first isolated in the laboratory. More recently, William Pickles (1885–1969), a general practitioner in Wensleydale, Yorkshire, was able to elucidate many of the epidemiological characteristics of hepatitis and other infections well before microbiological advances were to confirm his observations.

From these beginnings the surveillance of infection has assumed national and international proportions. In the UK, information on microbial disease is collated in England and Wales by the Communicable Disease Surveillance Centre at the Central Public Health Laboratory, London, and in Scotland by the Communicable Diseases (Scotland) Unit at Ruchill Hospital, Glasgow. The Royal College of General Practitioners also undertakes regular recording of disease voluntarily reported by various practices. Elsewhere, national surveillance is carried out in different countries

(e.g. at the Centers for Disease Control in the USA). On a world-wide basis the World Health Organization (WHO) provides important liaison and support. This international co-operation is vital as 'germs do not recognize boundaries'.

The most outstanding achievement of international surveillance was the development of a programme for smallpox eradication. The multi-disciplinary approach adopted by the WHO, in which programmes were community based with measurable goals and constant monitoring, resulted in the last outbreak being recorded in October 1977; smallpox was officially declared eradicated in December 1979.

EPIDEMIOLOGY: DEFINITIONS AND PRINCIPLES

Epidemiology is usually defined as *the study of the nature, distribution, causation, mode of transfer, prevention and control of disease*. It has also been regarded as 'the natural history of disease' or as 'the human face of ecology'. Closely linked with the study of epidemiology is the concept of surveillance which is the most effective infection control technique available. Surveillance is defined as: *the epidemiological study of a disease as a dynamic process involving the ecology of the infectious agent, the host, the reservoirs, the vectors as well as the complex mechanisms concerned in the spread of infection and the extent to which this spread will occur.* The three main elements of surveillance of infection are:

1. The systematic collection of pertinent data
2. The orderly consolidation and evaluation of the data
3. The prompt dissemination of the findings, especially to those who can take appropriate action.

Surveillance provides for the recognition of acute problems requiring immediate local, national or international action, and for the assessment of specific problems by revealing trends or facilitating forecasts. It also provides a rational basis for planning and implementing efficient control measures and for their evaluation and continuing assessment. Although particularly appropriate to the study of infectious diseases, epidemiological principles are also used to elucidate the causes of non-communicable diseases.

The infectious process is a dynamic state involving three main factors: the micro-organism, the host and the environment (Fig. 66.1).

The micro-organism

Since few micro-organisms are harmful to humans the concept of *virulence* (i.e. the degree of pathogenicity of an infectious agent indicated by fatality rates and/or its ability to invade and damage the tissues of the host) must be recognized. The degree of virulence depends on *invasiveness* (i.e. the capacity of the organism to spread widely through the body) and *toxigenicity* (i.e. the toxin-producing property of the organism) (see Chapter 8). A second variable is the *dosage* of the organism and this is closely related to the virulence. A small number of organisms of high virulence is usually sufficient to cause disease in a susceptible person, whereas if the organism is of low virulence it often fails to cause disease. A third variable is the *portal of entry*. Many organisms have a predilection for a particular tissue or organ. For example, the causal organism of typhoid fever, *Salmonella typhi*, usually causes typhoid only when it enters the human body through the mouth in food or water.

The host

The reaction of the host to a micro-organism will depend on the ability to resist infection. The individual may not possess sufficient resistance against a particular pathogenic agent to prevent contraction of infection when exposed to the organism. Alternatively, the individual may possess specific protective antibodies or cellular immunity as a result of previous infection or immunization. However, immunity is relative and may be overwhelmed by an excessive dose of the infectious agent or if the person is infected via an unusual portal of entry; it may also be impaired by immunosuppressive drug therapy, concurrent disease, or the ageing process.

Herd immunity

Herd immunity is an important element in the balance between the host population and the micro-organism and represents the degree to which the community is susceptible or not to an infectious disease as a result of members of the population having acquired active immunity from either previous infection or prophylactic immunization (see Chapter 68). Herd immunity can be measured:

1. *Indirectly* from the age distribution and incidence pattern of the disease if the disease is clinically distinct and reasonably common. This is an insensitive and inadequate method for those infections which manifest themselves subclinically.

2. *Directly* from assessments of immunity in defined population groups by antibody surveys (sero-epidemiology) or skin tests; these may show 'immunity gaps' and provide an early warning of susceptibility in the population. Although it may be difficult to interpret the data in absolute terms of immunity and susceptibility, the observations can be standardized and reveal trends and differences between various defined population groups in place and time.

The decision whether to introduce herd immunity artificially by immunization against a particular disease will depend on several epidemiological principles:

1. The disease must carry a substantial risk
2. The risk of contracting the disease must be considerable

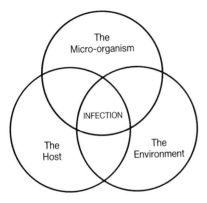

Fig. 66.1   The three main factors involved in the infectious process

3. The vaccine must be effective
4. The vaccine must be safe.

The effectiveness and safety of immunization programmes is monitored by observing the expected and actual effects of such programmes on disease transmission patterns in the community by appropriate epidemiological techniques.

The environment

The environment plays a major role in the causation, spread and control of infection. In the UK, the virtual disappearance of relapsing fever, plague and cholera, the rarity of indigenous typhoid fever and the relative infrequency of tuberculosis and bacillary dysentery are all indications of the improvements which have taken place in environmental conditions. The decrease in overcrowding and infestation together with the demand for cleaner water supplies and better sanitation have been of paramount importance in producing these dramatic advances. This is well illustrated in the case of tuberculosis, which was declining before the availability of chemotherapy and mass BCG vaccination in countries where socio-economic conditions were improving (Fig. 66.2). Paradoxically, better living conditions may unexpectedly create new problems; for example, poliovirus infection, previously experienced mainly in early childhood, is usually postponed in more favoured communities to older ages when paralysis is a more likely complication unless there is an adequate immunization programme.

THE SPREAD OF INFECTION

Infection spreads in well-defined epidemiological patterns. A knowledge of these will lead to an understanding of the best methods of control, or even eradication, and enables an estimate to be made of the likelihood of this happening.

Infection spread directly from one person to another

Among this group can be included such highly infectious diseases as measles. Infection is passed directly from a person with the disease to a susceptible contact. Diseases in this category are usually clinically apparent and healthy carriers are not a feature. When it is possible to diminish the number of susceptibles in the target population then eradication becomes feasible, as has happened with smallpox.

Infection in which healthy carriers are involved

Because apparently healthy individuals may harbour the bacilli responsible for such diseases as

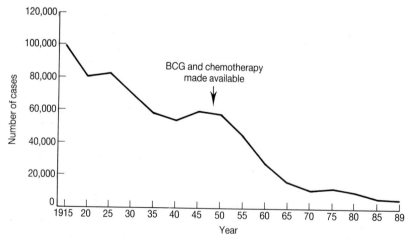

Fig. 66.2 Notifications of tuberculosis in England, Wales and Scotland, 1915–1989

typhoid, paratyphoid and diphtheria, often for long periods after having acquired the infection, it is possible for such infections to be transmitted to others and the source remains undetected.

Infection in which persons harbour the organism before the onset of clinical illness

Organisms such as *Streptococcus pneumoniae* may not cause the person any harm until an event such as a skull fracture allows the transfer of the bacterium from the middle ear to the cerebrospinal space where it can cause a potentially lethal meningitis.

Infection derived from animal sources

Diseases derived from animals, such as leptospirosis, Q fever, anthrax, rabies and brucellosis are known as *zoonoses*. These diseases are spread by direct contact with the animal concerned or indirectly by such means as the ingestion of infected milk, contact with infected bone products, etc.

Infections derived from environmental sources

The spread of legionellae from cooling towers and air conditioning units to cause Legionnaires' disease is an example of illness derived from an infected environment. By dealing appropriately with the infected source the population is protected.

OUTBREAKS OF INFECTION

The crowding together of humans (or for that matter animals, fish or birds) provides the necessary conditions to allow micro-organisms to multiply and spread. When humans led nomadic lives there was less opportunity for outbreaks to occur; the main opportunities came when large numbers gathered for a pilgrimage or had other reasons for a meeting. These clusterings facilitated the spread of infection, resulting in outbreaks; the subsequent dispersal of the group enabled the causative organism to be carried elsewhere.

The threat of outbreaks in overcrowded and difficult conditions is particularly well illustrated in military history; on many occasions the germ has been as important in determining the outcome of a campaign as the sword or gun. The typhoid bacillus caused severe effects during both the American Civil War (1861–65) and the Boer War (1899–1902). The use of typhoid vaccine in the latter years of the First World War meant that the main impact of typhoid in this war subsided after 1916. Similarly, typhus was rife in the Civil War in Britain (1642–49), when both the Parliamentary and the Royalist armies were affected. The pandemic of influenza in 1918–19, in which about 700 million people were affected with approximately 22 million deaths, was a scourge of military camps and affected many servicemen returning home from the First World War.

Nomenclature of outbreaks

The term *outbreak* is often confused with other epidemiological terms used to enumerate infection.

1. *Sporadic case*: a person whose illness is not apparently connected with similar illnesses in another person.
2. *Outbreak*: the occurrence of cases of a disease associated in time or location among a group of persons. A *household outbreak* involves two or more persons resident in the same private household and not apparently connected with any other case or outbreak. A *general outbreak* involves two or more persons who are not confined to one private household.
3. *Epidemic*: the large-scale temporary increase in the occurrence of a disease in a community or region which is clearly in excess of normal expectancy.
4. *Pandemic*: the occurrence of a disease which is clearly in excess of normal expectancy and is spread over a whole geographical area, usually crossing national boundaries.

Types of outbreak

There are three main patterns of outbreak which may be revealed by the construction of graphs of occurrence of cases over time.

1. *The explosive outbreak.* This is characterized by the occurrence of a large proportion of cases in a relatively short period of time (Fig. 66.3); there is a sharp rise and fall in the number of infected persons, since the usual cause of such an event is a common source which infects the people concerned. This type of outbreak is also frequently termed *a common source outbreak* or a *point source outbreak.* This pattern of infection is often discovered when water or food becomes contaminated, although other vehicles of infection can also be responsible for this type of outbreak.

2. *Person-to-person spread.* Outbreaks caused by infections which are spread from person to person have a more protracted course taking longer than explosive outbreaks to build up and to subside.

An infective agent may be passed from person to person by a variety of routes. Diseases such as dysentery, hepatitis type A and gastro-enteritis which are usually spread by the faecal–oral route often follow this pattern of spread (Fig. 66.4).

3. *Explosive outbreaks with subsequent person-to-person spread.* This pattern is often apparent when there is contamination of a common water or food source and the initial cases subsequently infect their contacts. Thus, the pattern of the outbreak is a combination of that seen with an explosive outbreak, but followed by a slower decline (Fig. 66.5).

Analysis of outbreaks

The investigation of an outbreak should be approached in a logical and methodical way. The cause may be elucidated by determining details of the *persons* involved, the *place* where they had

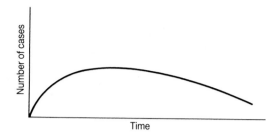

Fig. 66.4 Epidemic curve apparent when there is person-to-person spread of infection

been and the *time* when they became ill.

The fundamental pieces of information which should be sought whenever an outbreak occurs are as follows:

1. *WHO gets infected?* What is their age? For example, if a possible food-borne outbreak mainly affects children, could the source be milk or ice-cream?

2. *WHERE were those who became infected?* Where have they recently been? For example, in a hospital outbreak were they all in the same surgical ward? Could a member of the operating staff be a carrier of a pathogen? In a community outbreak of Legionnaires' disease were those affected living downwind from a contaminated source of infection? (See Fig. 66.6).

3. *WHEN did the infection occur?* By knowing the incubation period of the infection it may be possible to trace back to an event which was attended by all those affected.

4. *WHAT was the common factor?* For example, in a food poisoning episode, the ingestion of an

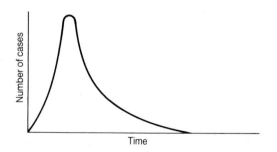

Fig. 66.3 Epidemic curve apparent when there is an explosive (common or point source) outbreak

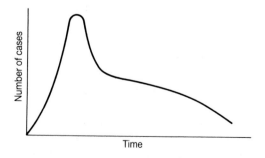

Fig. 66.5 Epidemic curve apparent when there is person-to-person spread subsequent to a common source outbreak

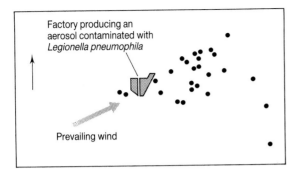

Fig. 66.6 Occurrence of Legionnaires' disease in persons living downwind from a factory with an evaporative condenser contaminated with *Legionella pneumophila*

article of food by most of those affected but not by those unaffected may be a vital piece of evidence.

5. *HOW did those involved become infected?* For example, abscess formation among recently immunized persons might be due to contaminated vaccine.

6. *WHY did the infection occur?* For example, the reheating of meat is often the cause of a *Clostridium perfringens* food poisoning outbreak.

Investigation of outbreaks

In the investigation of outbreaks it is important to have a standardized approach to the various steps involved. Such an approach might have the following as a basis:

1. *Verify the diagnosis.* It is always prudent to confirm that the clinical history is compatible with the diagnosis. Occasional 'pseudo-epidemics' can occur, sometimes resulting from contamination of specimens.

2. *Establish the existence of an outbreak.* The increased interest of an investigator can sometimes result in an increase in the number of reports of illness. It is important to check the previous level of investigation of a clinical entity.

3. *Establish the extent of an outbreak.* Often the number of cases notified is only a proportion of the total number of those affected. It is necessary to seek out the additional cases or vital information may be lost.

4. *Identify common characteristics of experiences of the affected persons.* An individual history from each confirmed or suspected case is required in order to detect any common factor among those affected (e.g. eating the same item of food).

5. *Investigate the source and vehicle of infection.* In addition to ascertaining the general characteristics of the material suspected as being the source or vehicle of infection, appropriate laboratory investigation will often have to be done. Good co-operation with the laboratory staff is vitally important.

6. *Analyse the findings.* The data should be analysed by the various epidemiological criteria, especially persons, time and place. Denominators should be obtained in order to calculate attack rates.

7. *Construct an hypothesis.* On the basis of the evidence an hypothesis should be constructed concerning the origin of the outbreak. This may be confirmed by laboratory findings but action to control the outbreak may be needed in advance of such findings.

Control of outbreaks

The investigation of an outbreak should be carried out as swiftly as possible so that adequate control measures can be started without delay. Knowledge of the *source of infection*, the *route of transmission* and the *persons at risk* should allow appropriate action to be taken in order to achieve success.

Sources of infection

These may be:

1. Human cases or carriers
2. Animal cases or carriers
3. The environment.

If the initial cases have readily identifiable clinical features (e.g. measles) then control is often easier as it is much more likely that the index case will be located. On the other hand, it is more difficult to control diseases in which apparently healthy carriers are responsible, as it is necessary to search for an infected person who may be asymptomatic.

It may be important to isolate the case or carrier, and possibly to institute appropriate treatment, until the patient is no longer infectious. The degree of isolation will depend on the type of disease as not all infections require strict isolation. For example, a patient with a highly infectious disease may require very strict isolation whereas the salmonella excreter will usually need only to cease food handling activities and observe a high standard of personal hygiene until free from infection. In contrast to 'isolation' the term 'quarantine' applies to restrictions on the healthy contacts of an infectious disease.

If an animal reservoir is responsible, action has to be directed at ensuring that the source of infection is eradicated, withdrawn from consumption, or rendered harmless (e.g. by the pasteurization of milk or the adequate cooking of meat).

When the environment is the source of an outbreak the control measures required will depend on the nature of infection and the mode of spread. In recent years, water-borne spread of Legionnaires' disease (e.g. from shower heads, air-conditioning systems, or droplet spread from cooling towers) has become increasingly recognized (Fig. 66.7). Environmental measures, such as the use of biocides, can destroy the causative legionellae at their source and so prevent further cases.

The hospital setting is particularly dangerous since the presence of compromised patients can result in tragic consequences. Moreover, the in-creasing use of invasive techniques and the appearance of antibiotic-resistant strains of micro-organisms further compound the problem. In a survey of hospital patients in England and Wales 9% of all patients acquired infection while in hospital. The early detection of infection by effective surveillance, the emphasis on the cleanest possible environment and awareness among the staff of potential problems are among the measures that need to be stressed in order to control infection among hospital patients (see Chapter 67).

Route of transmission

Infection may be spread by:

1. Direct or indirect contact
2. Air-borne transmission
3. Percutaneous transmission
4. Food- and water-borne transmission
5. Insect-borne transmission
6. Transplacental transmission.

There are various ways in which the routes of transmission occurring during an outbreak may be blocked by measures appropriate to the route involved: effective hand washing; disinfection or disposal, if necessary, of the patient's belongings; and strict adherence to high standards of personal hygiene by the *contacts* of a case are important measures. When the disease is air-borne, over-crowding should be avoided and, where appropriate, dormitory or ward beds should be well spaced out. The acquired immune deficiency syndrome (AIDS) is a good example of a disease which can be spread *percutaneously* via contaminated needles as well as by other routes. *Food* and *water* should be as free as possible from infection as these are major causes of outbreaks. To deal with *insect-borne transmission*, eradication policies and repellents should be considered. The *transplacental* route is important in the spread of diseases such as hepatitis B.

Persons at risk

Where indicated and feasible, susceptible persons at risk should be protected as soon as possible. Among the measures available the following may need to be considered:

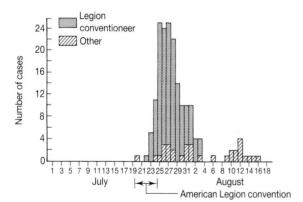

Fig. 66.7 Legionnaires' disease among those associated with a convention in a hotel in Philadelphia (July to August 1976): an example of an explosive outbreak

1. Immunization
2. Chemoprophylaxis for close contacts.

Immunity against several infectious diseases can be obtained either by active or passive immunization (Chapter 68). Examples of rapid effective protection of communities by active immunization are the 'ring vaccination' policy used to protect close contacts of poliomyelitis and so stop more widespread dissemination of poliovirus, and the early (within 72 h of exposure) administration of measles vaccine to close contacts in an institution. Passive immunization, usually by means of human normal immunoglobulin or human specific immunoglobulin, gives rapid protection to contacts of hepatitis A and some other infections, although protection is short lived. Chemoprophylaxis is effective in the protection of close contacts of meningococcal infections and diphtheria.

MATHEMATICAL MODELS

Mathematical modelling techniques attempt to define by use of relatively simple estimates and assumptions, the conditions governing transmission of communicable agents. Details of the multiplication and growth rates of micro-organisms and the spread of infection under natural or experimental conditions need to be known. Measurable factors include: the number of infective persons or sources of introduction of infection; the proportion of susceptible persons in a community at risk; the duration of immunity; the introduction of new susceptibles; the removal rate of infective persons (by isolation, immunity or death); and the response to vaccines and chemotherapeutic agents. Mathematical models can be used to predict institutional outbreaks and epidemics. This approach has been used to forecast the number of cases of AIDS that are likely to occur.

ASSOCIATION AND CAUSATION OF INFECTION

A problem commonly encountered by microbiologists and epidemiologists is the attribution of an infectious disease to a particular micro-organism.

How do we determine if the relationship is one of causation or merely a chance association? Koch addressed this when he formulated his 'postulates' in 1891. These state that:

1. The organism must always be found in the given disease
2. The organism must be isolated in pure culture
3. The organism must reproduce the given disease after inoculation of a pure culture into a susceptible animal
4. The organism must be recoverable from the animal so inoculated.

For many organisms pathogenic to man it is not possible to fulfil Koch's postulates; moreover, they are not applicable to the study of the transmission of infection within a population. For this purpose it is more appropriate to consider the following factors, suggested by the medical statistician Bradford Hill, in order to establish whether a disease is caused by a particular infectious agent:

1. *Strength.* What is the strength of the association? During the cholera epidemic in London in 1854 John Snow compared the death rates among persons drinking the sewage-polluted drinking water of the Southwark and Vauxhall Company and those receiving the purer water of the Lambeth Company; he discovered that the rate in the former was 14 times higher (Table 66.2). This strength of association allowed Snow to consider that polluted water was a cause of cholera, although at that time the causative organism itself had not been identified.

2. *Consistency.* Similar observations, made by different people at different times in different places,

Table 66.2 Deaths in London during the cholera epidemic of 1854 according to source of water supply

Water source	Number of houses supplied	Deaths
Southwark and Vauxhall Company (polluted)	10 000	71
Lambeth Company (non-polluted)	10 000	5

add confidence to a conclusion that causation is likely.

3. *Specificity*. If the association is limited to a specific group of persons, with a specific type of illness, who have all been subjected to the same specific infection, then a cause and effect relationship can be more strongly suspected.

4. *Temporality*. This can be of especial importance when persons in particular occupations become infected (e.g. leptospirosis in fishworkers). The history of working in a particular environment *before* infection rather than vice versa is particularly relevant.

5. *Biological gradient*. If a dose–response curve is apparent then the evidence for causation is much stronger.

6. *Plausibility*. Is the possibility biologically plausible? The likelihood of veterinary surgeons becoming infected with *Brucella abortus* from ill cattle which they have recently been treating seems biologically plausible.

7. *Coherence*. If all the evidence is coherent (e.g. if the same micro-organism is isolated from the index case, the vehicle of transmission and from the victims) this is strong support for causation.

8. *Experiment*. Is the frequency of infection reduced if certain preventative measures are taken? The beneficial effects of the pasteurization of milk to diminish the number of cases of milk-borne salmonellosis is presumptive evidence of a zoonotic relationship.

9. *Analogy*. Has there been similar evidence in the past? The known capacity of the rubella virus to cause congenital abnormalities in the infants of infected mothers makes it easier to accept the possibility of other viruses causing similar problems if maternal infection occurs.

CONCLUSION

Because of the multifactorial causation of infection it is usually necessary to study the epidemiology of infection in a *multidisciplinary* manner. The microbiologist, the clinician, the epidemiologist, the infection control nurse, the veterinarian, the environmentalist, and other appropriate personnel, must all be involved; the extent of the involvement will depend on the nature of the infection. Success will depend on the expertise and co-operation of these members of the team.

RECOMMENDED READING

Benenson A S (ed) 1990 *Control of Communicable Diseases in Man*, 15th edn. American Public Health Association, Washington, DC

Campbell D M, Paixao M T, Reid D 1988 Influenza and the "spotter" general practitioner. *Journal of the Royal College of General Practitioners* 38; 418–421

Christie A B 1987 *Infectious Diseases. Epidemiology and Clinical Practice*, 4th edn. Churchill Livingstone, Edinburgh

Eylenbosch W J, Noah N D 1988 *Surveillance in Health and Disease*. Oxford University Press, Oxford

Grist N R, Ho Yen D O, Walker E, Williams G R 1987 *Diseases of Infection*. Oxford University Press, Oxford

Last J M (ed) 1983 *A Dictionary of Epidemiology*. Oxford University Press, Oxford

Mims C A 1982 *The Pathogenesis of Infectious Disease*, 2nd edn. Academic Press, London

Noah N D, Reid D 1979 Sources of data on infectious diseases in England, Wales and Scotland. *Journal of Infection* 1: 259–298

Reid D, Grist N R, Pinkerton I W 1986 *Infections in Current Medical Practice*. Butterworths: Update, London

Pickles W N 1939 *Epidemiology in Country Practice*. Wright, Bristol (re-issued 1972 by the Devonshire Press, Torquay)

Tyrrell D A J 1982 *The Abolition of Infection. Hope or Illusion? Rock Carling Fellowship Lecture*. Nuffield Provincial Hospitals Trust, London

Velimirovic B, Greco D, Grist N R, Mollaret H, Piergentili P, Zampieri A 1984 *Infectious Disease in Europe. A Fresh Look*. World Health Organization Regional Office for Europe, Copenhagen

67

Hospital infection

R. A. Simpson

Historically, hospitals have a notorious reputation for infection. The hazards of puerperal sepsis and the horrors of septic infection in the pre-Listerian era have been well documented; admission to hospital in the mid-19th century was associated with the fear of gangrene and death.

Since that time, surgical and medical techniques have developed dramatically, basic standards of building and hygiene have greatly improved and the identification and treatment of infecting micro-organisms have become possible in most cases. Despite such significant changes, infection acquired in hospitals still remains one of the main causes of morbidity and mortality, leading directly or indirectly to an enormous increase in the cost of hospital care and to the emergence of new health hazards for the community. Advances in biomedical technology and therapeutics are producing greater numbers of highly susceptible patients requiring treatment in hospitals and this is aggravated by the occurrence of transferable resistance to antibiotics in pathogenic bacteria and the emergence of new pathogens transmitted by a variety of routes.

CLASSIFICATION

In determining the extent of hospital infection, the following categories should be considered:

1. Infections contracted and developing outside hospitals which require admission of the patient (e.g. pneumonia).

2. Infections contracted outside hospital which become clinically apparent when the patient is in hospital (e.g. measles).

3. Infections contracted and developing within hospital (e.g. postoperative wound infection).

4. Infections contracted in hospital but not becoming clinically apparent until after the patient has been discharged (e.g. breast abscess).

5. Infections contracted by hospital staff as a consequence of their work, whether or not this involves direct contact with patients (e.g. hepatitis B).

On average, 5–10% of all hospital patients will develop an infection as a result of their stay in hospital. Urinary, respiratory and wound infections are the most common.

FACTORS THAT INFLUENCE INFECTION

Hospital infection, also known as *nosocomial infection*, may be exogenous or endogenous in origin. The exogenous source may be another person in the hospital (*cross-infection*) or a contaminated item of equipment or building service (*environmental infection*). A high proportion of infections that are clinically apparent in hospital are endogenous or *self-infection*, the infecting organism being derived from the patient's own skin, gastro-intestinal or upper respiratory flora.

Most infections acquired in hospital are caused by micro-organisms that are commonly present in the general population, in whom they cause disease less often and usually in a milder form than in hospital patients. Thus, contact with micro-organisms is seldom the sole or main event predisposing to infection. Various risk factors, alone or in combination, influence the frequency and nature of hospital infection.

Susceptibility to infection

Natural resistance to infection is lower in infants and the elderly, who often comprise the majority of hospital patients. Pre-existing disease, such as diabetes, or other conditions for which the patient was admitted to hospital and the medical or surgical treatment, including immunosuppressive drugs, radiotherapy or splenectomy, may also reduce the patient's natural resistance to disease. Moreover, the natural defence mechanisms of the body surfaces may be bypassed either by injury or by procedures such as surgery, insertion of an indwelling catheter, tracheostomy, or ventilatory support.

CONTACT WITH OTHER PATIENTS AND STAFF

In common with any larger institution or workplace, the patients and staff of a hospital share many facilities in close or crowded conditions. Thus, outbreaks of diarrhoeal and food-borne disease may be traced to a common source via the hospital water or food supplies. The specific role of hospitals in admitting infected patients or carriers for treatment or isolation clearly serves as a potential source of infection for others. Patients with comparable susceptibility to infection tend to be concentrated in the same area, e.g. in neonatal units, burns units or urological wards, where infected and non-infected patients may be cared for by the same staff, thus creating numerous opportunities for the spread of micro-organisms by direct contact.

Inanimate reservoirs of infection

Equipment and materials in use in hospitals often become contaminated with micro-organisms which may subsequently be transferred to susceptible body sites on patients. Gram-positive cocci, derived from the body flora of the hospital population, are found in the air, dust and on surfaces where they may survive along with fungal and bacterial spores of environmental origin. Gram-negative aerobic bacilli are common in moist situations and in fluids, where they often survive for long periods, and may even multiply in the presence of minimal nutrients. Awareness of the common reservoirs of environmental and contaminating hospital micro-organisms provides the basis for maintaining standards of hygiene (cleaning, disinfection, sterilization) throughout the hospital.

Role of antibiotic treatment

At least 30% of hospital patients receive antibiotics and this exerts strong selective pressures on the microbial flora. Sensitive species or strains of micro-organisms which normally maintain a protective function on the skin and other mucosal surfaces, tend to be eliminated, whereas those that are more resistant survive and become endemic in the hospital population. This may restrict the range of agents available for treatment and may lead to the transmission of plasmid-mediated antibiotic resistance into strains that show increased virulence, survival and spread within the hospital.

MICRO-ORGANISMS CAUSING HOSPITAL INFECTION

The most important micro-organisms responsible for hospital infection are listed in Table 67.1. Several trends have been observed over the last few decades. The explosive outbreaks of *Staphylococcus aureus* infection that were frequently seen in surgical wards and maternity units up to the mid-1970s demonstrates the infectious potential of strains exhibiting particular virulence and colonizing capabilities. When combined with resistance to antibiotics, as has occurred throughout the 1980s in epidemic or pandemic strains characterized by resistance to methicillin (MRSA), the challenge for outbreak control is even more daunting. In contrast, other strains of MRSA persisting in some UK hospitals appear better able to colonize patients or staff than to produce

Table 67.1 Commonly occurring micro-organisms in hospital infection

Urinary tract infections	*Escherichia coli* *Klebsiella, Serratia, Proteus* spp. *Pseudomonas aeruginosa* Faecal streptococci *Candida albicans*
Respiratory infections	*Haemophilus influenzae* *Streptococcus pneumoniae* *Staphylococcus aureus* Enterobacteriaceae Respiratory viruses
Wounds and skin sepsis	*Staphylococcus aureus* *Escherichia coli* *Proteus* spp. Anaerobes Faecal streptococci Coagulase-negative staphylococci
Gastro-intestinal infections	*Salmonella* spp. *Shigella sonnei* Viruses

systemic disease. This illustrates the adaptation and evolutionary changes possible within common hospital bacteria revealed by careful epidemiological typing and observation. The changing patterns may be related to particular events and infection control measures, so that lessons can be learnt for future control and prevention.

With the advent of more elaborate surgery and intensive care, combined with the use of broad-spectrum antibiotics and immunosuppressive drugs, the Gram-negative bacteria have risen in importance.

Presently, about 60% of hospital-acquired infections are caused by aerobic Gram-negative rods and about 30% by Gram-positive cocci. Many Gram-negative bacilli such as *Pseudomonas aeruginosa* are *opportunists* capable of causing infection in compromised patients.

Such organisms may be found in the patient's own flora, or in damp environmental sites, including patient equipment and medicaments. They may exhibit natural resistance to many antibiotics and antiseptics and the ability to colonize traumatized skin such as burns and bedsores.

In recent years, groups of micro-organisms which formerly played no recognized part in hospital infection have emerged. These include the coagulase-negative staphylococci present in normal skin flora (see Chapter 15). Viral or fungal infection, particularly of the immunocompromised patient, has become more important. *Legionella pneumophila*, disseminated from environmental sources such as cooling towers, causes sporadic cases or outbreaks of respiratory infection in the hospital community. Awareness of the risks of blood-borne viruses, including hepatitis B, human immunodeficiency virus (HIV) and cytomegalovirus has increased in patients and in staff.

ROUTES OF TRANSMISSION

The hospital offers many opportunities for the exchange of microbes, many of which are harmless and a normal part of the balance between man and his environment. For there to be a significant risk of infection, a number of factors, including the right susceptible host and the appropriate inoculum of infecting micro-organism, must be linked via an appropriate route of transmission. Understanding of the sources and transmission routes of hospital infection enables efforts to be concentrated in more effective preventive measures.

Common routes of transmission for different micro-organisms are shown in Table 67.2.

Airborne transmission

Infections may be spread by air-borne transmission from the respiratory tract (talking, coughing, sneezing), from the skin by natural shedding of skin scales, during wound dressing or bed making and by aerosols from equipment such as respiratory apparatus and air-conditioning plants. Infectious agents may be dispersed as small particles or droplets over long distances (Fig. 67.1). Staphylococci survive well on mucosal secretions, skin scales and dried pus and may be redistributed in the air after initial settlement during periods of increased activity (Fig. 67.2). Gram-negative bacilli do not generally survive desiccation in air and this route of transmission is therefore limited to conditions of high humidity such as ventilatory equipment.

Table 67.2 Hospital infection: sources and spread

Route	Source	Example of disease
I. Aerial (from persons)		
Droplets	Mouth	Measles, Tuberculosis Lower respiratory tract/Pneumonia
Skin scales	Nose Skin exudate Infected lesion	Staphylococcal sepsis Streptococcal sepsis
II. Aerial (from inanimate sources)		
Particles	Respiratory equipment Air-conditioning plant	Gram-negative respiratory infection Legionnaires' disease Fungal infections
III. Contact (from persons)		
Direct spread	Respiratory secretions	Staphylococcal and streptococcal sepsis
Indirect via equipment	Faeces/urine Skin and wound exudate	Enterobacterial diarrhoea *Pseudomonas aeruginosa* sepsis
IV. Contact (environmental sources)		
	Equipment Food Medicaments Fluids	Enterobacterial sepsis (*Klebsiella, Serratia, Enterobacter* spp.) *Ps. aeruginosa* and other pseudomonads
V. Direct contact		
Into blood, tissue or body fluid	Sharp injury Blood products	Hepatitis B, AIDS

Contact spread

The most common routes of transmission for hospital infection are by *direct* contact spread

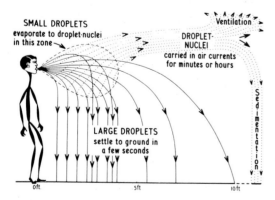

Fig. 67.1 Spread of respiratory infections by droplets and droplet nuclei.

from person to person or by *indirect* contact spread via contaminated hands or equipment. Faeces, urine or pus as well as contaminated dust particles or fluids may be carried on thermometers, bed-pans, bed-linen, cutlery or other shared items. Hands and, to a lesser extent, clothing of hospital staff serve as vectors of Gram-negative and Gram-positive infection around a busy theatre or ward. Procedures involving contact with mucosal surfaces, e.g. insertion of a urinary catheter, may introduce micro-organisms from the contaminated hands of the operator or from the patient's own urethral flora into the normally sterile bladder. Similarly, intravenous fluids and topical medicaments have direct contact with vulnerable sites for infection.

Food-borne infection may occur from any food source available in the hospital, including those prepared in the hospital kitchen, special diets,

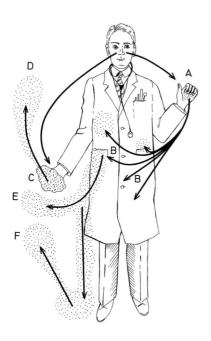

Fig. 67.2 Infection of the air with dust particles derived from nasal and oral secretions contaminating hands, handkerchief, clothing and surrounding surfaces:
A Hand soiled with secretions from lips or nose-picking; **B** clothing contaminated by hand; **C** soiled handkerchief; **D** infected dust from handkerchief; **E** dust from clothing (e.g. from near handkerchief pocket); **F** infected dust raised after settling on floor.

infant feeds, kitchen or commercial supply. Deteriorating hygiene standards may support the proliferation of flies, cockroaches and other insects or rodents which damage stored products and act as carriers of microbes. Of special note is the accidental transmission of predominantly blood-borne infections such as hepatitis B by needle-stick or contaminated 'sharp' injury.

Self-infection and cross-infection

The interaction between different sources of infection may be illustrated by the example of a patient undergoing lower bowel surgery. *Self-infection* may occur due to transfer into the wound of staphylococci (or occasionally streptococci) carried by the patient in his nose and distributed over his skin, or of coliform bacilli and anaerobes released from his bowel during surgery. Alter-

natively, *cross-infection* may result from staphylococci or coliform bacilli derived from other patients or healthy staff carriers: the organisms may be transferred into the wound *during operation* through the surgeon's punctured gloves or moistened gown, on imperfectly sterilized surgical instruments and materials, or by air-borne theatre dust; or *postoperatively* in the ward from contaminated bed-linen, by air-borne ward dust or in consequence of a faulty wound dressing technique.

Of all the possible routes, by far the most likely in this example is self-infection from the patient's own bowel flora and it is therefore against this route that most specific preventive measures in colorectal surgery are directed. Understanding of possible sources of infection and the methods available to block transmission to susceptible sites forms the basis of hospital infection control.

The site and extent of infection and the time it was first recognized after the date of operation often help to establish whether cross-infection occurred during operation or postoperatively in the ward: clustering of cases according to a common surgical team or location in the ward may suggest a common source and may be the first firm indication of an outbreak of hospital infection.

Cross-infection from other patients or from staff carriers is especially dangerous because the causal organisms are often strains that have been selected in the hospital population for high infectivity and resistance to antibiotics. They are, however, potentially preventable by the practice of basic hygienic precautions.

Soon after admission to hospital, individuals commonly become contaminated with the 'hospital flora'. This has been shown with *Staph. aureus* in studies of patients before and during hospital treatment. Patients who need to stay longer in hospital, e.g. those requiring intensive care or the elderly, are less able to withstand infection and the risks of hospital infection are greater.

PREVENTION AND CONTROL
The infection control policy

The establishment of an effective infection control organization is the responsibility of good management of any hospital. There will normally be two parts:

1. An *infection control committee*, meeting regularly to formulate and update policy for the whole hospital on matters having implications for infection control and to manage outbreaks of nosocomial infection.

2. A team of workers, headed by the infection control doctor (usually the microbiologist), to take day-to-day responsibility for this policy.

The functions of the *infection control team* include surveillance and control of infection and monitoring of hygiene practices, advising the infection control committee on matters of policy relating to the prevention of infection and the education of all staff in the microbiologically safe performance of procedures. The *infection control nurse* is a key member of this team. Close working links between the microbiology laboratory, infection control nurse and the different clinical specialties and support services (including sterile services, laundry, pharmacy, engineering) are important to establish and maintain the infection control policy, and to ensure that it is rationally based and that

the recommended procedures are practicable. Some of the control measures in which the infection control team should be involved are shown in Fig. 67.3.

Sterilization

The provision of sterile instruments, dressings and fluids is of fundamental importance in hospital practice. By the end of the 19th century, heat processing of instruments, dressings, surgical gloves, face-masks and theatre clothing began to supersede the phenol antiseptic soaks of the Lister era. Sterilization in autoclaves and hot air ovens became accepted hospital practice. The development of automatic, high-vacuum sterilizers for processing wrapped goods facilitated the provision of a centralized service of sterile supply to wards, complementing the existing theatre service. In recent years, the availability of a wide range of prepacked single-use items (syringes, needles, catheters, drainage bags) sterilized commercially by gamma irradiation or ethylene oxide

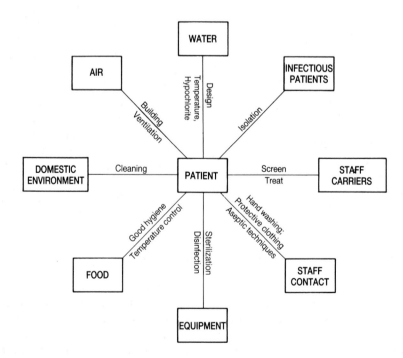

Fig. 67.3 Control measures to reduce exogenous hospital-acquired infection.

has further improved aseptic procedures and removed the need for reprocessing items that are difficult to clean and therefore impossible to sterilize.

Most fluids for topical use or intravenous administration are now prepared commercially or in regional units where standards of quality control and efficiency for bulk processes are more readily achieved than in individual hospital pharmacies.

Aseptic techniques

The provision of sterile equipment will not prevent the spread of infection if there is carelessness in its use. Wherever possible *no touch* techniques must be used, coupled with strict personal hygiene on the part of the operator. These routines are rigidly laid down in operating theatre practice and may be modified as required for other procedures such as wound dressing and insertion of intravenous catheters.

Cleaning and disinfection

The general hospital environment can be kept in good order by attention to basic cleaning, waste disposal and laundry. The use of chemical disinfectants for walls, floors and furniture is unnecessary other than in special instances such as spillages of body fluids from patients with blood-borne virus infections. Ward equipment such as bedpan washer/disinfectors and dishwashers should be monitored to ensure reliable performance and cleaning materials such as mop-heads and cloths should be heat disinfected and stored dry after use. Pre-cleaning of contaminated instruments and equipment, preferably by means of an automatic washing process with an ultrasonicator, is an essential step before disinfection or sterilization.

Skin disinfection and antiseptics

The ease of acquisition and transfer of transient hospital contaminants, particularly Gram-negative bacilli via the hands of staff, is an important factor in the spread of hospital infection. Thorough hand washing after any procedure involving nursing care or close contact with the patient is essential.

Gloves may be worn for many dirty contact procedures, such as emptying a urinary drainage bag or bed-pan, although it should not be forgotten that the gloved hand may also become colonized by transient hospital flora.

Procedures for pre-operative disinfection of the patient's skin and for surgical scrubs are mandatory within the operating theatre. The use of antiseptics for irrigation of the wound site at operation or for other mucosal surfaces such as the bladder after urological surgery in catheterized patients or the peritoneum during dialysis may also be beneficial. Dilute 'in-use' solutions of antiseptics may readily become colonized with Gram-negative bacteria and should be replaced regularly. Ideally, *single-use* preparations should be used. Restriction should be placed on the indiscriminate use of antiseptics and disinfectants by means of a *disinfectant policy* agreed by pharmacists, microbiologists and key users, such as theatre staff.

Prophylactic antibiotics

Although widespread and haphazard use of antibiotics hastens the emergence of antibiotic-resistant bacteria and increases both the incidence of toxic side-effects and the cost of treatment, there is good evidence that rational antibiotic prophylaxis plays an important role in infection control. Specific indications include peri-operative prophylaxis in gastro-intestinal and gynaecological surgery directed predominantly against anaerobic infection and for patients known to have bacteriuria at the time of urological surgery or instrumentation, directed against the urine isolate. An *antibiotic policy* which limits the choice of broad-spectrum agents is important both for prophylaxis and treatment (see Chapter 65).

Protective clothing

Different activities within the hospital require different degrees of protection to staff and patients. In operating theatres the wearing of sterile gowns, sterile gloves, headgear and face-masks minimizes the shed of micro-organisms. The properties of fabrics available for theatre use have improved and now include close-weave ventile fabrics that are comfortable to wear and allow evaporation of moisture. 'Total protection' of the operating site may be considered for certain high-risk clean surgery such as hip replacements, during which the surgical team may wear exhaust-ventilated suits rather like spacesuits and operate under conditions of ultraclean laminar airflow.

For many ward procedures in which there may be soiling, or for simple *barrier nursing* of patients with communicable diseases, plastic aprons and gloves are used. Gloves, face-masks and goggles are also indicated for specific procedures when blood contact is likely through splashes or aerosols, such as dental procedures.

Isolation

The isolation policy should list facilities and procedures needed to prevent the spread of specific infections to other patients (*source isolation*) and to protect susceptible or immunocompromised patients (*protective isolation*). Effective isolation demands a highly disciplined approach by all staff to ensure that none of the barriers to transmission (air-borne, direct and indirect contact) are breached. Multibedded rooms may be used, and even wards converted during hospital outbreaks, but the simplest solution wherever possible is to use single rooms.

'Cubicle' isolation, by which the patient is nursed alone in a room separated by a door and corridor from other patients, confers a substantial measure of protection. Preferably, each isolation room has its own toilet and washing facility. Clean, filtered air is supplied to the room, which should be at negative pressure (*exhaust ventilated*) to the corridor for source isolation or at positive pressure (*pressure ventilated*) to the corridor for protective isolation. If, however, there is a small airlock vestibule separating the room from the outer corridor then exhaust ventilation of the airlock will give effective isolation for either situation. The vestibule or lobby should contain a washbasin and include space for gowning and equipment.

In some critical situations such as bone marrow transplant units, where air-borne contamination with environmental fungal spores is a problem, the efficiency of air filtration may be increased and laminar airflow maintained as a barrier around the patient. Stringent isolation, such as a plastic tent or 'Trexler' isolator, is required only for patients with highly contagious infections, such as those due to Lassa, Marburg and Ebola viruses, who are nursed in a *high-security isolation unit*.

Hospital building and design

The routine maintenance of the hospital building is important, ensuring that surfaces wherever possible are smooth, impervious and easy to clean. Major rebuilding works on or near the hospital site may generate dust containing fungal and bacterial spores with implications for specialized units serving immunocompromised patients. Close communications with the works department and hospital administration are necessary to co-ordinate any protective action. When a new hospital or modification of existing building is planned, the infection control team should be closely involved in discussing the plans. In many countries, guidance on new building design exists to minimize potential hospital-acquired infection. Areas requiring special attention include operating theatres, kitchens, acute wards, laboratories and air-conditioning systems. The risk of Legionnaires' disease is reduced by installing water supplies that circulate below 20°C for the cold and above 60°C for the hot circuit.

Equipment

Any object or item of equipment for clinical use should be assessed to determine the appropriate method, frequency and site of decontamination. Wherever possible, heat processes are the preferred choice although this may be precluded for certain thermolabile items such as fibre-optic endoscopes (see Chapter 5).

Personnel

An occupational health service in hospitals should screen staff pre-employment and offer appropriate immunization. Hepatitis B vaccine should be given to those at special risk, such as those working in renal dialysis units and dental practice. All staff (including medical students) should receive general health protection. The notification and screening of staff with specific infections such as diarrhoeal disease or following needlestick injury should be understood within the infection control policy.

Monitoring

Routine microbiological monitoring of the environment is of little benefit, although monitoring of the physical performance of air-conditioning plants and machinery used for disinfection and sterilization is important. In the event of an outbreak of hospital infection, more specific monitoring targeted at the known or likely causative microorganism should be considered.

The microbiological screening of staff or patients is not undertaken routinely but may be needed for specific purposes, such as before cardiac surgery, to eliminate *Staph. aureus* from carriage sites which may otherwise cause self-infection, or for detection of staff carriers in critical areas such as dialysis units (hepatitis B).

Surveillance and the role of the laboratory

The detection and characterization of hospital infection incidents or outbreaks relies on laboratory data that alert the infection control team to unusual clusters of infection, or to the sporadic appearance of organisms that may present a particular infection risk or management problem. Bacterial typing schemes and antibiograms (see Chapter 4) are very important in this regard. Regular visits to the wards are also important to record data on infected patients for whom specimens have not been received and to respond to problems as they occur. Such visits also serve to provide opportunities for practical teaching, which is another important element of the infection control team's responsibility.

EFFICACY OF INFECTION CONTROL

There is acceptable proof of efficacy for only a few infection control measures. These include sterilization, handwashing, closed-drainage systems for urinary catheters, intravenous catheter care, peri-operative antibiotic prophylaxis for contaminated wounds and techniques for the care of equipment used in respiratory therapy. Isolation techniques, while not proven by objective study, are also assumed reasonable as suggested by experience or inference. Other measures which have been introduced, but are now considered to be ineffective, include the chemical disinfection of floors, walls, sinks and routine environmental monitoring.

A major study on the efficacy of nosocomial infection control in the USA has confirmed the importance of effective surveillance, control methods and an infection control team in the reduction of infection rates. One important role of the team is to monitor compliance with practices known to be effective and to eliminate the many rituals or less effective practices which may even increase the incidence or cost of cross-infection. As further advances occur in medical care and limited health care resources are spread across hospital and community needs, innovations in infection control will need to be evaluated for efficacy and cost effectiveness. With this understanding it is possible that hospital infection can be controlled and largely prevented. The dictum of Florence Nightingale, made over a century ago, that 'the very first requirement in a hospital is that it should do the sick no harm', remains the goal.

RECOMMENDED READING

Ayliffe G A J, Collins, B J, Taylor L J 1990 *Hospital Acquired Infection*, 2nd edn. Wright, Bristol

British Medical Association 1989 *A code of practice for sterilisation of instruments and control of cross infection*. Edward Arnold, London

Freeman R, Gould F K 1987 *Infection in Cardiothoracic Intensive Care*. Edward Arnold, London

Lowbury E J L, Ayliffe G A J, Geddes A M, Williams J D 1981 *Control of Hospital Infection*, 2nd edn. Chapman and Hall, London

Maurer I M 1985 *Hospital Hygiene*, 3rd edn. Edward Arnold, London

Meers PD, Ayliffe G A J, Emmerson A M, Leigh D A, Mayon-White R T, Mackintosh C A, Stronge J L 1981 Report on the national survey of infection in hospitals. *Journal of Hospital Infection* 2(supplement)

Wenzel R P (ed) 1987 *Prevention and Control of Hospital Infection*. Williams and Wilkins, Baltimore

68

Prophylactic immunization

J. G. Collee

Prophylactic immunization is only one of the measures that may be used for the control of infectious diseases. Its cost and efficacy must be assessed against other forms of defence such as: environmental sanitation; safe sewage disposal; a secure water supply; food hygiene; clean air and adequate ventilation; good animal husbandry with effective quarantine arrangements where necessary; insect vector control; and improved nutrition.

Other aspects of community defence against infection include: the surveillance of infectious diseases; early detection; prompt and adequate treatment; and isolation facilities, when appropriate, with proper measures to control cross-infection and transmission (Table 68.1). A detailed knowledge of the epidemiology of infections, and of the correct use of antimicrobial drugs and immunological products for therapy or prophylaxis, is crucial.

Table 68.1 Approaches to the prevention of infectious disease: an indication of priorities

Preventive engineering: water, sewage, ventilation, food production and food processing

Surveillance and diagnostic awareness

Prompt management: recognition, treatment, isolation and contact tracing where necessary

Improvement and maintenance of good socio-economic conditions: housing, nutrition, education, medical and social care

Increased resistance to infection by appropriate active immunization policies and in some special circumstances by passive immunization

Much of the morbidity and mortality of infection is still either not assuredly preventable by immunization or presents great difficulties. For example, many of the diarrhoeal diseases and respiratory infections that take a heavy toll of life and health among young children in poor and overcrowded communities are not amenable to control by specific vaccines. Nor are the common bacterial infections associated with haemolytic streptococci, staphylococci and coliform bacilli, or many virus infections. However, some spectacular successes can be claimed, and encouraging efforts are being made to extend the range of success.

RATIONALE OF IMMUNIZATION

The objective is to produce, without harm to the recipient, a degree of resistance sufficient to prevent a clinical attack of the natural infection. The degree of resistance conferred may not protect against an overwhelming challenge, and other control measures must operate in concert with any immunization policy, as discussed above.

PASSIVE IMMUNIZATION
Homologous and heterologous sera

Artificial passive immunization is used in clinical practice when it is considered necessary to protect a patient at short notice and for a limited period. Antibodies, which may be antitoxic, antibacterial or antiviral, in preparations of human or animal serum are injected to give temporary protection. Human preparations are referred to as *homologous* and are much less likely to give rise to the adverse reactions occasionally associated with the injection of animal (*heterologous*) sera. An additional advantage of homologous antisera is that, although they do not confer durable protection, their effect may persist for 3–6 months, whereas the protection afforded by a heterologous serum is likely to last for only a few weeks.

Equine antitoxins

Antiserum raised in the horse against diphtheria toxin (*equine diphtheria antitoxin*) is available for the prophylaxis and treatment of diphtheria. A similar heterologous antiserum is available for emergency use in cases of suspected botulism and to protect those thought to be at risk. Equine tetanus antitoxin is still used in some countries, but it should be abandoned in favour of human tetanus immunoglobulin (p. 288). It is most important to give an intended recipient of equine serum a prior test dose to exclude hypersensitive subjects who may have been sensitized by a previous dose of equine serum.

Pooled immunoglobulins

Protective levels of antibody to a range of diseases are present in pooled normal human serum. *Human normal immunoglobulin* (HNIG) is available in the UK and elsewhere for the short-term prophylaxis of hepatitis A in contacts or travellers who intend to visit countries where hepatitis A is common. HNIG also protects an immunocompromised child temporarily against measles if given promptly after contact with a case. However, HNIG does not give reliable post-exposure protection against mumps or rubella.

Specific immunoglobulins

Preparations of specific immunoglobulins are available in the UK for passive immunization against tetanus (human tetanus immunoglobulin; HTIG), Hepatitis B (HBIG), rabies (HRIG), varicella–zoster (ZIG) and vaccinia (AVIG).

ACTIVE IMMUNIZATION
Types of vaccine
Toxoids

If the signs and symptoms of a disease can be attributed essentially to the effects of a single toxin, a modified form of the toxin that preserves its antigenicity but has lost its toxicity (a *toxoid*) provides the key to successful active immunization against the disease. This has been spectacularly successful with tetanus and diphtheria.

Inactivated vaccines

If the disease is not mediated by a single toxin, it may be possible to stimulate the production of protective antibodies by using the killed (inactivated) organisms. This is done as a routine with vaccines against pertussis (whooping cough), typhoid and influenza. There is also an inactivated polio vaccine.

Attenuated live vaccines

In some cases, the inactivation procedure to make a killed vaccine destroys or modifies the protective antigenicity (*immunogenicity*) of the organisms. Hence, another approach is to use suspensions of living organisms that are reduced in their virulence (*attenuated*) but still immunogenic. This strategy has yielded: oral (live) polio vaccine; mumps, measles and rubella vaccines (now combined); and yellow fever vaccine.

Sometimes it is possible to use a related organism with shared antigens. Thus, the vaccinia virus vaccine was used to eradicate smallpox, and a bovine tubercle bacillus was modified by Calmette and Guérin to make bacille Calmette–Guérin (BCG) which protects man against tuberculosis.

Special procedures

Some vaccines, such as influenza vaccine, can be refined by a process that removes unwanted protein and other reactive material but retains the important protective antigens. Some others must be conjugated to proteins to render them immunogenic. Some vaccines, such as hepatitis B vaccine, can be bio-engineered, and there is much current interest in the possibility of developing *subunit vaccines* consisting of purified fragments of the major immunogenic components of micro-organisms, particularly viruses.

Immune response

Antibodies against the agents of some bacterial and viral infections may be present in the mother's blood and be passively acquired by the baby. This gives some protection to the infant at a time when it is poorly equipped to produce specific antibodies, but it may interfere to a varying extent with the infant's capacity to respond to the stimulus of injected or ingested vaccines in the very early months of life. Although the capacity of the infant to produce specific antibody to injected antigens is poorly developed in the first few months of life, this problem can often be resolved by the use of *adjuvants*. Thus, effective responses are produced to powerful antigens such as alum-adsorbed toxoids. Pertussis whole-cell vaccines have an adjuvant effect of their own, so the combination of adsorbed toxoids and whole-cell pertussis vaccine (the triple DTP vaccine) is an effective immunizing complex that can be given at 2, 3 and 4 months of age to cover the period when the lethal potential of pertussis is greatest (see Chapter 33). The tissues of the newborn respond effectively to BCG vaccine because the protection here is cell mediated. The use of a high-potency measles vaccine at 6 months of age is likely to be exploited in countries where measles kills or severely injures the very young.

When a good specific antibody response is being sought to a toxoid or a killed antigen, the usual procedure is to give three doses of the antigen at spaced intervals. The first or 'priming' dose evokes a low level of antibody after a latent period of about 2 weeks, but the second dose elicits a much greater (secondary) antibody response, and this is further boosted by the third dose. The efficacy of injected antigen preparations can be enhanced by slow-release agents such as mineral carriers which have adjuvant effects. With most antigens, the response is better if the first two doses are separated by an interval of a month or two. A third dose is

generally recommended at some time thereafter, and further booster doses may be given to maintain immunity.

Duration of immunity

After an effective course of active immunization, a protective amount of antibody may persist in the blood for some years and a subsequent booster injection may maintain protection for a further decade. Much depends upon circumstances that will vary for different vaccines and different groups of people. The duration of active protection cannot be absolutely equated with the presence of demonstrable antibody because factors such as the sensitivity of the test and the actual protective role of the antigen detected have to be taken into consideration.

Age of commencement of active immunization

This must take account of the immaturity of the antibody-forming system in the very early months (see above) and the infectious challenges that a child may encounter early in life and in later years. The start of any immunization programme must be adjusted to the known epidemiology of the diseases that are prevalent in the country in which it is to be instituted, and it must also be related to any serious infective challenges that may be imported from time to time. Poliomyelitis is a good example of a disease that has been largely eradicated from many communities; however, the disease is quick to strike back if the immunization shield is lowered.

CONTROLLED STUDIES OF PROPHYLACTIC VACCINES

Combined field and laboratory studies aim to provide confidence in the efficacy of vaccines. A field trial can show only whether or not the actual preparation of vaccine used was successful under the circumstances prevailing at the time. Accordingly, trials require very sophisticated design and much care in their execution. They are very expensive. In order to satisfy the requirement for reproducibility, the method of preparation of the vaccine must be meticulously described and controlled. Much work continues to define and to refine laboratory tests for the protectiveness of a particular vaccine that might be correlated with its efficacy in field trials. The laboratory test that gives results most closely corresponding to the protective value in the field trials may then be adopted as the test for standardizing future batches of vaccine.

Manufacturers of vaccines for commercial use are required in the UK and in many other countries to satisfy certain standards relating to the purity, safety, potency and stability of their products. In addition, the World Health Organization has established internationally agreed requirements. At the national level, a system for continuing surveillance of the efficacy of prophylactic vaccines with continuing notification of any suspected adverse reactions is essential.

CONTRA-INDICATIONS TO THE USE OF VACCINES

The delivery of an important immunization programme should not be unwisely prejudiced by catch-all statements that take a legalistic view of theoretical hazards and thus err on the side of opting out. The risk of opting out of an immunization schedule should be clearly appreciated.

It is difficult to make valid generalizations about contra-indications to vaccination, but there are some useful general principles: do not give a vaccine to a patient with an acute illness, but do be sure that the postponed immunization is subsequently given. Do not give a live vaccine to a pregnant woman, unless there is a clear balance of risk in favour of vaccination; in general, avoid giving any vaccine in the first trimester of pregnancy. Do not give live vaccines to patients receiving immunosuppressive drugs or irradiation, or to patients suffering from malignant conditions of the reticulo-endothelial system — delay until after successful therapy when they are in remission.

Experience with human immunodeficiency virus (HIV) antibody-positive patients with or without the signs and symptoms of acquired immune deficiency syndrome (AIDS) indicates so far that measles, mumps, rubella and polio (live virus) vaccines can be given, but that BCG vaccine should not be given. Inactivated vaccines are not contra-indicated.

Hazards of immunization

Possible adverse reactions to active immunization with an injected preparation generally range from mild or moderate pain at the site of injection, to fever and malaise for a day or two after. Anaphylactic reactions are very rare; as they may be fatal, doctors and nurses should be aware of the possibility and should be prepared for such an emergency. No death of a child attributed to an anaphylactic reaction to an active immunizing agent was notified in the UK in the decade 1979–89. This is reassuring, but it is also a challenge to maintain our collective and individual vigilance.

During the first few years of life when many vaccines are given, children tend to have various health problems that include occasional febrile convulsions and may, sadly, include an unexplained cot death or other tragedy. It is inevitable that some of these events will coincide with the period shortly after a vaccine was given to a child and the possibility of a causal relationship will be entertained. The probability of such a link certainly deserves to be considered, but it is most important to bear in mind that the issue is emotive and that ill-balanced or ill-informed adverse publicity can do irreparable harm to an immunization programme. For example, annual notifications of whooping cough in England and Wales dropped from more than 100 000 in the early 1950s to some tens of thousands in the late 1950s as the vaccine gained ground. By the early 1970s (and after modification of the vaccine to take account of a possible deficiency in its protective cover), whooping cough was largely controlled in the UK with about 75% of children immunized. In the late 1970s, after some ill-informed adverse publicity, acceptance rates for the vaccine fell steeply to 30% or lower, and the uptake of other vaccines was also affected. Epidemics of whooping cough followed in the UK in 1978 and 1982 with tens of thousands of children affected. It should be remembered that the morbidity associated with whooping cough is still very considerable and very young children still die of the disease or are severely injured by it (see Chapter 33). Deaths attributable to whooping cough averaged seven per year in the 5 years from 1976 to 1981. In the UK epidemic of 1978–80, 0.02% of notified cases died.

As a result of efforts to restore confidence in pertussis vaccine, uptake figures increased in the 1980s and the disease again began to be brought under control.

Children who are most vulnerable are likely to be least protected. Pertussis, polio and measles spread most effectively when living conditions are overcrowded and unhygienic. To some extent, these diseases depend upon population density for their spread. Some underprivileged groups in a community are in very real danger when the average rate of vaccine uptake falls, because they often represent the extreme end of the fall in vaccine cover.

In view of the stringency of the regulations that control the quality and efficacy of vaccines, the probability of error lies more with the vaccinator than with the producer. There is a special obligation to ensure that a vaccine is properly stored, properly reconstituted (if relevant) and properly administered (Table 68.2). The appropriate instructions should be followed in detail. *An injectable vaccine must be given with a sterile syringe and needle, and a separate sterile syringe and needle must be used for each injection.* (The only possible exception to this rule is the use of a special jet injector which does not employ a skin-penetrating needle.) The skin over the injection site should be clean and disinfected with an aqueous solution of 70% alcohol which should be allowed to dry before the injection is given. Immunization should be postponed if there is skin sepsis.

Site of injection

This will vary with the vaccine to be given. Specific instructions should be followed. In general, and with the exception of BCG, injectable vaccines are given by intramuscular or deep subcutaneous injection. The anterolateral aspect of the thigh or upper arm is the preferred site for infants.

Table 68.2 Safety considerations

Use a separate sterile syringe and needle
Avoid errors: check the vial personally
Consider the patient's history: note pregnancy and various contra-indications
Keep careful records

Some doctors and nurses use the upper outer quadrant of the buttock, but fat in this area may interfere with the efficacy of the vaccine.

HERD IMMUNITY

This is an important concept. When most of the people in a community are immune to a particular infection that is spread from person to person, the natural transmission of the infection is effectively inhibited. Thus, if almost all children in a residential school have been immunized against measles, the school is most unlikely to have an outbreak of measles; even the few children who have not been immunized will enjoy a measure of protection afforded by the general herd immunity in that they will not be challenged within the school. This will only apply so long as the school population is largely composed of immune pupils and a non-immune pupil does not encounter a visitor who is infected with measles. If there is an influx of non-immunes, the level of herd immunity will fall and the general protection will be lost. When the pupils go into other communities at holiday times, the non-immune individuals are liable to get measles at their first contact with an infective case.

For herd immunity to operate well in a community or a country, vaccine uptake rates must exceed 90%. For some highly transmissible infections, uptake rates above 95% are the target. Bear in mind that herd immunity operates only for infections transmitted from person to person. Tetanus is not transmitted in this way; a non-immune person is fully vulnerable to tetanus even if he or she is surrounded by fully immunized colleagues in a closed community (Fig. 68.1).

IMMUNIZATION PROGRAMMES

An immunization campaign carried out without provision for its continuation as a routine proce-

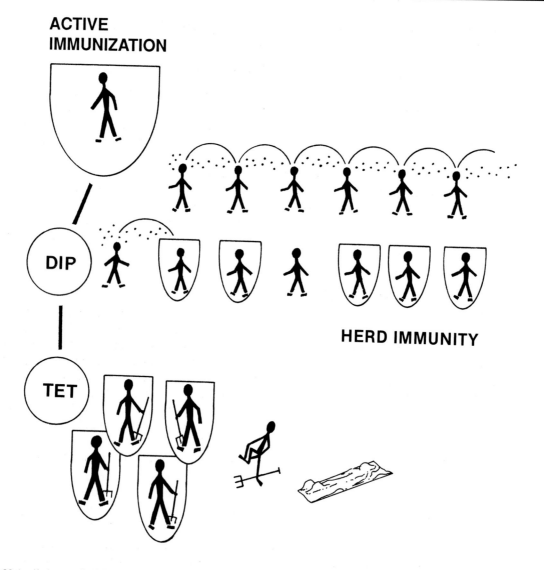

Fig. 68.1 If almost all of the members of a community receive active immunization against a disease that is normally transmitted from person to person, the resulting herd immunity confers some advantage even upon an occasional non-immune member because rapid transmission of the disease through the community is prevented. This is true for diphtheria, but not for tetanus, which is not dependent on person-to-person spread.

dure will not give satisfactory results unless complete eradication of the disease is achieved. Thus, in planning immunization schedules, consideration must be given to ensuring that the general public is receptive and understands the policy. It is essential to secure the trust and co-operation of parents who have to bring their children to the doctor or clinic for a series of inoculations and who will undoubtedly seek reassurance that the

benefits are considerable and the risks negligible. Note that parental consent must be obtained for each immunization.

In the planning and execution of a programme, immunological points that merit special attention are:

1. The use of combined antigens and the simultaneous administration of killed and live vaccines

2. The incorporation of adjuvants in killed vaccines and toxoids
3. The age of commencement
4. The dosage and spacing of antigens.

IMMUNIZATION SCHEDULES

The provision of a programme of active immunization to a community should be governed by considerations of need, efficacy, safety and ease of administration. An over-riding consideration is the cost and the availability of skilled manpower. Circumstances vary widely in different countries, and priorities vary.

In the UK, it is generally agreed that protection of the susceptible population against diphtheria, whooping cough, and tetanus (with a triple vaccine), poliomyelitis (with a live vaccine), and mumps, measles and rubella (with a combined live vaccine) merit priority in the very early years of life. BCG vaccine is offered to tuberculin-negative children at 10–14 years. In the UK it is now recommended that the DTP triple vaccine and oral polio vaccine are started early, at 2 months, with further doses at 3 months and 4 months (Table 68.3). This secures earlier protection against pertussis in the months when the disease is most dangerous to the young child.

NOTES ON SOME VACCINES IN COMMON USE

Adsorbed tetanus toxoid

The preparation in routine use in the UK is adsorbed onto an aluminium salt; it is is more effective and less reactive than simple toxoid. It is a component of the triple DTP vaccine. A course of three injections given at intervals of about 6 weeks and 6 months immunizes for at least 5 years. A booster dose at school entry then protects for 10 years, and booster doses can be given thereafter at intervals of 10 years. Prevention of tetanus should be considered in relation to the management of wounds (see p. 287).

Diphtheria toxoid

The adsorbed preparation used in the UK and incorporated into the triple DTP vaccine contains aluminium phosphate and affords good protection which is boosted at school entry age. This preparation is not used for adults; a dilute adsorbed diphtheria vaccine preparation is used for people who are more than 10 years old. Active immunization of adults against diphtheria is not practised in the UK as a routine, unless there is a potentially high occupational risk of encountering

Table 68.3 Schedule of immunization for children in the UK: a model for countries with adequate public health services

Age	Vaccine	Notes
During year 1	Diphtheria Tetanus Pertussis }	Start at 2 months; second dose at 3 months and third dose at 4 months by intramuscular or deep subcutaneous injection
	Oral polio vaccine	Give at the same times as the DTP injections
During year 2	Measles Mumps Rubella	Give one injection of the combined live vaccine at age 12–18 months
At 4–5 years	Diphtheria Tetanus }	Booster
	Oral polio vaccine	Booster
At 10–14 years	Rubella[a] BCG vaccine[a]	For girls only For tuberculin-negative children
At 15–18 years	Tetanus Oral polio	Booster Booster

[a] Allow an interval of at least 3 weeks between rubella and BCG.

the organism in laboratory or clinical work, or unless a person has been in contact with a case of diphtheria and protection is deemed necessary. A course of erythromycin gives further protection to a close contact and this has replaced the use of diphtheria antitoxin in contacts. The falling level of immunity to diphtheria among adults in communities that regard themselves as having good preventive medical services gives some cause for concern and calls for continuing vigilance.

The Schick test (p. 233) can be used to check the immunity of those recruited to work where there is an occupational hazard of diphtheria.

Pertussis vaccine

The vaccines in general use in 1990 are whole-cell preparations of killed *Bordetella pertussis*. Acellular vaccines containing antigenic components of the organism have been developed and are being assessed for their protective potency. Meanwhile, the protection afforded by the whole-cell vaccines is acknowledged to be considerable. Three injections are given at intervals of 1 month or more. Whole-cell pertussis vaccine is a component of the DTP triple vaccine and it has the added advantage of being an adjuvant in that combination.

Adverse reactions that may be associated with pertussis vaccine include soreness at the site of injection, irritability and pyrexia. Other reactions such as persistent screaming, shock, vomiting and convulsions have been reported, but the association with pertussis vaccine is not invariably clear. Sometimes an association with a different vaccine is claimed, and sometimes there is no history of recent vaccination. Thus, whilst there may be a causal association, in some cases there seems to be a considerable chance that the association is casual and not attributable to the vaccine. Particular attention has been paid to a possible association of convulsions and encephalopathy and cerebral damage. It should be noted that unexplained convulsions occur in young children, especially during the period when the immunization programme is set, and that such an incident may occur by chance shortly after a vaccine has been given. Moreover, the age at which certain cases of cerebral damage begin to be apparent coincides with this age range. Accordingly, we are quite uncertain if there is a risk of permanent brain damage associated with pertussis vaccine; if there is, it must be very small and it must be greatly outweighed by the known risk of neurological and other damage that may be life-threatening when the natural disease occurs.

Poliomyelitis vaccines

The control of poliomyelitis is one of the great success stories of active immunization. The Salk vaccine came first; this is a killed mixture of the three types of poliovirus (1, 2, 3). A course of three injections is given at appropriate intervals.

The polio vaccine favoured in the UK and many other countries is the live attenuated form developed by Sabin. This is a mixture of the three types and it is given orally on three occasions, usually at the same time as the triple DTP vaccine is given in the early months. Note that the oral polio vaccine (OPV) is not given by injection. As it is a live preparation, the vaccine must be stored and held according to the manufacturer's instructions and not allowed to become inactivated in a bottle on the desk. OPV colonizes the gut and gives rise to local and humoral antibodies. The faeces contain live virus for some time, and poliomyelitis caused by a vaccine strain is a rare, but recognized hazard. Any non-immune contact in the household should be advised to be immunized at the same time, but difficulties in arranging this should not delay the primary job of getting the baby immunized. It is important to advise on the hygienic handling of the baby's nappies during the period of excretion of the virus (and at any other time, for that matter!).

Measles, mumps and rubella (MMR) vaccine

This is a mixture of live attenuated strains of these three viruses in freeze-dried form; it has to be stored at 2–8°C (not frozen), reconstituted according to the manufacturer's instructions and used promptly. One injection of the mixture is given in the 2nd year of life in the UK schedule.

The measles component may give rise to fever or malaise and sometimes a rash about a week after inoculation. The mumps component may cause some parotid swelling seen about 3 weeks after inoculation. Very occasional cases of mumps vaccine-associated meningoencephalitis are being reported; these also occur at 3 weeks and follow a generally benign course, but there may be confusion with other non-benign syndromes in this age group. The rubella component is not usually associated with reactions in this age group, though temporary malaise, mild fever and arthralgia occurring about the 9th day after vaccination have been noted in some older recipients of rubella vaccine.

It is hoped that the incorporation of MMR vaccine in the UK schedule will eradicate measles, mumps and rubella in this country. Much depends upon an adequate uptake of the vaccine, as these diseases are highly transmissible. Meanwhile, a booster dose of rubella vaccine alone will be offered to girls aged 10–14 years and the vaccine is offered to all seronegative women of child-bearing age and to professional attendants who might come into contact with pregnant women at clinics, etc. Although rubella vaccine is not thought to be teratogenic, any woman of child-bearing age who is given the vaccine should avoid pregnancy for a month.

BCG

The attenuated strain of bovine tubercle bacillus known as bacille Calmette–Guérin (BCG) produces cross-immunity to human tuberculosis and has significantly contributed to the control of the disease in many countries. An intradermal injection of the live attenuated vaccine is given on the lateral aspect of the arm at the level of the deltoid insertion, but not higher, or on the upper lateral surface of the thigh. Instruction on the reconstitution of the freeze-dried vaccine, the dosage and the detailed technique of giving a truly intradermal injection should be most carefully observed. With the exception of newborn children, any recipient of BCG vaccination should have been tested for hypersensitivity to tuberculin and found to be negative. Tuberculin tests include the *Mantoux test* in which diluted tuberculin is injected intradermally, and the *Heaf test*, which is done with a multiple puncture apparatus (see Chapter 19). Be sure to appreciate the difference between the tuberculin test and a BCG vaccination; and note that attention to detail in the sterilization of the Heaf apparatus is of crucial importance.

Hepatitis B vaccine

The first vaccine for the protection of groups of people considered to be at special risk of acquiring hepatitis B was an inactivated plasma-derived vaccine, but a bio-engineered vaccine is now in common use. A course of three injections of either of these vaccines is given by intramuscular injection (not into the buttock) at intervals of 1 and 5 months; thus, it takes 6 months to complete the course, and this is of practical importance. Protective antibody responses are generally achieved in about 90% of those given the vaccine with a range of responses from weak to strong, but there is a worrying minority of non-responders (10–15% in the over-40 years age group). Non-response rates are particularly worrying among patients on maintenance haemodialysis. In the general population, the protection afforded to responders is thought to last for about 5 years, when a booster dose of vaccine may be given. Established policy must await further experience with hepatitis vaccines.

Other vaccines

Various vaccines are available for the protection of special groups of people or for individuals in special circumstances (Table 68.4). The reader is referred to the appropriate chapters for more detailed consideration of such topics as: the

Table 68.4 Vaccines for active immunization of people at special risk

Anthrax	Q fever
Cholera	Rabies
Haemophilus influenzae infection*	Smallpox (vaccinia vaccine)
Hepatitis B	Typhoid
Influenza*	Typhus
Japanese B encephalitis	Varicella–zoster*
Meningococcal infection*	Yellow fever
Plague	
Pneumococcal infection*	

The asterisk indicates that there are some problems (see text).

prevention of tetanus in wounded patients; the indications for pneumococcal vaccine; the management of rabies; and the control of Q fever.

PROTECTING THE TRAVELLER

An intending traveller to another country should seek advice in advance about the prevailing diseases and the precautions that should be taken. Advice on immunization is unlikely to be of much help if the traveller unwisely runs the risk of drinking raw water or eating uncooked salads and vegetables in a country where sanitation is inadequate and water supplies are insecure.

In advising travellers about exotic diseases, do not forget that diseases once common in countries with developed medical services may still be common in countries that lack such services. Thus, a booster dose of poliomyelitis vaccine may be appropriate, for example. If work in a hospital or health clinic is envisaged, include the risk of diphtheria in your list. Do not forget that tetanus is still a major killer on a global scale. Remember that tuberculosis is still common in some countries. If the traveller is going to Central Africa or Central America, bear in mind the need for protection against yellow fever. Other vaccines that may be indicated include those that will afford some protection against typhoid. Some of the special vaccines listed in Table 68.4 may also merit inclusion, especially if the traveller's activities when abroad are likely to expose him or her to the relevant diseases.

Active immunization against hepatitis A and other forms of viral hepatitis (excluding yellow fever) is not yet possible. Passive protection against hepatitis A is conferred by the injection of human normal immunoglobulin (HNIG, p. 792). A traveller to an endemic area can be protected for some months in this way. Give the injection shortly before your patient sets off, but not so late that the patient still has sore buttocks while in transit.

An effective malaria vaccine has been sought for many years, but none is yet available. Consequently, it is essential to ensure that any traveller to (or through) a malarious zone is adequately protected by relevant advice and by the proper prophylactic drugs (see Chapter 61).

UNRESOLVED PROBLEMS

Nothing is perfect (see Table 68.5). Some vaccines are more imperfect than others, and some circumstances pose special problems. The influenza virus has shifts and drifts in its antigenic pattern, so vaccines must be frequently updated. Then decisions have to be made on the patients who merit this special protection. As these include many old people and many patients with respiratory or cardiovascular impairment, the decisions are quite difficult.

Cholera vaccines have had a chequered record with very little evidence of real efficacy for the traveller who is much better protected by a basic knowledge of hygiene. Some new developments are a little more promising.

Acute purulent (bacterial) meningitis is a dramatic clinical problem. A vaccine that affords some protection against groups A and C of the meningococcus is available, but a group B vaccine is not available at the time of writing (1990) and group B strains cause a lot of trouble. Similarly, a vaccine to protect against *Haemophilus influenzae* type b is not yet generally available, although haemophilus meningitis rivals meningococcal meningitis in frequency. The problem is that vaccines made from the type b capsular polysaccharide of *H. influenzae* are poorly immunogenic. However, effective protein-conjugate vaccines have been developed and are now coming into use.

We are still quite unclear about the place of pneumococcal vaccine (see Chapter 17). A vaccine produced against 23 types of pneumococci is recommended, particularly for the protection of patients who do not have a spleen or are about to be splenectomized in the course of therapy. It is also suggested that the vaccine may be of use for

Table 68.5 Properties of an ideal vaccine

Promotes effective immunity
Confers lifelong protection
Safe (no side effects)
Stable
Cheap
Seen to be good and effective (protected from adverse publicity by regular appraisal and informed comment)

the protection of various groups of patients against pneumococcal infections.

Typhoid vaccine is associated with reactions of pyrexia and malaise attributable to the lipopolysaccharide endotoxin content of the presently available preparation. An attenuated strain, Ty21a, has been developed with a built-in metabolic error which is the basis for a new live vaccine given by the oral route. This is presently under trial.

Several vaccines have been developed against various herpesviruses including herpes simplex, varicella–zoster and Epstein–Barr viruses. So far, they have run into difficulties.

A vaccine effective against HIV is being urgently sought in the fight against AIDS. There have been many disappointments, but there are some recent grounds for hope.

RECOMMENDED READING

Anonymous. Immunological products and vaccines. In: *British National Formulary*. British Medical Association and Royal Pharmaceutical Society of Great Britain, London (revised at intervals of about 6 months)
Department of Health, Welsh Office, Scottish Home and Health Department 1990 *Immunisation against Infectious Disease*. Her Majesty's Stationery Office, London
Nicholl A, Rudd P (eds) 1989 *British Paediatric Association Manual on Infections and Immunizations in Children*.
Oxford University Press, Oxford
Reid D, Grist N R 1987 Tetanus immunization. *Update* 34: 149–156
Root R K, Warren K S, Griffiss J M, Sande M A 1989 *Immunization*. Churchill Livingstone, New York.

The health authorities of some countries issue useful booklets with guidelines appropriate to the local conditions

Index